Management *of the* Mechanically Ventilated Patient

Management *of the* Mechanically Ventilated Patient

Lynelle N.B. Pierce, RN, MS, CCRN
Clinical Nurse Specialist, Critical Care
University of Kansas Hospital
Kansas City, Kansas

SECOND EDITION

Illustrated

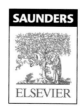

SAUNDERS

ELSEVIER

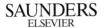

SAUNDERS
ELSEVIER

11830 Westline Industrial Drive
St. Louis, Missouri 63146

Management of the Mechanically Ventilated Patient

ISBN-13: 978-0-7216-0397-1
ISBN-10: 0-7216-0397-1

Previous edition copyrighted 1995

ISBN-13: 978-0-7216-0397-1
ISBN-10: 0-7216-0397-1

Executive Publisher: Barbara Nelson Cullen
Senior Developmental Editor: Jennifer Ehlers
Publishing Services Manager: Deborah L. Vogel
Senior Project Manager: Ann E. Rogers
Design Direction: Bill Drone

Working together to grow
libraries in developing countries

www.elsevier.com | www.bookaid.org | www.sabre.org

ELSEVIER   BOOK AID International   Sabre Foundation

Printed in the United States of America

Last digit is the print number: 9   8   7   6   5   4   3   2   1

To my husband Greg
My companion and helper.

To my daughters—
Amanda and Natalie Naema
They offer a fresh view on life, and their expanding minds
teach me something new every day.

Contributors

Marge Barnett, ARPN, BC-PCM
Palliative Care Team
Clinical Nurse Specialist
University of Kansas Medical Center
Kansas City, Kansas
Appendix IV: Ventilator Withdrawal at End of Life

Suzanne M. Burns, RN, MSN, RRT, ACNP, CCRN, FAAN, FCCM, FAANP
Professor of Nursing
Acute and Specialty Care
University of Virginia Health System
Charlottesville, Virginia
Chapter 11: Weaning from Mechanical Ventilation

Michael A. Gentile, AS, BS
Laboratory Research Coordinator
Duke University Medical Center
Durham, North Carolina
Chapter 12: Nonconventional Modes and Alternative Methods of Mechanical Ventilation

Sherry Nelles, RN, BSN, CCRN
Clinical Nurse IV, MICU
Duke University Medical Center
Durham, North Carolina
Chapter 12: Nonconventional Modes and Alternative Methods of Mechanical Ventilation

Dana Oakes, BA, RRT-NPS
Educational Consultant
Author of Best-Selling Oakes' Books
Respiratorybooks.com
Orono, Maine

Linda A. Perkins, RN, BS, CCRN

Staff Nurse
Intensive Care Unit
Eastern Maine Medical Center
Bangor, Maine
Chapter 8: Ventilator Graphics and Waveform Analysis

Lisa Riggs, RN, MSN, APRN, BC, CC

Clinical Nurse Specialist
St. Luke's Hospital
Kansas City, Missouri
Appendix II: Drugs Used in Intensive Respiratory Care

Sean P. Shortall, RRT-NPS, RPFT

Clinical Educator
Respiratory Medicine Department
Eastern Maine Medical Center
Bangor, Maine
Chapter 8: Ventilator Graphics and Waveform Analysis

Reviewers

Nancy Ames, RN, MSN, CCRN
Adult Clinical Nurse Specialist
Critical Care Medicine Department
National Institutes of Health
Bethesda, Maryland

Nader Habashi, MD
Department of Trauma Critical Care Medicine
R Adams Cowley Shock Trauma Center
Baltimore, Maryland

Karen Johnson, PhD, RN, CCRN
Assistant Professor
Department of Organizational Systems and Adult Health
University of Maryland School of Nursing
Baltimore, Maryland

Lisa Riggs, RN, MSN, APRN, BC, CC
Clinical Nurse Specialist
St. Luke's Hospital
Kansas City, Missouri

Foreword

It is not every day that a respiratory therapist is asked to write the Foreword for a nursing book. I am delighted and honored to have been asked to do this.

First, let me say that this is simply the best book I have ever seen covering the topic of *mechanical ventilation* and *intensive respiratory care* specifically for nurses. I have had the opportunity to research dozens upon dozens of books in preparation for writing my own, and this book rises head and shoulders above others in its comprehensiveness, quality, accuracy, and attention to detail. It is, honestly, unrivaled within its niche.

Second, let me say something about Lynelle Pierce. To me, Lynelle is one of the greatest the nursing profession has to offer. Her love for her profession is evident throughout the book, and her dedication to nurses being the "best of the best" is exemplified on every page.

I am also particularly excited that nurses and respiratory therapists have collaborated on this project. These two professions have long worked toward what has always been a common goal: unparalleled quality patient care. Lynelle's motivation to achieve this goal is clearly evident.

Mechanical ventilation and respiratory care is one of the most significant aspects of critical care, and yet, for the most part, nurses in North America receive little more than cursory training in this area. In a field that is changing faster than the average person can keep up, *Management of the Mechanically Ventilated Patient,* 2nd edition, not only fills the gap for these educational needs, but it also identifies, teaches, and solidifies nursing standards within the area of respiratory care.

My hat goes off to Lynelle and to all the contributors. This book should become a "must have" for every critical care nurse.

Dana Oakes, BA, RRT-NPS
Author of Best-Selling Oakes' Books
Respiratorybooks.com
Orono, Maine

Preface

Management of the Mechanically Ventilated Patient is both an educational manual and a clinical reference for those involved in monitoring, managing, and delivering care to patients requiring respiratory intervention or mechanical ventilation. The second edition carries on the tradition of the first in that topics, ranging from the simple to complex, are addressed in an easy-to-read and understandable manner. The range of coverage and practical approach make this guide valuable to the beginning student and advanced practitioner in critical care.

This book is written for nurses, including nurse anesthetists and acute care nurse practitioners, physicians, and respiratory therapists. My vision is collaborative practice among these disciplines in the respiratory care of the patient. Truly collaborative practice improves patient outcomes and requires mutual respect for the knowledge base, perspective, and contributions that each brings to the care of the patient. Within the scope of practice for the nurse, respiratory therapist, and physician are the interventions required to care for the mechanically ventilated patient. Respiratory care belongs collaboratively to these fields. Therefore, being knowledgeable and responsible for that care includes understanding the therapy. The goal of this book is to provide understanding.

Ten years have passed since the first edition. Patient care has evolved significantly, requiring substantial updating of all content. In this edition, each chapter has been carefully reviewed and revised to reflect current knowledge of respiratory care. Content markedly expanded includes patient positioning, lung expansion techniques, noninvasive ventilation or ventilation without an endotracheal tube, lung protective ventilatory strategies, ventilatory adjuncts such as nitric oxide, prevention of complications of mechanical ventilation such as pneumonia and ventilator-induced lung injury, and ventilator withdrawal at end of life.

The first edition I wrote entirely; however, with this edition I invited contributors from the disciplines of respiratory therapy and nursing. These authors bring their expertise to the entirely new Chapter 8, "Ventilator Graphics and Waveform Analysis" and Appendix IV, "Ventilator Withdrawal at End of Life" and to the rewritten chapters "Weaning from Mechanical Ventilation" and "Specialized Techniques in Mechanical Ventilation."

The foundation for management of the mechanically ventilated patient is in the opening chapters: anatomy basics and practical physiology. These chapters provide a scientific basis for patient care and for interpreting complex data. The chapters that follow progress to aspects of intermediate and intensive respiratory care. Airway maintenance, an essential facet of patient care, is covered in detail. The practitioner is provided with complete and easy-to-reference information on administration of oxygen, humidification and aerosol therapy, lung expansion, positioning, and secretion-clearance techniques. Clinical application continues throughout the text, which is full of pertinent facts relevant to patient management.

The heart of the text, Chapters 6 to 12, details both fundamental and advanced (but still practical) information about mechanical ventilation. These chapters evolved from lectures repeatedly delivered to diverse audiences and from bedside teaching. Every attempt has been made to answer the most commonly asked questions. Mechanical ventilation is covered from the beginning decision-making process as to whom it should be applied and continues with how the ventilator performs the respiratory cycle, choosing the appropriate mode and settings, regulating ventilator settings based on objective patient-ventilator data, and adjusting alarm parameters. Chapters then proceed into essential information about complications of mechanical ventilation, a systematic approach to monitoring the patient-ventilator system, how to troubleshoot and respond to alarms, and in-depth information on how to intervene with patient and/or ventilator problems.

Chapter 10 reviews the array of invasive and noninvasive techniques of patient monitoring used for gathering real-time physiologic data and managing the patient's respiratory care. Also covered are modifications of the traditional physical examination when assessing the mechanically ventilated patient and treatment of tissue oxygenation imbalances, because the ultimate goal of the respiratory system is to maintain adequate oxygenation to all of the tissues of the body.

Expanding beyond the traditional modes, nonconventional modes, such as independent lung ventilation and high-frequency oscillatory ventilation, and ventilatory adjuncts such as heliox, inhaled nitric oxide, and extracorporeal membrane oxygenation are described, including their advantages and disadvantages. Unlike most texts, detail is provided about the unique facets of patient monitoring and intervention when a specific technique is applied. This information is particularly useful for practitioners responsible for establishing practice guidelines or standards of practice.

In the dramatically changing health care arena, the critical care practitioner is challenged to become competent in an ever-broadening array of skills and constantly requires the acquisition of new and advanced knowledge. Respiratory care professionals retain a unique, expanding, and highly technological respiratory care knowledge base of their own. However, other disciplines are being called upon to understand more fully, to intervene, and to communicate more effectively the patient's respiratory care needs. The intent of this book is to assist, challenge, and inspire you to competence in caring for the critically ill patient requiring respiratory care and mechanical ventilatory support. These people trust in your constant surveillance and in your wisdom as you deliver care.

Acknowledgments

My deepest appreciation to my husband Greg and my beautiful daughters, Amanda and Natalie. They deserve to share in my tremendous sense of accomplishment in completing this second edition. Though I alone could put the words to paper to create this book, they were my support staff in every respect.

I wish to express my gratitude to my family—my father who taught me about perseverance and commitment, and my mother who taught me patience and tenderness. You two are the foundation of who I am as daughter, wife, mom, author, speaker, nurse, teacher, and sister. For their unwavering love and support, I thank my brother Joe and my sisters Debbie and Cheryl. Also my father- and mother-in-law Georgia and Weslie Pierce. Though all of your lives are busy you always took a moment to ask about the book.

To the contributors, thank you. I was given a gift when I found each of you and your incredible expertise. Working with you has been a pleasure.

I gratefully acknowledge others who have supported the development of this book, including the many manufacturers of respiratory care products and others in the industry for their willing support in the form of reference material, photos, and artwork. Also, to the entire staff at Elsevier for their characteristic quality editorial and production work. I am especially appreciative to my Editor, Barbara Nelson Cullen, who provided me with this opportunity and has supported and represented me through both editions.

My sincere appreciation to the many colleagues and mentors who have both challenged and assisted me to grow as an educator and practitioner in critical care and the subspecialty of pulmonary care. I am so grateful to the many students I have had the opportunity to teach. This material was refined through their questioning, enticing me to learn more.

Finally I wish to acknowledge the members of the health care team, especially the nurses who, with knowledge and compassion, care for the critically ill.

Lynelle N. B. Pierce

Contents

5 Lung Expansion, Positioning, and Secretion Clearance, 140

6 Mechanical Ventilation: Indications, Ventilator Performance of the Respiratory Cycle, and Initiation, 181

8 Ventilator Graphics and Waveform Analysis, 266

Sean P. Shortall and Linda A. Perkins

9 Complications of Mechanical Ventilation and Troubleshooting the Patient-Ventilator System, 288

10 Noninvasive Respiratory Monitoring and Invasive Monitoring of Direct and Derived Tissue Oxygenation Variables, 331

APPENDIXES

I Pulmonary Symbols and Abbreviations, 457

IV Removal of Mechanical Ventilation at End of Life, 477

Margaret L. Barnett

Management *of the* Mechanically Ventilated Patient

Pulmonary Anatomy

The respiratory system is both remarkable and complicated. Its overall function is to provide life-sustaining oxygen to all the cells of the body and to remove the byproduct of cellular metabolism, carbon dioxide. Therefore the efficient pulmonary system, along with the cardiovascular system, is intimately related to the body's metabolic processes. This becomes even more evident with an understanding of humoral control of ventilation. Knowledge of pulmonary anatomy provides a sound foundation for understanding the complex processes of respiration.

UPPER AIRWAY

The upper airway consists of the nasal passages, the sinuses, the pharynx, the epiglottis, and the larynx. Its functions are to conduct air to the lower airway, to protect the lower airway from foreign matter, and to warm, filter, and humidify the inspired air.

Nasal Passages

Beyond the olfactory function, the nose warms, filters, and moistens inspired air. The structure of the nose, with its two nasal cavities, turbinates, and rich vasculature, provides maximum contact between inspired air and the nasal mucosa (Fig. 1-1). Temperature adjustment and humidification begin as soon as air hits the anterior nasal cavity; thus, by the time inspired air reaches the alveoli, it is 100% saturated with water vapor. The nose clears debris from the inspired air in two ways. Strong hairs at the entry of the nostril trap the debris. Then nasal cilia, which are very fine microscopic hair-like projections, sway together in waves to move trapped particles posteriorly. When an artificial airway is in place, these functions of warming, filtering, and humidification of inspired air are bypassed and must be provided for the patient.

Sinuses

Sinuses are spaces that decrease the weight of the skull, provide mucus for the nasal cavity, and are important as resonance chambers of the voice. Named for the bone in which they lie, they are present in four of the cranial bones and one facial bone. The sinuses are divided into two groups: the paranasal (Fig. 1-2) and the mastoid sinuses. The paranasal sinuses are paired and include the frontal, ethmoid, sphenoid, and maxillary sinuses. All are lined with ciliated mucus-producing cells and have small pathways that communicate with the nasal cavity, the pathway meatus lying underneath the nasal turbinates. Occlusion of the meatus causes fluid to accumulate in the sinuses, potentially leading to a sinus infection. Inflammation within the sinuses is

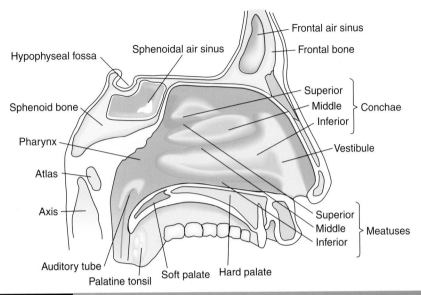

FIGURE 1-1

Lateral view of nasal cavity with nasal septum removed. Within the nasal cavity, convolutions of cartilaginous tissue known as turbinates provide an increased surface area for the warming, humidification, and filtering of inspired air. *(Modified from Jacob S, et al. Structure and Function in Man, 5th ed. Philadelphia: Saunders, 1982.)*

called sinusitis. The mastoid sinus communicates with the middle ear. Lining the mastoid sinus is a mucous membrane that is continuous with the nasopharynx. Inflammation of this lining is called mastoiditis.

Pharynx

Air passes from the nasal cavity into the space behind the nasal cavity and the mouth called the pharynx. The pharynx extends to the point where the airway (larynx) and the digestive tube (esophagus) divide. There are three divisions of the pharynx: the nasopharynx, oropharynx, and laryngeal pharynx (or hypopharynx) (Fig. 1-3). The nasopharynx begins at the base of the nasal cavities and extends to the soft palate. It contains the eustachian tubes and the lymphoid mass known as the adenoids. The eustachian tubes form a connection to the middle ear. During swallowing, they open to equalize pressure across the middle ear. The oropharynx extends from the soft palate and uvula to the epiglottis and is visible with the mouth open and the tongue depressed. Two sets of tonsils are contained in the oropharynx: the palatine and the lingual. The laryngopharynx contains the larynx and is the critical dividing point of solids and liquids from air.

Larynx

The larynx contains the vocal cords for phonation and is also an organ with sphincter functions that help prevent aspiration. The principal cartilages of the larynx are the thyroid, arytenoid, and cricoid (Fig. 1-4). The largest and most superior of the

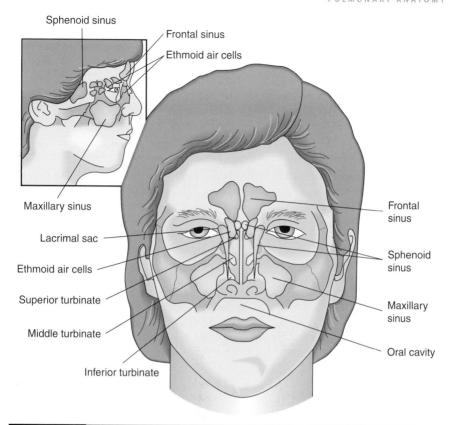

Sphenoid sinus
Frontal sinus
Ethmoid air cells

Maxillary sinus
Lacrimal sac
Ethmoid air cells
Superior turbinate
Middle turbinate
Inferior turbinate

Frontal sinus
Sphenoid sinus
Maxillary sinus
Oral cavity

FIGURE 1-2

Anterior view of the head showing the frontal, ethmoid, sphenoid, and maxillary sinuses. *(Modified from Thibodeau GS, Patton KT. Anatomy and Physiology, 5th ed. St. Louis: Mosby, 2003, p. 688.)*

cartilages is the thyroid (meaning "shieldlike"), which is commonly referred to as the Adam's apple. The cricoid cartilage lies just below the thyroid and is attached to it by the cricothyroid membrane. It is this membrane that is incised to perform an emergency procedure, the cricothyroidotomy, for upper airway obstruction. The arytenoid cartilage serves as the attachment of the vocal cord ligaments. It swings in and out from a fixed point, thus opening and closing the space between the vocal cords, actions that are necessary to vary the pitch of sounds. Sound intensity is affected by the amount of air passing between the vocal cords. Thus, when an artificial airway is in place, the patient is unable to phonate.

The mucous membrane lining the pharynx forms two pairs of folds that project inward. The first fold forms the false vocal cords because they play no part in vocalization. They come together to protect the lower airway and act with the true vocal cords to close so sufficient intrathoracic pressure can be developed to generate a cough. The vocal cords are thin white borders on the lower pair of mucosal folds. The vocal cords and the space between are known as the glottis (Fig. 1-5). The cords

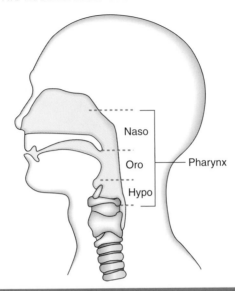

FIGURE 1-3

The three anatomic divisions of the pharynx are named for the respiratory structures that lie next to them. The hypopharynx is also known as the laryngeal pharynx. *(Modified from Spearman CB, Sheldon RL. Egan's Fundamentals of Respiratory Therapy, 4th ed. St. Louis: Mosby, 1982.)*

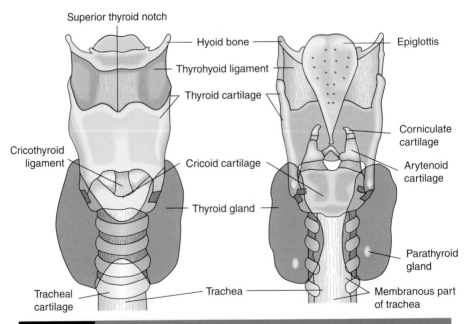

FIGURE 1-4

Anatomy of the larynx. **A,** Anterior view. **B,** Posterior view. The structure is primarily cartilage, not bone. *(Modified from Thibodeau GS, Patton KT. Anatomy and Physiology, 5th ed. St. Louis: Mosby, 2003, p. 690.)*

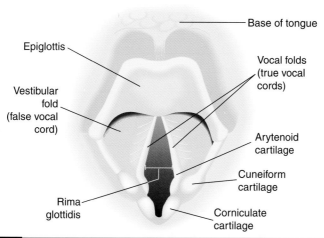

FIGURE 1-5

The vocal cords. *(Modified from Thibodeau GS, Patton KT. Anatomy and Physiology, 5th ed. St. Louis: Mosby, 2003, p. 691.)*

are drawn apart during inspiration and relax toward midline during expiration. The epiglottis is a leaf-shaped cartilaginous structure extending from the base of the tongue and attached to the thyroid cartilage by ligaments. It projects upward and posteriorly. During swallowing the epiglottis flaps down to direct swallowed material into the esophagus, thus guarding the opening of the larynx.

LOWER AIRWAY

The lower airway consists of a series of tubes that divide like the branches of a tree, becoming narrower, shorter, and more numerous as they penetrate deeper into the lung. Its functions are to conduct air, provide mucociliary defense, and, most important, perform external gas exchange.

Conducting Airways: Nonalveolate Region

Approximately the first 16 divisions of the tracheobronchial tree take no direct part in gas exchange and are thus designated the conducting zone (Fig. 1-6). The volume is approximately 150 mL and is known as the anatomic dead space.

The trachea, which is made of 16 to 20 C-shaped rings of cartilage, extends from the cricoid cartilage in the larynx to the point where the right and left main-stem bronchi divide: the carina. The average adult trachea is 10 to 12 cm in length and 2.0 to 2.5 cm in diameter. The posterior portion of the trachea is made of smooth muscle and lies adjacent to the esophagus (Fig. 1-7). Excessive pressure on this smooth muscle by the cuff of an artificial airway can lead to erosion and tracheoesophageal fistula. The lining of the trachea consists of ciliated epithelium and mucus-producing goblet cells.

The main-stem bronchi consist of circumferential smooth muscle and plates of cartilage that irregularly encircle the airway. The smooth muscle constricts in

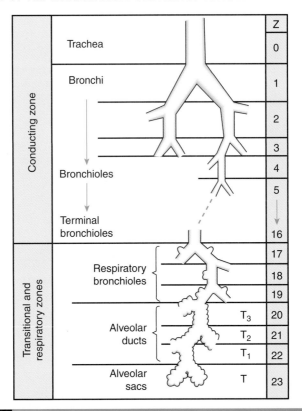

FIGURE 1-6

The 23 divisions of the tracheobronchial tree. Each time the airways branch, a new division, or generation, arises. *(Modified from Weibel E. Design and structure of the human lung. In A Fishman [ed.], Assessment of Pulmonary Function. New York: McGraw-Hill, 1980.)*

response to certain stimuli. Lining the bronchi are ciliated epithelium and more mucus-producing goblet cells. Progressing distally in the airways there is a loss of cartilage, mucus-secreting cells, and cilia.

The trachea divides into the main-stem bronchi. The right main-stem bronchus angles 20 to 30 degrees from the midline and therefore lies almost vertical to the trachea. This position promotes both a greater incidence of aspiration into the right lung in the upright individual and accidental right main-stem intubation when an endotracheal tube is advanced too far into the airway. The left main-stem bronchus is shorter and narrower and angles off more sharply at 45 to 55 degrees; therefore it lies more horizontal to the trachea. The point where the bronchi, nerves, lymphatic vessels, and blood supply leave the mediastinum and enter the lung is known as the hilum.

After penetrating the lung, the right main-stem bronchus divides into three lobar bronchi that supply the upper, middle, and lower right lung lobes. Two lobar divisions of the left main-stem bronchus supply the two lobes of the left lung: the upper and the lower. The lobar bronchi then bifurcate and trifurcate into segmental

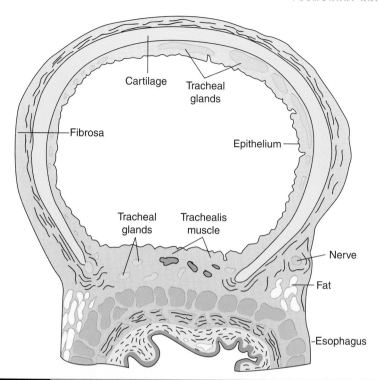

Cartilage

Tracheal glands

Fibrosa

Epithelium

Tracheal glands

Trachealis muscle

Nerve

Fat

Esophagus

FIGURE 1-7

The trachea, which lies adjacent to the esophagus, is made of C-shaped rings of cartilage closed posteriorly by the trachealis muscularis muscle. *(Modified from Kelly EE, Wood RL, Enders AC. Bailey's Textbook of Microscopic Anatomy, 18th ed. Baltimore: Williams & Wilkins, 1984.)*

bronchioles or terminal bronchioles that supply the lung segments on the left and right. The bronchioles lack cartilage and are made of connective tissue that contains elastic fibers and limited smooth muscle. Bronchioles, which are 1 to 2 mm in diameter, are held open by radial traction from the elastic recoil forces of the lung tissue. With the lack of supporting cartilage, these airways are susceptible to bronchospasm.

Respiratory Zone: Alveolate Region
Alveolar buds begin to appear on the walls of the transitional airways, or respiratory bronchioles, which make up the seventeenth through nineteenth generations of airway branches. The terminal respiratory unit, or acinus, is that portion of the lung arising from a single terminal bronchiole. The acinus is the primary gas-exchanging unit of the lung, consisting of the respiratory bronchiole, alveolar ducts, alveolar sacs, and the alveoli (Fig. 1-8). The number of airway divisions, or generations, from the trachea to the alveolar sac is generally 23. The distance from the terminal bronchiole to the most distant alveolus is only about 5 mm, but the respiratory zone makes up most of the lung; its volume is approximately 3000 mL.

Bronchiole   Alveolar duct   Alveoli

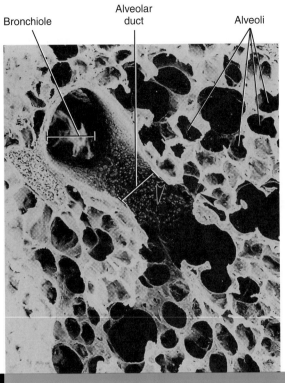

FIGURE 1-8

Scanning electron micrograph of a bronchiole, alveolar duct, and surrounding alveoli. The structure of the acinus, the site of external gas exchange in the lung, is made visible to the human eye. *Arrowhead* indicates opening of the alveoli into the alveolar duct. *(From Thibodeau GS, Patton KT. Anatomy and Physiology, 5th ed. St. Louis: Mosby, 2003.)*

Approximately 300 million alveolar-capillary units are in the adult lung. The total surface area of the lung parenchyma is 50 to 100 m², about the size of a tennis court. The distance between the alveolus and the capillary is less than the diameter of a single red blood cell. The alveoli are surrounded by capillaries so dense that, when fully recruited, they form almost a complete sheet of blood.

The cellular makeup of the alveolus makes it an efficient gas exchanger. Type I alveolar cells are squamous epithelium one cell layer thick that are structured to promote gas exchange and prevent fluid transudation into the alveolus. They are particularly sensitive to oxygen and inhaled agents. Type II cells differentiate into type I cells as needed and produce surfactant, a lipoprotein that reduces the surface tension within the alveolus. The alveolar macrophages, free-moving scavenger cells, phagocytize foreign materials that have evaded the cough reflex and the mucociliary clearance system.

Surfactant prevents the alveoli and bronchioles from collapsing, especially during expiration, by reducing surface tension. Surface tension is caused by the

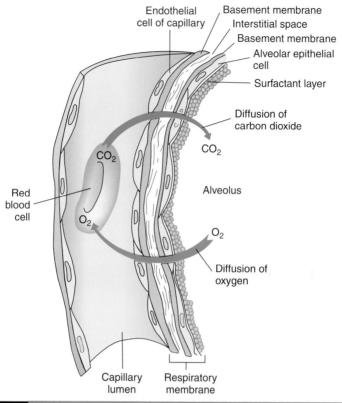

Endothelial
cell of capillary

Basement membrane
Interstitial space
Basement membrane
Alveolar epithelial
cell
Surfactant layer

Diffusion of
carbon dioxide

CO_2

CO_2

Red
blood
cell

Alveolus

O_2

O_2

Diffusion of
oxygen

Capillary
lumen

Respiratory
membrane

FIGURE 1-9

The pathway molecules of gas must travel for gas exchange to occur at the alveolar-capillary membrane. *(Modified from Sexton DL. Nursing Care of the Respiratory Patient. Norwalk, Conn.: Appleton & Lange, 1990.)*

liquid lining the alveoli. This liquid develops a cohesive force that tends to collapse the alveoli. The lung therefore consists of hundreds of millions of relatively unstable bubbles, each 0.3 mm in diameter. Surfactant makes it easier to expand the lung (increases compliance), thereby reducing the work associated with breathing. Surfactant and alveolar stability may be lost in some surfactant-deficient disease states; this loss leads to atelectasis, impaired gas exchange, and increased work of breathing. Exogenous surfactants are now being used for the treatment or prevention of respiratory distress syndrome in the newborn, a condition in which there is a lack of pulmonary surfactant because of lung immaturity.

Gas exchange occurs remarkably efficiently at the alveolar-capillary membrane. Figure 1-9 illustrates the pathway of a gas molecule beginning from inside the alveolus. Blood passes through the capillaries in approximately a half second at rest. However, it is estimated that gas exchange is completed when the blood has traversed only a fourth of the capillary distance. This efficiency provides for gas exchange reserve during disease and exercise states. Diffusion distance and time may be increased in alveolar congestion, interstitial or alveolar edema, or pulmonary fibrosis. Gas exchange at the alveolar-capillary membrane is known as *external respiration*, whereas the exchange of oxygen and carbon dioxide between the systemic capillaries and the cells of the various organ systems is known as *internal respiration*.

COLLATERAL VENTILATION

Collateral ventilation is the process in which one portion of the lung is ventilated via another. These alternative pathways to ventilation are present at the level of the respiratory bronchiole, terminal bronchiole, and the alveoli. Small holes, the *pores of Kohn*, that are present in the walls of the alveoli provide for even gas distribution among the alveoli of an alveolar sac. There are 1 to 7 in each alveolus. Two additional pathways are also present. *Lambert's canals* are intercommunicating channels that connect terminal and respiratory bronchioles with adjacent peribronchial alveoli. These are accessory channels for airflow into and out of the distant alveoli. Finally, the third and largest pathway for collateral ventilation, the *channels of Martin*, connect respiratory bronchioles to each other, serving as side roads or alternate pathways to reaching a distant alveolus (Fig. 1-10). Collateral channels of ventilation may serve to prevent absorption collapse when air is retained in a distant lung portion but cannot be exhaled because of partial airway obstruction. They may also serve to promote ventilation of alveoli when their supplying airways are obstructed by secretions or a foreign body, therefore sustaining gas exchange. Getting gas into the distal alveoli is also essential to the cough mechanism, which relies on the expulsion of the obstructive material to maintain airway patency. These pathways may facilitate even distribution during breathing and assist the lung to respond to structural damage caused by disease.

Airway Innervation

The tracheobronchial tree is innervated by both sympathetic and parasympathetic nerve fibers. Parasympathetic innervation is supplied by the vagus nerve. Stimulation of the vagus nerve by laryngeal irritation results in weak bronchoconstriction, primarily of the larger airways. Sympathetic receptors are primarily the β-2 type. When these adrenergic receptors are stimulated by either of two catecholamines, epinephrine or norepinephrine, the result is bronchodilation. Patients with reversible airflow obstruction—such as in asthma, emphysema, bronchitis, and other obstructive diseases—may obtain relief by using drugs that induce bronchial dilation by either stimulating the β-adrenergic receptors or blocking the effects of vagal nerve stimulation (see Appendix II, Drugs Used in Intensive Respiratory Care).

VASCULAR SUPPLY

Bronchial Circulation

The lung has two different circulatory systems: the bronchial and the pulmonary. The bronchial circulation provides arterial blood to the lung, bronchi, and bronchioles as far as the distal portion of the terminal bronchioles. As a division of the systemic circulation, the bronchial arteries arise from the upper intercostals, subclavian, or internal mammary artery, and then traverse the bronchi and drain into the

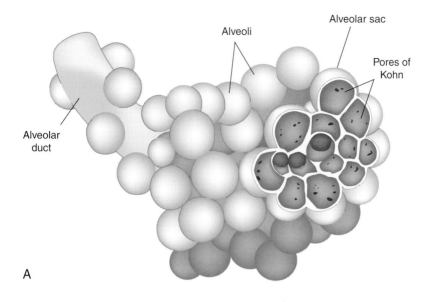

Alveoli

Alveolar sac

Pores of Kohn

Alveolar duct

A

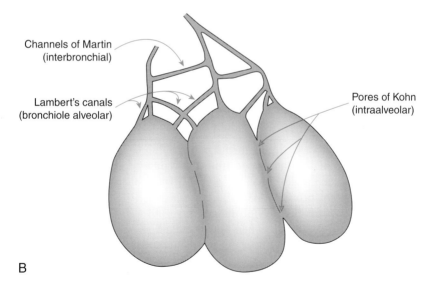

Channels of Martin (interbronchial)

Lambert's canals (bronchiole alveolar)

Pores of Kohn (intraalveolar)

B

FIGURE 1-10

A, The pores of Kohn are small holes in the walls of the alveoli that provide for collateral airflow between the alveoli. Ventilation through these pores contributes to the synchronous ventilation of alveolar units that are receiving less gas because of airway obstruction. **B,** In addition to the pores of Kohn, there are two other known collateral channels of ventilation: the channels of Martin and Lambert's canals. (**B,** Modified from Frawley PM, Habashi NM. Airway pressure release ventilation: theory and practice. AACN Clinical Issues 2001; 12:239.)

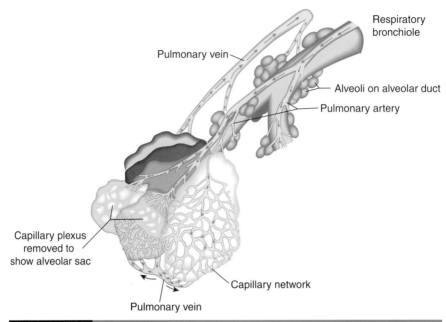

Pulmonary vein

Respiratory bronchiole

Alveoli on alveolar duct

Pulmonary artery

Capillary plexus removed to show alveolar sac

Capillary network

Pulmonary vein

FIGURE 1-11

Alveoli are encased in a meshwork of pulmonary capillaries, which promotes extreme efficiency in gas exchange. *(Modified from Wilkins RL, Sheldon RL, Krider SJ. Clinical Assessment in Respiratory Care, 4th ed. St. Louis: Mosby, 2000.)*

pulmonary veins. This circulation receives only approximately 2% of the cardiac output because the metabolic needs of the lung are low and the lung parenchyma is also oxygenated by direct contact with inspired gas.

Pulmonary Circulation

The pulmonary circulation begins in the main pulmonary artery, which receives oxygen-depleted, mixed venous blood from the right side of the heart. The main pulmonary artery then divides into right and left pulmonary arteries at the point where the main-stem bronchi divide in the hilum. The arteries further divide, running parallel to each division of the airways until they finally terminate in a capillary network so dense that, when fully recruited, the alveoli are nearly coated with blood (Fig. 1-11). The walls of the pulmonary arteries are very thin. They contain smooth muscle but are much less muscular than the arteries of the systemic circulation. The oxygenated blood is collected by the pulmonary veins, which unite with other veins, eventually forming the four large pulmonary veins that drain into the left atrium. Unlike the systemic circulation, the pulmonary arteries carry venous blood and the pulmonary veins carry oxygenated blood.

Lymphatic System

The functions of the pulmonary lymphatic tissue are to maintain fluid homeostasis and to play a role in immunologic defense. The lymphatic system, made up of

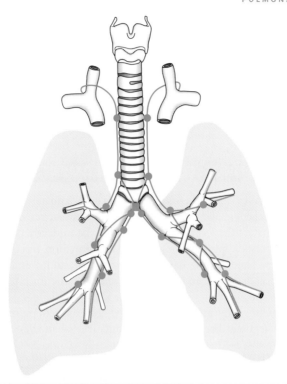

FIGURE 1-12

The main lymphatic channels course along the bronchial tree. Lymph nodes, which filter the lymph, are scattered along the channels. *(Modified from Weibel E. Design and structure of the human lung. In A Fishman [ed.], Assessment of Pulmonary Function. New York: McGraw-Hill, 1980.)*

channels and lymph nodes, the tonsils, thymus, and spleen, reabsorbs excess fluid in the lung interstitium and the peribronchial and pleural spaces and returns to the circulation the serum, escaped plasma protein, and products of cellular metabolism that cannot be absorbed by the capillaries. By reducing interstitial protein concentration, the lymphatic system decreases interstitial colloid oncotic pressure and assists in the prevention of pulmonary edema formation. The immunologic function of the lymphatic system is to filter out bacteria and other harmful substances that have escaped the mucociliary escalator. Filtering is performed in the lymph nodes before the lymphatic fluid is returned to the general circulation, thereby protecting the body from dissemination of foreign material.

Lymphatic vessels are present superficially around the lungs, just beneath the visceral pleura and in the peribronchial and perivascular spaces, forming networks around the blood vessels that they accompany in the thoracic cavity. The channels contain valves that promote unidirectional lymph flow. Lymph is fluid that is formed by the normal processes of interstitial fluid development. Its flow is from the periphery toward the main lymphatic channels along the bronchial tree (Fig. 1-12), toward the lymph nodes clustered about each hilus, and from there onward to either the thoracic or the right lymphatic ducts, which drain into the right and left subclavian veins. Lymph nodes are scattered throughout the course of the lymphatic channels. These nodes are lymph-filtering stations; large particulate matter may therefore be deposited in them. The lymphatic vessels are not typically visualized on the chest radiograph except in certain disease processes such as histoplasmosis, a fungal infection spread in the droppings of fowl, bats, and birds. When the lymphatic system is unable to remove excess fluid, pleural effusion or pulmonary edema may develop.

LUNGS: LOBES AND SEGMENTS

The lungs are conical in shape, their apices arising approximately 2 to 4 cm above the inner third of the clavicle and their bases resting on the upper diaphragm surface, which is approximately the level of the sixth rib at the midclavicular line. The right lung, which accounts for approximately 55% of lung function, has three lobes: upper, middle, and lower. The left lung has two lobes: upper and lower. However, the left upper lobe has a superior and an inferior division. The inferior portion is known as the lingula and is considered comparable to the right middle lobe.

The lobes of the lung are further divided into bronchopulmonary segments (Fig. 1-13). Each segment has its own airway and arterial and venous blood supply, which allows any diseased segment to be surgically removed. Understanding the location of the various pulmonary segments is useful in applying the pulmonary hygiene techniques of postural drainage, percussion, and vibration and for anatomically defining and describing areas of abnormality.

PLEURA AND PLEURAL SPACE

The lungs and the thoracic cavity are lined with the pleura, a continuous sheet of elastic and collagenous fibers that is described in two portions: the visceral pleura and the parietal pleura (Fig. 1-14). The visceral pleura is a thin, delicate lining around the lungs, lung fissures, and hilar bronchi and vessels. The parietal pleura lines the inner surface of the thoracic cavity. The parietal pleura has nerve receptors for pain, but the visceral pleura does not. A mucous solution is produced by the cells of the pleura. This solution, which is probably less than 10 mL, lubricates the pleural surfaces, allowing for smooth movement of the surfaces over one another. It also holds the two pleurae together by means of surface tension forces; thus the pleurae move in unison with the thoracic cage on inspiration. Surface tension is an attractive force between adjacent liquid molecules. This force preserves the integrity of the surface, preventing it from separating. It is the surface tension between the two pleurae, opposing the tendency of the lung to want to collapse because of its elastic recoil, that leads to the existence of a pressure of approximately negative 5 mm Hg within the intrapleural space.

The pleural space is essentially a potential space between the two pleural surfaces. If excessive fluid (pleural effusion, hemothorax, etc.) or air (pneumothorax) enters this space, lung expansion may be inhibited. If the decreased expansion is significant enough to compromise respiration, a chest tube may be needed (see

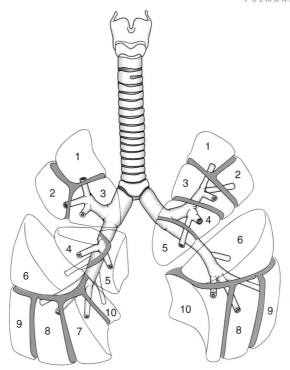

FIGURE 1-13

Divisions of the tracheobronchial tree and the bronchopulmonary segments. *(Modified from Weibel E. Design and structure of the human lung. In A Fishman [ed.], Assessment of Pulmonary Function. New York: McGraw-Hill, 1980.)*

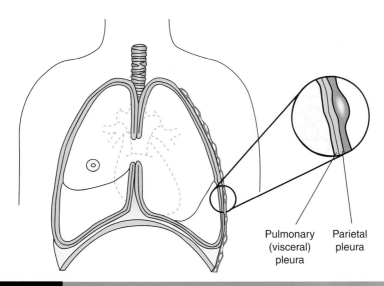

Pulmonary (visceral) pleura   Parietal pleura

FIGURE 1-14

Pleural linings of the lungs. *(Modified from Carroll P. Understanding Chest Drainage. Fall River, Mass.: Deknatel, Inc., 1992.)*

Appendix III, Chest Drainage Systems). Because the right and left parietal and visceral pleurae are entirely separate, pleural space disease may exist in one hemithorax and be absent in the other.

THORACIC CAGE

The lungs are housed in the thoracic cage, which is bordered posteriorly by the vertebral column, anteriorly by the sternum, and laterally by the ribs. Its floor is formed by the dome-shaped diaphragm. The ribs, 24 in number, 12 on each side, attach posteriorly to the spinal column and then extend around and down, under the arms, where they turn upward again and extend, not as bone but as cartilage, to the sternum (Fig. 1-15). These resilient bars of cartilage, the costal cartilages, extend from all the ribs, except the last two pairs, toward the sternum. The first seven pairs of ribs, the true ribs, have cartilage that actually reaches the sternum. The last five pairs are the false ribs. Of the false ribs, numbers 8, 9, and 10 have costal cartilages that turn up and join the rib above. Ribs 11 and 12 are floating ribs in that they have no anterior attachment. The ribs provide not only protection of the lungs but also an

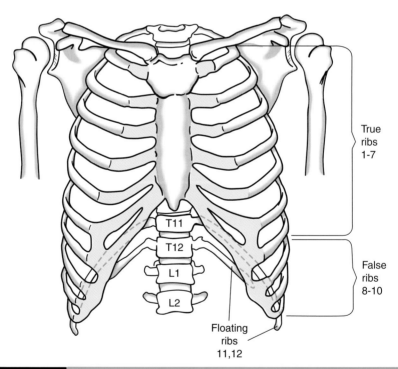

FIGURE 1-15

The bony thorax.

attachment for the respiratory muscles. On the underside of each rib the costal groove contains an intercostal artery, nerve, and vein. When needles or tubes are placed in the intercostal space, the inferior margin of the rib must be avoided to prevent damage to these structures.

The sternum has three parts: the manubrium above, the body in the middle, and the xiphoid process below. The point where the manubrium and the body articulate, the angle of Louis, is a prominent ridge that can be felt under the skin. At this point, the second rib articulates with the sternum and is a landmark for both the point where the trachea divides into the left and right main stem and for counting the ribs and the intercostal spaces (ICSs). The ICSs are numbered according to the number of ribs above; therefore the space above the second rib is the first ICS.

RESPIRATORY MUSCLES

Inspiratory Muscles

The principal muscle of respiration is the *diaphragm*. The central portion is composed of fibrous tissue and is known as the central tendon. The muscular portion of the diaphragm attaches to the xiphoid process, the costal margins of the lower six ribs, and the vertebral column. The muscle fiber composition of the diaphragm makes it highly suited to the type of endurance work it must perform. When high-resistance workloads, which require strength, not especially endurance, are placed on the diaphragm, the muscle fibers may fatigue quickly if energy demands exceed supply. The diaphragm can adapt with time to high-resistance workloads placed on it by some disease states.

In the resting position, the diaphragm is dome shaped. On inspiration the diaphragm contracts, flattening the dome. This action increases the superior-inferior dimension of the thoracic cavity, forces the abdominal contents downward, and elevates the lower ribs. The diaphragm normally accounts for approximately 70% of the tidal volume. The diaphragm also assists in generating high abdominal pressures in maneuvers such as coughing, vomiting, sneezing, and defecation.

Playing a lesser role in inspiratory activities are the *external intercostal muscles*. These muscles arise from the lower border of the first 11 ribs and have fibers that extend downward and forward to the upper border of the rib below. On inspiration, the external intercostal muscles contract, elevating the ribs and increasing the anterior-posterior dimension of the thoracic cavity.

The accessory muscles of respiration are called into play with increased effort breathing. During inspiration the *scalene muscle*, which extends from the cervical vertebrae to the first two ribs, contracts to elevate the first two ribs. The *sternocleidomastoid muscle*, which extends from the jawline to the sternum, assists in elevating the sternum. Both muscles therefore attempt to increase the anterior-posterior diameter of the thorax. Figure 1-16 illustrates the ventilatory muscles.

Expiratory Muscles

Expiration during normal quiet ventilation is a passive activity that occurs because of relaxation of the inspiratory muscles and recoil of the lung parenchyma. During

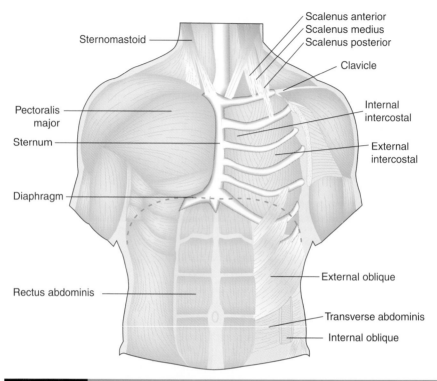

FIGURE 1-16

The muscles of ventilation. See text for description. *(Modified from Wilkins RL, Stoller JK, Scanlan CL, et al. Egan's Fundamentals of Respiratory Care, 8th ed. St. Louis: Mosby, 2003, p 161.)*

forceful expiration the *internal intercostal muscles* contract, decreasing the anterior-posterior diameter of the thorax by pulling the ribs downward and inward. These muscles lie under the external intercostals and have similar points of attachment but differ in that they have fibers that pass downward and backward.

The abdominal muscles used for increased effort expiration include the *internal and external oblique muscles*, the *rectus muscle*, and the *transverse abdominis muscle*. When contracted, these muscles force the diaphragm upward and depress the lower ribs, decreasing the superior-inferior diameter of the thorax.

Innervation of the Ventilatory Muscles

Knowledge regarding the nervous innervation of the muscles of respiration (Fig. 1-17 and Table 1-1) provides a basis for understanding the respiratory effects of neuromuscular disease. This knowledge is particularly valuable when caring for patients with neuromuscular disorders or spinal cord injury because one can detect ventilatory failure early, determine what respiratory muscle function has been lost or spared, and develop a rehabilitation plan.

TABLE 1-1 Innervation of the Muscles of Ventilation

Muscles	Innervating Nerves
Diaphragm	Phrenic nerve. Arises from the cervical spinal cord, roots C3, C4, and C5. Susceptibility to injury to one or both phrenic nerves is increased during thoracic surgery or trauma because of course of nerve down the thoracic cavity. High cervical spinal cord injury may result in immediate loss of diaphragm function and death. Patients with high spinal cord lesions develop hypertrophy of sternocleidomastoid and trapezius muscles, which are spared because of innervation by cranial nerve XI.
External and internal intercostal muscles	Intercostal nerves. Arise from thoracic spinal nerves 1 to 12. Patient with thoracic spinal cord injury may learn to breathe without a ventilator by using diaphragm and neck muscles. Expiratory muscle paralysis results in reduced cough effectiveness and impaired secretion clearance.
Abdominal	Spinal nerves. Arise from T7 through L1. Reduced expiratory effort therefore results in less effective cough and secretion clearance.
Scalene	Spinal nerves C4 through C8. Function is lost in high-level spinal cord lesions.
Sternocleidomastoid	Cranial nerve XI, spinal accessory. Spared in cervical spinal cord injury.
Trapezius	Spinal nerves C3 and C4 and cranial nerve XI, spinal accessory. Partially spared in cervical spinal cord injury.

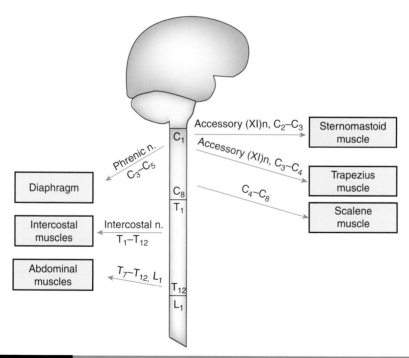

FIGURE 1-17

Motor innervation of ventilatory muscle groups. (*Modified from Tobin MJ. Respiratory muscles in disease. Clin Chest Med 9(2):277, 1988.*)

PROTECTIVE MECHANISMS

Cough

The coughing response represents an important protective mechanism for the body and utilizes forced expiration as the basic pattern for expelling foreign objects from the respiratory passages. The cougher inspires, closes the glottis and vigorously contracts the expiratory muscles in a Valsalva maneuver, and then suddenly opens the glottis. Because air is momentarily prevented from leaving the lungs, intrapleural and intrapulmonic pressures are built to maximum levels. On the sudden opening of the glottis, a blast of air is forced through the trachea, effectively ejecting the foreign object or mucous deposit from the airway. Mechanical, chemical, or physical stimuli initiate a cough, which is a cholinergic vagal reflex, whose receptors are primarily located in the larynx, trachea, and larger bronchi. When an endotracheal tube is in place, the mechanics of coughing are disrupted in that the glottis cannot close normally, potentially leading to a less efficient cough.

Sneeze

A sneeze is elicited by irritation of the mucous membranes of the nose by mechanical, physical, or chemical stimuli. It results when the sensory receptors of the trigeminal or olfactory nerves are stimulated. A deep inhalation is initiated, followed by a violent exhalation through the nose.

Mucociliary Clearance System

The mucociliary clearance system, consisting of mucus and ciliated cells, functions to trap and transport airborne particles not filtered in the nose and larger airways. Normal production of mucus in the lungs is approximately 100 mL/day. Mucus comes from two sources: the surface goblet cells and the submucosal glands, which produce a mixed serous and mucous secretion. The submucosal glands respond to vagal stimulation with increased output. Output is therefore decreased with vagal blocking agents (see Appendix II, Drugs Used in Intensive Respiratory Care) or pulmonary denervation, as in pulmonary transplantation. Conversely, increased production of mucus, as in bronchitis or cystic fibrosis, can overwhelm the mucociliary system.

Ciliated epithelium is present from the upper airways down to the terminal bronchioles. Each cell contains an estimated 200 to 275 cilia, each approximately 6 to 7 mm long that beat upward in a coordinated, wavelike fashion projecting mucus upward, or in the case of the nose, backward toward the pharynx, at a velocity of 10 to 20 mm/min. Once the secretions reach the oropharynx, they are eliminated by expectoration or swallowing. Many factors may affect the function of the mucociliary clearance system (Box 1-1).

Immunoglobulins and enzymes are also found in the mucous blanket of the lungs. IgA is the principal antibody found in normal mucous secretions. Immunoglobulin deficiencies may lead to a predisposition to respiratory infection.

BOX 1-1 Factors Adversely Affecting Mucociliary Function

Cigarette smoke
Hyperoxia and hypoxia
Hypercapnia
Lack of, or low, humidity in inspired air
Systemic dehydration
Artificial airways
Inhalation anesthetics
Narcotics
Sedatives
Alcohol
Acute respiratory tract infections
Cellular destruction caused by tracheal suctioning
Smoke inhalation
Denervation as a result of lung transplantation
Increasing age
Sleep

Enzymes play a role in the destruction of bacteria. Considering that the respiratory tract is in constant contact with the environment, it is truly remarkable that the lower respiratory tract is almost sterile. Working together to achieve this feat are the mucociliary clearance system, enzymes, alveolar macrophages, the pulmonary lymphatic system, and immunoglobulins.

CONTROL OF VENTILATION

Ventilation is controlled through an interplay of many complex processes to ensure that adequate oxygen is available for metabolism and that the byproduct of cellular metabolism, carbon dioxide, is removed and acid–base homeostasis is maintained. Despite many years of study, our understanding of the control of ventilation is incomplete. Breathing is primarily controlled humorally, through the action of chemical stimuli on regulatory centers in the brain stem.

Voluntary Control: Cortical Centers

Although breathing continues rhythmically without our conscious effort, such as when sleeping or concentrating on work, conscious control of breathing is possible. Conscious regulation of breathing is mediated by the cerebral cortex, specifically in the motor cortex of the frontal lobe and the limbic area. An individual may voluntarily hyperventilate, hold his breath, or alter his breathing pattern to sniff, sing, speak, hum, or perform isometric work such as straining to have a bowel movement or lift a heavy object. However, the ability of the cerebral cortex to override other central regulatory centers for breathing is limited. For example, holding one's breath to the point of unconsciousness is limited by carbon dioxide stimulation of spontaneous breathing.

Involuntary Control: Medullary, Pontine, and Peripheral Centers

Both peripheral and central centers take part in the involuntary control of breathing. Ventilatory centers are named according to their location within or outside the central nervous system (Fig. 1-18). Within the central nervous system the primary centers for the control of breathing are in the medulla oblongata and pons. Only recently have physiologists become aware that there is no single group of pacemaker cells for inspiration or expiration that fire by self-excitation. Nor are there distinct groups of inspiratory and expiratory cells that mutually inhibit one another, resulting in rhythmic breathing. Instead, within the medulla are groups of respiratory neurons: the dorsal respiratory group (DRG) and the ventral respiratory group (VRG), both of

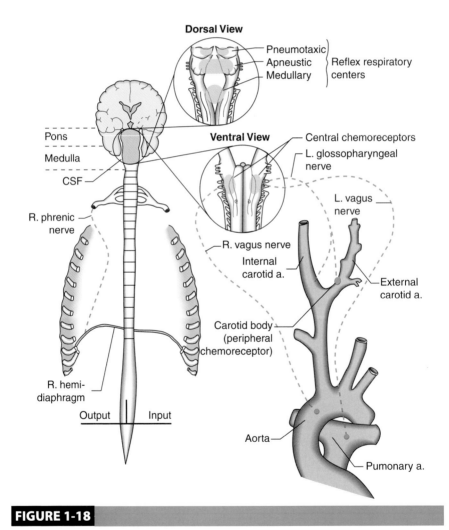

FIGURE 1-18

Central and peripheral centers responsible for the control of ventilation. *(Modified from Slonim NB, Chapin JL. Respiratory Physiology. St. Louis: Mosby, 1967.)*

which contain inspiratory and expiratory neurons that work together to modify the basic breathing pattern.

The DRG are mainly inspiratory neurons that send impulses through the phrenic and thoracic nerves to the external intercostal muscles and the diaphragm. VRG neurons contain both inspiratory and expiratory neurons. From the VRG, motor impulses are sent via the vagus nerve to the laryngeal and pharyngeal muscles, resulting in abduction of the vocal cords, widening the glottic opening. Other VRG inspiratory neurons send messages to the diaphragm and external intercostals while expiratory VRG neurons send impulses to the internal intercostals and abdominal muscles. Input to these centers comes via the glossopharyngeal and vagus nerves from the lungs, airways, joint proprioceptors, and peripheral chemoreceptors.

The two pontine centers, the apneustic and the pneumotaxic, modify the output of the medullary centers. The apneustic center acts on the medulla to promote deep and prolonged inspiration. Injury to the pons can lead to an abnormal breathing pattern known as apneustic breathing, which is a gasping type of ventilation with maximal inspiratory effort. Output from the apneustic center is limited by the pneumotaxic center, which acts to inhibit inspiration by sending impulses to the medulla. The pneumotaxic center, therefore, controls the inspiratory endpoint. It switches off inspiration. Strong pneumotaxic impulses result in a fast respiratory rate, whereas weak impulses prolong inspiratory time. How the pneumotaxic and apneustic centers exactly work together remains to be determined.

Humoral Control of Ventilation

Ventilation is primarily controlled by feedback mechanisms in which oxygen, carbon dioxide, and hydrogen ions serve as chemical stimuli. Chemoreceptors in the brain stem and the periphery are sensitive to blood levels of oxygen, carbon dioxide, and hydrogen ions and respond to hypercapnia, acidemia, and hypoxemia by sending impulses to the medulla to increase ventilation (Table 1-2).

CENTRAL CHEMORECEPTORS

Chemoreceptors located in the medulla are primarily influenced by the hydrogen ion concentration (pH) of the cerebrospinal fluid (CSF). An increase in partial pressure of carbon dioxide in arterial blood (Pa_{CO_2}) causes maximal increases in the hydrogen

TABLE 1-2	Location and Response of the Chemoreceptors Involved in the Control of Ventilation			
Location	**Category**	**Stimulus**		**Response**
Medulla	Central	Increased hydrogen ion concentration of cerebrospinal fluid (decreased pH)		Strong stimulus to increase the rate and depth of ventilation
Aortic arch and bifurcation of the carotid arteries	Peripheral	Decreased Pa_{O_2}		Increase in the rate and depth of ventilation
		Increased Pa_{CO_2} or decreased pH		Mild increase in ventilation

ion concentration of the CSF because it lacks the protein hydrogen buffers found in the blood. Central chemoreceptors, when stimulated by a decreasing pH because of increasing H^+ ion concentration, increase the depth and rate of respiration. A low concentration of CSF hydrogen ion, alkalosis, retards ventilation. Central chemo-receptors do not respond to a low partial pressure of oxygen in arterial blood (PaO_2).

PERIPHERAL CHEMORECEPTORS

Peripheral chemoreceptors are small, highly vascular structures called the carotid and aortic bodies. They are located on the aortic arch and at the bifurcation of the internal and external carotid arteries. Afferent impulses from the carotid bodies to the medulla are sent via the glossopharyngeal nerve (cranial nerve IX) and from the aortic bodies via the vagus nerve (cranial nerve X). Peripheral chemoreceptors are extremely sensitive to decreases in blood oxygen tension. Hypoxemia increases the activity of the peripheral receptors, leading to an increase in the rate and depth of ventilation, especially when the PaO_2 falls below 60 mm Hg. The peripheral chemo-receptors also respond to increases in $PaCO_2$ and hydrogen ion concentration with an increase in ventilation, but they do so less sensitively than the central receptors.

Mechanical Reflexes

STRETCH RECEPTORS

Stretch receptors are located in bronchial smooth muscle. When they are stimulated by lung hyperinflation, impulses are sent to the respiratory center, via the vagus nerve, to limit further inflation and increase expiratory time. This is known as the Hering-Breuer inflation reflex. The Hering-Breuer deflation reflex initiates inspi-ratory activity at very low lung volumes.

IRRITANT RECEPTORS

Activity of the irritant receptors, which lie between the epithelial cells of the airway, is mediated by the vagus nerve. When stimulated by inhaled particles such as cigarette smoke or cold air, the reflex response is bronchoconstriction and increased respiratory rate.

J RECEPTORS

Receptors located in the alveolar walls near the capillary are appropriately named juxtacapillary receptors, or J receptors. They are innervated by the vagus nerve and, when stimulated, cause rapid, shallow breathing, a sensation of dyspnea, and narrow-ing of the glottis during expiration. Stimulants include fluid in the alveoli and distention of the pulmonary capillaries, conditions that are present in adult respira-tory distress syndrome, left heart failure, pneumonia, and pulmonary edema.

OTHER RECEPTORS

Proprioceptors in the joints are believed to be responsible for the increase in rate and depth of ventilation with increased movement of the joint, which occurs with exercise or even during passive range of motion. Gamma receptors in the intercostal muscles and the diaphragm muscle spindles may be responsible for the sensation of dyspnea when increased respiratory effort is required. An increase in body temperature or stimulation of pain receptors can lead to hyperventilation. In addition, stimulation of the carotid and aortic baroreceptors, by an increase in blood pressure, may cause reflex hypoventilation or apnea, whereas a decrease in blood pressure may result in hyperventilation.

RECOMMENDED READINGS

Corrin B. Normal lung structure. In B. Corrin (ed.), *Pathology of the Lungs* (pp. 1–34). London: Churchill Livingstone, 2000.

Des Jardins T. *Cardiopulmonary Anatomy and Physiology*. Australia: Delmar, 2002.

Guyton AC. *Textbook of Medical Physiology*. Philadelphia: Saunders, 2000.

Thibodeau GS, Patton KT. *Anatomy and Physiology*, 5th ed. St. Louis: Mosby, 2003.

Tobin MJ. Respiratory muscles in disease. *Clin Chest Med* 1988; 9(2):263–286.

Weibel E. Design and structure of the human lung. In A. Fishman (ed.), *Assessment of Pulmonary Function* (pp. 18–68). New York: McGraw-Hill, 1980.

Wilkins RL, Stoller JK, Scanlan CL, et al. The respiratory system. In RL Wilkins, JK Stoller, CL Scanlan et al. (eds.), *Egan's Fundamentals of Respiratory Care,* 8th ed. (pp. 137–186). St. Louis: Mosby, 2003.

Wilkins RL, Stoller JK, Scanlan CL, et al. Ventilation. In RL Wilkins, JK Stoller, CL Scanlan et al. (eds.), *Egan's Fundamentals of Respiratory Care,* 8th ed. (pp. 207–227). St. Louis: Mosby, 2003.

CHAPTER 2

Practical Physiology of the Pulmonary System

Practice in many clinical arenas requires a strong understanding of physiologic processes. Physiology is utilized as the basis to interpret knowledgeably the large amounts of data gathered in patient care settings. It is from this physiologic vantage point that we interpret the cause of findings (e.g., high airway pressures, hypoxemia, hypercapnia) and therefore choose the appropriate therapy. We then evaluate the effects of therapies, using physiologic measures that provide quantifiable gauges of whether or not the patient is improving. For example, serial measures of oxygenation or ventilation, percentage shunt, compliance, and resistance help us in reevaluating our therapies. Finally, physiology helps us understand the positive or adverse effects of therapies, such as the effects of changing the body position on ventilation/perfusion relationships and thus oxygenation, the effects of positive end-expiratory pressure (PEEP), and how to treat adverse PEEP effects. The foundation for caring for the patient supported by a mechanical ventilator begins with an understanding of how spontaneous ventilation is achieved.

VENTILATORY CONCEPTS

Mechanics of Spontaneous Ventilation

The purpose of ventilation is to supply fresh gas to the lungs, to be exchanged at the alveolar-capillary membrane. The basic principle underlying the movement of gas is that it travels from an area of higher to lower pressure. Physiologic pressures related to the flow of gases into and out of the lung are atmospheric pressure, intrapulmonary (or intraalveolar) pressure, and intrapleural (or intrathoracic) pressure. The difference between two pressures is called a pressure gradient. The three important pressure gradients related to ventilation are transrespiratory, transpulmonary, and transthoracic pressure (Table 2-1).

At rest, the pressure within the alveoli is atmospheric, or 0 cm H_2O (Fig. 2-1). When a spontaneous inspiration is initiated, muscular effort is exerted by the contraction of the diaphragm and the external intercostal muscles. Inspiration is thus an active process that requires the expenditure of energy. Contraction of the inspiratory muscles enlarges the thoracic cavity. The lungs expand because they are pulled outward, along with the movement of the thoracic wall. The lungs move with the chest wall because of surface tension created by the small amount of fluid between the visceral and parietal pleurae. Negative pressure normally within the intrapleural space becomes even more negative on inspiration (from –5 cm H_2O to

TABLE 2-1 Pressures and Pressure Gradients Related to Ventilation

Pressure/Definition	Abbreviation	Alternate Terms	Explanation
Pressure at the body surface	Pbs	Atmospheric pressure	Atmospheric pressure is the pressure exerted by the surrounding air on the earth's surface and is equal to 760 mm Hg or 1034 cm H_2O. Airway pressures are measured relative to atmospheric; therefore Pbs is the zero pressure reference to which all other airway pressures are measured
Pressure at the airway opening	Pao	Mouth pressure	Zero unless positive pressure is applied
Alveolar pressure: pressure within the alveoli	Palv	Intrapulmonary	Varies during the breathing cycle
Intrapleural pressure: pressure within the pleural space	Ppl	Intrathoracic	Subatmospheric (negative) because of the tendency of the lungs to want to collapse. Elastic recoil of the lungs continuously exerts a pull on the thoracic wall
PRESSURE GRADIENTS (THE DIFFERENCE BETWEEN TWO PRESSURES)			
Transrespiratory pressure gradient Prs = Palv – Pao	Prs	Pressure difference down the airway	Responsible for gas flow into and out of the lungs
Transpulmonary pressure gradient P_L = Palv – Ppl	P_L	Pressure difference across the lung. Also known as transmural pressure	Created entirely by the elasticity of the lung. Maintains alveolar inflation or volume
Transthoracic pressure gradient Pw = Ppl – Pbs	Pw	Difference in pressure between the pleural space and the body surface. Pressure difference across the chest wall	Total pressure necessary to expand or contract the lungs and chest wall together

*Pressures are measured in cm H_2O and are expressed relative to atmospheric pressure. Therefore, a pressure of 2 cm H_2O is atmospheric (1034 cm H_2O) plus 2 cm H_2O.

–8 cm H_2O); thus the transpulmonary pressure gradient (P_L) widens, causing the alveoli to expand. As the alveoli expand, intraalveolar pressure also becomes subatmospheric (–1 cm H_2O); therefore air at atmospheric pressure flows into the lung. Inspiration continues until intraalveolar pressure rises to equal atmospheric pressure. Air does not have to be drawn, or sucked, into the lung. Air simply moves from an area of high pressure to one of low pressure.

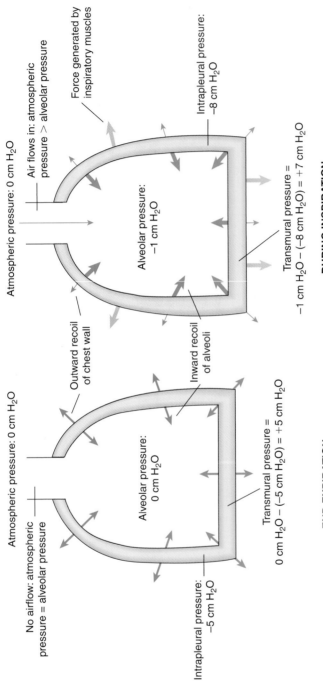

FIGURE 2-1

Pressure changes within the thoracic cavity during spontaneous ventilation. (*Left*) At end-expiration the muscles of respiration are relaxed. Lung volume is determined by the competing forces of elastic recoil of the lung and thorax. No airflow occurs because atmospheric and alveolar pressures are equal. (*Right*) Contraction of the respiratory muscles on inspiration enlarges the thoracic cavity. The lung is pulled outward with the chest wall and intrapleural pressure becomes more negative. Alveolar pressure drops below atmospheric pressure, and air, because of its tendency to move to an area of less pressure, flows into the lungs. (*Modified from Levitsky MG. Pulmonary Physiology, 6th ed. New York: McGraw-Hill, 2003.*)

Expiration is a passive process that occurs because of the elastic recoil of the lung. When contraction of the inspiratory muscles ceases, the thoracic cage and lungs recoil to their original size. Intrapleural pressure becomes less negative. Intraalveolar pressure becomes slightly positive on expiration, which ends when intraalveolar and atmospheric pressures equalize. In the spontaneously breathing individual, lung volume attained at end expiration is determined by the competing forces of elastic recoil and thoracic cage stiffness.

The increased negativity of the intrapleural pressure during inspiration is important for bringing air into the lungs and for promoting venous return to the right side of the heart (preload) by expanding the great veins. When an individual is placed on a positive-pressure ventilator, the normally low intrathoracic pressures are disrupted in that they become positive. Positive pressure within the thorax affects the distribution of gases and may also lead to hemodynamic embarrassment, primarily through a reduction in right heart preload (see Chapter 9).

Lung Volumes and Capacities: Spirometry

Air within the lung can be measured with an instrument called a spirometer. Total air is divided into subdivisions called *volumes*. When two or more volumes are added, they are called a lung *capacity* (Fig. 2-2). Measurement of lung volumes is useful because many pathophysiologic states alter lung volumes. The effect of therapies utilized specifically to enhance particular lung volumes can also be evaluated. The following definitions are relevant.

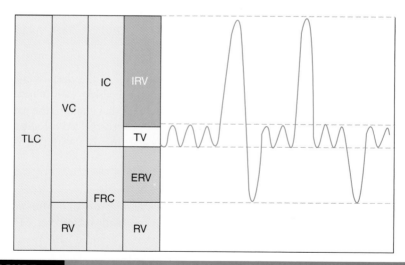

FIGURE 2-2

Measurement of lung volumes and capacities with a spirometer. *(Modified from Bonner JT, Hall JR. Respiratory Intensive Care of the Adult Surgical Patient. St. Louis: Mosby, 1985.)*

TIDAL VOLUME (VT)

The tidal volume (VT) is the volume of gas moved into or out of the lung in a single normal inspiration or expiration. It averages 500 mL, or 5 to 8 mL/kg. It represents the volume reaching the alveoli, approximately 350 mL, plus the volume in the conducting airways, known as the anatomic dead space, which is approximately 150 mL, or 2 mL/kg.

INSPIRATORY RESERVE VOLUME (IRV)

The inspiratory reserve volume (IRV) is the volume of air that can be inspired at the end of a normal tidal inspiration. It is appropriately titled "reserve" volume. The IRV is called on when increased tidal breathing is necessary, as in exercise.

EXPIRATORY RESERVE VOLUME (ERV)

The expiratory reserve volume (ERV) is the maximal volume of gas that can be exhaled after a normal exhalation.

RESIDUAL VOLUME (RV)

The residual volume (RV) is the volume of gas remaining in the lungs after a maximal expiration. This volume cannot be measured with spirometry. It is obtained indirectly by using the helium dilution test, nitrogen washout method, or body plethysmography to determine the functional residual capacity (FRC). The formula RV = FRC − ERV is then used to determine RV.

INSPIRATORY CAPACITY (IC) = IRV + VT

The inspiratory capacity (IC) is the maximal volume of gas that can be inspired after a normal exhalation. Measurement of the IC as a determinant of maximal tidal volume capability is a more useful and accurate measurement than the IRV because when the IRV is measured, deciding when the tidal volume (VT) ends is extremely subjective.

VITAL CAPACITY (VC) = IRV + VT + ERV

The vital capacity (VC) is the volume of gas exhaled after the deepest possible inspiration. This measurement can be obtained at the bedside with a handheld spirometer in a cooperative patient. It is clinically useful in that it tells us the patient's maximal ventilatory capability. VC may be measured and trended as an indicator of a patient's ventilatory capability when respiratory muscles are compromised, as they may be after a new spinal cord injury.

FUNCTIONAL RESIDUAL CAPACITY (FRC) = ERV + RV

The FRC is the volume of air remaining in the lungs at the end of a normal expiration. This is the volume where gas exchange is constantly taking place. The VT can be thought of as the dilutional volume. Tidal breaths bring in fresh gas to mix with the volume already present in the lungs, the FRC, where steady-state gas exchange is occurring. In many pathologic conditions, such as atelectasis, secretion or fluid collection in the lungs, or pleural effusion, the FRC is reduced and thus gas exchange is affected. Direct measurement of the FRC cannot be performed with spirometry (see the definition of residual volume).

TABLE 2-2 Lung Volumes and Capacities	
Measurement	**Volume* (mL)**
Tidal volume (VT)	500
Inspiratory reserve volume (IRV)	3000
Expiratory reserve volume (ERV)	1200
Residual volume (RV)	1300
Inspiratory capacity (IC) = IRV + VT	3500
Vital capacity (VC) = IRV + VT + ERV	4700
Functional residual capacity (FRC) = ERV + RV	2500
Total lung capacity (TLC) = IC + FRC	6000

*Average volume in a 70-kg young adult. There is a range of normal values that varies by age, height, body size, and gender. Volumes are less in women than men when height and age are equal.

TOTAL LUNG CAPACITY (TLC) = IC + FRC

The total lung capacity (TLC) is the maximal volume of air in the lungs after a maximal inspiration. TLC is the sum of all lung volumes (Table 2-2).

Closing Volume

The closing volume (CV) is that volume on expiration where small airways in the lung base begin to close. Expressed as a percentage of the VC, it is normally 10% but may increase with age and in disease processes that lead to a loss of lung elasticity. CV may actually exceed FRC in some diseases, which leads to impaired gas exchange. CV cannot be measured with a spirometer.

The airways in the basilar portion of the lung close sooner than those above because the PL, transpulmonary pressure gradient, is less at the base. The reason is that intrapleural pressure is less negative at the lung bases because of the weight of the lungs hanging within the thorax. When lung elasticity or volume decreases, the intrapleural pressure at the base of the lungs may actually become positive, compressing the lung. Under these conditions, CV increases and alveolar ventilation decreases. These changes become evident in the patient's blood gases.

FACTORS AFFECTING VENTILATION

Compliance

Compliance is a measurement of the distensibility of the respiratory tissue. The elasticity of the pulmonary tissues is primarily due to its interstitial makeup of elastin and collagen fibers. This interstitial network provides crucial support for airways, alveoli, and capillaries. In some disease states, these fibers become less elastic, leading to so-called stiff lungs.

Elastic recoil refers to the return of tissue to its resting position after being stretched. For example, pantyhose and rubber bands are both made of elastic fibers that should return to their resting state when an applied stretch is removed. Likewise, the lungs have very strong elastic recoil that makes them want to return continually to their resting state. Indeed, if the negative pressure in the intrapleural space (the pressure that opposes the lung's elastic recoil) is disrupted, the lungs collapse.

Distensibility refers to the stretchability of the lung, that is, the relative ease with which the lung can be stretched with a given force. Compliance is a measurement of the lung's distensibility. It is defined and measured as the volume change per unit of pressure change. The compliance of both the chest wall and the lung tissue is known as total lung compliance. The following is the physiologic formula for total lung compliance (CTL):

$$\text{CTL} = \frac{\text{Change in volume}}{\text{Change in pressure}}$$

Various pathologic conditions such as acute respiratory distress syndrome (ARDS), pneumonia, pulmonary edema, pulmonary fibrosis, pneumothorax, and hemothorax lead to low compliance, or stiff lungs. Pathologic conditions that affect total compliance generally fall into three categories: disease of the lung interstitium, disease of the intrapleural space, and disease of the chest wall.

A decrease in compliance affects ventilation. As an example, if the patient is not able to increase the *work* required to generate greater muscular effort to expand the thorax and overcome the stiffer elastic recoil of the lung, a decrease in VT results. The distribution of ventilation is also affected in that it will be uneven. Ventilation will be preferentially distributed to the areas of best compliance.

In the clinical setting, treatments that improve compliance can be implemented. Measures of compliance are then used to evaluate the effectiveness of the chosen therapy and to decide whether the patient is progressing. These serial measures actually quantify whether a treatment is decreasing the abnormality and improving the compliance.

Begin by gathering assessment data and determining whether they are suggestive of disease processes that adversely affect compliance (e.g., congestive heart failure [crackles, rales], pneumothorax, atelectasis, infiltrates, pleural effusion, lobar collapse). If a consolidative or infiltrative disease process is present, then the patient will need therapies designed to mobilize secretions, such as chest physiotherapy (CPT); suctioning; and turning, coughing, and deep breathing. The diuresing of edema, however, may also be a choice. If the patient has pleural space disease, therapies should be directed toward evacuating the pleural effusion, pneumothorax, hemothorax, or empyema and then maintaining the chest tube drainage system. If the reduction in compliance is caused by a decrease in chest wall movement, then the therapies may include pain control, sedating the patient to promote synchrony with the ventilator, or, in the case of a circumferential chest burn, an escharotomy.

Two forms of compliance—static and dynamic—can be measured. In settings that use microprocessor ventilators, the ventilator easily performs measurements of respiratory mechanics after the operator inputs only a few simple commands. Static compliance is the truest measure of the compliance of the *lung* tissue. It is measured while there are no gases flowing into or out of the lungs. The following is the physiologic formula for static compliance (CST):

$$C_{ST} = \frac{\text{Exhaled tidal volume}}{\text{Plateau pressure} - \text{PEEP}}$$

During care of a patient who requires a ventilator, the measurements of exhaled tidal volume, plateau pressure, and PEEP are easily obtained. The exhaled tidal volume is the most accurate measure of the volume actually in the lungs at the time the pressure measurement was taken; therefore it should be utilized as the volume measurement (see the discussion in Chapter 6 of exhaled tidal volume). The plateau pressure is obtained by instituting a 2-second inspiratory pause at the peak of inspiration. This pause creates the condition of no gases flowing into the lungs. At the point at which no gases are flowing, and with the glottis open, the pressure within the alveoli is obtainable in the form of the plateau pressure. The reading taken during the inspiratory pause, the plateau pressure, reflects pressure, due to the elastic recoil forces of the lung tissue alone, on the volume of gas in the lungs. No pressure resulting from the flow of gases is measured. When the calculation is performed, any artificial pressure placed in the airway, such as PEEP, must be subtracted from the plateau pressure. When a patient does not have an endotracheal tube in place, measurement of static compliance is still possible. This is achieved by measuring pleural pressure, which reflects alveolar pressure, with an esophageal balloon.

A normal value for static compliance is 70 to 100 mL/cm H_2O. This means that for every 1 cm H_2O pressure change in the lungs, there is a change in volume of 70 to 100 mL of gas. A decrease in static compliance implies abnormalities of the lung parenchyma, pleural space, or chest wall. An increase in compliance from normal, although it may sound good, is a significant problem. Increased compliance occurs in disease processes that destroy the lung's elastic tissues, such as emphysema. Deteriorating elasticity leads to a decrease in the transpulmonary pressure, the force that holds small airways open. Small airways decrease in size and may even collapse, airway resistance increases, and expiratory flow decreases. The inspiratory work of breathing also increases when the transpulmonary pressure decreases because a greater force is required to achieve a change in pressure that will promote sufficient inspiratory flow.

Dynamic compliance is a measurement taken while gases are moving in the lungs; therefore it measures not only compliance of the lung tissue but also resistance to gas flow. It may be used as a measurement of compliance. It is somewhat easier to obtain than static compliance because it does not require the use of the inspiratory hold maneuver. However, dynamic compliance is not a pure measurement of lung compliance. The following is the physiologic formula for dynamic compliance (C_{DYN}):

$$C_{DYN} = \frac{\text{Exhaled tidal volume}}{\text{Peak inspiratory pressure} - \text{PEEP}}$$

Again, the exhaled tidal volume should be used as the numerator because it is the most accurate measurement of the volume actually in the lungs at the time the pressure measurement was taken. The exhaled tidal volume is then divided by the pressure in the airway at the peak of inspiration. At this point, gases are still flowing in the lungs, and some pressure measured is caused by the movement of the gas particles (resistance). Any artificial pressure, such as PEEP, must be subtracted from the pressure measurement when the calculation is performed.

The normal value for dynamic compliance is 50 to 80 mL/cm H_2O. Dynamic compliance measures are always smaller than static compliance because peak airway pressure is always greater than plateau pressure. A decrease in dynamic compliance may indicate a decrease in lung compliance or an increase in airway resistance.

No single value of compliance is as useful as a trend of the variable with time. Measures are used to quantify the extent of the compliance problem and monitor patient progress after therapy is instituted.

Resistance

Resistance is a measurement of the opposition to the flow of gases through the airways. There are two types of resistance: tissue and airway. Tissue resistance, which is caused by tissue friction during inspiration and expiration, normally makes up approximately 20% of total resistance. Airway resistance (Raw) is the opposition to the flow of gases caused by friction between the walls of the airway and the gas molecules, as well as viscous friction between the gas molecules themselves. Resistance to gas flow is measured in the clinical setting with the following physiologic formula:

$$Raw = \frac{Peak\ pressure - Plateau\ pressure}{Flow}$$

Airway resistance is driving pressure divided by flow rate. Driving pressure is the difference in the pressure between the beginning of the circuit, the mouth (peak pressure), and the end of the circuit, the alveoli (plateau pressure). Flow rate is the speed at which a gas travels, or to look at it another way, the volume of gas delivered in a given amount of time. Its unit of measure is liters per minute. The normal value for airway resistance is 0.5 to 3.0 cm H_2O/L/sec, measured at a standard flow rate of 0.5 L/sec.

Factors that affect airway resistance include *airway length, radius*, and *flow rate*. If the length of the airway is increased, the resistance to flow is increased. This is one of the reasons that ventilator tubing length is standardized. Moreover, a lengthy endotracheal tube creates higher resistance than a tracheostomy tube of the same diameter. Airway radius affects resistance in that, if the size of an airway is doubled, resistance decreases 16-fold. Likewise, if the airway radius is decreased, the resistance to gas flow is increased. Therefore the flow of gas into the lungs is decreased. The airway radius can be variable in clinical situations. This is an important concept to remember when an artificial airway is chosen or in the management of a disease that decreases the diameter of the airways, such as asthma. Airway radius may also be affected by such factors as a mucous plug or fluid in the ventilator tubing.

Flow rate and the pattern of flow also affect resistance. If the flow rate is increased, pressure in the airway increases and therefore resistance also increases. This becomes easier to understand using the analogy of a garden hose. Begin with a garden hose of a given radius and length. You turn on the water at the spigot at a certain flow rate, and a degree of pressure (which you can think of as resistance) is created in the hose. Now turn up the flow rate of water running through the hose.

What is going to happen? The pressure (and thus resistance to flow) within the hose increases. The same is true for the flow of gases through the airways. At higher flow rates, airway pressures rise and resistance increases. This occurs during rapid breathing and in the mechanically ventilated patient when high flow rates are required (see the discussion of flow rate in Chapter 6).

Pressure in the airway rises with increasing flow rates primarily because of the patterns of flow created (Fig. 2-3). Laminar flow is characterized by parallel lines of gas traveling together; it is streamlined and low pressure. Turbulent flow is disorganized; there are eddies and whorls that create friction between the molecules of gas. Turbulent flow, which occurs more often when the flow rate is high, causes higher airway resistance. Transitional flow is a mixture of laminar and turbulent flow.

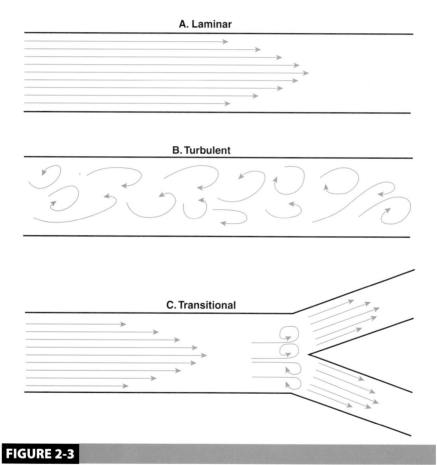

FIGURE 2-3

Patterns of airflow within the respiratory tract. (**A**) represents laminar flow, which creates an olive-shaped velocity head. This smooth, rounded velocity head eases into even the smallest airways while creating minimal pressure. (**B**) represents turbulent flow, which creates higher pressure and greater shearing forces on the walls of the airways. (**C**) represents a transitional pattern created when orderly flow is disrupted at points where the airways bifurcate. *(Modified from Levitsky MG. Pulmonary Physiology, 6th ed. New York: McGraw-Hill, 2003.)*

When a patient is being mechanically ventilated, the number used to roughly assess resistance is the peak inspiratory pressure. This can be read on the airway pressure gauge manometer. For a more thorough discussion of interpreting airway pressures in terms of compliance and resistance, see Chapter 9.

High airway resistance may be caused either by patient factors or by the factors related to ventilator circuitry. Examples of patient-related factors include bronchoconstriction, secretions in the airway, or bronchial mucosal edema, as in thermal injury. Examples of ventilator circuit factors are as follows: biting or kinking of the endotracheal tube, kinking of the vent tubing between the bed rail and the mattress, and water in the ventilator tubing. In all these conditions that cause increased resistance, gas flow into the lungs is decreased if the pressure getting the air into the lungs is not increased. Increased airway resistance therefore decreases the patient's tidal volume and alveolar ventilation. It also increases the amount of pressure required to get air into the lungs. Finally, the distribution of ventilation is affected in that it becomes uneven. The areas of the lung that have the least resistance are ventilated better than high-resistance areas.

Time Constants for Lung Elasticity

It should now be clear that uneven distribution of ventilation in the lung may be caused by regional differences in compliance or resistance. These regional differences may be expressed as a time constant (the product of airway resistance and lung compliance) whose formula is as follows:

$$\text{Time constant (seconds)} = \text{Resistance} \times \text{Compliance}$$

The time constant is the time required, in seconds, to inflate a lung region to 60% of its filling capacity if the filling pressure was to remain constant. Different time constants may exist for different regions of the lung. Areas of the lung that have either increased resistance or decreased compliance will have a longer time constant. Lung units with longer time constants require a longer inspiratory time to inflate to 60% of their potential filling volume (Fig. 2-4). If the respiratory rate (RR) is high, then only lung units with short time constants inflate fully. The overall results are regional maldistribution of gases and decreased alveolar ventilation. An understanding of time constants is useful in the application of lung recruitment maneuvers and forms of mechanical ventilation using prolonged inverse inspiratory-to-expiratory (I:E) ratios. Prolonged I:E ratios and lung recruitment maneuvers are designed to improve the distribution of gases within the lung, and thus alveolar ventilation, by improving ventilation to lung units with longer time constants.

Work of Breathing

Breathing requires mechanical work, which is performed by the respiratory muscles, and metabolic work, which is the expenditure of energy and is reflected by the oxygen consumption of the respiratory muscles. Mechanical work is defined as force times distance, meaning that work is performed whenever an applied force causes an object to move. In the lung, mechanical work equals pressure (force) times volume (distance factor). The total work of breathing (WOB) is the sum of physiologic work plus the work imposed by the breathing apparatus. Components of physiologic

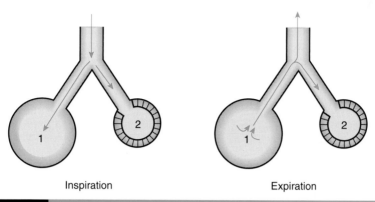

Inspiration   Expiration

FIGURE 2-4

Effect of uneven time constants on the distribution of ventilation. Compartment 2 has a long time constant because of poor compliance or increased resistance. During inspiration, gas is slow to enter compartment 2, and therefore it does not fill as well as the lung unit with a normal time constant (compartment 1). At expiration the abnormal units may still be inhaling, although the lung units with normal time constants have begun to exhale.

work are the work to expand the chest wall and the work to expand the lung. The work that the respiratory muscles must perform to expand the lung is that which will overcome elastic and nonelastic forces: compliance and resistance, respectively. When compliance decreases or resistance increases, a greater force is required to move volume in the lung. That is, the WOB increases. The WOB imposed by the breathing apparatus consists of work imposed by the circuit and work imposed by the endotracheal tube. These factors must not be underestimated and should be modified as much as possible through appropriate choice of ventilator settings (inspiratory pressure support, flow-by, etc.) and choice of airway.

The WOB is calculated by determining the area under a pressure volume curve of the lung. The WOB is an important factor to take into account when considering initiating mechanical ventilation, choosing an appropriate mode of ventilation, altering ventilator settings, weaning a patient from a ventilator, or advancing a patient's activity level. That is, this question must be asked: Does the patient have sufficient muscle strength to maintain the WOB, given the compliance and resistance of the pulmonary tissue, the work imposed by the ventilator circuitry, and the ventilatory demands?

Physical assessment of the patient may provide some of the most useful clues as to patient tolerance of imposed ventilatory demands. If the WOB is manageable, the respiratory examination reveals a normal RR, absence of the use of accessory muscles of respiration, and no abnormal thoracoabdominal movement such as respiratory alternans or abdominal paradox. Moreover, the patient demonstrates no increase in blood pressure or heart rate from baseline, barring any concurrent processes that could account for such changes.

Also clinically meaningful is the WOB expressed in metabolic terms, commonly called the oxygen cost of breathing. Normal quiet breathing requires only approximately 5% of the total resting oxygen consumption. In disease processes in which compliance or resistance is affected, the oxygen cost of breathing can increase markedly, to as much as 25% to 30% of total oxygen consumption. A considerable portion of the total body energy expenditure may be required to maintain respiratory efforts, carbon dioxide production may exceed alveolar ventilation, and respiratory acidosis may ensue.

PERFUSION

Distribution of Perfusion in the Lung

It is commonly believed that the distribution of perfusion is even throughout the lung, but this is not true. Two significant factors lead to the natural uneven distribution of perfusion within the lung. These factors are the interplay of arterial, venous, and alveolar pressures within the pulmonary system and gravitational forces.

When a human being is standing upright, blood flow increases linearly down the lung, in such a way that it is greatest in the bases. This changes with alterations in body position; thus, when one is lying supine, blood flow is greatest in the posterior lung zones, and when one is lying on one's side, blood flow is greatest in the dependent lung (Fig. 2-5). Blood flow is therefore gravity dependent in nature, and

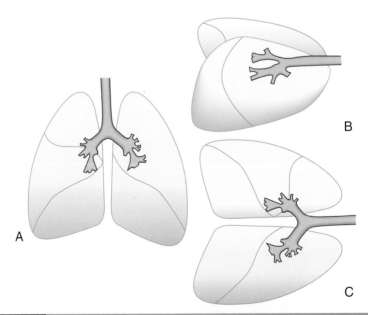

FIGURE 2-5

Blood flow in the lung is gravity dependent in nature. The greatest percentage of blood is in the most dependent lung regions. This is true regardless of body position, as shown in the erect (**A**), supine (**B**), and lateral decubitus (**C**) positions. *(Modified from Shapiro BA, et al. Clinical Application of Blood Gases, 4th ed. Chicago: Year Book, 1989.)*

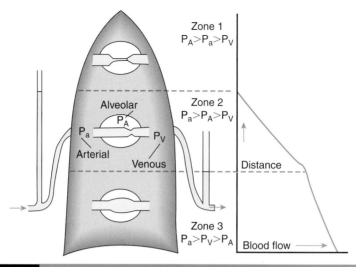

FIGURE 2-6

Three-zone model of the lung, which explains the uneven distribution of blood flow in the lung. The basis of this model is that both alveolar and pulmonary venous pressures affect capillary perfusion pressure. In the patient who is lying supine, the three lung zones, obeying gravitational laws, occur at right angles to that shown above. See text for explanation. *(Modified from West JB. Respiratory Physiology: The Essentials, 7th ed. Philadelphia: Lippincott Williams & Wilkins, 2004.)*

the hydrostatic pressure differences within the blood vessels explain the regional differences in perfusion distribution. Understanding these pressure differences and their effect on perfusion distribution is explained in a model of three lung zones described by West (Fig. 2-6).

An underlying principle of West's model is that uneven distribution of blood flow is explained by hydrostatic pressure differences in the pulmonary arterial system from the base to the apex of the lung. Pressure within the alveoli easily influences the adjacent pulmonary capillaries because they have such thin walls. Indeed, the capillaries may actually become compressed during mechanical ventilation when alveolar pressure is high, as when tidal volumes are too large or maldistributed or inflating pressures are high, causing overinflation of alveoli.

The apices of the lungs represent zone I, a region above the heart and therefore not well perfused. In this region, alveolar pressure may exceed arterial pressure; however, typically pulmonary artery pressure is just sufficient to raise blood to the top of the lung. If alveolar pressure rises, as may occur with positive-pressure ventilation, or if arterial pressure falls, as in hemorrhage or other causes of decreased perfusion pressure, then no flow occurs in zone I. The absence of flow in areas where ventilation is intact is known as alveolar dead space, or wasted ventilation.

Zone II is the middle portion of the lung. Perfusion through zone II lung areas is dependent on the pressure difference between the pulmonary arteries and the alveolar pressure, not the typical arterial-venous pressure difference. Because hydrostatic forces are greater and perfusion is now occurring at the level of the heart, pulmonary arterial pressures are higher and should exceed alveolar pressure.

In zone III, venous pressure exceeds alveolar pressure; perfusion is therefore determined by the usual mechanism of the arterial-venous pressure difference. Perfusion is greatest in zone III because of gravitational, or hydrostatic, forces.

Overall lung perfusion increases during exercise or other causes of increased cardiac output. The distribution of perfusion is also influenced by several therapies used in critically ill patients, such as PEEP, vasodilators, and inotropic agents.

Pulmonary Vascular Resistance

The pulmonary circulation is a high-volume, low-pressure system. The entire cardiac output is received into the pulmonary circulation from the right side of the heart at a systolic pressure of 25 mm Hg and a diastolic pressure of 8 mm Hg. The result is a mean perfusion pressure of 15 mm Hg, compared with a mean systemic pressure of 100 mm Hg. The resistance in the pulmonary circuit is only one tenth that of the systemic circuit. As a result of this low-pressure system, the work of the right side of the heart is kept small and the entire cardiac output is perfused with minimal pressure over the vast vascular surface area of the pulmonary circulation.

Pulmonary vascular resistance (PVR) can be calculated if the patient has a pulmonary artery catheter in place. Resistance in the pulmonary vasculature is determined by measuring the pressure at the beginning of the circuit (mean pulmonary artery pressure) minus the pressure at the end of the circuit (pulmonary capillary wedge pressure) and dividing by flow rate (cardiac output):

$$\text{Pulmonary vascular resistance (PVR)} = \frac{\text{PA} - \text{PCWP}}{\text{CO}} \times 80$$

$$\text{Normal} = <250 \text{ dynes} \cdot \text{sec} \cdot \text{cm}^{-5}$$

where
PA = mean pulmonary artery pressure
PCWP = pulmonary capillary wedge pressure
80 = factor used to convert units of measure from mm Hg/L/min to dynes/sec/cm^{-5}
CO = cardiac output

Regulation of the PVR occurs even though the pulmonary capillaries do not contain a significant amount of muscle. Recall that in a resting state all the pulmonary capillaries are not perfused. Alteration in the number of vessels perfused (capillary recruitment) and alteration in the amount of perfusion that any given vessel receives (capillary distention) are two main mechanisms of maintaining a low pressure in the pulmonary vascular system (Fig. 2-7).

Hypoxic Vasoconstriction

A second unique characteristic of the pulmonary circulation is its response to changing respiratory gas tensions. The response to alveolar hypoxia is potent pulmonary vasoconstriction, known as hypoxic pulmonary vasoconstriction. This response

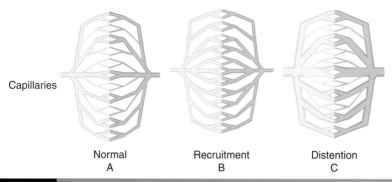

Capillaries

Normal	Recruitment	Distention
A	B	C

FIGURE 2-7

Physiologic mechanisms that assist in maintaining a low pulmonary vascular resistance (PVR). **A,** In the normal lung, some capillaries are minimally perfused. **B,** The mechanism of *recruitment* calls in more capillaries to conduct blood when the pulmonary artery pressure rises. This is the main mechanism for decreasing PVR. **C,** Capillary *distention* occurs with increasing pressure or cardiac output. A distended capillary offers less resistance to blood flow. *(Modified from Dettenmeir PA. Pulmonary Nursing Care. St. Louis: Mosby, 1992.)*

increases pulmonary vascular resistance and can significantly increase the work of the right side of the heart. That is, the right heart afterload is increased. However, this mechanism is important in maintaining homeostasis in gas exchange. Vasoconstriction, in areas of low alveolar P_{O_2}, diverts blood flow toward alveoli with more optimal oxygen tensions, thereby better matching perfusion to the well-ventilated areas. The overall result is improved gas exchange. For example, if a patient has a left lower lobe (LLL) pneumonia, ventilation to this area of the lung is decreased and alveolar oxygen tension in the LLL is therefore decreased. Hypoxic vasoconstriction occurs in this lung region, diverting blood flow to areas of adequate alveolar ventilation and thus improving overall gas exchange. Box 2-1 outlines other humoral factors that may affect pulmonary vascular tone.

BOX 2-1 Factors Affecting Pulmonary Vascular Resistance

Increase (Pulmonary Constrictors)	**Decrease (Pulmonary Dilators)**
Low alveolar oxygen tension	Oxygen
Hypercapnia	Hypocapnia
Acidosis	Alkalosis
Hypothermia	β-Adrenergic agonists
Sympathetic stimulation	Isoproterenol
α-Adrenergic agonists	Dobutamine
Norepinephrine	Sodium nitroprusside
Increased pulmonary blood flow	Nitroglycerin
Increased airway pressure	Prostaglandin E_1
Pulmonary embolism	Theophylline
Angiotensin II	Prostacyclin

DIFFUSION

Once the gas reaches the alveoli, the next process of external respiration, diffusion, begins. Diffusion is the movement of gas molecules from an area of relatively high partial pressure to one of low partial pressure. The driving force for the molecules is the pressure gradient of the gases across the alveolar-capillary (A-C) membrane. The normal pathway that gas molecules must travel at the A-C membrane is illustrated in Chapter 1 (Fig. 1-9). Factors affecting diffusion include the total surface area of the A-C membrane, the thickness of the tissue through which the gases must diffuse, the diffusion coefficient of the gas (how readily the gas diffuses relative to the other gases in the solution), and the difference in partial pressure of the gases between the two sides of the membrane.

Factors that decrease surface area, such as significant pulmonary vascular disease or lobectomy, may decrease the diffusion of gases. However, the lung has a tremendous surface area for gas exchange, approximately 70 m². Disease processes that increase the thickness of the A-C membrane, and thus increase the diffusion distance for gases, include pulmonary edema and chronic lung conditions that cause fibrotic changes.

Both oxygen and carbon dioxide diffuse readily across the A-C membrane. Carbon dioxide diffuses 20 times more readily than oxygen; factors that adversely affect diffusion are therefore less likely to affect the diffusion of carbon dioxide than that of oxygen. Despite the many factors that may affect diffusion, gas exchange is completed by the time the red blood cell is only a third of the way along the capillary: approximately 0.3 to 0.4 second. Because the red blood cell is in the pulmonary capillary almost a full second at rest, there is an enormous reserve time for gas exchange to take place. Only when accompanied by other factors that adversely affect diffusion, such as illness or exercise, do very high cardiac output states adversely affect diffusion.

The final factor that affects diffusion, the partial pressure of gases across the A-C membrane, warrants further discussion. To understand diffusion gradients, one must become familiar with the normal partial pressures of gas in the inspired air, the alveolus, and the pulmonary capillary (Fig. 2-8).

Inspired air at sea level has a total pressure of 760 mm Hg. Each gas in inspired air—oxygen, carbon dioxide, and nitrogen—exerts a partial pressure, which is determined by the percentage of that gas in relation to the total gases. For example, oxygen, which is 21% of inspired air, exerts a partial pressure of 159 mm Hg. Once the air is inspired, it is warmed and humidified by the upper airway, and the partial pressure of the water vapor becomes 47 mm Hg. Because the total partial pressure can still be only 760 mm Hg, the partial pressure of all the other gases must change by the time they become alveolar gases. Furthermore, the partial pressure of alveolar gases (PA) is affected by the fact that inspired air is mixed with gases already in the alveoli because exhalation does not result in complete emptying of the alveolus.

Respiratory gases in the pulmonary blood exert partial pressures as well. Venous blood returning from the tissue beds of the body normally has partial pressures of gases that reflect tissue use of oxygen and excretion of carbon dioxide: $Pv_{O_2} = 40$ mm Hg, $Pv_{CO_2} = 46$ mm Hg, pH = 7.36, and $Sv_{O_2} = 75\%$.

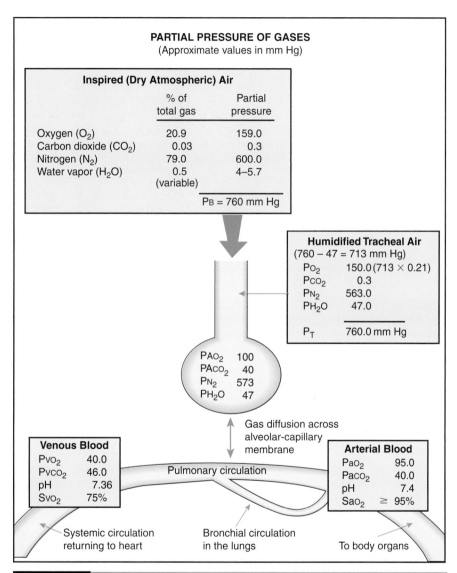

PARTIAL PRESSURE OF GASES
(Approximate values in mm Hg)

Inspired (Dry Atmospheric) Air

	% of total gas	Partial pressure
Oxygen (O_2)	20.9	159.0
Carbon dioxide (CO_2)	0.03	0.3
Nitrogen (N_2)	79.0	600.0
Water vapor (H_2O)	0.5 (variable)	4–5.7

$P_B = 760$ mm Hg

Humidified Tracheal Air
$(760 - 47 = 713$ mm Hg$)$

P_{O_2}	150.0 (713×0.21)
P_{CO_2}	0.3
P_{N_2}	563.0
P_{H_2O}	47.0
P_T	760.0 mm Hg

P_{AO_2}	100
P_{ACO_2}	40
P_{N_2}	573
P_{H_2O}	47

Gas diffusion across alveolar-capillary membrane

Venous Blood

P_{vO_2}	40.0
P_{vCO_2}	46.0
pH	7.36
S_{vO_2}	75%

Pulmonary circulation

Arterial Blood

P_{aO_2}	95.0
P_{aCO_2}	40.0
pH	7.4
S_{aO_2}	$\geq$ 95%

Systemic circulation returning to heart

Bronchial circulation in the lungs

To body organs

FIGURE 2-8

Partial pressures of dry inspired and humidified tracheal and alveolar gases. Alveolar pressures are in millimeters of mercury at sea level under BTPS conditions (body temperature of 37° C, ambient pressure, and saturated with water vapor). Also shown are the partial pressures of gases in the venous and arterial blood. *(From Kersten LD. Comprehensive Respiratory Nursing. Philadelphia: Saunders, 1989.)*

This review of the partial pressures of gases in the alveolus and the pulmonary capillary shows that a pressure gradient exists for the movement of oxygen from the alveolus into the pulmonary capillary and for the movement of carbon dioxide from the capillary into the alveolus. Under normal conditions, complete equilibration of gases occurs at the A-C membrane; the partial pressures of alveolar and arterial gases are therefore assumed to be the same.

The blood, after traversing the pulmonary capillaries, travels to the left atrium. There the venous blood from the bronchial circulation, which is not oxygenated, is mixed with the arterialized blood, which is in equilibrium with the alveolar gas. This has the effect of decreasing the partial pressure of oxygen in arterial blood relative to that in the alveolus. This alveolar-arterial gradient (A-a gradient), called the anatomic shunt, is normally 10 mm Hg in healthy individuals.

Although many factors can affect the diffusion of gases at the A-C membrane, the lung has significant diffusion reserve, which promotes remarkable function even in disease. Some factors that may cause diffusion defects include thickening of the alveolar wall (alveolar fibrosis), alveolar-capillary destruction (emphysema), alveolar consolidation (pneumonia), and interstitial and alveolar edema. However, ventilation/perfusion inequalities are the major contributors to abnormal gas exchange in the lung.

VENTILATION/PERFUSION RELATIONSHIPS

Distribution of Ventilation and Perfusion in the Lung

The ratio of alveolar ventilation ($\dot{V}$) to pulmonary blood flow ($\dot{Q}$) determines the composition of the gas leaving the lung. Ideally, each alveolus would be matched to well-perfused capillaries, leading to a $\dot{V}/\dot{Q}$ ratio of 1.0; however, ventilation and perfusion are not equally distributed throughout the lung. Recall that perfusion is greater at the base than at the apex of the lung. This is due to hydrostatic and gravitational forces. Therefore, if the patient changes body position, blood flow is always greatest in the most dependent lung regions.

Ventilation also increases linearly down the lung in the spontaneously breathing individual. This is due to regional differences in lung compliance that result from regional differences in intrapleural pressure. The lung hangs in the thoracic cavity in such a way that the weight of the lung is greatest at its base. The result is an intrapleural pressure of approximately -10 cm H_2O at the apex of the lung and approximately -2 cm H_2O at the base (Fig. 2-9). The alveoli at the apex are far more expanded and have a larger resting volume, so that with inspiration there is relatively less change in volume in these apical alveoli. At the base of the lung, the alveoli have a smaller resting volume and, on inspiration, the transpulmonary pressure change is greater. Therefore more volume is distributed to the base of the lung.

Regional differences in ventilation and perfusion result in relatively greater ventilation than perfusion at the apex of the lung, making the $\dot{V}/\dot{Q}$ ratio high (3.0). Perfusion, however, is relatively greater than ventilation at the bases, making the $\dot{V}/\dot{Q}$ ratio low (0.6).

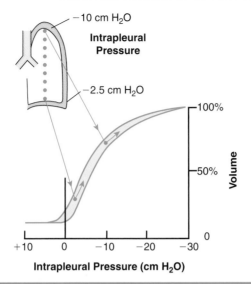

FIGURE 2-9

Ventilation down the lung and the reason it varies regionally. The weight of the lung hanging in the thorax creates greater negative pressure at the apex than at the base. At the apex there is less change in transpulmonary pressure on inspiration, relative to the base, and consequently less change in volume. Therefore, in spontaneously breathing humans, ventilation is preferentially distributed to the base of the lung. This is true regardless of body position. *(From West JB. Respiratory Physiology: The Essentials, 7th ed. Philadelphia: Lippincott Williams & Wilkins, 2004.)*

Normal V̇/Q̇ Ratio

The *overall* V̇/Q̇ ratio represents an average of all the ratios throughout the lung. Normally, alveolar ventilation is 4 L/min, whereas cardiac output is 5 L/min. The V̇/Q̇ ratio for the whole lung, then, averages 4/5, or 0.8, despite regional differences. Normal pulmonary gas exchange is dependent on this ratio of ventilation to perfusion in the lung. Disturbances in this V̇/Q̇ ratio, which include shunt and dead-space units, account for the abnormal arterial blood gas values in most respiratory disorders (Fig. 2-10).

V̇/Q̇ INEQUALITIES

Low V̇/Q̇: Shunt (Q̇s/Q̇T)

One type of V̇/Q̇ inequality is known as shunt. Shunt occurs when blood enters the arterial system without perfusing ventilated areas of the lung. There are two types of shunt: anatomic and physiologic. Anatomic shunt was discussed previously. It is the 2% to 5% of the cardiac output that normally bypasses the pulmonary arterial system. This blood is part of the bronchial, pleural, and coronary circulations. *Physiologic shunt* occurs when pulmonary blood flow is adequate but the alveolus is not well ventilated. In effect, perfusion is wasted.

45

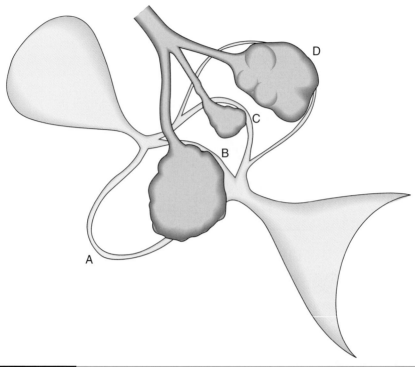

FIGURE 2-10

Spectrum of ventilation/perfusion matching in the lung. **A,** Anatomic shunt: blood flow through nonventilated areas. **B,** Normal matching of ventilation and perfusion. **C,** Shunt: perfusion in excess of ventilation. **D,** Dead space: ventilation in excess of perfusion. *(Modified from Wilkins RL, Sheldon RL, Krider SJ. Clinical Assessment in Respiratory Care, 4th ed. St. Louis: Mosby, 2000.)*

Shunt is the most common cause of hypoxemia in the critical care setting. This hypoxemia results in increased myocardial and ventilatory work. Blood passes through the lungs; however, in some lung regions it never interfaces with well-ventilated alveoli and therefore is not oxygenated. It is for this reason that in pure shunt the administration of supplemental oxygen does not result in an increase in PaO_2. Increasing the PO_2 to those alveoli that are well ventilated does not help either because the hemoglobin molecules traversing these alveoli are already carrying their maximum capacity of oxygen. Causes of shunt include atelectasis, consolidative-infiltrative disease processes, bronchospasm, and the use of vasodilators, which overcome hypoxic vasoconstriction when this compensatory mechanism is in place.

It is possible to quantify the percentage of shunt in the clinical setting. Calculation of this percentage can be useful as a baseline measure. Then, after the abnormality causing the shunt is determined and treatment initiated, additional measures can facilitate evaluation of the effects of therapy, and plotting the trend of measures can help guide the therapeutic plan and its revision, if necessary.

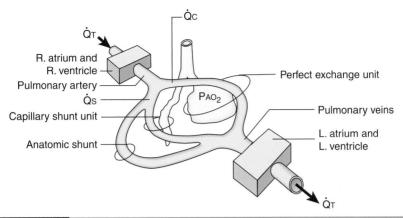

FIGURE 2-11

Calculation of intrapulmonary shunt using arterial and mixed venous blood samples:

$$\dot{Q}s/\dot{Q}_T = \frac{(Cco_2 - Cao_2)}{(Cco_2 - C\overline{v}o_2)}$$

Where Cco_2 = oxygen content of pulmonary capillary blood, which mathematically
represents the portion of the cardiac output that exchanges perfectly
with alveolar air

Cao_2 = oxygen content of arterial blood

$C\overline{v}o_2$ = oxygen content of mixed venous blood

Shunted blood ($\dot{Q}s$) is expressed as a ratio of the total blood flow ($\dot{Q}_T$). Normal value = 2% to 5%.
A percentage shunt of 28%, for example, would indicate that 28% of the cardiac output traveled
through the lungs without the occurrence of oxygenation. *(Modified from Shapiro BA, et al. Clinical
Application of Blood Gases, 5th ed. St. Louis: Mosby, 1994.)*

The form of shunt that is caused by $\dot{V}/\dot{Q}$ mismatching because of disease, and
the one we want to measure, is physiologic shunt. There are several methods of measuring shunt. The shunt equation, however, is the gold standard, the truest measure
of physiologic shunt (Fig. 2-11). It requires a pulmonary artery (PA) catheter to
determine oxygen content of mixed venous blood. The use of a PA catheter is not
indicated in all patients, and therefore the estimated shunt equation (see below) was
developed as an alternative method of trending the changes in the physiologic shunt.
In this equation the arterial-venous oxygen content difference (a-vDo$_2$) is assumed
to be 3.5 vol%. This value is representative of the a-vDo$_2$ of the critically ill patient
with an adequate cardiovascular reserve.

$$\dot{Q}s/\dot{Q}_T = \frac{(Cco_2 - Cao_2)}{3.5 + (Cco_2 - Cao_2)}$$

This equation is useful when the patient does not have a PA catheter in place.
The equation assumes cardiovascular stability. The estimated shunt has a stronger
correlation to the measured shunt than other shunt indices primarily because the
calculation utilizes oxygen content rather than tension.

In an effort to try to find an equation that can be used when the patient does not have a PA catheter, gas exchange indices that use oxygen tension rather than oxygen content measures were developed. Shunt calculations using oxygen tension variables only estimate the shunt and may be unreliable with changes in the fraction of oxygen in inspired gas (FIO_2). If this fact is kept in mind, then the use of these equations has its place in the clinical setting. The use of oxygen tension (PaO_2) in calculating shunt is based on comparing what the PaO_2 should be, on a particular FIO_2, with its actual value. Box 2-2 provides examples of these equations.

In some settings, as part of the assessment of the adequacy of oxygenation, the alveolar-arterial gradient (PA-aO_2) is calculated. The normal value, 10 mm Hg when a patient is breathing room air and 100 mm Hg when breathing 100% oxygen, is due to normal $\dot{V}/\dot{Q}$ differences down the lung and the normal small physiologic shunt. The normal value increases with age because of airway closure at the bases in older individuals, caused by loss of elastic recoil, and can be calculated by the following equation: $2.5 + (0.43 \times age)$. An increase in the A-a gradient is strictly an indication that there is a defect in oxygenation ability. It is not a specific measure of shunt. In fact, of the estimated shunt equations, the A-a gradient is the weakest predictor. The gradient also changes unpredictably with changes in FIO_2.

If the A-a gradient is normal in the presence of hypoxemia, the cause is hypoventilation. If hypoxemia is accompanied by an increase in the gradient, the cause may be anatomic right-to-left shunt, diffusion limitation, or $\dot{V}/\dot{Q}$ inequality. Therefore an increase in the A-a gradient signals a problem in oxygenation; however, the cause of the problem may fall within any of the previously mentioned categories. If the problem is shunt and the FIO_2 is increased, there may be no change in the PaO_2, whereas the PaO_2 should increase in a diffusion defect.

One clinical use of the A-a gradient is to determine whether the cause of hypoxemia accompanied by hypercapnia is simply because of hypoventilation alone, or to hypoventilation complicated by another disease process affecting pulmonary function. In the patient with both hypoxemia and hypercapnia, if the A-a gradient is normal, the cause is hypoventilation alone. If the A-a gradient is increased, a complicating process such as pneumonia, pulmonary edema, or atelectasis is present.

High $\dot{V}/\dot{Q}$: Dead Space (V_D/V_T)

In the second type of $\dot{V}/\dot{Q}$ inequality, ventilation is present but the alveoli are poorly perfused; in effect, ventilation is wasted. This is known as dead-space ventilation. There are two types of dead space: anatomic and physiologic. Anatomic dead space, as discussed previously, is the amount of air in the conducting airways. It is normally about 2 mL/kg, or approximately 150 mL. Although the anatomic dead space in any one individual is a fixed volume, in shallow breathing a greater percentage of the inspired volume is ventilation to the anatomic dead space. Physiologic dead space occurs when ventilation is normal but perfusion to some alveoli is reduced or absent. Either there is not enough blood or the blood is blocked from reaching the alveoli. Causes of physiologic dead space include pulmonary embolus; decreased pulmonary perfusion, as in low cardiac output or acute pulmonary hypertension; mechanical

BOX 2-2 Gas Exchange Indices Used to Estimate Physiologic Shunt

1. Arterial/alveolar ratio (a/A ratio)

$$\frac{Pao_2}{PAo_2}$$

PAo_2 is calculated by the alveolar air equation:

$$PAo_2 = Fio_2 (PB - PH_2O) - Paco_2/0.8$$

where PB = barometric pressure
 PH_2O = vapor pressure of water at 37° C (whose value is 47 mm Hg)
 0.8 = assumed respiratory quotient (ratio of CO_2 production to O_2 consumption)

Normal value for the a/A ratio is 0.8, meaning that 80% of the alveolar oxygen is reaching the arterial system.

Moderate shunt = 0.50 – 0.80
Significant shunt = 0.25 – 0.50
Critical shunt = <0.25

The a/A ratio remains relatively stable with changes in the Fio_2. Calculation can be used to predict the Fio_2 required for a desired Pao_2.

2. Pao_2/Fio_2 ratio

Normal ratio is 550 (a person breathing Fio_2 of 1.0 at sea level should have a Pao_2 of 550 to 600 mm Hg). The obtained value is subtracted from the normal value (550), and for every difference of 100, the shunt is 5%.

Example:

Pao_2 of 68 on Fio_2 of 0.4,
68 mm Hg/0.4 Fio_2 = 1.7, then
 1.7 × 100 = 170 (estimation of Pao_2 on 100% oxygen)
550 – 170 = 380, then
380/100 = 3.8, then
3.8 × 5 = 19% shunt

The percentage shunt can also be roughly estimated from the Pao_2/Fio_2 ratio as follows:

500: ~5% shunt
300: ~15% shunt
200: ~20% shunt

3. A-a gradient (on 100% oxygen)

$$PAo_2 - Pao_2$$

where PAo_2 is calculated by the alveolar air equation previously presented

The patient must receive 100% oxygen for at least 15 minutes to eliminate all other causes of A-a gradient other than shunt. Ideally, the PAo_2 would be near 670, with the Pao_2 close to 550. Every 20 mm Hg difference is equal to a 1% shunt.

ventilation with large tidal volumes or pressures that overdistend the alveoli to such a degree that alveolar pressure exceeds capillary pressure; extrinsic pressure on the pulmonary vessels such as pneumothorax or hydrothorax or presence of tumor; and diseases in which extensive capillary damage and intravascular coagulation occur, such as sepsis, burns, or ARDS. Dead space increases the $Paco_2$ because the

BOX 2-3 Measurements of Dead-Space Ventilation

1. Arterial/Alveolar P_{CO_2} Gradient (a-A P_{CO_2})

$$\text{Arterial } P_{CO_2} - \text{Alveolar } P_{CO_2}$$

where Alveolar P_{CO_2} is measured by means of end-tidal P_{CO_2}

Normal gradient is an alveolar P_{CO_2} 2 mm Hg less than arterial. Acute increase reflects increase in physiologic dead space.

2. Minute Ventilation ($\dot{V}_E$) – Pa_{CO_2} Disparity

When an increase in the $\dot{V}_E$ is not associated with the expected decrease in Pa_{CO_2}, dead-space ventilation should be suspected. An increase in the metabolic rate (and thus production of carbon dioxide) must be ruled out. This is useful clinically because it does not require measurement of exhaled carbon dioxide.

3. Dead Space/Tidal Volume Ratio

$$V_D/V_T = \frac{Pa_{CO_2} - P_{ECO_2}}{Pa_{CO_2}}$$

where Pa_{CO_2} = partial pressure of CO_2 in arterial blood
              P_{ECO_2} = partial pressure of CO_2 in expired air
         normal value = 0.25 – 0.40 (25% – 40%)

The total exhaled gases must be collected into a large balloon for a 5-minute period. The patient must have a constant respiratory pattern; therefore, this measurement is most accurately taken when controlled modes of ventilation are used. The metabolic rate must be in a steady state. If the V_D/V_T ratio is 0.6 or greater, an attempt to wean the patient from the ventilator is usually unsuccessful because ventilatory reserve generally is exceeded by the necessary increase in $\dot{V}_E$.

---

blood carrying the carbon dioxide back from the tissues does not interface with the alveolus. Increased dead space demands increased minute ventilation and therefore an increase in the work of breathing if a normal Pa_{CO_2} is to be maintained.

Box 2-3 illustrates measurements of dead-space ventilation that can be performed in the clinical setting. Measurement of end-tidal carbon dioxide, required in the first equation in Box 2-3, is further explained in Chapter 10.

EFFECT OF BODY POSITION ON $\dot{V}/\dot{Q}$ MATCHING

Body position may affect gas exchange by altering the matching of ventilation to perfusion in the lung. Postural variations in gas exchange may be clinically significant, particularly in patients with unilateral or asymmetric lung disease. Improved oxygenation has been demonstrated in patients with predominantly unilateral lung disease from various causes by positioning the patient in the lateral decubitus position, where the healthier lung is dependent (good lung down). Improved oxygenation is attributed to positionally induced enhancement of the matching of ventilation to perfusion. This conclusion is supported by investigators who demonstrated a decrease in the percentage of shunt when the patient is positioned with the good lung down. Therefore an awareness of the effect of changes in position on pulmonary ventilation and perfusion may permit therapeutic application of patient positioning.

Perfusion, being gravity dependent in nature, is greatest to the less diseased lung when that lung is placed in the dependent position. Ventilation, because it is preferentially distributed to areas of best compliance and least resistance, is also best in the dependent lung. The duration of the immediate effect of body position on gas exchange is unpredictable. A patient with unilateral disease who initially shows enhanced oxygenation with the good lung down may demonstrate a gradual fall in oxygenation during a period in which the position is maintained. The mechanism responsible for this deterioration is atelectasis and airway closure by secretions that gradually migrate from the upper lung into the more dependent, and previously relatively less diseased, lung; this leads to a fall in PaO_2. In the mechanically ventilated patient, hypoventilation related to three factors may also contribute to a decreasing oxygenation status when the patient is placed in the lateral decubitus position. These three factors are decreased dependent lung motion from mediastinal weight, dependent diaphragm elevation as a result of the weight of the abdominal contents, and relative immobility of the dependent chest wall. Therefore the use of body position to achieve optimal oxygenation requires careful evaluation of individual patient response over time.

There are several clinical implications for the use of therapeutic positioning to enhance oxygenation in patients with predominantly unilateral lung disease. First, having the patient lie in a position with the good lung down allows ventilation with lower levels of FIO_2 and PEEP. Second, recognition of the phenomenon should help prevent the diagnostic error of overall worsening respiratory status when, in fact, the arterial blood gas was possibly obtained when the patient was positioned in the less favorable lateral position. Third, changing body position without considering its possible ill effects may be life-threatening in patients with severe respiratory insufficiency and unilateral involvement.

The efficacy of position changes is widely recognized. In the critical care setting, position changes are often difficult to accomplish effectively because of various tubes, catheters, and other technologic apparatuses that are impediments to movement. Additionally, patients are often required to remain in the supine position for extended periods so that data gathering and treatments may be employed. Nonetheless, even though turning a patient may be cumbersome, if done properly it has far fewer detrimental effects on the patient than relative immobility. In the patient with predominantly unilateral lung disease, the incorporation of chest x-ray interpretation data into the decision to perform the routine patient care intervention of turning the patient ascribes an additional patient benefit to the maneuver: enhancement of oxygenation. Therefore, in selected cases in the intensive care setting, the physiologic basis for turning patients may be related to the distribution of ventilation and perfusion in the lung. Selected therapies applying this concept are discussed further in Chapter 5.

OXYGEN TRANSPORT IN THE BLOOD

Oxygen is transported in the blood in two ways: dissolved in the serum and in combination with hemoglobin. The oxygen dissolved in the serum is measured as the PaO_2. The PaO_2 constitutes only 2% to 3% of the total oxygen transported in the body. There is 0.0031 mL of oxygen dissolved in each 100 mL blood for each 1 mm Hg partial pressure of oxygen. Thus, at a PaO_2 of 100 mm Hg, only 0.3 mL of oxygen would be carried per 100 mL of plasma. This is only a very small part of the total oxygen content of the blood. If this were the only method of carrying oxygen in the blood, then the cardiac output would have to be almost 160 L/min to deliver enough oxygen to the tissues to meet resting metabolic needs!

Most oxygen in the body (97% to 98%) is transported to the cells in combination with hemoglobin and measured as the percentage of oxygen saturation (SaO_2). The percentage of saturation of blood is that portion of the total hemoglobin saturated with oxygen. It is a relationship between the amount of oxygen that is carried and the amount that can be carried. Each gram of hemoglobin can transport 1.34 mL of oxygen per 100 mL of blood.

Oxygen binds loosely and reversibly with the heme portion of the hemoglobin molecule. When the PO_2 is high, as it is at the alveolar-capillary membrane, oxygen readily binds to hemoglobin, forming oxyhemoglobin. At the capillary level, where tissue partial pressures of oxygen are low, hemoglobin readily releases oxygen. The relationship between the PaO_2 and the SaO_2 is expressed in an S-shaped curve of great physiologic significance: the oxyhemoglobin dissociation curve (Fig. 2-12).

The affinity, or strength of the bond, between hemoglobin and oxygen is affected by various physiologic states that cause the curve to shift to the right or left. The clinical significance is in an awareness of how these factors affect the patient's ability to unload oxygen at the tissue level. The affinity of hemoglobin is expressed as the PaO_2 value at which 50% of the hemoglobin is saturated (P_{50}). Under standard conditions on the normal curve, the PaO_2 is 27 mm Hg at P_{50}.

Factors that cause a shift of the curve to the left (increase oxygen affinity to hemoglobin) include a decreased H^+ ion concentration, alkalemia, decreased body temperature, and decreased 2,3-diphosphoglycerate (2,3-DPG), which is an intermediate metabolite of glucose that facilitates dissociation of oxygen from hemoglobin at the tissues. A shift to the left results in a lower P_{50}; that is, less oxygen tension is required to saturate 50% of the hemoglobin. Thus, for any given SaO_2, the PaO_2 is lower than it would be on the normal curve. Hemoglobin is not giving up oxygen readily at the tissues.

Factors that cause a shift of the curve to the right (decrease oxygen affinity to hemoglobin) include an increased H^+ ion concentration, acidemia, increased body temperature, and increased 2,3-DPG. A shift to the right results in a higher P_{50} value, meaning that it takes a higher PaO_2 to saturate 50% of the hemoglobin. When the curve has a right shift, for any given SaO_2 the PaO_2 is higher than it would be on the normal curve because hemoglobin is readily giving up oxygen to the tissues. Under the conditions just listed, especially increased body temperature and acidemia, the ready release of oxygen by hemoglobin is favorable because, under these conditions, oxygen demand at the tissues is higher than normal.

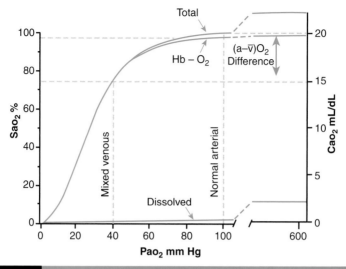

FIGURE 2-12

Oxyhemoglobin dissociation curve, relating the partial pressure of oxygen in arterial blood (Pa_{O_2}) to the percentage of hemoglobin saturated with oxygen in the arterial blood (Sa_{O_2}). The upper, flat part of the curve is the arterial portion, whereas the steeper part is the venous dissociation portion. The lower line represents oxygen dissolved in the blood. Note that dissolved oxygen contributes very little to total oxygen content (Ca_{O_2}). The middle line depicts oxygen bound to hemoglobin at that Pa_{O_2}, and the upper line shows a combination of oxygen bound to hemoglobin and dissolved in the blood. *(From Luce JM, Pierson DJ, Tyler ML. Intensive Respiratory Care. Philadelphia: Saunders, 1993.)*

RESPIRATORY CHEMISTRY: ACID-BASE REGULATION

The respiratory and renal systems work constantly to keep the body within a normal acid-base balance that provides a milieu for the optimal function of metabolic processes. Acid-base balance is a reflection of H^+ ion concentration in the body, which is represented by the pH. The pH is the negative logarithm of the concentration of H^+ ions; therefore, as the H^+ ion concentration increases, the pH decreases and vice versa.

The normal pH (7.35 to 7.45) is maintained by a balance of acid to base in the body. An acid is a substance that liberates H^+ ions when it dissociates in solution. A base is a substance that can bind or accept H^+ ions. Normally, the body has 20 acid ions for every base ion. This relationship can be calculated with the Henderson-Hasselbalch equation:

$$pH = pK + \log \frac{[HCO_3^-]}{Pa_{CO_2}}, \text{ or } \frac{Kidneys}{Lungs}, \text{ or } \frac{20}{1}$$

where pK = a constant of 6.1

The Henderson-Hasselbalch equation defines the relation among pH, P_{CO_2}, and bicarbonate (HCO_3^-). Bicarbonate is regulated mainly by the kidney, and carbon

53

dioxide is regulated by the lung. The ratio of bases to acids must remain at 20:1 to maintain a normal pH. When this ratio becomes imbalanced, resulting in an increase in H^+ ions, the pH decreases (becomes <7.35), and the patient is said to have acidemia. The *process* of becoming acidemic is called acidosis (e.g., diabetic ketoacidosis). Conversely, if the ratio of acids to bases in the body is imbalanced in that there is an excess of bases, the pH increases (becomes >7.45), and the patient is said to have alkalemia. The process of becoming alkalemic is correctly termed *alkalosis.*

Hydrogen ions are added to body fluids as a byproduct of metabolic processes. These acids must be eliminated or neutralized by the body so the patient does not develop acidemia. The hydrogen ion or acid produced is either fixed or volatile. Carbon dioxide is a volatile acid that is eliminated through the respiratory system by means of adequate alveolar ventilation. Fixed acids, such as hydrochloric acid and carbonic acid, must be excreted by the kidney. Therefore the lungs and the kidneys are primary organs in maintaining acid-base regulation.

To some extent, both volatile and fixed acids are neutralized in the body through combination with a base. Conversely, strong bases may be neutralized through combination with weak acids. These processes are called chemical buffering. Chemical buffers, therefore, are substances that minimize changes in pH when either acids or bases are added. Buffer systems occupy various locations in the body. Proteins and phosphates are buffers in the cells, hemoglobin is a buffer in the red blood cells, and bicarbonate, and proteins again, are buffers in the extracellular fluid. The combination of all the buffer systems is called the total buffer base. By far the most important buffer system is the bicarbonate buffer system (Fig. 2-13) because it accounts for more than half of total buffering.

The respiratory system controls the carbon dioxide tension of the blood by regulating alveolar ventilation, a process that may very quickly correct an acid-base disturbance. Alveolar ventilation (VA) is the volume of gas within the respiratory bronchioles and alveolar ducts (i.e., the respiratory zone of the lung). The VA does not reflect the volume of gas moved into and out of the mouth. The volume of gas moved into and out of the mouth per minute, the minute ventilation ($\dot{V}E$), consists of the alveolar ventilation plus the dead-space ventilation. Therefore, VA = $\dot{V}E$ – VD. VA strives to maintain the Pa_{CO_2} at 35 to 45 mm Hg (eucapnia).

Hypoventilation, or decreased alveolar ventilation, results in excessive acid. When the Pa_{CO_2} is more than 45 mm Hg, hypercapnia is present. If the pH is less than 7.35 and the Pa_{CO_2} is more than 45 mm Hg, the patient is said to have *respiratory*

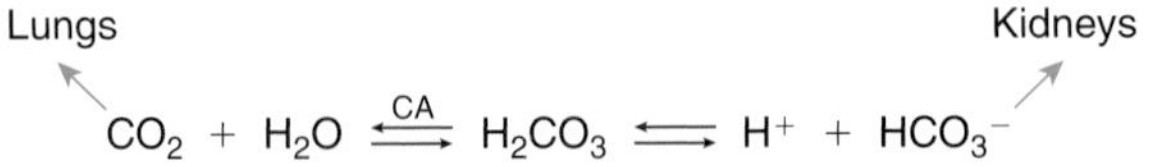

Lungs   Kidneys

$$CO_2 + H_2O \overset{CA}{\rightleftharpoons} H_2CO_3 \rightleftharpoons H^+ + HCO_3^-$$

FIGURE 2-13

Bicarbonate buffer system. Carbonic acid (H_2CO_3) is formed by the combination of carbon dioxide (CO_2) to water (H_2O) in the presence of the enzyme carbonic anhydrase (CA). Carbonic acid then quickly dissociates into hydrogen and bicarbonate (HCO_3^-). The bicarbonate buffering system then operates by using the lungs to regulate CO_2 and the kidneys to regulate HCO_3^-.

acidosis. Hyperventilation, or increased alveolar ventilation, causes acids to be blown off. When the $PaCO_2$ is less than 35 mm Hg, hypocapnia is present, a condition known as *respiratory alkalosis* when the pH is more than 7.45. It is important to note that hyperventilation is not synonymous with a rapid RR. For example, the patient may be breathing 40 times per minute and still have a $PaCO_2$ of 50 mm Hg.

The kidneys defend blood pH by controlling bicarbonate concentration. This is accomplished by excretion of hydrogen ions in the urine when the blood is too acidic and excretion of bicarbonate in the urine when the blood is too alkaline. It may take hours to days for the kidney to affect pH.

If there is an abnormal rise in HCO_3^- concentration in the serum or a significant loss of hydrogen ions, accompanied by a pH of more than 7.45, the patient is said to have *metabolic alkalosis.* Conversely, if there is a loss of bicarbonate or a rise in hydrogen ions or both, accompanied by a pH of less than 7.35, the patient has *metabolic acidosis.* Table 2-3 shows the causes, symptoms, and treatment of respiratory and metabolic acidosis and alkalosis.

Compensation refers to a return of the blood pH back to normal by the lungs or the kidneys. The system, respiratory or renal, opposite the primary disorder attempts the compensation. For example, in respiratory alkalosis the body first attempts to compensate by decreasing alveolar ventilation. However, hypoventilation cannot occur to a significant degree because hypoxemia eventually stimulates the drive to breathe. The renal system then attempts to compensate for the respiratory acid-base imbalance by excreting HCO_3^-. If the compensation is *complete,* the pH is returned to normal. If the compensation is *partial,* then the pH works its way toward normal. The body does not overcompensate.

INTERPRETATION OF ARTERIAL BLOOD GASES

Using the information about respiratory chemistry just presented, and given an arterial blood gas (ABG) measurement, one should be able to determine whether the primary disturbance of acid-base imbalance is respiratory or metabolic. An ABG measurement provides more information than just the acid-base balance. It also enables the assessment of the adequacy of oxygenation and ventilation. Before proceeding to the determination of abnormalities, it is essential to know the normal values of the variables obtained with an ABG measurement.

Oxygenation is assessed with the PaO_2, whose normal value is 80 to 100 mm Hg in adults. Hypoxemia is a state in which the PaO_2 is less than 60 mm Hg, whereas hypoxia is a state in which there is inadequate oxygen at the tissue level. Factors affecting PaO_2 that must be considered in an interpretation of the value include age and altitude, both of which decrease the PaO_2, and the administration of supplemental oxygen. Oxygenation may be further assessed with the SaO_2, whose normal value is 92% to 100%. At 92% saturation, the PaO_2 is approximately 60 mm Hg; a lower value indicates hypoxemia (see oxyhemoglobin dissociation curve, Fig. 2-12).

Ventilation is assessed with the $PaCO_2$. Normal values were discussed previously and are reiterated later. Acid-base status is assessed with the pH, $PaCO_2$, HCO_3^-, and the base excess (BE). The BE reflects an increase or decrease in the total buffer base. It is an indicator of the metabolic makeup of acid-base disturbances. A decrease in

TABLE 2-3 Causes, Symptoms, and Treatment of Acid-Base Disturbances

Disturbance	Causes	Symptoms	Treatment
Respiratory acidosis	Hypoventilation, acute process aggravating chronic lung disease, severe obesity, respiratory center depression (e.g., stroke, head trauma, drug overdose), respiratory neuromuscular disease, airway obstruction	Acute CO_2 retention: confusion, lethargy, stupor, coma	Decrease hypoventilation: treat underlying cause; cough and deep breathing, IPPB, incentive spirometry, bronchodilators, noninvasive ventilation, intubation, and mechanical ventilation
Respiratory alkalosis	Hyperventilation, hypoxemia, anxiety reaction, CNS irritation (e.g., central hyperventilation), metabolic acidosis, excessive artificial ventilation	Complaints of shortness of breath, anxiety, muscle cramps, tetany, perioral tingling, seizures	Decrease alveolar ventilation: sedation, improve oxygenation, rebreather bag, change ventilator settings (decrease RR or tidal volume)
Metabolic acidosis	Excessive acids: diabetic ketoacidosis, renal failure, lactic acidosis, starvation, salicylate overdose, ethylene glycol	Kussmaul respirations (deep, rapid), disorientation, restlessness, coma	Treat underlying abnormality
	Bicarbonate loss: diarrhea, pancreatic, biliary, or small bowel fluid loss; renal disease		Replace HCO_3^-
Metabolic alkalosis	Loss of acids: emesis, nasogastric suction (chloride is lost as well)	Apathy, mental confusion, shallow breathing, tetany, spastic muscles	Control emesis or GI losses; if unable to control, replace chloride with Ringer's lactate solution or sodium chloride. Chloride replacement allows HCO_3^- to exit the cell to be excreted. Reduce use of alkaline antacids; monitor diuretic use, administer acetazolamide to increase renal HCO_3^- excretion, correct potassium depletion
	Excessive base: overuse of antacids, milk of magnesia, or $NaHCO_3^-$; citrate in blood transfusions, lactate in hyperalimentation		
	Diuretic therapy resulting in K^+, Na^+, and Cl^- losses; H^+ moves into cell, HCO_3^- concentration increases		

CNS, Central nervous system; GI, gastrointestinal; IPPB, intermittent positive-pressure breathing, RR, respiratory rate.

the BE indicates loss of base and metabolic acidosis, whereas an increase in BE indicates metabolic alkalosis. Normal values for the ABG variables are shown in the following table:

		Acidemia	Alkalemia	Hypoxemia
pH	: 7.35-7.45	↓	↑	
Pa_{O_2}	: 80-100 mm Hg			Mild: <80 mm Hg Moderate: <70 mm Hg Severe: <60 mm Hg
Pa_{CO_2}	: 35-45 mm Hg	↑	↓	
HCO_3^-	: 22-26 mEq/L	↓	↑	
BE	: −2 to +2 mEq/L	↓	↑	
Sa_{O_2}	: 92%-100%			<92%

Systematic analysis of ABG values involves five steps:
1. Begin by looking at each number individually and labeling it. Decide whether the value is high, low, or normal, and label the finding; for example, a pH of 7.50 would be high and labeled as alkalemia.
2. Describe the adequacy of oxygenation by assessing the Pa_{O_2} and the Sa_{O_2}.
3. Determine acid-base status by assessing the pH.
4. Decide whether the acid-base disorder is respiratory or metabolic. Check the Pa_{CO_2} (respiratory) and the HCO_3^- (metabolic) to see which one is altering in the same manner as the pH. Use the BE to confirm your interpretation, especially when the disorder is mixed. In a mixed disturbance, there is an acid-base imbalance in both systems.
5. Determine the extent of compensation.
   a. Look at the system (respiratory or metabolic) that does not match the pH to determine whether it is moving out of its normal range in an effort to correct the acid-base disturbance.
   b. *Absent:* The value of the opposite system is normal, indicating that no compensation is occurring. The pH is assumed to be abnormal.
   c. *Partial:* If the value that does not match the pH status is above or below the normal range and the pH is still outside the normal range, then partial compensation has occurred.
   d. *Complete:* The value that does not match the pH is above or below normal and the pH is normal.

Examples of Arterial Blood Gases

EXAMPLE 1

pH	7.34	(acidemia)
Pa_{O_2}	129	(adequate oxygenation)
Pa_{CO_2}	48	(acidemia)
HCO_3^-	26	(normal)
BE	+1	(normal)
Sa_{O_2}	99%	(normal)

Interpretation: Respiratory acidosis with no compensation; adequate oxygenation.

EXAMPLE 2

Patient with chronic bronchitis, emphysema, and cor pulmonale, treated with digitalis and diuretics.

pH	7.40	(normal pH)
PaO_2	57	(hypoxemia)
$PaCO_2$	58	(acidemia)
HCO_3^-	35	(alkalemia)
BE	+9	(alkalemia; use to determine whether the primary disorder is respiratory or metabolic)
SaO_2	89%	(hypoxemia)

Interpretation: Metabolic alkalosis with complete respiratory compensation; hypoxemia.

EXAMPLE 3

Sixty-two-year-old man with history of cancer; status: post–abdominal surgery for drainage of abscess.

pH	7.29	(acidemia)
PaO_2	192	(normal)
$PaCO_2$	40	(normal)
HCO_3^-	19	(acidemia)
BE	−5.6	(acidemia)
SaO_2	97.5%	(normal)

Interpretation: Metabolic acidosis with no compensation; adequate oxygenation.

EXAMPLE 4

Thirty-four-year-old man; status: post-85% total body surface area burn in a house fire. Initially presented with a pH of 7.18. Resuscitated with 40 L lactated Ringer's solution and 6 ampules of $NaHCO_3^-$. The patient is sedated, medically paralyzed, and being mechanically ventilated with a $\dot{V}E$ of 17 L/min.

pH	7.37	(normal)
PaO_2	126	(normal)
$PaCO_2$	40	(normal)
HCO_3^-	20	(acidemia)
BE	−3.1	(acidemia)
SaO_2	98%	(normal)

Interpretation: Fully compensated metabolic acidosis; adequate oxygenation.

Interpreting Arterial Blood Gases in Terms of $\dot{V}/\dot{Q}$ Mismatches

Abnormalities in $\dot{V}/\dot{Q}$ matching are evident in the patient's ABG values. Low $\dot{V}/\dot{Q}$ units, shunt, cause hypoxemia, whereas high $\dot{V}/\dot{Q}$ units, dead space, result in a rising $PaCO_2$. The patient's clinical presentation also provides significant information regarding the possible presence of a $\dot{V}/\dot{Q}$ mismatch.

The patient who initially has an increasing $\dot{V}E$ and a rising $PaCO_2$ may have a hypermetabolic or other state resulting in carbon dioxide production that exceeds the patient's ventilatory capabilities, or the patient may have increasing dead space. Possible causes of increased dead space were delineated previously. When dead space increases, the ventilatory demand increases. Of concern to the clinician is what is causing the increased V_D/V_T and whether the patient has sufficient ventilatory reserve to meet the increased demand. In the following example, both patients have an increased $\dot{V}_E$ as a result of increased V_D/V_T.

	Compensated Patient	**Uncompensated Patient**
$\dot{V}_E$	18	16
Pa_{CO_2}	40	55
pH	7.40	7.33

Only one patient is able to maintain acid-base balance. Both patients are at risk of developing fatigue and ventilatory failure because of the high demands placed on their systems, so they need to be monitored carefully. However, the uncompensated patient is at higher risk of developing ventilatory failure and likely needs mechanical ventilation. The underlying mechanism resulting in increased V_D/V_T (e.g., pulmonary embolus, decreased cardiac output) needs to be determined and appropriate therapy implemented. Treatments of pulmonary emboli include (but are not limited to) heparin therapy, inferior vena cava interruption of emboli with an umbrella or a bird's nest, and thrombolytic therapy. If the decreased pulmonary perfusion is caused by low cardiac output, therapies need to be implemented that will achieve an optimal hemodynamic state. Alveolar overdistention caused by overzealous mechanical ventilation is managed by adjustment of the ventilator settings. Changes may include decreasing the V_T or changing the flow pattern or ventilatory mode in an effort to decrease the inspiratory pressures.

The patient who has hypoxemia despite supplemental oxygen likely has increasing shunt. Recall that shunt is the most common cause of hypoxemia in the intensive care unit. Many therapies may be implemented in an effort to decrease shunt. Pulmonary hygiene interventions range from cough and deep breathing to therapeutic bronchoscopy; pulmonary edema may be managed partly with diuresis, and bronchospasm with a bronchodilator. If mechanical ventilation is used, PEEP may be used to reexpand the alveoli and decrease physiologic shunt. It must always be remembered, however, that the ventilator serves as a mechanism to support oxygenation and ventilation, not as a primary treatment for ventilation/perfusion abnormalities. Returning the patient to health requires identification and management of the underlying pathology, application of physiologic measures to monitor patient progress, and dynamic revision of the plan of care.

RECOMMENDED READINGS

Beachey W. Acid-base balance. In RL Wilkins, JK Stoller, CL Scanlan (eds.), *Egan's Fundamentals of Respiratory Care*, 8th ed. (pp. 271–295). St. Louis: Mosby, 2003.

Des Jardins T. *Cardiopulmonary Anatomy and Physiology: Essentials for Respiratory Care*, 4th ed. Australia: Delmar Thomson Learning, 2002.

Dupuis YG. Work of breathing. In YG Dupuis (ed.), *Ventilators: Theory and Clinical Application*, 2nd ed. (pp. 209–216). St. Louis: Mosby, 1992.

Hess DR, Medoff BD, Fessler MB. Pulmonary mechanics and graphics during positive pressure ventilation. *Int Anesthesiol Clin* 1999; 37(3):1–34.

Jubran A. Monitoring patient mechanics during mechanical ventilation. *Crit Care Clin* 1998; 14(4):629–653.

Levitsky MG. *Pulmonary Physiology,* 6th ed. New York: McGraw-Hill, 2003.

Ruppel GL. Ventilation. In RL Wilkins, JK Stoller, CL Scanlan (eds.), *Egan's Fundamentals of Respiratory Care*, 8th ed. (pp. 207–228). St. Louis: Mosby, 2003.

Ruppel G, Blonshine S, Foss CM, et al. AARC Clinical Practice Guideline, Static Lung Volumes: 2001 Revision and update. *Respir Care* 2001; 46(5):531–539.

Scanlan CL, Wilkins RL. Gas exchange and transport. In RL Wilkins, JK Stoller, CL Scanlan (eds.), *Egan's Fundamentals of Respiratory Care*, 8th ed. (pp. 229–270). St. Louis: Mosby, 2003.

Shapiro BA, Harrison RA, Cane RD, et al. *Clinical Application of Blood Gases,* 4th ed. Chicago: Year Book, 1989.

West JB. *Respiratory Physiology: The Essentials,* 7th ed. Philadelphia: Lippincott Williams & Wilkins, 2004.

Wilkins RL. Interpretation of blood gases. In RL Wilkins, SJ Krider, RL Sheldon (eds.), *Clinical Assessment in Respiratory Care* (pp. 119–139). St. Louis: Mosby, 2000.

CHAPTER 3

Airway Maintenance

The purpose of airway maintenance is to ensure adequate ventilation. Artificial airways may be used to establish patency and control of the airway. Vigilant airway monitoring and possible use of an airway adjunct are indicated in the following circumstances:

- Partial or complete upper airway obstruction
- Prevention of aspiration when upper airway protective reflexes are inadequate
- Facilitation of secretion removal
- Provision of a closed system for the initiation of mechanical ventilation

Assess the patient for adequacy of ventilation. The patient may be making respiratory efforts but not moving sufficient air through the upper airway. There are many causes of upper airway complete or partial obstruction, such as the presence of food, vomitus, secretions, blood, expanding hematoma, and edema. In the patient with a depressed level of consciousness, muscle tone of the upper airway itself may be lost, resulting in an anatomic obstruction.

In partial airway obstruction, the patient may present with increased respiratory effort and changes in voice tone. Signs and symptoms may progress to hoarseness and to complaints of difficulty in obtaining enough air. Complete obstruction is an emergency. Patients may grab at their throats and be extremely agitated, or they may have a depressed level of consciousness. The work of breathing is dramatically increased, and suprasternal and intercostal retractions may be noted. A classic sign of severe upper airway obstruction is stridor, a shrill, crowing sound made on inspiration.

Many airways are available for airway maintenance. The appropriateness of one over another depends on the specific indications and individual patient considerations. The limitations and complications of each airway must also be considered.

HEAD-TILT TECHNIQUE, WITH CHIN-LIFT OR JAW-THRUST MANEUVER

Indications

When loss of tone in the natural airway is the cause of loss of patency, the head-tilt technique, with the chin-lift or jaw-thrust maneuver, is indicated. When the mandibular muscles lose tone, the tongue falls back, obstructing the pharynx, and the epiglottis may occlude the airway at the level of the pharynx. Positioning of the head and jaw reinstates a patent airway. The head-tilt position is contraindicated in trauma patients for whom the stability of the cervical spine is not yet determined. In these patients, only the chin-lift or jaw-thrust maneuver should be used. If a patent airway is still not established, an airway adjunct should be used.

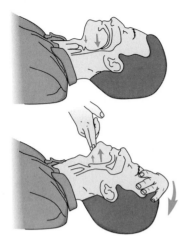

FIGURE 3-1

Opening the airway. *(Top)* When patients are unconscious, upper airway muscle tone is decreased, which leads to obstruction of the airway by the tongue and epiglottis. *(Bottom)* Relief of obstruction by the head-tilt technique with the chin-lift maneuver.
(Reproduced with permission. From Textbook of Advanced Cardiac Life Support, 1987, 1990. Copyright American Heart Association.)

Technique

The basic technique is to extend the patient's neck, or tilt the head backward into the so-called sniffing position. This position is achieved by firmly placing the palm of one hand on the forehead and tilting the head backward. The chin is then brought forward either by lifting it with two fingers or by thrusting the jaw forward with the fingers placed behind the mandible (Fig. 3-1). When pulling the chin forward, the fingers should not jut into the soft tissue under the chin, causing the tongue to be pushed farther back into the airway.

OROPHARYNGEAL AIRWAY

The oropharyngeal airway, most commonly made of plastic, holds the tongue away from the posterior portion of the pharynx when it is properly placed. When the device is in position, it curves over the tongue, with its tip in the posterior pharynx (Fig. 3-2).

Indications

The use of the oropharyngeal airway is indicated when the patient has a depressed level of consciousness resulting in loss of muscle tone and airway obstruction. It may make bag-valve-mask ventilation more effective. The device is also used to prevent biting, and thus occlusion, of an endotracheal tube. It is contraindicated in an awake and alert patient because it may stimulate the gag reflex, creating patient discomfort with possible emesis and aspiration.

Technique

The proper size oropharyngeal airway is chosen by measuring the airway on the patient. When the tip of the oropharyngeal airway is placed at the edge of the patient's mouth, it should extend to the bottom of the ear. An airway that is too short forces

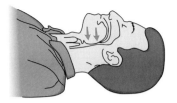

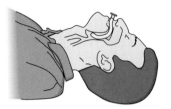

FIGURE 3-2

When correctly placed, the oropharyngeal airway holds the tongue away from the posterior portion of the pharynx, relieving airway obstruction. *(Top)* Obstructed airway, with incorrect head position. *(Bottom)* Correct head-tilt position and placement or oropharyngeal airway. *(Modified from Textbook of Advanced Cardiac Life Support, 1987, 1990. Copyright American Heart Association.)*

the patient's tongue back into the pharynx. An airway that is too long stimulates the gag reflex.

There are two methods of insertion. The airway may be inserted "upside down," with its tip against the hard palate. The airway is slid into the mouth until the soft palate is reached, at which point it is rotated so its curvature matches that of the tongue. The tip is advanced to the back of the mouth to ensure its position in the posterior portion of the pharynx. The end of the airway should rest between the teeth but not compress the lips against the teeth, which leads to mucosal trauma. The second method of insertion utilizes a tongue blade to depress the patient's tongue while inserting the airway, matching its curvature with that of the natural curvature of the tongue.

Management Principles

After insertion of the airway, the adequacy of ventilation must be assessed by observation and auscultation of the breath sounds. The chin-lift maneuver should accompany the use of the oropharyngeal airway, if its use is not contraindicated, to provide optimal airway control.

NASOPHARYNGEAL AIRWAY

The nasopharyngeal airway, a soft tube made of rubber or soft latex, is placed in the nose and extends to the posterior portion of the pharynx. It is sometimes called a nasal trumpet (Fig. 3-3).

Indications

The use of a nasopharyngeal airway is indicated when the patient has a depressed level of consciousness resulting in loss of muscle tone and airway obstruction and

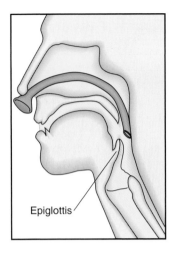

Epiglottis

FIGURE 3-3

The nasopharyngeal airway is used to relieve upper airway obstruction and to facilitate passage of a suction catheter. *(Modified from Luce JM, Pierson DJ, and Tyler ML. Intensive Respiratory Care. Philadelphia, Saunders, 1993.)*

when an oropharyngeal airway would be contraindicated or technically difficult to place. Examples include distortion of the oral cavity because of trauma, tight closure of the jaw during a seizure, or closure of the jaw with wire for stabilization post injury. The nasopharyngeal airway is also used to facilitate the passage of a suction catheter, thus reducing nasal trauma when nasopharyngeal suctioning is indicated. This airway may be contraindicated in the presence of coagulopathy because severe epistaxis may result.

Technique

The proper length of the nasopharyngeal tube is chosen by measuring from the nostril to the earlobe or angle of the jaw. The internal diameter of the tube varies with tube length. A tube that is too long may enter into the esophagus and cause gastric distention. If a tube is too short to enter into the posterior portion of the pharynx, a patent airway cannot be established.

To insert the airway, lubricate it with a water-soluble lubricant or water. The correct nostril is chosen by positioning the beveled tip to the patient's midline. Insert the airway along the floor of the nose for minimal trauma to the turbinates and minimal discomfort to the patient. Gentle, steady pressure should be used. If resistance is met, then the use of the other nostril or a smaller tube should be attempted. When the airway is properly positioned, the flanged portion of the airway will rest against the nostril.

Management Principles

Assess the condition of the nares and prevent skin breakdown by pressure necrosis. Immediately after insertion, assess the adequacy of ventilation. Suction the airway if necessary to remove from the lumen any secretions or blood. If adequate ventilation is not established, recheck head and jaw positions. Use a pocket face mask or manual resuscitation bag and mask to deliver positive-pressure ventilation if necessary.

POCKET FACE MASK

The pocket face mask provides a method of ventilating a patient's lungs that is more aesthetic than mouth-to-mouth ventilation. It does not establish a patent airway and may need to be used with the oropharyngeal or nasopharyngeal airway and/or the head-tilt and chin-lift maneuvers. The pocket face mask is made of a soft plastic material that allows the mask to be compressed into a flat position for storage. When needed, the mask is popped up into its expanded position (Fig. 3-4). Its use eliminates the need for direct contact with the patient's mouth and nose. It provides effective ventilation, placement and technique are easy to teach to individuals of variable skill levels, and some models allow for the supplemental administration of oxygen. For these reasons, placement of a pocket face mask in strategic locations in patient care areas is strongly recommended.

Technique

Pop the mask up into its fully expanded position. Connect the one-way valve and filter to the mask to prevent exposure to exhaled gases. The ideal position from which to approach the patient is from the top of the patient's head. Use the head-tilt maneuver and place the mask over the patient's mouth and nose. Grasp the jaw with your fingers and apply upward pressure while using the thumb side of your palms to press downward and hold the mask in place. Finally, blow into the opening of the mask. The air going from the rescuer to the victim is filtered. During expiration the one-way valve closes, diverting filtered, expired air away from the rescuer.

Management Principles

Observe the rise and fall of the patient's chest to determine the adequacy of ventilation. Limitations to adequate ventilation include a small rescuer vital capacity,

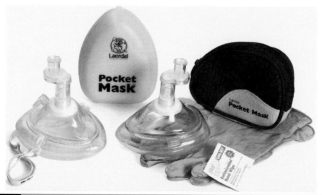

FIGURE 3-4

Laerdal pocket face mask in its fully expanded position with filter in place. *(Courtesy of Laerdal Medical Corporation, Wappingers Falls, NY.)*

loss of volume because of an inadequate seal around the patient's mouth and nose, and inability to ventilate because of an obstruction of the airway by mucus, emesis, blood, or a foreign object.

ENDOTRACHEAL INTUBATION

Endotracheal intubation is accomplished by placing a tube, either nasally or orally (Table 3-1), through the larynx and into the trachea.

Indications

The following are indications for the use of endotracheal intubation: (1) airway obstruction/compromise that persists despite the use of previously discussed methods (i.e., airway edema), (2) secretion management because an endotracheal tube provides a conduit for suctioning, (3) airway protection from regurgitation or aspiration in patients with a depressed level of consciousness or ineffective upper airway reflexes, and (4) the need for high concentrations of oxygen, mechanical ventilation, or general anesthesia.

TABLE 3-1 Nasal Versus Oral Endotracheal Intubation

	Nasal	Oral
Indications	Nonemergent, elective intubation Suspected or known cervical spine injury	Emergency airway Technically difficult with suspected cervical spine injury
Advantages	Situations in which oral access is difficult or impossible, such as oral trauma, maxillomandibular wiring More comfortable for patient Easier to stabilize and maintain good oral hygiene Less gagging Communication by mouthing of words possibly enhanced	Allows passage of larger tube: less airway resistance to gas flow, improved secretion removal Less kinking Easier to insert Preferred method; less sinusitis and otitis media
Disadvantages	More difficult to place Requires use of smaller lumen tube: greater airway resistance to gas flow, more difficult secretion removal Kinks more easily Epistaxis possible during insertion Contributes to development of sinusitis, otitis media	Less comfortable for patient: may cause gagging and stimulate oral secretion production More difficult to stabilize Patient may bite down on airway, reducing gas flow More difficult to maintain good oral hygiene and to communicate by mouthing words

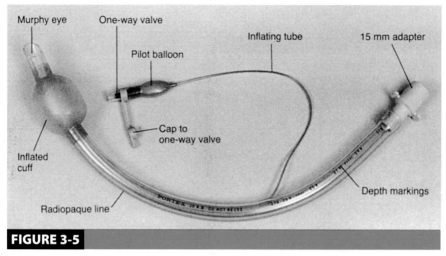

FIGURE 3-5

Basic design features of the endotracheal tube.

Tube Design

The basic design of the endotracheal tube (ETT) is standardized (Fig. 3-5). The *connector* fits into the tube at the proximal end. It has a standard 15-mm outside diameter that permits universal connection to respiratory therapy or anesthesia equipment. The *tube body* has a standard curvature, centimeter markings that allow for the determination of depth of insertion, and radiopaque markings either running the length of the tube or at the distal end, so that the tube can be located on a chest x-ray film. The *distal tip* of the ETT has a beveled edge, which allows for easier passage of the tube through the glottic slit. A Magill type of ETT has an opening only at the distal end of the tube, whereas a Murphy type of tube also has a small hole opening opposite the beveled edge. This hole allows for gas flow in the event that the bevel becomes lodged against the tracheal wall or otherwise occluded. Adult ETTs are equipped with a *cuff*, which when inflated seals the trachea, allowing for the application of positive-pressure ventilation and minimizing aspiration (see the section Monitoring and Managing Cuffs, later). Finally, the *inflating system* is a small-bore tube fused within the wall of the ETT, which allows for inflation of the cuff. At the proximal end of this small lumen is a spring-loaded valve that is activated by inserting a syringe. Air can then be inserted into the cuff. The valve closes when the syringe is removed, thus preventing the escape of air from the cuff. Adjacent to this valve is the *pilot balloon*, a small balloon that, when felt for air pressure, indicates the general inflation state of the cuff.

Endotracheal tubes come in different sizes. The tube size is determined by the internal diameter (ID) of the lumen and is measured in millimeters. The ID is marked on the outside of the tube. Tube size increases in increments of 0.5 mm. The risk of glottic injury is reduced by using a tube that approximates the patient's glottic dimensions. Glottic size is related to sex, not height, weight, or body surface area. The usual size of a tube needed for an adult woman is 7.0 or 7.5 and for an adult man is 8.0 or 8.5. In an emergency situation, an 8.0-mm ID tube serves as a good standard-sized tube.

Technique

INTUBATION EQUIPMENT

Intubation must be performed only by persons trained in this difficult skill. Endotracheal intubation is most often facilitated by direct laryngoscopy. Laryngoscopy, which is the direct visualization of the vocal cords or glottic slit, is performed with the use of a laryngoscope. The laryngoscope consists of two basic parts: the handle and the blade (Fig. 3-6). The handle, which is textured to allow for a good grip, houses batteries to supply power to the built-in light source on the blade. The indentation of the blade fits into the bar on the handle, and the light is illuminated when it is properly snapped into its right-angle position. Laryngoscope blades may be either curved (MacIntosh) or straight (Miller) and come in a variety of sizes to allow for variation in patient size. The laryngoscope handles and blades should be checked periodically and batteries and lights changed as necessary to keep the equipment in a ready state.

Equipment necessary for endotracheal intubation includes the following:
- The ETT
- Suction equipment in good working order, along with a rigid-tip suction catheter (Yankauer) and a suction catheter
- Oxygen source, connecting tube, and a manual resuscitation bag and mask
- Water-soluble lubricant
- A 10-mL syringe for cuff inflation
- Tape or other device for stabilization of the tube
- Magill forceps for directing the tube into the larynx or removing foreign material
- A plastic-coated malleable stylet that can be inserted into the tube to make it more rigid, thus facilitating insertion

The individual who assists with an intubation, especially in an emergency situation, should ensure that all equipment is ready, anticipate the needs of the intubationist, and assist in patient positioning, teaching, and medication administration as necessary. A good assistant is always appreciated and helps to achieve the common goal: the establishment of either an oral or a nasal patent airway (Fig. 3-7).

ORAL ENDOTRACHEAL INTUBATION

Assemble all equipment and check the tube cuff for patency and symmetry by inflating it with air. Lubricate the tube. Explain the procedure to the patient and provide sedation as necessary. Position is a key factor that can affect success. The bed should be moved away from the wall and the height raised and the patient moved up to the head as much as possible. Position the patient supine, with a towel or

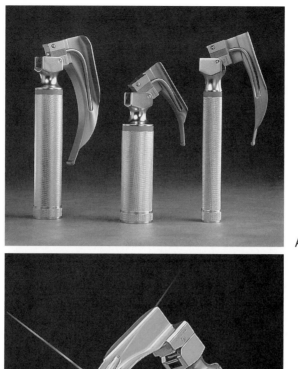

A

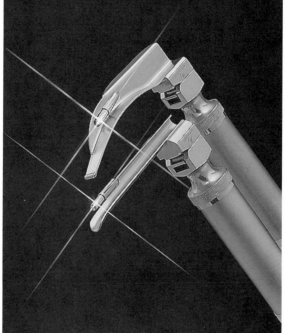

B

FIGURE 3-6

Laryngoscope, used during endotracheal intubation for direct visualization of the vocal cords. **A,** The two basic parts of the laryngoscope: the handle and the blade. **B,** The U-shaped indentation on the base of the blade hooks over the bar on the laryngoscope handle. The blade is then snapped upward into place. When the blade forms a 90-degree angle with the handle, it is correctly placed.

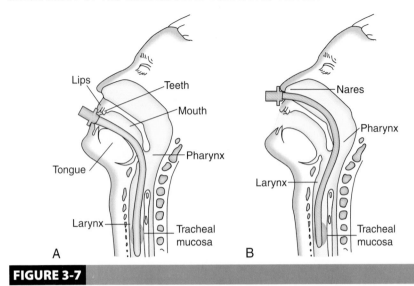

FIGURE 3-7

Endotracheal intubation may be performed (**A**) orally or (**B**) nasally. *(Modified from GA Traver [ed.], Respiratory Nursing: The Science and the Art. New York, John Wiley & Sons. 1982. Copyright © 1982 John Wiley & Sons.)*

blanket under the head, to achieve the sniffing position, which facilitates viewing of the glottis. Preoxygenate the patient with 100% oxygen. The laryngoscope is inserted into the right side of the mouth and the tongue is displaced to the left. The tip of the curved blade is inserted into the vallecula, which is the space between the base of the tongue and the epiglottis. The tip of the straight blade is inserted under the epiglottis. Upward traction is then exerted to expose the glottic opening. (Care must be taken to avoid using the upper teeth as a fulcrum.) The tube is then inserted through the vocal cords and slightly beyond (5 to 6 cm), into the trachea. The stylet is used to shape the curvature of the tube when there is difficulty passing the tube into the trachea. The laryngoscope is removed, the stylet is removed, and the cuff is inflated. Breath sounds are immediately auscultated while the patient's lungs are ventilated with a manual resuscitation bag to determine whether the procedure was successful. The tube should then be stabilized without delay, and a chest x-ray obtained to confirm placement. If an attempt at intubation is prolonged (>30 seconds) or if the oxygen saturation drops significantly, the heart rate or rhythm changes, or cyanosis develops, then the procedure should be interrupted and the patient oxygenated with 100% oxygen with a manual resuscitation bag and mask device.

NASAL ENDOTRACHEAL INTUBATION

Assemble all equipment and check the tube cuff for patency and symmetry by inflating it with air. Lubricate the tube. Explain the procedure to the patient and provide sedation as necessary. Position the patient according to the intubationist's preference: semi-Fowler's, high Fowler's, or supine. Nasal intubation is usually performed blindly; that is, no laryngoscope is used to visualize the vocal cords, no hyperextension is utilized, and the head remains in the midline position. The tube is inserted into the nostril that appears to have the greatest patency after a topical anesthetic is liberally applied. While the tube is gently advanced along the floor of the nostril, breath sounds are listened for at the proximal tube end. At the time of inspiration, the intubationist advances the tube through the open vocal cords. If the tube was placed correctly, a vapor column (cloudiness) is visible in the endotracheal tube. In nasal endotracheal intubation in which a laryngoscope blade is used, Magill forceps may also be used to assist in advancing the tube through the glottic slit once it is visualized. Once the tube is in place, the cuff is inflated, and while the patient is undergoing ventilation with a manual resuscitation bag, breath sounds are immediately auscultated to ascertain the presence of bilaterally equal breath sounds. The tube is then stabilized, with caution exercised to prevent upward pressure on the nares. A chest x-ray should be obtained immediately to confirm placement.

Assessment of Tube Placement

Assessment of tube placement must be performed immediately after inflation of the cuff. Methods include auscultation of breath sounds high in each axilla, to decrease the chance of being misled by breath sounds referred from the opposite lung; auscultation over the stomach, where the presence of gurgling sounds or air movement indicates possible esophageal intubation; and auscultation over both lung fields. Simultaneously, the chest wall should be observed for equal, bilateral expansion. Esophageal intubation can also be detected using capnography. If the tube is in the trachea, the capnographic carbon dioxide level should rapidly rise. Colorimetric carbon dioxide analysis is considered by many the standard for detection of esophageal intubation. The device is placed on the end of the ETT and the patient is given six full breaths. At end-expiration on the sixth breath, the color is read. The indicator paper changes colors if carbon dioxide is detected (Fig. 3-8). Colorimetric devices are less expensive than capnography; are portable, which makes them easy to stock with intubation supplies; and are single-use disposable items. Capnography and colorimetric devices both assist in the detection of esophageal intubation. However, in patients in cardiac arrest, poor pulmonary perfusion results in low exhaled carbon dioxide levels, which may yield a false-negative result. Other methods for assessing tube position include fiberoptic laryngoscopy, esophageal detection devices, evaluation of oxygenation using pulse oximetry, and of course portable chest x-ray. The ideal position of the ETT is in the mid-trachea, 5 cm from the carina, with the head in a neutral position. Once tube placement is confirmed, the depth marking at the teeth or naris should be noted in the medical record.

Complications

Endotracheal intubation is a highly technical skill that is not without complications (Box 3-1). Vigilant monitoring and care of the patient prevents many complications.

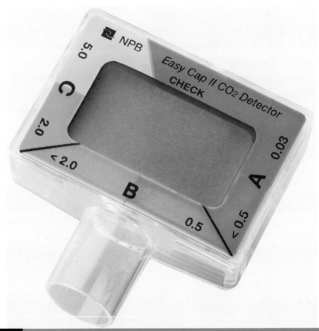

FIGURE 3-8

Disposable colorimetric carbon dioxide (CO_2) detector for confirming endotracheal tube placement. When CO_2 is detected, the color of the indicator changes from purple to yellow. Detection of CO_2 confirms tube placement in the lungs because the only source of CO_2 is the alveoli. *(Courtesy Nellcor Puritan Bennett Inc., Pleasanton, Calif.)*

Tube Stabilization Techniques

Each time the patient is assessed, the security of the airway should be viewed as the highest of priorities. Endotracheal tubes may be secured with either tape or harnesses specially designed for this purpose (Fig. 3-9). Whenever an ETT-securing device is removed, two persons must be present, one to hold the airway to prevent dislodgment if the patient coughs or gags and the other to perform oral and nares care and stabilize the tube. Inflation of the cuff should never be viewed as a method of tube stabilization.

There are several techniques for securing an ETT. General principles common to each technique include the following:

- Device/tape should go completely around the patient's head to provide stabilization superior to that of tape placed only across the cheeks.
- Secure an oral endotracheal tube to the upper lip, not to the mandible, which moves with talking.
- Reposition oral ETTs once every 24 hours to prevent pressure necrosis.
- Secure a nasal endotracheal tube to the upper lip, not to the bridge of the nose, so as to reduce traction on the nares.

BOX 3-1 Complications Associated with Endotracheal Intubation

DURING THE INTUBATION PROCEDURE
Vomiting with possible aspiration
Trauma: laryngeal, pharyngeal, tracheal, dental, nasal
Bradycardia caused by vagal stimulation
Hypoxemia caused by delay in procedure
Cardiac arrhythmias
Right main-stem intubation
Esophageal intubation

WHILE THE TUBE IS IN PLACE
Tube malposition: too high, too low
Right main-stem intubation
Laryngeal or tracheal necrosis, erosion
Pharyngeal edema
Mouth, lip, or nares pressure-sore development
Inadequate ventilation or oxygenation as a result of tube obstruction or kinking
Loss of cuff integrity
Unplanned (self) extubation
Aspiration
Sinus effusions, sinusitis, otitis media

AFTER EXTUBATION
Sore throat, hoarseness
Laryngeal edema or spasm potentially leading to airway obstruction, stridor
Laryngeal incompetence because of sensory deficit, possible aspiration
Vocal cord immobility, paresis, or paralysis, potentially resulting in aspiration

LATE COMPLICATIONS AFTER EXTUBATION
Tracheal stenosis
Laryngeal or tracheal granuloma
Laryngeal stenosis: glottic or subglottic

- Avoid securing multiple tubes together (e.g., an endotracheal tube and a nasogastric tube) because if the patient pulls on one, both tubes will be dislodged.
- Prevent the patient's hair from sticking to tape by placing a second piece of tape, 6 to 8 inches long (sticky sides together), along that portion of the tape that will be at the patient's occiput.
- Fold the end of the tape to create a pull tab and thus promote easier removal for tape changes.

The quest for an optimal method of stabilizing ETTs led to the production of harness devices that are widely used in critical care units. The device should be removed at least once daily for oral care and assessment of the mouth for pressure areas. Some harness models have a built-in bite block. A combination headgear and faceplate holds the tube securely and reduces tube movement, thus easing frictional trauma to the mouth and trachea. Such devices are more costly than cloth tape; however, they can be washed and reused. Although these devices cannot eradicate unplanned extubation, in patients who tongue at their tubes in an attempt to dislodge them, the harness holds the tube more securely than tape.

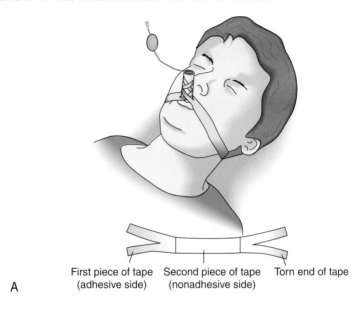

First piece of tape   Second piece of tape   Torn end of tape
(adhesive side)   (nonadhesive side)

A

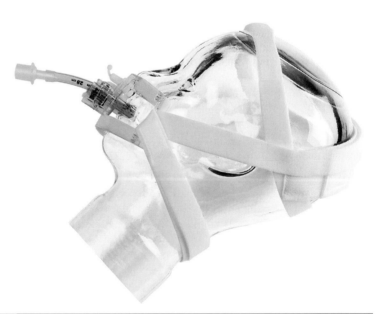

B

FIGURE 3-9

Two methods of securing the endotracheal tube: (**A**) tape and (**B**) harness device. Harness device shown is the SecureEasy Endotracheal Tube Holder. Its nonelastic headgear reduces the risk of self-extubation without putting excessive pressure on the patient's face. A soft bite-block comfortably prevents tube occlusion. (*A, Modified from Hess DR, MacIntyre NR, Mishoe SC, et al. Respiratory Care: Principles and Practice. Philadelphia, Saunders, 2002, p 710. B, Courtesy Medex, Carlsbad, Calif.*)

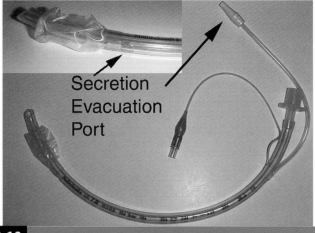

Secretion
Evacuation
Port

FIGURE 3-10

The Hi-Lo Evac tube has a port for suctioning subglottic secretions. The lumen opening is just above the cuff on the dorsal portion of the tube. The tube is used as one measure for reducing bacterial health-care-acquired pneumonia associated with mechanical ventilation. *(From Cairo JM, Pilbeam SP. Mosby's Respiratory Care Equipment, 7th ed, St. Louis, Mosby, 2004.)*

Special-Purpose Endotracheal Tubes

A variety of special-purpose ETTs are manufactured. There are tubes with preformed curves and wire reinforcement to help prevent kinking, double-lumen tubes for dual lung ventilation, and flexible metal tubes designed with water-filled cuffs to prevent fire hazard during laser surgery. Of special interest is an ETT with a port located above the cuff for the evacuation of subglottic secretions (Fig. 3-10).

Secretion-clearing endotracheal tubes decrease the incidence of ventilator-associated pneumonia (VAP) by nearly 50%. Bacteria-laden secretions slip past the glottis into the trachea and pool in the subglottic space above the ETT cuff. These secretions leak past the cuff and are aspirated into and contaminate the lower respiratory tract, causing pneumonia. By applying continuous or intermittent suction to a port attached to a dorsal lumen that opens just above the cuff, subglottic secretions are removed. Use of this tube is recommended by the Centers for Disease Control and Prevention (CDC) as part of a strategy to reduce health-care-associated bacterial pneumonia. The recommendation is category II, which means it is suggested for implementation and supported by suggestive clinical or epidemiologic studies or by a strong theoretical rationale. The addition of a subglottic secretion removal lumen increases the outer diameter of the tube 0.7 to 0.8 mm as compared to a standard tube.

With the addition of a suction port to the ETT come additional airway management responsibilities. The suction lumen must have the appropriate level of vacuum applied. The manufacturer recommends continuous low-pressure suction not exceeding -20 mm Hg, which requires that an additional suction regulator be available at the bedside. This could prove to be a potential hidden cost or pragmatic issue affecting ease of use and should be given forethought prior to implementation of the tube. The patency of the suction lumen must be frequently assessed. If no secretions are being aspirated, this may be an indication that either there are no secretions in the subglottic space or the evacuation port is blocked by secretions, blood, etc. A blockage is cleared by administering a bolus of air using a syringe, into the suction lumen. Routine administration of a bolus of air every 4 hours may prevent blockage and ensure continuous patency. Very recent improvements in tube design, including a larger distal opening to the suction lumen, reportedly reduce difficulties in maintaining patency and enhance secretion removal. If suction is discontinued for patient transport or some other reason, then the suction port should be capped off with the suction lumen cap. The cap prevents contaminants from leaking out of or from entering the lumen. Safety dictates that the suction lumen be clearly marked to avoid confusion with other tubes (such as feeding tubes) coming from the patient's mouth or nares. Standards of practice need to clearly define the responsibility of the nurse versus the respiratory therapist in the collaborative management of the airway.

The finding that a secretion-clearing ETT reduces VAP would seem to dictate their use in all patients. However, the benefits of using such a tube must be weighed against the increased cost. Patients for whom intubation is anticipated to be a very brief experience (e.g., surgery and recovery) may not be appropriate candidates for such a tube. Whereas patients with higher known VAP rates, such as those requiring mechanical ventilation for more than 72 hours, are a more appropriate target population but not always easy to predict. Institutions should review the available evidence, including the cost of health-care-acquired pneumonia in terms of dollars and lives, and develop specific guidelines for appropriate use of this airway for their patient populations.

TRACHEOSTOMY TUBES

Tracheostomy tubes provide an airway directly into the anterior portion of the neck, usually at the level of the second or fourth tracheal rings. The tracheotomy procedure is performed by a surgeon, either at the bedside or in the controlled setting of the operating room.

Indications/Advantages

Tracheostomy tubes are indicated (1) for long-term secretion management, (2) to reduce dead-space ventilation and airway resistance (in comparison with endotracheal tubes) and therefore to reduce the work of breathing, (3) for protection of the airway from aspiration, (4) when upper airway obstruction prevents placement of an endotracheal tube, and (5) when prolonged mechanical ventilation is necessary. Tracheostomy tubes are better tolerated; therefore, the patient may require less sedation or restraint use and create less airflow resistance than oral or nasal ETTs, allow for oral intake and better oral hygiene, and, in the case of some tube designs, even allow for talking. They prevent further laryngeal injury by the translaryngeal tube, are more securely fixed and thus decrease the incidence of accidental extubation and improve patient mobility, and often facilitate the transfer of the patient from the intensive care unit. In trauma patients, tracheostomy is associated with a decreased incidence of health-care-acquired pneumonia.

There are no existing clear-cut data that delineate the ideal timing of tracheostomy in patients with an ETT in place for mechanical ventilation. Each case must be reviewed individually, and the potential risks and benefits weighed carefully. Whether a tracheostomy should be performed must be discussed early in the clinical course and revisited often. Heffner suggests that critical care teams use flexibility in their decision making and avoid overly simplistic rules that promote tracheostomy after a set number of days of intubation. If the team projects that the length of time that mechanical ventilation or an artificial airway will be required may be prolonged, then the decision should be made to perform the tracheostomy. In this case, the benefits of a tracheostomy may outweigh the risks and costs of the procedure, whereas for a patient with an acute exacerbation of chronic obstructive pulmonary disease, early intervention and evidence of improvement may not have the same projected benefit. Finally, a patient with a grave prognosis may never be considered for such an intervention. Additional investigation is needed that examines the benefits of tracheostomy performed at different times during the course of critical illness in varying patient populations.

Percutaneous Dilational Tracheostomy

Percutaneous dilation tracheostomy (PDT) is a procedure that can be performed by surgeons and nonsurgeons at the bedside in the intensive care unit (ICU) to achieve a secure airway in the trachea. Originally developed in 1985, it has gained wider acceptance in the ICU. A small incision is made in the neck and trachea, and using the Seldinger technique the opening is enlarged using specialized dilators until the desired tube size fits into the opening. Advantages include that no operating room or general anesthesia is required and there is no need to move high-risk patients. Compared to surgical tracheostomy, there is a decreased incidence of pneumothorax, bleeding, and stenosis. According to Durbin, patients for whom surgical tracheostomy may still be a better option include patients with coagulation abnormalities because bleeding vessels are more easily controlled under direct vision; those on high levels of support (i.e., >70% oxygen and ≥10 PEEP); and patients with unstable cervical spines and those with unfavorable neck anatomy, including obesity, previous surgery, and poor neck mobility). However, those with recent surgical repair of neck injuries may benefit from PDT because of its lower wound infection rate.

Collaboratively, the nurse and respiratory therapist monitor the patient and assist during the procedure. The patient should be properly positioned and the height of the bed adjusted relative to the individual performing the procedure. Prior to the draping and prepping of the patient, it is important to ensure the intravenous access lines are accessible so sufficient sedation and analgesia may be administered. Sterile supplies are gathered and sterility maintained throughout. Physiologic parameters are monitored continuously and documented minimally at 15-minute intervals throughout the procedure and the subsequent hour. The most significant peri-operative risk is accidental decannulation. When a patient undergoes a surgical tracheostomy, the trachea is surgically attached to the skin. This promotes prompt identification of the tract and reinsertion of the tracheal tube should it become

BOX 3-2	Complications Associated with Tracheostomy

DURING THE TRACHEOSTOMY OPERATION
Placement of tube in false passage
Moderate bleeding or hemorrhage
Pneumothorax and subcutaneous emphysema

WHILE THE TRACHEOSTOMY TUBE IS IN PLACE
Tube dislodgement or decannulation
Stomal cellulitis or infection
Tracheal injury: necrosis, erosion, tracheovascular fistula
Inadequate ventilation or oxygenation as a result of tube obstruction
Loss of cuff integrity
Unplanned (self) extubation
Aspiration

DURING DECANNULATION
Difficult removal of tube because of tight stoma

LATE COMPLICATIONS AFTER EXTUBATION
Tracheal granuloma, stenosis, dilation
Poor wound healing: scar, keloid, persistent stoma

dislodged and need replacing. With a PDT, the trachea is not secured in this fashion and a mature tract takes approximately 2 weeks to form. Accidental decannulation and attempted reinsertion of the airway during this time may result in difficulty securing the airway, bleeding, tracheal injury, and death. Oral intubation may be required if the airway becomes dislodged or needs replacing.

Complications

Tracheostomy is not without complications (Box 3-2). Vigilant monitoring and care of the patient prevents many complications. Tracheovascular fistula is a rare but catastrophic complication of tracheostomy. Vascular injuries occur at the stoma or the cuff and may present as profuse bleeding if thyroid or innominate artery erosion has occurred. Patients with neck malignancy or radiation therapy are at greatest risk. If the bleeding is not rapidly controlled, exsanguination or suffocation caused by blood aspiration may occur. In the patient with a tracheotomy, a gloved finger should be inserted into the stoma and an attempt made to compress the bleeding artery digitally against the posterior portion of the sternum. Definitive therapy involves emergency surgical repair. Fortunately, tracheovascular complications are rare.

Tracheostomy Tube Designs

Tracheostomy tubes are available in a variety of sizes, styles, and materials. Primarily they are made of either plastic or metal. General design features (Fig. 3-11) include the *neck flange*, which should lie flush against the patient's neck. The flange has holes on either end in which tracheostomy ties are inserted for securing of the airway. Some tracheostomy tubes have flanges that are adjustable so the extratracheal portion of the tube can be made shorter or longer, a useful feature when soft tissue

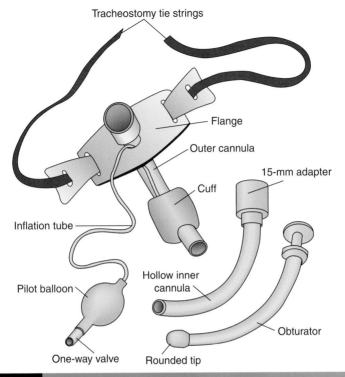

Tracheostomy tie strings

Flange

Outer cannula

15-mm adapter

Cuff

Inflation tube

Hollow inner cannula

Pilot balloon

Obturator

One-way valve   Rounded tip

FIGURE 3-11

General design features of the tracheostomy tube. *(Modified from Wilkins RL, Stoller JK, Scanlan CL., et al. Egan's Fundamentals of Respiratory Care, 8th ed. St. Louis, Mosby, 2003, p 667.)*

swelling is present or when the patient has a large thick neck. The flange should lie securely against the patient's skin so that movement of the tube into and out of the stoma, and thus airway trauma, are minimized. The *tube body* has both extratracheal and intratracheal portions, divided by the neck flange. A radiopaque marker is located on the body. Near the end of the body is the *cuff* (uncuffed tubes are also available). When inflated, the cuff seals the trachea, allowing for the application of positive-pressure ventilation and minimizing aspiration. Finally, the *inflating system*, a small-bore tube fused within the wall of the tracheostomy tube, allows for the inflation of the cuff. At the proximal end of this small lumen is a spring-loaded valve that can be opened by inserting a syringe to allow air to be inserted into the cuff. The valve closes when the syringe is removed, thus preventing the escape of air from the cuff. Adjacent to this valve is the *pilot balloon*, a small balloon that, when felt for air pressure, indicates the general inflation state of the cuff. The *obturator* is inserted into the lumen of the tracheostomy tube, its rounded end extending slightly farther than the body. The obturator creates a smooth tube tip, which prevents injury to the tracheal wall when the tube is initially inserted. It must always be removed after the tube is inserted to allow for the passage of air and should be kept in a visible place at the patient's bedside should emergency reinsertion of a misplaced tube be necessary.

Tracheostomy tubes are available in standard length or extra length. The extra-length tubes may be proximal (horizontal extra length) or distal (vertical extra length). Extra proximal length facilitates tracheostomy tube placement in patients with a large neck such as an obese individual. Extra distal length facilitates placement in patients with tracheal malacia or tracheal anomalies. An adjustable flange design is also available to allow bedside adjustments to meet extra length needs. The practitioner is cautioned that these tubes are usually temporary and should be replaced with a tube with a fixed flange because the flange may slip over time, resulting in a misplaced airway.

CUFFED VERSUS UNCUFFED TUBES

The choice of a cuffed tube over an uncuffed tube is made if the patient will require mechanical ventilation or if aspiration may be a problem. Cuffed tubes are most often used in the acute care setting. Uncuffed tubes are useful in long-term care settings when the patient has competent glottic function and aspiration is therefore not a problem. Uncuffed tubes are also used in the pediatric population.

SINGLE VERSUS DOUBLE CANNULAS

Tracheostomy tubes may be single or double cannula. The cannulas of the double-cannula tube are referred to as the inner cannula and the outer cannula. The inner cannula is removable to facilitate cleaning of the inner tracheal lumen, a useful feature because tracheal tubes tend to be left in place for prolonged periods and accumulation of secretions may become a problem. When the inner cannula is not in place, the ventilator usually cannot be connected to the tracheostomy because the outer lumen is not the same size as a standard-size connector. Therefore, if the patient cannot tolerate being off the ventilator, a spare inner cannula must be available for use when tracheostomy care is being performed.

The inner cannula is secured to the outer cannula by various mechanisms. Some cannulas twist to lock into place, others snap-lock into place, and still others have a hinge on the outer cannula that swings to lock over and thus secure the inner cannula. Caregivers must ensure that they know how to secure and remove the inner cannula.

Inner cannulas may be reusable or disposable. Reusable cannulas are washed and replaced, whereas disposable ones are used only once and then discarded. Disposable inner cannulas (DICs) reduce the time required for performing tracheostomy care and reduce the possibility of caregiver contamination by splashing, which can occur when an inner cannula is cleaned. Whether DICs are more or less cost effective than reusable inner cannulas is unknown (Fig. 3-12).

METAL TUBES

Metal tubes are indicated for long-term use in chronic care populations because of the durability of the metal. Metal tubes are also used for weaning patients from their tracheostomy in preparation for decannulation (see section on decannulation, later).

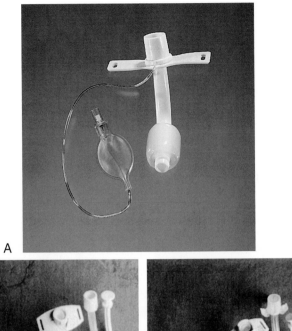

A

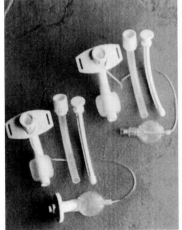

B

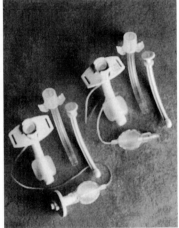

C

FIGURE 3-12

Tracheostomy tubes. **A,** Single cannula. **B,** Double cannula with reusable inner cannula. **C,** Double cannula with disposable inner cannula. *(Courtesy Nellcor Puritan Bennett Inc., Pleasanton, Calif.)*

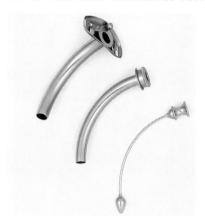

A

B

FIGURE 3-13

A, Metal tracheostomy tube, which is uncuffed, comes with an obturator and a reusable inner cannula. Fitting a manual resuscitation bag (MRB) to this tube requires a special adapter. The end of the adapter, which fits to the MRB, has a standard 15-mm connector; the other end, which fits into the inner cannula of the tracheostomy tube, is much smaller and varies by tube size. **B,** Metal tracheostomy tube with 15-mm adapter incorporated into the inner cannula. *(Courtesy Pilling Surgical, Research Triangle Park, NC.)*

The most commonly used metal tube is the Jackson tube. Made of sterling silver or, more commonly, stainless steel, it is an uncuffed tube with an inner cannula and a metal obturator (Fig. 3-13). Dr. Chevalier Jackson originally developed the silver tracheostomy tube and the sizing system (e.g., sizes 00, 0, 1, and 2). Within the industry there is no standard for tracheostomy tube sizing. This means that tubes of the same numeric size from different companies may not have the same internal or external diameters.

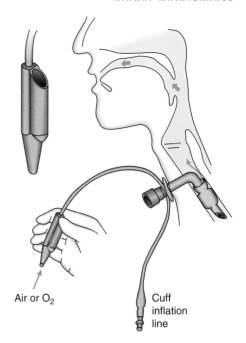

FIGURE 3-14

"Talking" tracheostomy tube. Air or oxygen, which is instilled through a special channel, exits from holes above the cuff, allowing for phonation. *(Modified from Luce JM, Pierson DJ, and Tyler ML. Intensive Respiratory Care. Philadelphia, Saunders, 1993.)*

Air or O$_2$

Cuff inflation line

A second important principle in the management of the patient with a metal tracheostomy tube concerns ensuring adequate manual ventilation when necessary. The standard 15-mm connector on a manual resuscitation bag (MRB) does not fit onto a metal tracheostomy tube. An adapter, which is standard in size at one end, can be used to mate the tracheostomy tube to the MRB. One end of this adapter narrows to a smaller lumen that fits into the inner lumen of the metal tube, allowing for a closed system for manual ventilation. The adapter must be the appropriate size for the size of the metal tube. In the clinical setting, an adapter of the appropriate size must be readily available at the bedside. Alternatively, metal tracheostomy tubes may be fit with an inner cannula with a 15-mm connector.

SPEAKING TRACHEOSTOMY TUBES

A tracheostomy tube that allows for speech is indicated to provide the patient with a mechanism for voice communication, thereby reducing frustration, improving patient and caregiver understanding, cultivating adaptation to illness, and promoting increased independence and self-esteem.

Communication mechanisms include either specially made tracheostomy tubes or a valve attached to the patient's tracheostomy tube. The special "talking" tracheostomy tubes have a channel through which air flows, exiting above the cuff and allowing for speech when the cuff is inflated (Fig. 3-14). This extra channel is attached to a standard air or oxygen flowmeter by a supply tube. A thumb valve on the air line controls the flow of gas. The practitioner needs to assist the patient in

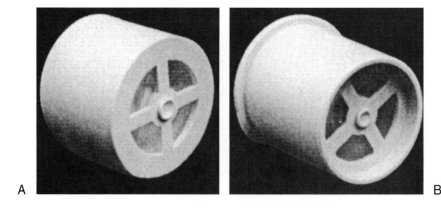

A   B

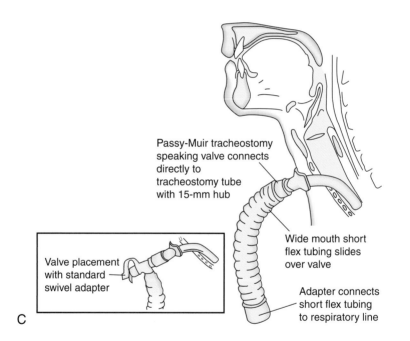

Passy-Muir tracheostomy speaking valve connects directly to tracheostomy tube with 15-mm hub

Wide mouth short flex tubing slides over valve

Adapter connects short flex tubing to respiratory line

Valve placement with standard swivel adapter

C

FIGURE 3-15

Two examples of the Passy-Muir tracheostomy speaking valve. Valve designs are for (**A**) patients who are not undergoing mechanical ventilation and (**B**) patients who are being mechanically ventilated. **C,** Options for valve placement within the ventilator circuitry. *(Courtesy Passy-Muir Inc., Irvine, Calif.)*

learning how to use the thumb valve to control the flow of gas. The flowmeter should be adjusted to provide the degree of flow needed for comfortable, audible speech (usually 4 to 6 L/min). For prevention of drying of the upper airway, the air source should be disconnected when not in use. Talking tracheostomy tubes that work by this mechanism can be used without interrupting mechanical ventilation.

The Passy-Muir Tracheostomy Speaking Valve (Fig. 3-15) is a one-way valve that attaches to a standard tracheostomy tube. At the end of inspiration the valve closes so that, on exhalation, air is forced up through the vocal cords. An added advantage is that secretions are also forced into the oral cavity for expectoration. The patient must be carefully assessed for tolerance because the work of breathing is increased with the use of the valve. Valves are available for use both when a patient is using a ventilator and when he or she is not. When the valve is attached, the cuff must be deflated.

Before the Passy-Muir valve is used, a thorough assessment of several issues must be performed. Successful use of the valve requires the patient to be able to exhale efficiently around the tracheostomy tube and through the mouth and nose. Glottal patency assessment may be performed by deflating the cuff and instructing the patient to attempt vocalization on expiration. The cuff should be deflated slowly over a 2- to 5-minute period. This allows the patient's oropharyngeal muscles to adjust to the sensation of airflow. The patient should also be assessed for hemodynamic stability, sufficient pulmonary compliance to maintain an effective functional residual capacity, intact cognitive function, and ability to handle secretions. Assessment for the presence of contraindications should also be performed. Contraindications include use of a foam-cuffed tube, presence of an artificial airway that is too large to allow for adequate air passage around its perimeter, thick and copious secretions, and severe airway obstruction that may prevent complete exhalation. The device is not intended for use with endotracheal tubes.

When the Passy-Muir valve is used on mechanically ventilated patients, adjustment of the ventilator settings is necessary to compensate for air leak around the deflated tracheostomy cuff that is escaping through the upper airway and not entering the lungs. When an increase in tidal volume is necessary, it should be made in small increments to avoid overcompensation that may result in an increase in peak inspiratory pressure. When pressure support ventilation is used, the inspiratory pressure will need to be adjusted. The inspiratory flow rate may also have to be increased if a larger tidal volume is used or if a longer expiratory vocalization period is needed. The set PEEP should be reduced because the valve creates auto-PEEP. Ventilator alarms that need to be turned off are the exhaled tidal volume and minute ventilation alarms because the tidal volume will no longer be returning to the ventilator.

While the valve is in place, the patient should be carefully monitored for respiratory stability and tolerance. Monitoring should include oxygen saturation, skin color, heart rate, respiratory rate, blood pressure, patient perception of the experience, anxiety, work of breathing, and secretion management. The amount of time that the valve is in place should be gradually increased. Eventually some patients may even learn to place the valve themselves, increasing their independence. The valve can be tethered to the tracheal tube flange for easy patient access. The valve should be removed while the patient is sleeping and during respiratory therapy treatments.

In the absence of a specially designed tube or valve, the patient may still be able to speak. The patient needs to be taught to use a finger to occlude the tracheostomy lumen on exhalation so air can be redirected up through the vocal cords. This technique is particularly easy to use with uncuffed tubes because if the tube has a cuff, it must be let down. Problems with finger occlusion include contamination from the patient and the environment, difficulty with hand control, patient embarrassment because finger occlusion is conspicuous, and limited duration of vocalizations. With finger occlusion the patient generally can speak only in phrases, whereas with a device such as the Passy-Muir valve, the patient can communicate in complete sentences.

FENESTRATED TUBES

The fenestrated tube has one or more pea-sized holes (fenestrae) in the upper one-third posterior portion of the outer cannula. When the inner cannula is removed, air flows out of this hole and up through the vocal cords so that phonation can occur (Fig. 3-16). Increasing the airflow through the upper airway also possibly helps to reduce the patient's psychological dependence on the tube before weaning. The inner cannula is removed to facilitate talking, and then the patient is instructed to hold a finger over the tracheal lumen on expiration to promote flow of air through the fenestration and vocal cords. Another method is to let the cuff down, remove the inner cannula, and place a plug over the tracheal opening. The patient is then ventilating both through the fenestration and around the tracheostomy. With the use of either method, a fair amount of resistance to ventilation is created; however, this may be tolerated long enough to allow the patient the opportunity to speak. When the inner cannula is replaced, mechanical ventilation and pulmonary treatments may be readily applied. Table 3-2 provides guidelines for the state of the cuff and the inner cannula during suctioning, talking, and eating.

TABLE 3-2	Guidelines for the State of the Cuff and Nonfenestrated Inner Cannula on a Fenestrated Tracheostomy Tube		
	Cuff Inflated	**Cuff Deflated**	**Inner Cannula**
Suctioning	X		In
Talking		X	Out
Eating	X		In

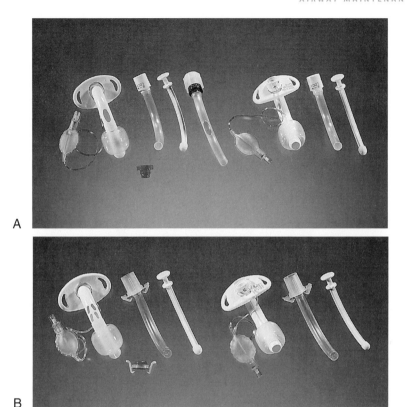

FIGURE 3-16

Fenestrated tracheostomy tubes. **A,** Reusable inner cannula. **B,** Disposable inner cannula. Removal of the inner cannula allows for phonation. Removal of the inner cannula with the cuff down and the decannulation plug in place facilitates air movement not only around but through the tube, preparing the patient for breathing through the natural airway. *(Courtesy of Nellcor Puritan Bennett Inc., Pleasanton, Calif.)*

TRACHEOSTOMY BUTTONS

Tracheostomy buttons are small cannulas that extend only from the skin to the anterior surface of the trachea. They are generally made of plastic.

Indications

Buttons are used to prevent stoma closure and ensure easy access to the airway in the event that it becomes necessary to provide an airway on an occasional basis, suction the airway, or possibly reinstitute mechanical ventilation. Examples of patients that may need an intermittent airway are burn and trauma patients requiring repeated trips to the operating room. Use of the tracheostomy button may also be the final step in weaning a patient from a tracheostomy to the natural airway.

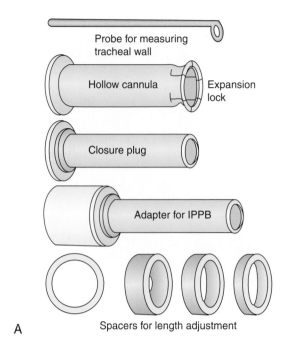

Probe for measuring tracheal wall

Hollow cannula

Expansion lock

Closure plug

Adapter for IPPB

A   Spacers for length adjustment

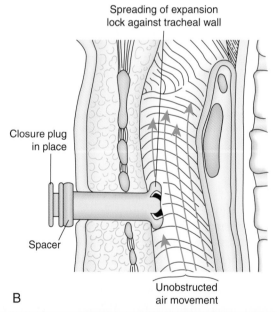

Spreading of expansion lock against tracheal wall

Closure plug in place

Spacer

B

Unobstructed air movement

FIGURE 3-17

Olympic tracheostomy button. **A,** Individual parts. **B,** Breathing with the closure plug in place. Insertion of the closure plug, or intermittent positive-pressure breathing (IPPB) adapter spreads the flanged tip of the button. The flanged tip is known as the expansion lock. *(Modified from Kersten LD. Comprehensive Respiratory Nursing. Philadelphia, Saunders, 1989.)*

Management Principles

The button, if sized and inserted properly, creates very little resistance to gas flow through the trachea. The distal end should be snug against the anterior surface of the trachea. Ensure that the button is not protruding into the trachea. Spacers, which look like washers, may be applied between the patient's neck and the proximal end of the button to ensure proper fit. If the button is too short, its distal end lies in the anterior cervical tissue. This leads to premature stoma closure or accidental dislodgment by the patient during coughing.

The Kistner button comes in a fixed length with a spacer that is used to customize patient fit. The proximal end may be either covered with a one-way valve attachment or plugged. The one-way valve allows air to flow in during inspiration but closes during expiration. If the valve becomes moist, it may stick and should be replaced. If the proximal end is fitted with a plug, the patient breathes completely through the natural airway.

The Olympic button (Fig. 3-17), which may have both outer and inner cannulas, comes in a variety of sizes and lengths. The appropriate size needed for a particular patient is determined with the use of a measuring probe. At the distal end, the outer cannula has flanges that should lie snug against the anterior tracheal wall to help secure the button in place. Spacer rings may be placed externally to prevent the button from extending too far into the trachea. Insertion of the inner cannula creates a standard-size external adapter for the institution of breathing treatments or for the use of a manual resuscitation bag. Alternatively, a closure plug may be inserted into the outer cannula, which allows the patient to breathe entirely by using the natural airway.

Tracheostomy Care

Routine tracheostomy care involves cleaning the stoma, the external portion of the tracheostomy tube, and the inner cannula. If dressings are being used, they also should be changed. The purpose of this procedure is to keep the tube free of mucus and other secretions that may be a source of infection or of encrustations that may impede airway patency. Tracheostomy ties must also be changed once a day, or more often if soiled.

Many facilities carry tracheostomy care kits (Fig. 3-18) that include all necessary supplies. These kits are particularly useful for cleaning the inner cannula because they contain sterile pipe cleaners or brushes. In general, the following supplies are needed: sterile basin, gloves, hydrogen peroxide, sterile saline solution, sterile cotton-tipped applicators, pipe cleaners or a brush, a replacement inner cannula, and a tracheal dressing. If the ties are to be changed, scissors and twill tape are also needed.

Immediately after a surgical procedure, the tracheostomy site should be assessed frequently. Some venous oozing is normal and may require dressing changes as often as every 2 hours to prevent collection of blood with possible aspiration. If bleeding is excessive, the surgeon may choose to pack the site. The surgeon may even suture the tracheostomy tube in place and prefer that these sutures not be disrupted for the first 48 hours. Even in these cases, it is still necessary to perform meticulous, sterile stoma care, as gently as possible, under the neck flange.

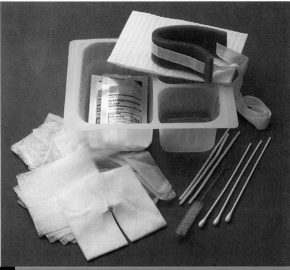

FIGURE 3-18

Equipment for tracheostomy care. Supplies may come prepackaged in a kit or be individually assembled. Supplies needed are hydrogen peroxide (H_2O_2), normal saline (NS), containers for H_2O_2 and NS, sterile precut tracheostomy dressing (sterile 4 × 4 gauze without cotton filler is also acceptable), clean tracheostomy tape, sterile gloves, cotton swabs, brush or pipe cleaners, sterile 4 × 4s. *(Not shown: scissors.)*

The frequency of tracheostomy care is a widely variable practice, and little data confirm what the practice should be. It is known that the presence of an artificial airway provides a portal for infection; however, it is not clear what infection risk is associated with cleaning or changing the inner cannula. The more frequently the ventilator circuit is changed, the greater the infection risk. Could it be extrapolated, therefore, that the more frequent the airway is entered to perform inner cannula changes or cleaning the greater the risk of entry of infectious agents? An additional potential risk associated with cannula change/cleaning practices is that patients requiring high levels of PEEP or FIO_2 may experience problems with gas exchange when the circuit is opened to perform this care. Burns and colleagues studied the extent of airway obstruction and colonization in 60 patients in the medical and surgical ICU who received inner cannula changes daily versus those who did not. Patients were entered into the study within 24 hours of receiving a surgical tracheostomy. The researchers checked the inner cannulas daily for obstruction and cultured on postoperative days 1 and 3. They found no statistically significant difference in colonization between protocols, and no obstructions were noted in either. This study suggests that the routine practice of changing inner cannulas in the ICU may be unnecessary, at least over a 3-day period.

Care of the single-cannula tracheostomy tube involves cleaning around the stoma and the external portion of the tube, changing the dressing, and changing the ties as necessary. When a double-cannula tube is used, care includes, in addition to the steps just described, the cleaning of the inner cannula. When the inner cannula is disposable, care involves removal of the inner cannula, replacement with a new cannula, and disposal of the old one. No attempt should be made to clean a disposable inner cannula, especially with the use of hydrogen peroxide, which disrupts the integrity of the structural material. Because hydrogen peroxide also causes pitting of a metal inner cannula, only sterile saline solution should be used for cleaning a metal tracheostomy tube. Reusable inner cannulas made of plastic may be cleaned with hydrogen peroxide, followed by rinsing with normal saline solution before reinsertion. Cleansing of the inner cannula is assisted with the use of a sterile pipe cleaner or brush.

When cleaning a reusable inner cannula on a patient who cannot tolerate disruption of mechanical ventilation, it is necessary to have two inner cannulas of identical size and type available. When the inner cannula that needs to be cleaned is removed, the spare is inserted. After the inner cannula is cleaned, it is stored in a container in readiness for the next care procedure.

Changing of tracheostomy ties is always a two-person procedure. One individual changes the tie, and the other holds the tracheostomy tube securely in place in case the patient coughs, gags, or simply makes a sudden movement during the procedure. Basic principles are, first, that the tie must be fastened with a knot, not a bow (which may be attractive but is impractical because it is not secure). Second, it should be tied firmly; that is, only one finger should be able to be inserted between the neck and the tie. A tie that is too loose allows tracheostomy tube movement, which could lead to erosion and possible dislodgement.

MONITORING AND MANAGING CUFFS

The purpose of cuffs on airways is twofold: to allow for the application of positive-pressure ventilation without a loss of tidal volume and to prevent aspiration of oral and gastric secretions. For the cuff to perform these two functions, it must exert some pressure against the tracheal wall. The pressure between the cuff and the tracheal wall is appropriately termed the cuff-to-tracheal wall (C/T) pressure. The C/T pressure should be as low as possible so that the cuff may perform its functions while the complications of excessive pressure are prevented. The cuff may be inflated with one of two techniques: the minimal leak technique (MLT) or the minimal occlusive volume (MOV) technique, also known as the minimal occlusive pressure or no-leak technique (Table 3-3). With either of these techniques the C/T pressure should be no higher than necessary to prevent excessive loss of volume, aspiration, and tracheal damage. Regardless of which technique is used to inflate the cuff, serial measurement of cuff pressure or volume is advised as a means of cuff monitoring (see Measuring Cuff Pressure and Measuring Cuff Volume, later).

Overinflation of a cuff creates excessive pressure on the tracheal wall. This constant pressure can lead to weakening of the tracheal muscles and softening of cartilage. The area of contact dilates, and volume must be added to the cuff to achieve an effective seal. The trachea may then further dilate, requiring more volume in the cuff, and a dangerous repetitive cycle is set up. This process is referred to as the "chasing" of the trachea by the cuff.

TABLE 3-3	Comparison of the Minimal Occlusive Volume (MOV) and Minimal Leak Techniques (MLT) of Cuff Inflation

Minimal Occlusive Volume	Minimal Leak Techniques
DEFINITION	
Sufficient air in cuff to abolish air leak on inspiration.	Sufficient air in cuff to allow small leak on inspiration.
PROCEDURE	
During auscultation over trachea, inject air into cuff until no leak is heard. Remove air until small leak is heard, usually 0.5 mL. Reinstill air until no leak is auscultated on inspiration.	During auscultation over trachea, inject air into cuff until no leak is heard. Remove air in 0.1-mL increments until small leak is heard.
ADVANTAGES	
Less potential for aspiration because trachea is sealed. No loss of tidal volume.	Avoidance of pooling of secretions above cuff because they either will be forced up by air passing around cuff or will drain into lungs to be coughed out. Potentially less injury to trachea because cuff-to-tracheal wall pressure will be less than in MOV.
DISADVANTAGES	
Greater potential for injury to tracheal wall than with MLT.	Aspiration caused by secretions filtering around cuff into lungs. Loss of tidal volume.

All cuffs made today are of low-pressure design; that is, they are made of softer materials than in the past (low-volume, high-pressure cuffs). When even high volumes are inserted into these low-pressure, compliant cuffs, less *pressure* is created than in a cuff made of a more rigid material. The softer materials of the low-pressure, high-volume cuffs are also malleable. They more easily conform to the varying (C, D, O, oval) shapes of the trachea and therefore keep the formation of cuff folds to a minimum. Cuff folds serve as potential sites for aspiration of secretions that pool above the inflated cuff. Even though the material used in modern cuffs substantially reduces the incidence of severe cuff site injury, the practitioner should not be lulled into a false belief that tracheal damage cannot occur just because improved material is used in today's cuffs. The C/T pressure may still become excessive if the tube is too small for the trachea or if the cuff is overinflated. In the past in some clinical settings, it was recommended that the cuff be let down for 5 minutes every 4 to 8 hours. This practice stemmed from the use of the high-pressure, low-volume cuffs and is no longer necessary with the newer cuffs.

Complications Associated with Cuffs

Most tracheal injury from endotracheal intubation is cuff site ulceration from lateral tracheal wall pressures exerted by the inflated cuff. Tracheal capillary arterial perfusion pressure is estimated to be approximately 22 mm, and lymphatic flow occurs at 5 mm Hg. The pathogenesis of tracheal injury begins when cuff pressure exceeds tracheal perfusion pressure. Ischemia and inflammation result and may progress to mucosal necrosis, ulceration, and hemorrhage. Mucosal injury through the healing process may result in granuloma and scar formation. After extubation or decannulation, these areas may cause stenosis or obstruction.

If tracheal cartilages are affected, the trachea may become dilated, as evidenced by the need for larger cuff volumes to seal the trachea, or tracheomalacia may develop. Erosion into adjacent structures may present as a tracheoesophageal or tracheovascular fistula, although these complications are rare with a soft cuff tube.

The goal is to keep the C/T pressure below capillary perfusion pressure. Maintaining cuff pressures below 20 to 22 mm Hg greatly reduces the risk of cuff site ischemia and injury. However, lower is not always better as evidenced by an increased risk of pneumonia when cuff pressures are maintained at 15 to 20 mm Hg. The dilemma is to keep cuff pressures high enough to reduce aspiration and pneumonia and low enough to prevent tracheal injury. According to Stauffer, available data suggest that an intracuff pressure in the narrow window of 18 to 22 mm Hg (25 to 30 cm H_2O) is the best compromise between the risk of aspiration and the risk of ischemia.

Measuring Cuff Pressure

Intracuff pressure provides an approximation of C/T pressure. The measurement of cuff pressure is therefore one mechanism advocated to prevent complications related to excessive C/T pressure. The maintenance of cuff pressure within the so-called normal range, however, does not ensure the prevention of tracheal damage. Ongoing evaluation of the pressure may nevertheless alert the clinician to a problematic situation and prompt troubleshooting.

As stated previously, the cuff should first be inflated by either the MLT or the MOV technique. Pressure may then be measured with a standard sphygmomanometer (Fig. 3-19), which measures pressure in mm Hg, or with an aneroid cuff-pressure manometer, which measures pressures in cm H_2O. The method for using a sphygmomanometer (Box 3-3) is useful when a device designed to measure cuff pressures is unavailable. However, with the removal of mercury from hospitals and the use of automatic blood pressure cuffs, finding a sphygmomanometer may prove to be a task in itself. A Cufflator or similar aneroid cuff-pressure manometer is a simple handheld instrument that should be utilized by following the manufacturer's guidelines (Fig. 3-20). The clinician should be aware these devices contain variable internal volumes that results in volume loss from the cuff at the time of the pressure measurement. The cuff pressure is maintained at 25 to 30 cm H_2O (18 to 22 mm Hg), which is below tracheal capillary perfusion pressure in the normotensive patient. Do not inflate the cuff to the "acceptable range" if the goals of the MLT or MOV can be achieved with a lower pressure.

The pressure should be monitored and recorded at least once per shift and more often if needed with ventilator or oxygen therapy equipment checks. Theoretically, the safest and most informative approach to routine cuff-pressure checks would be to measure and report both the preexisting cuff pressure and cuff pressure following adjustment. It is especially important to monitor cuff pressure if the MOV

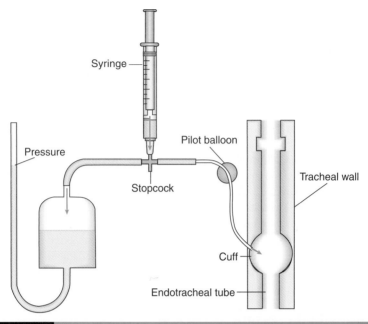

FIGURE 3-19

Setup for measuring cuff pressures with a standard sphygmomanometer (see Box 3-2 for procedure). *(Modified from Pilbeam SP. Mechanical Ventilation: Physiological and Clinical Applications, 2nd ed. St. Louis, Mosby–Year Book, 1992.)*

BOX 3-3 Measurement of Cuff Pressures with a Sphygmomanometer

1. Attach a three-way stopcock to the manometer tubing, a 10-mL syringe, and the pilot balloon. Ensure that the stopcock is turned off to the balloon to prevent the escape of air.

2. Prime the manometer tubing with enough air so that the pressure reads 10 mm Hg. Failure to prime the tubing causes some air from the cuff to fill the dead space of the tubing without registering pressure on the manometer. The 10 mm Hg pressure serves as the baseline pressure.

3. Turn the stopcock so that it is open from the cuff to the manometer (off to the syringe). Measure the pressure reading on the manometer.

4. Obtain the actual cuff pressure with the following formula:

$$\text{Manometer reading} \times 10 \text{ mm Hg} = \text{Cuff pressure}$$

5. Convert millimeters of mercury to centimeters of H_2O with the following formula:

$$\text{mm Hg} \times 1.36 = \text{cm } H_2O$$

$$\text{where 1 mm Hg} = 1.36 \text{ cm } H_2O, \text{ or 1 cm } H_2O = 0.74 \text{ mm Hg}$$

NOTE: If the volume in the cuff is increased or decreased with use of the 10-mL syringe (to achieve MOV or MLT), another pressure reading must be obtained. Even 0.5 mL of volume can make a significant difference in cuff pressure.

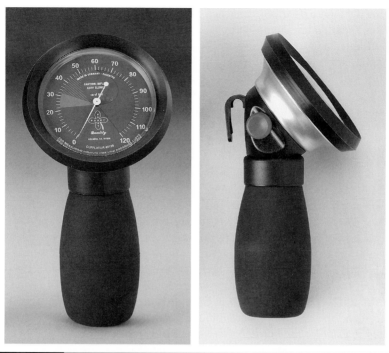

A   B

FIGURE 3-20

Aneroid pressure manometer. The bulb is squeezed to inflate the cuff. Depression of the thumb valve (shown in **B**) allows for deflation. Movement of a very small volume of air is possible. *(Courtesy J.T. Posey Company, Arcadia, Calif.)*

technique is used because a small increase in cuff volume can cause a precipitous rise in intracuff pressure. An attempt is made to control factors that can alter the parameter—primarily, high peak airway pressure and PEEP, patient position, and state of wakefulness. Wakefulness, and thus tracheal muscle tone, is altered by analgesics, sedatives, and so on.

Special Cuffs

FOME-CUF

In the attempt to alleviate problems associated with excessive or changing cuff pressures, the foam-filled cuff evolved (Fig. 3-21). The foam-filled cuff (FOME-CUF, Smiths Medical ASD, Keene, NH) allows for maintenance of low cuff pressures and adapts to a change in pressures, which can occur in air transport, in the operating room when nitrous oxide (which diffuses across the cuff) is used, and during positive-pressure ventilation.

Before insertion, the foam-filled cuff must be collapsed by active aspiration of all air. The collapse of the pilot port confirms that the cuff is in a collapsed state.

Plugging the pilot port with its attached stopper maintains the collapsed state. After insertion, the inflation line is left open and the cuff reexpands against the tracheal wall, self-inflating to ambient airway pressure. Because the natural tendency of the foam in the cuff is to expand, pressure in the cuff actually decreases as the volume in the foam cuff increases. Stretching of the trachea and the possibility of resultant injury are reduced. However, failure to recognize the paradoxical mechanism of inflation of the foam cuff, accompanied by injection of air into the cuff, may result in excessively high pressures.

The FOME-CUF device is a dynamic open system. It may be left open to atmospheric pressure or to ventilatory system pressure. The cuff is typically left open to atmospheric pressure during spontaneous respiration or high-frequency ventilation. Connecting the inflation line to a side-port adapter placed between the airway and the ventilator circuitry allows the cuff to inflate and deflate with cycling of the ventilator, ensuring a seal at peak inspiratory pressure. Typical applications of this setup include positive-pressure ventilation, except at high frequency and during anesthesia.

Air-filled cuffs require periodic assessment of cuff pressure, whereas the manufacturer of the FOME-CUF recommends periodic measurement of the *volume* of air in the cuff. If the volume of air in the cuff is *decreasing*, the foam is more fully expanded and the clinician is alerted to the possibility of tracheal dilation. Periodic deflation is also recommended to determine the integrity of the cuff and to prevent the silicone cuff from adhering to the tracheal mucosa.

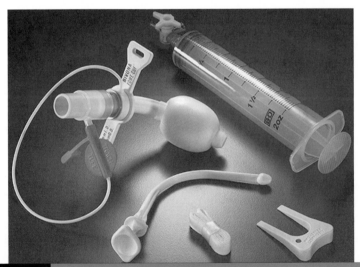

FIGURE 3-21

Foam-filled cuff tracheostomy tube. The cuff is actively deflated before insertion. The cuff then passively inflates to ambient pressure if left open to air. The pilot balloon shown here is attached to the nipple of the Sideport AutoControl airway connector. See text for explanation. *(Courtesy Smiths Medical ASD, Keene, NH.)*

MICROCUFF

Cuff material and design that reduce microaspiration is the focus of the new Microcuff ETT. The tube features an ultrathin (10 microns) polyurethane cuff membrane. The cuff length is also longer and more cylindrical than standard ETT cuffs (Fig. 3-22). In a study of pediatric patients, the Microcuff endotracheal tube was compared with four other conventional high-volume, low-pressure endotracheal tubes in respect to the cuff pressure required to prevent air leakage around the cuff. The Microcuff required a significantly lower pressure (mean 9.5 cm H_2O) to provide an effective seal that prevented air leakage than the conventional cuffs (mean 19.1 cm H_2O). This feature may lead to less damage to the trachea. An in vitro study compared the Microcuff to four other conventional ETTs regarding fluid leakage past the tube cuff. Fluid leakage past the tube cuff occurred in all conventional ETTs at cuff pressure from 10 to 60 cm H_2O. In the Microcuff tube, fluid leakage was observed within 10 minutes at 10 cm H_2O and within 60 minutes at 15 cm H_2O and was absent at pressures ranging from 20 to 60 cm H_2O. Results with the Microcuff were significantly better than all of the other tubes at cuff pressures ranging from 10 to 30 cm H_2O. In vivo studies will be required to confirm these findings and should extend beyond the 60-minute in vitro study period.

Conventional high-volume low-pressure cuffs create folds when inflated. Channels form and allow bacteria-laden secretions above the cuff to leak through the channels, past the cuff, and down into the lung. Microaspiration of potentially infectious secretions through gaps in the endotracheal tube cuff may lead to VAP. The microthin polyurethane cuff material of the Microcuff tube along with the cylindrical shape of the cuff was designed to prevent longitudinal folds, therefore preventing fluid and air leakage. This could potentially reduce VAP. Even though the polyurethane is thinner, it is twice as difficult to puncture and requires double the pressure to burst than standard cuff material. The Microcuff tube has been in use in Germany predominantly in pediatric patients and is new to the American market and adult populations. Further study in patient populations of this promising new technology is warranted.

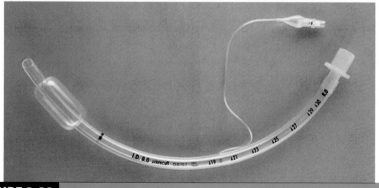

FIGURE 3-22

Adult Microcuff endotracheal tube. *(Courtesy Kimberly-Clark Healthcare, Roswell, Ga.)*

Managing Air Leaks

Possible sources of air loss are as follows:

- From around the cuff as a result of patient position changes
- From the cuff itself
- From a faulty one-way valve on the pilot balloon
- From a cracked or broken air inflation line

If it is determined that the leak is caused by position changes, repositioning the patient's head should correct the problem. If the leak is from the cuff or from a cracked or broken inflation line (often at the point of attachment to the airway), then call for assistance in reintubation. In the interim, if the patient is symptomatic, the methods of supporting ventilation include increasing the tidal volume delivered by the ventilator to compensate for the gas escaping through the upper airway, and increasing the FIO_2 to 1.0 to ensure adequate oxygenation. If the patient remains unstable, call for assistance and prepare for reintubation.

A leak may also occur because of a broken inflation line at the point where the pilot balloon attaches. Temporary repair may be achieved by cutting off the one-way valve–pilot balloon housing, inserting a 19- to 20-gauge blunt needle or intravenous catheter into the tubing, and attaching a three-way stopcock. Cuff inflation may then be maintained, thereby avoiding emergency reintubation.

Leaks in the one-way valve often occur because the valve sticks in the open position, allowing air to escape. To prevent further air loss, attach a Luer-Lok syringe or a stopcock turned off to the cuff to the end of the valve. Note that inserting a syringe into the valve with excessive force may result in a jammed or cracked valve.

Air leak may also be caused by an endotracheal or tracheostomy tube misplaced too high in the trachea. Before the tube is repositioned, any secretions that have collected above the cuff should be suctioned from the oropharynx. The cuff is then deflated and, with assistance, the tube is repositioned and stabilized.

SPECIAL CONCERNS

Unplanned Extubation

Unplanned extubation is defined as inadvertent removal of the endotracheal or tracheostomy tube, which is an unplanned event. Removal of the tube may be intentional or inadvertent. Unplanned extubation occurs in 3% to 20% of intubated patients and may result in serious cardiac or pulmonary complications. Reintubation after unplanned extubation ranges from 14% to 78%. Reintubation is associated with higher rates of VAP and even death. The rate of unplanned extubation can be reduced through quality improvement monitoring, which increases staff awareness of and vigilance for contributing factors, and through appropriate airway management practice guidelines. Monitoring unplanned extubation should be performed in the ICU to evaluate the quality of care and to provide a reference to determine if new interventions aimed at reducing incidence are effective.

The two most frequent methods by which self-extubation is accomplished is (1) by using the tongue and (2) by leaning forward and downward to the restrained hands and then manually removing the tube. Even the most vigilant caregivers

| TABLE 3-4 | Unplanned Extubation: Preventive Measures |

Measure	Rationale
Vigilant monitoring of all intubated patients	Interception of self-extubation attempt
Administration of sedation and analgesics, particularly to agitated patients or those with tenuous respiratory status	Improve patient comfort and control of patient in environment that may be perceived as intolerable
Application of soft restraints	Safety measure used until it can be ascertained that patient thoroughly understands airway's importance and demonstrates no periods of confusion or agitation
Use of arm immobilizers	Prevents arm from bending at elbow, making it difficult to get hand to airway
Use of "mitts" and restraint vests as necessary	Wrist restraints insufficient to prevent patient from leaning forward and grasping at airway
Positioning of ventilator circuitry and equipment attached to it (e.g., inline suction apparatus) up and over patient's shoulder	Deterrence of airway removal by pulling on its extensions
Nasal or orogastric tube not taped to endotracheal tube (ETT)	Deterrence of airway removal by pulling on equipment secured to it
ETT securely taped around patient's head	Greater stabilization provided than by taping only to the cheeks
ETT harness used to secure tube in high-risk patient (particularly helpful in patients who "tongue" at their tube)	Provision of greater stability than tape provides if applied properly. (Some models also provide bite block, making it more difficult to maneuver tube with tongue.)
Timely removal of ETT from patient ready for extubation	Avoidance of delay, which could lead to frustration and eventual intervention by patient

may sometimes find themselves with a patient who removed his or her airway intentionally. Conditions that place the patient at a high risk for self-extubation are as follows: agitation, inadequate sedation, patients with head trauma or with drugs or alcohol on board; change of shift, when patients may not have a direct caregiver in their room or nearby to observe them as closely; the night shift because there are fewer personnel to observe and interrupt an attempted self-extubation; and delay of patients who are ready for extubation but must wait "for the doctor's order, for the arterial blood gas values to come back," and so on. The best approach to the problem is to implement preventive measures (Table 3-4). Two fundamental components of guidelines aimed at reducing unplanned extubation are establishing standard methods of securing airways and close monitoring and appropriate management of agitation.

Laryngeal and Tracheal Injury

The primary sites of injury from artificial airways are the larynx and the trachea. Two major mechanisms are mainly responsible for airway damage: *tube movement*, which causes abrasion, and *pressure*, which causes necrosis. Duration of intubation also appears to play a significant role in glottic injury. Preventive measures should be implemented throughout the period of intubation in an effort to reduce the incidence of complications. Areas to focus on are head movement, tube size, cuff pressures, and duration of intubation.

Significant movement of the tube in the airway occurs as a result of head motion, especially flexion and extension. Flexion of the neck moves the tube toward the carina; extension pulls the tube toward the larynx. Head movement, therefore, should be kept to a minimum to reduce abrasive injury. Some patients may require sedation for effective reduction of excessive head movement.

Pressure injury can occur from the cuff and from the tube itself. Excessive C/T pressure may result in necrotic injury to the tissue as previously discussed; therefore, the cuff must be monitored and managed conscientiously. A tube of the appropriate size should be used in an effort to reduce the injury caused by larger tubes. Generally, this calls for a size 6.5 to 7.0 in female patients and a 7.5 to 8.0 in male patients when looking purely from the perspective of preserving the larynx. However, there is a fine line to walk regarding having a tube large enough to reduce the work of breathing related to the ETT and therefore promote extubation and a smaller tube that reduces laryngeal injury.

Injuries above the glottis are rare complications of intubation but unfortunately include potentially serious lacerations, hematomas, and edema of the pharynx or epiglottis. The vast majority of these injuries heal without sequelae.

Numerous investigations demonstrated that nearly all patients after prolonged intubation display laryngeal injury after extubation. Prolonged intubation generally was defined as greater than 1 week. Injuries at the level of the *glottis* are the most serious of the complications of intubation. Vocal cord erythema, edema, inflammation, abrasions, ulcerations, and granuloma formation occur most commonly at the point where the endotracheal tube makes contact with the vocal cords. Because the endotracheal tube lies in the posterior portion of the glottis, at the site of the arytenoid cartilages and the posterior commissure, these sites are most commonly injured. As a result, it is not uncommon for the laryngeal reflexes (cough, gag, swallow) to be blunted for a period after intubation or for the patient to have hoarseness. Vocal cord paralysis or paresis are injuries that result in impairment of the protective function of the glottis; therefore, the patient may aspirate. Chronic fibrosis and granuloma formation may occur with healing and result in impaired vocal cord function and loss of airway patency, particularly stenosis. Acid reflux management while the patient is intubated is also very important. Reflux of stomach acid that rests where the back of the endotracheal tube is resting on the mucosa causes granulation tissue that can fuse across the midline. As that matures a first-year scar band may form and the cords will not move because they are "fixed" and scarred into place.

Tracheal mucosa and cartilage injury occurs most commonly at the point of contact with the artificial airway cuff and where the tip of the tube contacts the tracheal wall. Two factors are primarily responsible: high C/T pressure and mechanical motion. Like injury to the glottis, injuries to the trachea range from mild to severe. Almost inevitable consequences of intubation are superficial mucosal inflammation, hyperemia, mild edema, and ciliostasis. The most concerning injuries are ulcerations secondary to ischemia and motion and dilation of the trachea, which are seen at the level of the cuff. Tracheal stenosis, which occurs with healing, may occur at any point along the length of mucosal contact with the artificial airway.

SWALLOWING EVALUATION

After intubation, especially if prolonged, the patient may be at increased risk for aspiration. Dysphagia following intubation is thought to be secondary to multiple factors such as muscle weakness or atrophy with disuse, impaired trigger of the swallowing reflex, and changes in sensation and proprioception from prolonged contact between the pharynx and the endotracheal tube. Ajemian and colleagues found that 56% of patients who were intubated for at least 48 hours had dysphagia, and 25% were silent aspirators when evaluated by fiberoptic endoscopic evaluation of swallowing (FEES) within 48 hours after extubation. This test is commonly referred to as a bedside video swallow. Other researchers noted that patients intubated for at least 24 hours have significantly delayed swallowing reflex; however, this was a transient finding almost entirely eliminated within 2 days after extubation. A study of trauma patients intubated for 48 hours showed a 45% incidence of aspiration, and 44% of them were silent aspirators. The majority (98%), however, were able to resume oral intake within 2 to 10 days.

Although clearly there is a risk for aspiration postextubation, no universally accepted guidelines are established regarding which patients should undergo formal swallowing evaluation. The index of suspicion should increase for any patient intubated for 48 hours or greater. Postextubation all patients should be monitored for possible aspiration or upper airway obstruction. An initial assessment of the patient postextubation may provide triggers to identify patients who may benefit from objective swallow testing. Immediately after extubation the patient should be assessed for vocal quality. The most common early symptoms of injury are hoarseness, gurgling, and inability to clear secretions in the upper airway. Persistent hoarseness and cough, especially when associated with liquid oral intake after extubation, are other warning signs that a swallowing evaluation may be indicated. However, coughing and gagging with intake are not reliable signs because patients with blunted sensory function often do not demonstrate these signs and are known as "silent aspirators."

In many institutions, speech therapy consultations serve as the mechanism to attain an evaluation of the effectiveness of the patient's swallow function. The speech pathologist can perform bedside evaluation of the swallow using a fiberoptic endoscope. The patient's swallow is evaluated with a series of liquids and foods of varying consistencies such as water, milk, applesauce, and a cracker. Addition of a small amount of dye assists with visualization of the bolus being swallowed. Most phases of the swallow (pre-swallow, post-swallow) can be visualized in this way; however, the exact moment of the swallow cannot be seen because the epiglottis obstructs the examiner's view. The therapist looks at lingual control of the food bolus, spillage into the glottis, stasis in the pyriform sinus or vallecula, and other details of the swallow. If a more thorough evaluation of the swallow is indicated, a fluoroscopic barium swallow can be performed in the radiology suite. Based on the results of their evaluation, the speech therapist provides instruction on what food volumes and consistencies may best be tolerated by the patient. They also provide instruction on methods of swallowing to reduce the incidence of aspiration (e.g., chin tuck) and exercises the patient should perform to improve the effectiveness of glottic closure.

Mouth Care

Meticulous mouth care should be performed in the intubated patient to prevent inoculation of the respiratory tract with bacteria that colonize the mouth, oropharynx, and dental plaque. VAP is thought to be related to aspiration of these bacteria-laden oral secretions. Frequent and aggressive oral care has been identified as a preventive measure to reduce the incidence of VAP. The CDC recommends the implementation of a comprehensive oral care program to reduce health-care-acquired pneumonia in the mechanically ventilated patient. Surveys of nurses in adult ICUs by Grap et al (2003) and Hanneman et al (2005) identify that nurses report more frequent oral care than is documented. Compliance with an evidence-based oral cleansing protocol by both nurses and respiratory therapists is improved, as demonstrated by Cutler and Davis when the regimen is clearly defined, supplies are readily available at the bedside, and a comprehensive education program is provided. Although the ideal frequency for oral care is not yet known, it is recommended that the teeth be brushed at least twice a day and the oral cavity including the gums and lips be swabbed and moisturized at 2- to 4-hour intervals in between brushing.

Before the procedure, ensure that the cuff is appropriately inflated. The patient's head should be positioned to the side, and the head of bed is elevated at least 30 degrees, if not contraindicated. If an oral airway is present, it should be removed and cleaned. Removing the oral airway ensures the entire oral cavity can be accessed. The teeth, gums, tongue, and palate should be gently brushed with a pediatric or soft toothbrush and a cleansing agent such as toothpaste. In between brushings the entire mouth, as stated earlier, should be gently cleaned with a sponge-tipped swab saturated in a 1.5% hydrogen peroxide solution, which is an effective antibacterial agent. Saliva serves a protective function because it reduces the buildup of plaque on the teeth. Unfortunately, when an ETT and possibly a gastric tube are both in the patient's mouth, it remains open for prolonged periods and may dry out. Drying of the oral cavity, known as xerostomia, is associated with cracks in the mucosa, mucositis, and gram-negative bacteria colonization. Following each cleaning, the mouth, gums, tongue, and lips should be moisturized, preferably with an agent that will not dry quickly.

Suctioning of the oral cavity and pharynx should be performed to prevent the accumulation of secretions in the posterior pharynx that can trickle down past the cuff and into the lungs. Suctioning is commonly performed with a Yankauer, covered Yankauer, or an oral saliva ejector. Between uses, a nondisposable oral suction catheter should be rinsed with sterile saline and allowed to air dry on a towel. Continuous subglottic suctioning using the special Hi-Lo Evac endotracheal tube discussed previously is associated with a reduction in VAP. Based on this finding it is recommended that when such a special endotracheal tube is not available or in use, supraglottic secretion removal should be performed using a single-use suction catheter minimally twice a day after brushing.

With each oral care episode, the oral cavity should be assessed for buildup of plaque on the teeth, ulcerations or sores in the mouth and on the lips, and overall appearance of the mucous membranes. The oral endotracheal tube should be repositioned if any signs of pressure ulceration of any stage are noted.

As a result of greater awareness of the benefits of an effective oral care regimen, a variety of oral care products are now available that contain the currently recommended products for oral care. Ensuring all of the proper equipment is readily available at the bedside may improve compliance with a comprehensive oral care regimen and make care more efficient.

REMOVAL OF THE ARTIFICIAL AIRWAY

Extubation

When the indications for intubation resolve and the patient is stable, extubation may be performed. Begin by explaining the procedure to the patient. Suction the patient one final time through the artificial airway and translaryngeally to remove secretions that may have pooled on top of the cuff. Remove the tape and deflate the cuff. Instruct the patient to take a deep breath while the tube is removed in one swift movement. If the patient cannot cooperate to time inhalation with tube removal, a positive pressure breath should be delivered with a manual resuscitation bag. The rationale for patient inhalation during extubation is to open the glottis maximally to prevent injury while the tube is removed. Immediately after extubation, ask the patient to cough and speak as you perform assessment of these functions. Supplemental humidified oxygen may be required. If the patient develops signs of upper airway obstruction, cool mist or racemic epinephrine nebulization and possibly intravenous dexamethasone is indicated to reduce edema. Observe the patient closely for obstruction.

Decannulation

Decannulation can be considered if the original upper airway obstruction is resolved, if airway secretions are controlled, and if mechanical ventilation is no longer needed. Decannulation is not an exact science. In general, the two methods are immediate decannulation and gradual decannulation. For the immediate procedure, after determination that the indications for tracheostomy are resolved and the patient is stable, the tracheostomy tube is removed and the patient immediately begins using the natural airway for gas exchange and secretion removal. In the gradual procedure, the tracheostomy tube is replaced at intervals by a tube of a smaller size (downsizing). This allows for gradual closure of the stoma, a transition period toward reuse by the patient of the natural airway for gas exchange and secretion removal, and assessment by the caregiver of the adequacy of these functions before tube removal. A tracheostomy button may be used after the tube is removed to maintain the stoma. After decannulation is performed, the stoma is covered with a dry dressing. If air loss is a problem, the stoma may be covered with petrolatum-impregnated gauze and then dry gauze. Stomal dressings should be changed twice a day and the site assessed for healing and complications.

SUMMARY

Management of the patient's airway is a significant part of the total care of the patient ventilator system. The prevention of adverse sequelae of the use of an artificial airway should serve as an outcome goal for practitioners caring for patients supported by mechanical ventilation. It is extremely rewarding when a patient who has had prolonged ventilatory support undergoes successful extubation/decannulation. How unfortunate it is, however, when this event is tainted by potentially preventable chronic morbidity for the patient.

RECOMMENDED READINGS

Ajemian MS, Nirmul GB, Anderson MT. Routine fiberoptic endoscopic evaluation of swallowing following prolonged intubation. *Arch Surg* 2001; 136:434–437.

Altobelli N. Airway care. In: RM Kacmarek, S Dimas, CW Mack (eds.), *The Essentials of Respiratory Care,* 4th ed. (pp. 672–687). St. Louis: Mosby, 2005.

Balon JA. Common factors of spontaneous self-extubation in a critical care setting. *Int J Trauma Nurs* 2001; 7(3):93–99.

Barnason S, Graham J, Wild C, et al. Comparison of two endotracheal tube securement techniques on unplanned extubation, oral mucosa, and facial skin integrity. *Heart & Lung* 1998; 27(6):409–417.

Bivona, Inc. *FOME-CUF User's Manual.* Gary, Ind: Bivona, Inc., 1991.

Blanch PB. Laboratory evaluation of 4 brands of endotracheal tube cuff inflator. *Respir Care* 2004; 49(2):166–173.

Burns SM, Spilman M, Wilmoth D, et al. Are frequent inner cannula changes necessary? A pilot study. *Heart & Lung* 1998; 27:58–62.

Carrion MI, Ayusa D, Marcos M, et al. Accidental removal of endotracheal and nasogastric tubes and intravascular catheters. *Crit Care Med* 2000; 28(1):63–66.

Centers for Disease Control and Prevention. Guidelines for preventing health-care associated pneumonia, 2003: Recommendations of CDC and the Healthcare Infection Control Practices Advisory Committee. *MMWR Morb Mortal Wkly Rep* 2004; 53(RR-3):1–40.

Cutler CJ, Davis N. Improving oral care in patients receiving mechanical ventilation. *Am J Crit Care* 2005; 14(50):389-394.

Dezfulian C, Shojania K, Collard HR, et al. Subglottic secretion drainage for preventing ventilator-associated pneumonia: A meta-analysis. *Am J Med* 2005; 118:11–18.

Dullenkopf A, Schmitz M, Frei AC, et al. Air leakage around endotracheal tube cuffs. *Eur J Anesth* 2004; 21:448–453.

Dullenkopf A, Gerber A, Weiss M. Fluid leakage past tracheal tube cuffs: Evaluation of the new Microcuff endotracheal tube. *Int Care Med* 2003; 29:1849–1853.

Durbin CG. Indications for and timing of tracheostomy. *Respir Care* 2005; 50(4):483–487.

Durbin CG. Techniques for performing tracheostomy. *Respir Care* 2005; 50(4):488–496.

Frutos-Vivar F, Esteban A, Apezteguia C, et al. Outcome of mechanically ventilated patients who require tracheostomy. *Crit Care Med* 2005; 33(2):290–298.

Grap MJ, Munro CL, Ashtiani B, et al. Oral care interventions in critical care: Frequency and documentation. *Am J Crit Care* 2003; 12:113–119.

Hanneman SK, Gusick GM. Frequency of oral care and positioning of patients: A replication study. *Am J Crit Care* 2005; 14(5):378–387.

Heffner JE. Tracheotomy: Indications and timing. *Respir Care* 1999; 44(7):807–815.

Hess DR. Managing the artificial airway. *Respir Care* 1999; 44(7):759–772.

Hess DR. Tracheostomy tubes and related appliances. *Respir Care* 2005; 50(4):497–510.

Hess DR. Facilitating speech in the patient with a tracheostomy. *Respir Care 2005*; 50(4):519–525.

Jaeger JM, Durbin CG. Special purpose endotracheal tubes. *Respir Care* 1999; 44(6):661–683.

Jevon P, Poonie JS. Practical procedures for nurses. Cardiopulmonary resuscitation: Tracheal intubation–1: Preparation. *Nurs Times* 2002; 98(2):43–44.

Jevon P, Poonie JS. Practical procedures for nurses. Cardiopulmonary resuscitation: Tracheal intubation–2: Procedure. *Nurs Times* 2002; 98(3):45–46.

Jevon P, Poonie JS. Practical procedures for nurses. Cardiopulmonary resuscitation: Tracheal intubation–1: Post intubation checks and management. *Nurs Times* 2002; 98(4):43–44.

Kapadia FN, Bajan KB, Raje KV. Airway accidents in intubated intensive care unit patients: An epidemiological study. *Crit Care Med* 2000; 28(3):659–664.

May RA, Bortner PL. Airway management. In D Hess, NR MacIntyre, SC Mishoe, et al. (eds.), *Respiratory Care: Principles & Practice* (pp. 694–727). Philadelphia: Saunders, 2002.

Munro CL, Grap MJ. Oral health and care in the intensive care unit: State of the science. *Am J Crit Care* 2004; 13(1):25–34.

Reibel JF. Decannulation: How and where. *Respir Care* 1999; 44(7):856–859.

Richmond AL, Jarog DL, Hanson VM. Unplanned extubation in adult critical care: Quality improvement and education payoff. *Crit Care Nurse* 2004; 24(1):32–37.

Rumbak MJ, Newton M, Truncale T, et al. A prospective, randomized, study comparing early percutaneous dilational tracheotomy to prolonged translaryngeal intubation (delayed tracheotomy) in critically ill medical patients. *Crit Care Med* 2004; 32:1689–1694.

Simmons KF, Scanlan CL. Airway management. In RL Wilkins, JK Stoller, CL Scanlon, et al. (eds.), *Egan's Fundamental of Respiratory Care*, 8th ed. (pp. 653–704). St. Louis: Mosby, 2003.

Skillings KN, Curtis BL. Tracheal tube cuff care. In DJ Lynn-McHale Wiegand, KK Carlson (eds.), *AACN Procedure Manual for Critical Care* (pp. 71–78). Philadelphia: Elsevier Saunders, 2005.

Smulders K, van der Hoeven H, Weers-Pothoff I, et al. A randomized clinical trial of intermittent subglottic secretion drainage in patients receiving mechanical ventilation. *Chest* 2002; 121:858–862.

Stauffer JL. Complications of endotracheal intubation and tracheotomy. *Respir Care* 1999; 44(7):828–843.

Tamburi LM. Care of the patient with a tracheostomy. *Orthop Nurs* 2000; 19(2):49–58.

CHAPTER 4

Administration of Oxygen, Humidification, and Aerosol Therapy

The delivery of supplemental oxygen may be necessary for the correction or prevention of hypoxemia. As shown in Chapter 2, in room air the fraction of inspired oxygen (FIO_2) is 0.21. That is, of all the air we inspire, 21% consists of oxygen molecules. Therefore, *supplemental oxygen administration* is the delivery of any oxygen concentration greater than 21%.

Indications
The need for supplemental oxygen should be determined through evaluation of the patient's arterial blood gas and clinical assessment findings (Table 4-1). In general, indications for oxygen therapy include the following:

■ Correction of hypoxemia, thereby decreasing the work of breathing and the myocardial workload it imposes, and promotion of adequate oxygen delivery to the tissues. The correction of hypoxemia alone does not ensure the sufficient delivery of oxygenated blood to the tissues. A competent cardiovascular system is also necessary for carrying the adequately oxygenated blood to the tissues.

■ Improvement of oxygenation in patients with decreased oxygen carrying capacity (e.g., those with anemia, sickle cell disease).

■ Acute myocardial infarction.

■ Short-term therapy to prevent hypoxemia such as after anesthesia.

■ Promotion of the reabsorption of air in body cavities (e.g., pneumocephalus, small pneumothorax).

Oxygen as a Drug
The administration of oxygen should be done with as much care and attention as the practitioner uses when administering any other drug. Oxygen, like most drugs, has safe dose ranges, adverse physiologic effects, and toxic manifestations that are associated with higher doses and prolonged use. For correction of hypoxemia, enough oxygen should be administered to saturate the hemoglobin 92% or

TABLE 4-1	Signs and Symptoms of Hypoxemia	
System	**Mild to Moderate**	**Severe**
Central nervous system	Confusion, agitation, combativeness	Lethargy and obtunded mental status
Cardiac	Tachycardia, ectopy	Bradycardia
	Hypertension	Hypotension
Respiratory	Dyspnea, tachypnea, shallow respirations, labored breathing	Increasing dyspnea and tachypnea, possible bradypnea or agonal respirations
Arterial blood gas	Pao_2: 60-80 mm Hg	Pao_2 < 60 mm Hg
Skin	Cool, clammy	Cyanosis

better. This safely achieves a Pao_2 of approximately 60 to 70 mm Hg. Administering additional supplemental oxygen, once the hemoglobin is fully saturated (99% to 100%), places the patient at risk of having toxic effects of this drug.

Complications Associated with Oxygen Use

HYPOVENTILATION AND CARBON DIOXIDE NARCOSIS

Oxygen-induced hypoventilation may occur because of suppression of the hypoxic respiratory drive. Normally, carbon dioxide is the primary stimulant driving the respiratory system. However, in patients with chronic hypercapnia ($Paco_2$ > 45 mm Hg), the central nervous system response to an elevated carbon dioxide level becomes blunted, and hypoxemia becomes the major ventilatory stimulus. Administration of oxygen-enriched gas to these individuals may result in hypoventilation, hypercapnia, and possibly apnea. Under these circumstances, oxygen should be administered in low concentrations (<30%) while the patient is observed for signs of respiratory depression. If oxygenation remains inadequate and respiratory depression occurs, then invasive or noninvasive mechanical ventilation is necessary.

ABSORPTION ATELECTASIS

Absorption atelectasis occurs when the alveoli collapse because the gas within them is absorbed into the bloodstream. Nitrogen, a relatively insoluble gas, normally maintains a residual volume within the alveolus. During the breathing of high concentrations of oxygen, nitrogen may be replaced, or "washed out" of the alveolus. When the alveolar oxygen is then absorbed into the pulmonary capillary, the alveolus partially to totally collapses. Absorption atelectasis is more likely to occur in areas where ventilation is decreased, such as in airways that are distal to partial obstruction, because the oxygen is absorbed into the blood at a faster rate than it is replaced.

PULMONARY OXYGEN TOXICITY

The exposure of the pulmonary tissues to a high oxygen tension can lead to pathologic parenchymal changes. The degree of injury is related to the duration of exposure and to the oxygen tension of the inspired air, not to the PaO_2. Generally, an FIO_2 of more than 0.5 is considered toxic. The first signs of oxygen toxicity are caused by the irritant effect of oxygen and reflect an acute tracheobronchitis. After only a few hours of breathing 100% oxygen, mucociliary function is depressed and clearance of mucus is impaired. Within 6 hours of the administration of 100% oxygen, nonproductive cough, substernal pain, and nasal stuffiness may develop. Symptoms such as malaise, nausea, anorexia, and headache may be reported. These changes are reversible on discontinuation of oxygen therapy.

More prolonged exposure to high oxygen tension may lead to changes in the lung that mimic acute respiratory distress syndrome (ARDS). Disruption of the endothelial lining of the pulmonary microcirculation results in leakage of proteinaceous fluid. An exudate consisting of edema, hemorrhage, and white blood cells forms in the lung. The damage to the lung may progress to cell death. The function of the pulmonary macrophage is also depressed, rendering the patient more susceptible to infection. The tissue injury in the lung caused by hyperoxia is generally agreed to be caused by the production of biochemically reactive, oxygen-derived free radicals that overwhelm the body's antioxidant defenses. Termination of exposure to toxic levels of oxygen allows cellular repair to begin; the repair may also result in varying degrees of pulmonary fibrosis, however.

Avoiding the use of high concentrations of oxygen for prolonged periods is the key to avoiding pulmonary injury from high oxygen tension. The lowest FIO_2 capable of generating a sufficient oxygen saturation serves as the best guide to oxygen therapy titration.

RETINOPATHY OF PREMATURITY

Retinopathy of prematurity, also known as retrolental fibroplasia, is a common complication in premature infants. Administration of excessive amounts of oxygen to premature infants may result in constriction of the immature retinal vessels, endothelial cell damage, retinal detachment, and possible blindness. However, increased exposure to high FIO_2 is believed to be only one of the contributing factors to this pathology. The amount of injury that occurs is related to the PaO_2; therefore, it is recommended that the PaO_2 be maintained at less than 80 mm Hg in neonates and that the time exposure to high FIO_2 be minimized, including during procedures such as suctioning, bronchoscopy, apneic spells, and intubation.

OXYGEN DELIVERY SYSTEMS

Many devices for administering supplemental oxygen are available. These devices are classified into two general categories: *low-flow systems* and *high-flow systems*. Whether a system is low or high flow does not determine its capability of delivering low versus high concentrations of oxygen. When choosing the appropriate technique for delivering supplemental oxygen, one must consider the device's advantages and disadvantages, the FIO_2 limits of the device, and its appropriateness for a particular patient (Box 4-1).

BOX 4-1 Oxygen Delivery Systems

LOW-FLOW SYSTEMS
Nasal cannula
Simple face mask
Partial rebreathing mask
Nonrebreathing mask

HIGH-FLOW SYSTEMS
Venturi masks

Large-Volume Aerosol Systems
High-humidity face mask
High-humidity face tent
High-humidity tracheostomy mask/collar
High-humidity T-piece (or "blow-by")

Low-Flow Systems

Low-flow systems, by definition, do not provide all the gas necessary to meet the patient's total minute ventilation. These systems require that the patient entrain, or draw in, room air while gas enriched with oxygen is also inspired from a reservoir. The reservoir of oxygen may be in the nasopharyngeal or oropharyngeal cavities, a mask, or a reservoir bag. With these systems, the FIO_2 delivered to the patient can only be estimated because the humidity, temperature, and actual FIO_2 cannot be precisely controlled. The FIO_2 is determined not only by the amount of oxygen delivered to the patient but also by the ventilatory pattern and thus by the amount of air the patient entrains. For example, if the patient's minute ventilation increases, the delivered FIO_2 *decreases* because the patient entrains a larger percentage of room air. Low-flow delivery systems include the nasal cannula, simple face mask, partial rebreathing mask, and nonrebreathing mask.

NASAL CANNULA
Description and Technique

Made of lightweight plastic, the nasal cannula consists of tubing and two prongs that fit into the nose (Fig. 4-1). To apply the device, direct the prongs inward, following the curvature of the nasal passages. Hook the tubing behind the patient's ears and adjust the strap under the chin. Correct use of a nasal cannula requires that the nose be free of obstruction and the cannula and prongs are correctly positioned. Mouth breathing is believed not to preclude the use of the nasal cannula, unless there is complete obstruction of the nares, because oxygen is drawn in from the anatomic reservoirs: the nasopharynx and oropharynx. However, the FIO_2 delivered is influenced by mouth breathing, and the patient's SaO_2 will help the clinician decide if another device is indicated. The nasal cannula is capable of delivering an FIO_2 ranging from 0.24 to 0.44, depending on the amount of flow (measured in liters) (Table 4-2). The maximal flow rate is 6 L/min because higher flow rates, although not affording an appreciably higher FIO_2, cause crusting of secretions, drying of the nasal mucosa, and epistaxis.

Advantages
- Inexpensive
- Well tolerated, comfortable

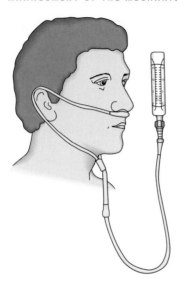

FIGURE 4-1

Nasal cannula in place, attached to an oxygen flowmeter.
(Modified from Kofke WA. Postoperative respiratory care techniques: Part III. Weaning from mechanical ventilation and oxygen therapy. Curr Rev PACN 1992; 13:161.)

TABLE 4-2 Estimated F_{IO_2} with Low-Flow Oxygen Delivery Devices*

100% O_2 Flow Rate (L/min)	F_{IO_2}
NASAL CANNULA	
1	0.24
2	0.28
3	0.32
4	0.36
5	0.40
6	0.44
SIMPLE OXYGEN MASK	
5-6	0.40
6-7	0.50
7-8	0.60
PARTIAL REBREATHER MASK†	
7	0.65
8-15	0.70-0.80†
NONREBREATHING MASK	
Set to prevent collapse of bag	0.85-1.0

*Exact F_{IO_2} delivered varies with changes in tidal volume, respiratory rate, minute ventilation, and ventilatory pattern.
†Flow rate should be set so reservoir bag only partially collapses on inspiration.

- Allows patient to eat and drink
- May be used with patients who have chronic obstructive pulmonary disease
- May be used with humidity

Disadvantages
- May cause pressure sores around ears and nose, which can be minimized by placing gauze padding between the tubing and the ears or face
- May dry and irritate nasal mucosa

SIMPLE FACE MASK
Description and Technique
The placing of a mask over the patient's face increases the size of the oxygen reservoir beyond the limits of the anatomic reservoir; therefore, a higher F_{IO_2} can be delivered. The oxygen flow must be run at a sufficient rate, usually 5 L/min or greater, to prevent collection, and thus rebreathing, of exhaled gases high in carbon dioxide. Flow rates greater than 10 L/min, however, do not appreciably increase the F_{IO_2} because the reservoir within the mask is filled.

The simple face mask (Fig. 4-2) has vent holes on the sides for the entrainment of room air and the release of exhaled gases. It has no valves or reservoir bag. Apply the mask securely over the patient's mouth, nose, and chin. Press the flexible metal pieces over the bridge of the nose to create a seal for prevention of gas loss. Adjust the strap around the patient's head, and instruct the patient in the importance of wearing the mask as applied. Intermittently clean the inside of the mask and remove accumulated water, particularly when humidity is used. Assess the skin for areas of pressure. Switch to a nasal cannula at mealtime.

Advantages
- Simple, lightweight
- Can be used with humidity
- Delivery of F_{IO_2} up to 0.60

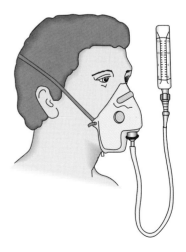

FIGURE 4-2

Simple face mask attached to an oxygen flowmeter.
(Modified from Kofke WA. Postoperative respiratory care techniques: Part III. Weaning from mechanical ventilation and oxygen therapy. Curr Rev PACN 1992; 13:161.)

Disadvantages

▓ May be considered confining by some patients, who may feel the need to remove the mask to speak
▓ Limitation of access to patient's face for expectoration of secretions, eating, drinking, oral or facial care, and other needs
▓ Possible aspiration of vomitus while mask in place
▓ Difficulty obtaining correct application when nasogastric or orogastric tube is in place
▓ Uncomfortable when facial trauma or burns are present
▓ May cause drying or irritation of the eyes

PARTIAL REBREATHING MASK

Description and Technique

The design of the partial rebreathing mask is similar to that of the simple face mask, with the addition of an oxygen reservoir bag (Fig. 4-3). Increasing the oxygen reservoir beyond the size of the anatomic reservoir allows the delivery of an FIO_2 greater than 0.60. The mask should fit snugly, and the oxygen flow rate should be adjusted so that the bag deflates by only about a third on inspiration. During inspiration the patient draws air from the mask, from the bag, and through the holes in the side of the mask. During exhalation the first third of exhaled gases flows back into the reservoir bag. This portion of exhaled gases comes from the anatomic dead space; therefore, it is still rich in oxygen, humidified, and warmed, and it contains little carbon dioxide. If oxygen flow to the system is high enough to keep the bag from deflating more than a third its volume during inhalation, then exhaled carbon dioxide does not accumulate in the reservoir bag. On the next breath the patient inspires part of the previously exhaled gas, along with 100% oxygen from the source. The bag is not a reservoir for carbon dioxide, a common misconception associated with the name *partial rebreather*.

Advantages

▓ FIO_2 >0.60 is delivered in moderate to severe hypoxia.
▓ Exhaled oxygen from the anatomic dead space is conserved.

Disadvantages

▓ Insufficient flow rate may lead to rebreathing of carbon dioxide.
▓ Mask over mouth may lead to feelings of claustrophobia in patients with severe hypoxemia.
▓ Mask prevents access to mouth for eating, drinking, expectorating.
▓ High oxygen flow rates may cause drying and irritation to the eyes.

NONREBREATHING MASK

Description and Technique

Nonrebreathing masks, like the partial rebreather, have a reservoir bag, but they also have one-way valves between the reservoir bag and the mask and over the exhalation ports of the mask (Fig. 4-4). The purpose of these valves is to prevent exhaled gases

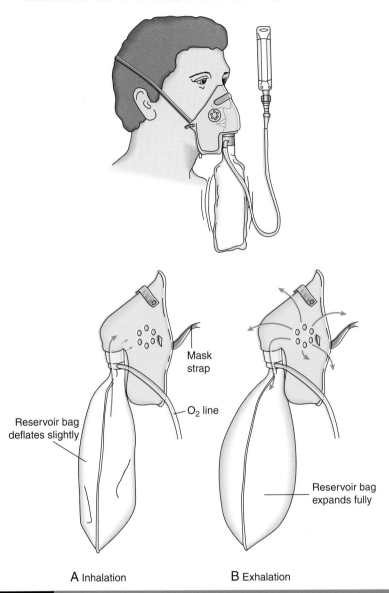

Mask
strap

O₂ line

Reservoir bag
deflates slightly

Reservoir bag
expands fully

A Inhalation   **B** Exhalation

FIGURE 4-3

(Top) Partial rebreathing mask correctly in place and attached to an oxygen flowmeter.
(Bottom) Arrows indicate the direction of gas movement on (**A**) inhalation and (**B**) exhalation.
*(Top, Modified from Kofke WA. Postoperative respiratory care techniques: Part III. Weaning from mechanical ventilation and oxygen therapy. Curr Rev PACN 1992; 13:161. **Bottom,** Modified from Kersten L.D. Comprehensive Respiratory Nursing. Philadelphia, Saunders, 1989.)*

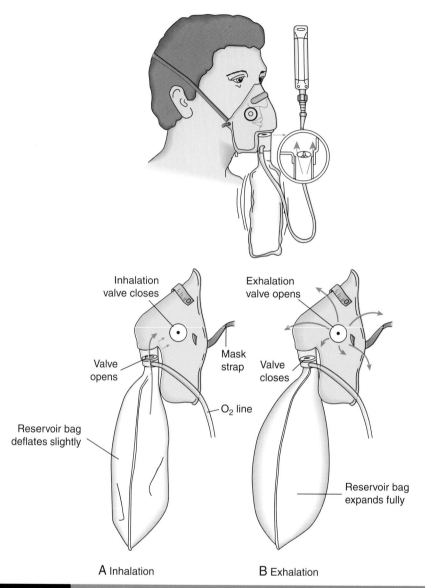

Inhalation
valve closes

Exhalation
valve opens

Valve
opens

Mask
strap

Valve
closes

O_2 line

Reservoir bag
deflates slightly

Reservoir bag
expands fully

A Inhalation

B Exhalation

FIGURE 4-4

(Top) Nonrebreathing mask correctly in place and attached to an oxygen flowmeter. *(Bottom)* Arrows indicate the direction of gas movement on (**A**) inhalation and (**B**) exhalation. *(Top, Modified from Kofke WA. Postoperative respiratory care techniques: Part III. Weaning from mechanical ventilation and oxygen therapy. Curr Rev PACN 1992; 13:161. **Bottom,** Modified from Kersten L.D. Comprehensive Respiratory Nursing. Philadelphia, Saunders, 1989.)*

from entering the bag and the entrainment of room air, respectively. On inspiration, the side port valves close and the valve between the bag and mask connection opens, allowing for inspiration of 100% oxygen. On expiration, the exhalation port valves open and the valve between the bag and mask closes, promoting the release of exhaled gases into the room and preventing their entry into the bag.

The flow rate should be set to prevent the reservoir bag from collapsing on inspiration (minimally 10 L/min). If the flow rate is set properly and if a tight fit is achieved, then theoretically the delivered FIO_2 is 1.0. However, in reality, the FIO_2 is usually nearer to 0.6 to 0.8. A tight fit is seldom achieved so room air is pulled in around the mask, and some manufacturers supply the mask with one of the exhalation valves removed. This is a safety measure, so that in the event of inadvertent discontinuation of the oxygen source the patient can still inspire room air. However, this action also decreases the delivered FIO_2 because when the valve is removed, more room air entrainment occurs.

Advantage
■ Delivery of high FIO_2

Disadvantages
■ Uncomfortable if tight fit, with possible feelings of claustrophobia
■ Limited access to mouth for eating, drinking, expectorating, oral or facial care
■ Possible sticking of valves, especially when moisture accumulates on them
■ Eye irritation from high flow rates of oxygen and improper fit at the nose

High-Flow Systems
In high-flow systems, the flow of gases is sufficient to meet all of the patient's minute ventilation requirements. These devices either have fixed air-to-oxygen entrainment ratios or reservoirs/flow rates that are adequate to provide all of the patient's inspired volume. In general, for delivery of a consistent FIO_2 to a patient with a variable (deep, irregular, shallow) ventilatory pattern, a high-flow system should be used. The FIO_2 remains fairly constant and is not affected by the patient's ventilatory pattern. Temperature and humidity can also be controlled. High-flow delivery systems include Venturi masks and large-volume aerosol systems, which include the high-humidity face mask, high-humidity face tent, high-humidity tracheostomy collar or mask, and high-humidity T-piece. The application of mechanical ventilation fits the definition of a high-flow system; however, it is placed in a class of its own.

AIR ENTRAINMENT MASK
Description and Technique
The air entrainment mask appears much like a simple face mask; however, it has a jet adapter placed between the mask and the tubing to the oxygen source. The jet adapters come in various sizes (and are often color coded) corresponding to various FIO_2 values. Sometimes called a Venturi mask, it operates on the Bernoulli principle of air entrainment (Fig. 4-5). As gas flows under pressure at a rapid flow rate through

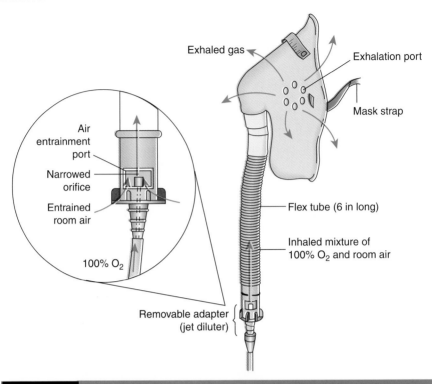

Exhaled gas

Exhalation port

Mask strap

Air entrainment port

Narrowed orifice

Entrained room air

100% O₂

Flex tube (6 in long)

Inhaled mixture of 100% O₂ and room air

Removable adapter (jet diluter)

FIGURE 4-5

Air entrainment (Venturi) mask. Air entrainment is explained by the Bernoulli principle. Gas flowing under pressure at a rapid flow rate through the narrowed orifice of the Venturi adapter creates an area of subatmospheric pressure laterally. A "jet drag" pulls (entrains) room air through side ports located on the adapter. FIO_2 is increased by either decreasing the size of the side ports or increasing the size of the jet orifice, both of which decrease the amount of room air entrained. *(Modified from Kersten L.D. Comprehensive Respiratory Nursing. Philadelphia, Saunders, 1989.)*

the narrowed orifice of the jet adapter, an area of subatmospheric pressure develops lateral to the small opening. This creates a "jet drag" that leads to the entrainment of room air through side ports located on the adapter. The FIO_2 is modified either by altering the size of the side ports or by altering the jet orifice diameter, both of which affect the amount of air entrained. The appropriate flow rate is usually inscribed on the jet adapter. Large volumes of air are entrained with this mask; volumes of oxygen-enriched gas (with a stable FIO_2), sufficient to meet even large minute ventilation needs, are therefore delivered with this device (Table 4-3).

Advantages
■ Delivery of a very predictable FIO_2
■ Useful in hypoxemic chronic obstructive pulmonary disease patients where delivery of excessive oxygen could depress the respiratory drive

TABLE 4-3	Air Entrainment Devices (Mask and Nebulizer) Delivered F_{IO_2}, Flow Settings, and Air-to-Oxygen Entrainment Ratios*		
F_{IO_2}	Flow Rate (L/min)	Air-to-Oxygen Entrainment Ratio	Total Liter Gas Flow (L/min)
0.24	4	25:1	104
0.28	6	10:1	66
0.35	8	5:1	48
0.40	8	3:1	32
0.60	12	1:1	Twice oxygen flow

*Flow rate settings and exact total number of liters of gas flow may vary slightly among products of different manufacturers. Consistency may also vary because products are generally plastic and mass produced.

Disadvantages

- Limited access to patient's mouth for eating, drinking, expectorating, etc
- Claustrophobic feeling generated by the mask
- Irritation to the eyes because of high flow rates

Large-Volume Aerosol Systems

The goal of adding humidity to the inspired gases is to minimize or eliminate the adverse effects to the patient from breathing a dry medical gas. Humidification assists in maintaining or improving the function of the normal mucociliary escalator (see Humidification/Nebulization, later). High-flow devices, used for administering humidified supplemental oxygen to patients who have an artificial airway, are the T-piece and the tracheostomy mask/collar. If the patient is breathing through the natural airway, the high-humidity face mask and the high-humidity face tent may be applied. Humidity may be added when various low-flow systems are used; however, the four systems just described are high-flow systems to which humidity may be applied.

With each of the following systems, after correct assembly and before application of the device, the F_{IO_2} must be chosen and the oxygen flow rate adjusted to ensure that it is operating like a high-flow system (i.e., that all of the patient's ventilatory needs are being met by the system). The desired F_{IO_2} is chosen by adjusting the air entrainment port on the nebulizer (Fig. 4-6). The initial flow rate is then set at 10 L/min. To ensure that the patient's entire minute ventilation needs are being met by the device, adjust the flow rate so that a constant mist can be seen coming from the extension tubing on the T-piece, from the exhalation port on the tracheostomy collar, from the exhalation ports on the face mask, and from over the top of the face tent. If the patient's ventilatory needs are high, and one flowmeter with nebulizer is therefore inadequate to deliver sufficient flow rates and support a constant mist, then utilize two. Use of a second nebulizer can be achieved by using a "Y" adapter.

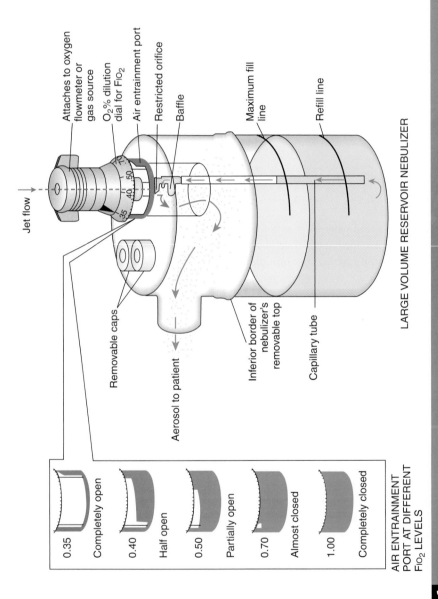

Jet flow →

Attaches to oxygen flowmeter or gas source

O_2% dilution dial for FiO_2

Air entrainment port

Restricted orifice

Baffle

Maximum fill line

Refill line

Removable caps

Aerosol to patient

Inferior border of nebulizer's removable top

Capillary tube

LARGE VOLUME RESERVOIR NEBULIZER

AIR ENTRAINMENT PORT AT DIFFERENT FiO_2 LEVELS

0.35 — Completely open

0.40 — Half open

0.50 — Partially open

0.70 — Almost closed

1.00 — Completely closed

FIGURE 4-6

Large-volume reservoir nebulizer. Alteration of the size of the air entrainment port adjusts the FiO_2. *(Modified from Kersten LD. Comprehensive Respiratory Nursing. Philadelphia, Saunders, 1989.)*

HIGH-HUMIDITY T-PIECE (OR "BLOW-BY")

Description and Technique

The high-humidity T-piece attaches to the endotracheal or tracheostomy tube to provide oxygen and humidification to a patient who is not using a mechanical ventilator. Corrugated tubing coming from the nebulizer attaches to one end of the T-piece. An extension (reservoir) of corrugated tubing is attached to the other end of the T-piece. The entire setup is connected to the patient's artificial airway (Fig. 4-7). The desired FIO_2, ranging from 0.28 to 1.0, is chosen by adjusting the air entrainment port on the nebulizer. The initial flow rate is set at 10 L/min. To ensure that the patient's entire minute ventilation needs are being met by the device, adjust the flow rate so that a constant mist, throughout inspiration, can be seen coming from the extension piece on the T-tube.

Advantages

▨ High humidity prevents airway drying and maintains mucociliary function.
▨ Device is lightweight.
▨ Precise FIO_2 can be delivered.

Disadvantages

▨ Tubing can become heavy with accumulated water and pull on the airway.
▨ When patient is changing body positions, accumulated water may accidentally drain into the patient's airway.
▨ Failure to regulate flow rate properly creates a low-flow system.

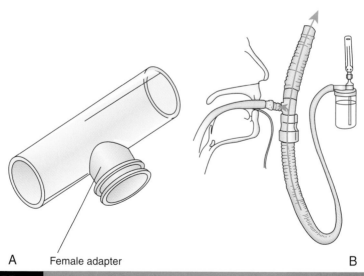

A   Female adapter   B

FIGURE 4-7

High-humidity T-piece. **A,** The T-piece, or T-tube, is connected to an endotracheal or tracheostomy tube to provide humidified oxygen. **B,** Use of a nebulizer provides humidity in an aerosol form.

(B, Modified from Kofke WA. Postoperative respiratory care techniques: Part III. Weaning from mechanical ventilation and oxygen therapy. Curr Rev PACN 1992; 13:161.)

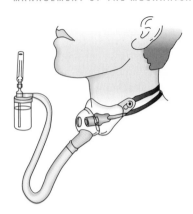

FIGURE 4-8

The high-humidity tracheostomy mask, or collar, fits over a tracheostomy or laryngectomy tube. The hole in the front of the mask is for exhalation. *(Modified from Kofke WA. Postoperative respiratory care techniques: Part III. Weaning from mechanical ventilation and oxygen therapy. Curr Rev PACN 1992; 13:161.)*

HIGH-HUMIDITY TRACHEOSTOMY MASK (TRACHEOSTOMY COLLAR)

Description and Technique

The tracheostomy mask, also known as the tracheostomy collar, is a clear mask designed to fit over a tracheostomy tube or a laryngectomy tube. The hole in the anterior portion of the collar-shaped mask is the exhalation port. It should be applied to the patient with the large-bore oxygen tubing connection at the bottom and the neck strap adjusted to ensure a snug fit (Fig. 4-8).

The desired FIO_2, ranging from 0.28 to 1.0, is chosen by adjusting the air entrainment port on the nebulizer. The initial flow rate is set at 10 L/min. To ensure that the patient's entire minute ventilation needs are being met by the device, adjust the flow rate so that a constant mist can be seen from the exhalation port throughout the entire respiratory cycle.

Advantages

- High humidity prevents airway drying and maintains mucociliary function.
- Device is lightweight and comfortable.
- Precise FIO_2 can be delivered.

Disadvantages

- Secretions can accumulate in the tracheostomy collar.
- Tubing can become heavy with accumulated water, dislodging collar from proper position and thus compromising accurate FIO_2 delivery.
- When patient is changing body positions, accumulated water may accidentally drain into the patient's airway.
- Failure to regulate flow rate properly creates a low-flow system.

HIGH-HUMIDITY FACE MASK

Description and Technique

The high-humidity face mask is similar in design to the simple face mask. Differences are that the high-humidity face mask is attached to a wide-bore oxygen tubing and nebulizer and that the exhalation ports are larger to accommodate larger

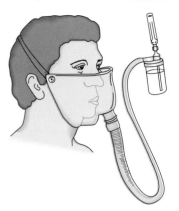

FIGURE 4-9

High-humidity face tent. *(Modified from Kofke WA. Postoperative respiratory care techniques: Part III. Weaning from mechanical ventilation and oxygen therapy. Curr Rev PACN 1992; 13:161.)*

aerosol particles and high water output. The mask should be applied as described previously in the discussion of the simple face mask. After the mask is applied, the FIO_2 is chosen by adjusting the dial at the top of the nebulizer. The initial flow rate is set at 10 L/min. To ensure that the patient's entire minute ventilation needs are being met by the device, adjust the flow rate so that a constant mist can be seen coming from the mask's side ports throughout inspiration.

Advantages
- High humidity prevents airway drying and maintains mucociliary function.
- Delivery of FIO_2 is more precise than with a simple face mask.

Disadvantages
- Mask is confining.
- Access to mouth for eating, drinking, expectoration, oral care, etc. is limited.
- Mask becomes uncomfortable because inside of mask and face rapidly become wet.
- Rushing air and gurgling water, collected in tubing, become noisy.
- Failure to regulate flow rate properly creates a low-flow system.

HIGH-HUMIDITY FACE TENT
Description and Technique
The face tent is a shell-shaped device that fits under the patient's chin, hugging the jaw, with the top arching over the patient's face (Fig. 4-9). The FIO_2 of the delivered gases is set by adjusting the air entrainment port on the nebulizer (range, 0.28 to 1.0). The initial flow rate on the nebulizer should be set at 10 L/min and then adjusted as necessary to produce a visible mist.

The volume of gas supplied by this device should meet the patient's entire minute ventilation needs; therefore, it fits the criteria for categorization of a high-flow system. Theoretically, a precise FIO_2 can be delivered by this device; however, because of the openness of the face tent and the ease with which it slips out of place, room air may be breathed at varying amounts, diluting the desired FIO_2.

Advantages

- High humidity prevents airway drying and maintains mucociliary function.
- Face tent is more comfortable than the simple or high-humidity face masks for the patient who has facial trauma or burns or who has undergone facial surgery.

Disadvantages

- Face tent is difficult to keep in place.
- Delivery of precisely prescribed FIO_2 is difficult.

MANUAL RESUSCITATION BAGS

Description

Manual resuscitation bags (MRBs) (Fig. 4-10) are used to provide oxygen and positive-pressure ventilation to a sealed airway such as a mask, endotracheal tube (ETT), or tracheostomy tube. MRBs consist of a self-inflating bag; an oxygen inlet valve, ideally capable of accepting an oxygen flow of 15 L/min; a nonrebreathing valve(s), which directs the flow of oxygen-enriched gas to the patient and prevents exhaled gases from entering the bag; in pediatric models, a pressure-release valve that opens when proximal airway pressure exceeds 40 cm H_2O; a standard-size (15 mm) adapter that enables the system to attach to a mask or directly to an artificial airway, and an oxygen reservoir. Additional accessories include positive end-expiratory pressure (PEEP) valves.

When the bag is squeezed to create inhalation, positive pressure opens the nonrebreathing valve, allowing the flow of oxygen from the bag into the mask or artificial airway and into the patient. If inspiratory pressures are high, a pop-off valve, if present, is activated. The pressure-release valve should be capable of being deactivated for adequate ventilation in patients with high airway resistance or low pulmonary compliance. On exhalation, the exhaled gases close the nonrebreathing valve and open a passage to the atmosphere, through which they escape.

MRBs are indicated for both oxygenation and ventilation of patients who have inadequate or absent spontaneous respirations in an arrest situation, who are being transported between departments or institutions (in the absence of a transport ventilator), and who require preoxygenation and ventilation between passes of a suction catheter.

MRBs provide positive-pressure ventilation and, because of the resistance to inspiration created by the nonrebreathing valve, are not intended to provide assisted ventilation in spontaneously breathing patients. The spontaneously breathing patient would have to be capable of generating sufficient negative pressure to open the valve and draw in the oxygen-enriched gas. Furthermore, when the MRB is used with a mask and spontaneous respirations resume, simply holding the setup loosely over the patient's mouth and intermittently squeezing the bag does not provide sufficient oxygen-enriched gas. Carbon dioxide may also be rebreathed because it collects in the mask. In a scenario of reliable and adequate spontaneous respiratory efforts, a tight-fitting mask is more appropriate than a MRB.

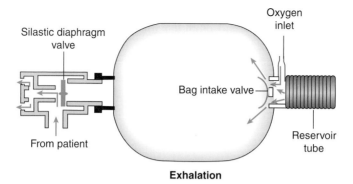

Exhalation

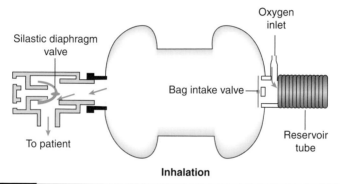

Inhalation

FIGURE 4-10

Manual resuscitator bag. Gas movement and valve action during both the inhalation-compression and exhalation-relaxation phases. The nonrebreathing valve is on the left, oxygen inlet and bag inlet valve to the right, and the oxygen reservoir to the far right. Changes in pressure during the inspiratory versus expiratory phases of ventilation result in alternate opening and closing of the nonrebreathing and oxygen inlet valves. *(Modified from Marshak AB. Emergency life support. In RL Wilkins, JK Stoller, C.L Scanlan, et al [eds.], Egan's Fundamentals of Respiratory Care, 8th ed. St. Louis, Mosby, 2003, p 727.)*

When spontaneous respirations are present and the use of a MRB is still indicated, the operator must ensure the simultaneous compression of the squeeze bag with the patient's inspiratory effort. Failure to synchronize manual ventilation with the patient's spontaneous effort may result in patient discomfort, complaints of dyspnea, and gastric distention (when the MRB is being used with a mask).

Factors that determine the F_{IO_2} delivered by an MRB include the oxygen flow rate, the ventilation rate and stroke volume, oxygen reservoir volume, and bag refill time. MRBs may be used with or without supplemental oxygen. In general, a higher F_{IO_2} is delivered when the oxygen flow rate is high (15 L/min) and the tidal volume and ventilatory rate are lower. Theoretically, 100% oxygen should be delivered when an oxygen reservoir is in place. Bench studies reveal variable performance in regard to the fraction of delivered oxygen in currently available models. To achieve the highest possible FIO_2, an oxygen reservoir should be used, oxygen input flow should be set maximally, and the stroke volume should be delivered in 2 seconds and allow for adequate refill time. A PEEP valve should be used if the patient is on 5 cm H_2O PEEP or greater. The PEEP valves may be built in or attachable and should be capable of generating PEEP up to 12 cm H_2O.

Volume delivery capability is affected by squeeze bag volume, whether one hand or two are used to compress the bag, hand size, and whether a complete seal was achieved at the MRB–patient interface. Volume delivery may also be affected eventually by operator fatigue. Hazards of MRB devices include gastric distention, especially when the bag is used with a mask. Gastric distention can be reduced by providing moderate to low inspiratory flows over a 2-second period. Another potential hazard is barotrauma from rapid respiratory rates and incomplete exhalation resulting in the development of auto-PEEP, too vigorous flows, and failure to use a pressure-relief valve in pediatric patients.

Technique

MANUAL RESUSCITATION BAG TO MASK

When using a bag-valve-mask (BVM) setup, employ a clear mask, if available, to visualize the airway and detect the presence of any vomitus or secretions that could be aspirated. The operator should be positioned at the head of the patient. An oral airway should be placed in the unconscious person to assist in maintaining a patent airway. For more optimal airway patency, use the head-tilt position if not contraindicated. The mask is applied over the mouth and nose and held securely in place by the thumb and forefinger placed in a C-shaped position on the top of the mask; the third, fourth, and fifth fingers are hooked under the edge of the mandible (Fig. 4-11). Firm pressure must be used to achieve a tight seal while ensuring that the fingers on the jawline are not exerting excessive pressure on the soft tissue under the jaw. The bag is then compressed while a tight seal is maintained, and the chest is observed for adequate respiratory excursion. Sufficient time for exhalation and BVM refill should be allowed before delivery of the next breath.

BVM ventilation is a difficult technique to master and should be performed only by those trained in the skill. Maintaining a seal and a patent airway is challenging because some of the tidal volume is often lost through leaks around the mask. Performance of the technique by two persons, one to hold the mask in position and the other to compress the bag, may provide more optimal results.

MANUAL RESUSCITATION BAG TO ARTIFICIAL AIRWAY

The MRB can be attached to an ETT or tracheostomy tube through the use of a standard-size (15 mm) adapter. The bag may then be squeezed using a one- or two-handed technique. Compression of the bag with two hands has been shown to deliver more optimal volumes. Use of only one hand may be necessary when only one operator is present and the second hand is needed to hold a sterile suction catheter or the airway so that excessive movement and irritation can be avoided.

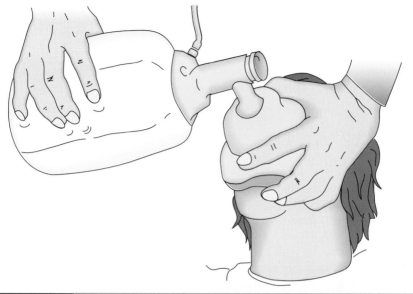

FIGURE 4-11

Technique of bag-valve-mask (BVM) ventilation. *(Modified from Wade JF. Comprehensive Respiratory Care. St. Louis, Mosby, 1982.)*

HUMIDIFICATION/NEBULIZATION

Recall from Chapter 1 that the nasal passages are remarkably efficient at humidifying all inspired gases. By the time air reaches the subglottic space, it is 98% to 100% humidified. Supplemental oxygen, however, is a dry gas. Its administration can lead to the drying of the respiratory passages, dehydration and thickening of the mucus in the airways, and therefore a decrease in the efficiency of the mucociliary system. Ciliary activity may be further retarded when oxygen concentrations are high. For maintenance of the normal function of the mucociliary system, it is agreed that supplemental inspired medical gases should be humidified when administered at flow rates greater than 4 L/min. Humidity, therefore, should be added to supplemental gases when the amount of humidity in that gas is less than normal. This principle *always* applies when the natural airway is bypassed by an endotracheal or tracheostomy tube, to prevent desiccation of the airways because the normal upper airway heat and moisture exchanging structures are bypassed.

The administration of aerosol, or high humidity, is recommended when secretions are thick and secretion retention, mucus plugging, or crusting is a problem. Bland aerosols, however, minimally affect the physical properties of mucus. Systemic hydration is the most effective method of reducing secretion viscosity. When there is bronchoconstriction or a history of airway hyperresponsiveness, irritation of

BOX 4-2 Definitions of Common Terms	
Humidification	Water evaporated in gas; water in its *gaseous* (vapor) form
Active Humidifier	Adds water vapor and heat to the inspired gases
Passive Humidifier	Uses exhaled heat and moisture to humidify inspired gases
Aerosol	Suspension of liquid or solid *particles* (water, medications) in gas
Nebulizer	System that produces aerosol particles that are then carried into the airways with the delivered gases

the airways can occur when high humidity is delivered. Conversely, inflammatory processes in the upper airway, such as tracheobronchitis, or postextubation laryngeal edema may benefit from the application of cool, bland aerosol. Humidity is also useful in the treatment of asthma, in which high flow rates of dry oxygen may exacerbate the disease. High humidity is also beneficial after inhalation anesthesia, when ciliary and surfactant activities are depressed.

Humidification can be provided without heating the inspired gases; however, raising the temperature increases the capacity for humidification. Heating of gases delivered into the airways may also serve the dual purpose of efficiently rewarming hypothermic patients. This principle is most often applied in the postoperative and emergency room arenas. High-flow gases delivered into the trachea by T-piece, tracheostomy collar, or mechanical ventilator should be heated.

In the next section, the principles of humidification and aerosol systems, as they relate to the humidification of supplemental oxygen therapy and the therapeutic use of aerosol medication administration, are reviewed (Box 4-2).

Humidification Devices
BUBBLE-THROUGH HUMIDIFIER
Description
The bubble-through or diffusion head humidifier (Fig. 4-12) is used with the nasal cannula, simple face mask, and reservoir masks. Bubble-through humidifiers vary in design. In the least efficient form, gas is simply forced down a tube to the base of the water reservoir. In a more efficient form, a diffuser at the end of the tube breaks the gas into bubbles, thereby increasing the surface area of gas and water, which promotes evaporation. The size of the bubbles varies with the design of the diffuser. The smaller the bubbles, the greater the content of water in the delivered gas because of the increase in the gas–water interface. Other factors that affect the amount of humidity are the water level and the flow rate of gas. Maximal gas–water contact is provided when the column of water through which the bubbles must pass is tall. Therefore, the water level should be checked frequently. Higher flow rates cool the water, decreasing its evaporative capacity and reducing contact time. Heating a bubble humidifier is not practical because the gases cool before reaching the patient, and any additional humidity gained is then lost again through condensation.

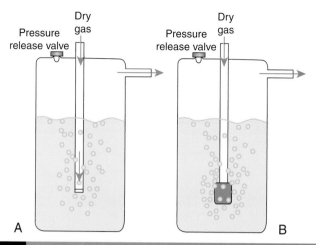

FIGURE 4-12

The bubble-through humidifier saturates gas with water vapor; it does not generate an aerosol.
A, Open lumen design. **B,** Diffuser type of end increases surface area of bubbles. *(Modified from Cairo J, and Pilbeam S [eds.], Mosby's Respiratory Care Equipment, 7th ed. St. Louis, Mosby, 2003, p. 93.)*

General Principles: Bubble-Through Humidifier

▨ Sterile water should be used in humidifiers to prevent nosocomial infection.

▨ Prevent blockage of small-bore oxygen delivery tubing by water that has spilled over into the tubing from the bubbling action within the humidifier.

▨ Devices have a positive-pressure release valve on the top. If the small-bore tubing becomes kinked or compressed, back pressure is released through this valve. When the valve is activated, a whistling sound is emitted, alerting the practitioner to investigation and corrective action so that oxygen flow to the patient can be resumed.

HEATED HIGH-FLOW HUMIDIFIERS

Description

Heated, high-flow humidifiers are most often used when gases are being delivered via an artificial airway and a mechanical ventilator. Heating the water causes a larger number of water molecules to gain sufficient kinetic energy to enter the gaseous state; therefore, the water vapor content of the inspired air is increased. The two basic designs, pass over and pass-over wick, allow the patient's entire inspiratory volume to be heated and humidified (Fig. 4-13).

Pass-Over Humidifier

The pass-over humidifier has a simple design, and its name explains the principle of operation. In this humidifier, gas passes over a heated water bath. Rising water vapor enters the gas, which is then transported to the patient.

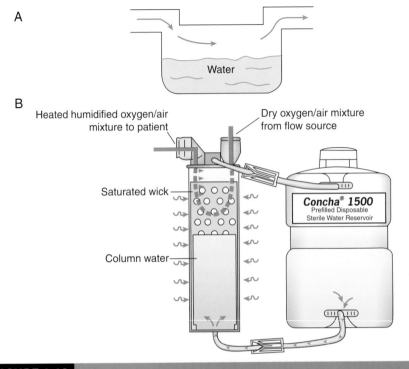

A

B

Heated humidified oxygen/air
mixture to patient

Dry oxygen/air mixture
from flow source

Water

Saturated wick

Column water

Concha® 1500
Prefilled Disposable
Sterile Water Reservoir

FIGURE 4-13

The two basic designs of heated mainstream humidifiers: pass over (**A**), and pass-over wick (**B**).
See text for details. (**B**, *Courtesy of Hudson Respiratory Care, Inc., Temecula, Calif.*)

Wick Humidifier

In the pass-over wick humidifier, some absorbent material, such as paper or composite, is partially submerged in the water. This material absorbs water from the reservoir using capillary action and serves as the wick. Gases are humidified as they circulate around or through the saturated wick.

General Principles: Heated Humidifiers

- A thermometer, preferably one of an inline design, should be used to determine that the desired temperature is reached and not exceeded. A reading slightly less than body temperature is appropriate. Overheated water should be drained and replaced because it can cause airway burns. Heed all temperature alarms.

- When a heating unit is described as servo-controlled, a microprocessor is working with the thermometer to maintain a constant temperature. Ensure that the temperature probe is appropriately applied and functioning.

- Accumulated water in the tubing should be emptied periodically and discarded. It should *never* be allowed to drain back into the humidifier or into the patient because it may be contaminated with bacteria. Excessive condensate also increases the FIO_2 delivered.

- Water in the tubing increases resistance to gas flow and reduces delivered tidal volume during use of pressure modes of ventilation and increases pressure in volume modes.

- Ensure the reservoir's water level is maintained to guarantee maximal humidification. Manual methods of adding water tend to increase the risk of reservoir contamination and cause fluctuations in temperature of gas delivered when cold water is added to the humidifier. Most models have a continuous, closed water-feed system. Be sure to install it correctly because overflowing water could flood the inspiratory circuit and be aspirated by the patient.

- Assess the patient for sputum character, breath sounds, and patency of artificial airway to determine whether there is adequate humidification.

HEAT AND MOISTURE EXCHANGERS

Heat and moisture exchangers (HMEs) are devices that fit between the airway and the ventilatory circuitry. They are commonly referred to as artificial noses. The principle behind the HME is a simple one. Exhaled gases pass through the HME, where water condenses on the inner surfaces and heat is retained. The retained heat and moisture are then added to the next inspired breath. Passive humidifiers often also have filtering characteristics. The moisture output of an HME is based on tidal volume (V_T), inspiratory time, respiratory rate, and temperature. A change in any one of these factors that increases the transit time through the HME reduces the ability of the device to remove moisture from exhaled gas and add moisture to inspired gas. Because the effectiveness of the HME also depends on how much heat and moisture are in the patient's exhaled gases, it should not be used on patients who are dehydrated or have hypothermia.

Lower rates of VAP are reported with the use of an HME as compared to heated humidifiers. However, there are additional important issues that must be weighed in the decision to use passive humidification. These include the dead space of the device, the difficulty in administering aerosol medications, and increase in resistance to gas flow. The larger the surface area within the HME, the more heat and moisture can be exchanged; however, dead-space volume (rebreathed gases) also increases. In patients with high minute ventilation demands, this increased dead space may be intolerable. As retained humidity increases in the HME, so does flow resistance increase and thus the work of breathing. The greatest concern with HME resistance is that the media can become occluded with secretions, blood, or fluid from a secondary source. Therefore, the HME must be removed prior to delivery of aerosolized medications and is contraindicated in patients with thick, copious, or bloody secretions or with heated humidification. When the exhaled V_T is less than 70% of the delivered V_T (ETT cuff leak, bronchopleural fistula), the HME is ineffective in exchanging moisture and therefore is contraindicated.

HMEs are simple to use, are cost effective, and provide freedom from potential electrical or thermal injury. There is also reduced concern that the patient will become overhydrated or will have condensate in the ventilator tubing inadvertently "dumped" into the airway during turning. The device should be firmly attached in place to avoid gas leakage at the connections and should be changed every

48 hours or more often if the technical performance is compromised. The device should be inspected frequently, and if three or more changes are required per day, a switch to heated humidification should be made.

AEROSOL THERAPY (NEBULIZERS)

Aerosol therapy is widely used in respiratory care. This section reviews the indications and generally accepted methods of administration of both large- and small-volume aerosol therapy.

Large-Volume Aerosol Delivery Systems (Nebulizers)

Large-volume aerosol delivery systems are used therapeutically in the presence of upper airway edema to humidify inspired medical gases, including when the upper airway is bypassed, and to induce sputum specimens. Edema of the airway may be treated with a cool bland aerosol (e.g., for subglottic edema, postextubation edema, laryngotracheobronchitis, and postoperative management of the upper airway). Heat bland aerosol is indicated primarily for minimizing humidity deficit when the upper airway is bypassed or high-flow oxygen is being administered. Hypertonic or hypotonic saline aerosol is used for sputum induction.

Two systems, the jet and the ultrasonic nebulizer, are used to increase the moisture content of gases administered by the high-humidity face mask, face tent, T-piece, or tracheostomy collar. Some confusion arises as a result of the use of the term *high humidity* in association with these systems because in reality an aerosol is delivered to the patient, as well as humidity. Aerosol therapy delivers water *particles*, not just water *vapor* (water in the gas phase) into the airways. The categories of nebulizers, jet and ultrasonic, describe the technique by which the aerosol is physically produced (Fig. 4-14). Aerosols may be cooled or heated.

JET NEBULIZER

The jet nebulizer is pneumatically driven, using the Venturi principle to create an aerosol. Gases from the flowmeter, delivered under high pressure, are passed through a jet. A capillary tube, with one end immersed under the liquid, intersects with the jet. Air pressure around the jet decreases, drawing water into the capillary tube. Water exits the capillary tube at the site of the jet flow and is shattered into small particles. This spray is further fragmented as it is blown against a baffle. A baffle, which may be a sphere, plate, or rod, for example, further reduces the size of the particles as they collide with it. After contact with the baffle, the aerosol is then delivered to the patient. The smaller the particle size, the greater its depth of penetration into the lung.

The orifice at the top of the nebulizer, which determines how much air will be entrained, is adjusted to achieve the desired FIO_2. The higher the FIO_2, the less mixing of room air is desired and thus the narrower is the opening. Aerosol content also decreases as the amount of entrained air decreases. Jet nebulizers may be heated or cooled.

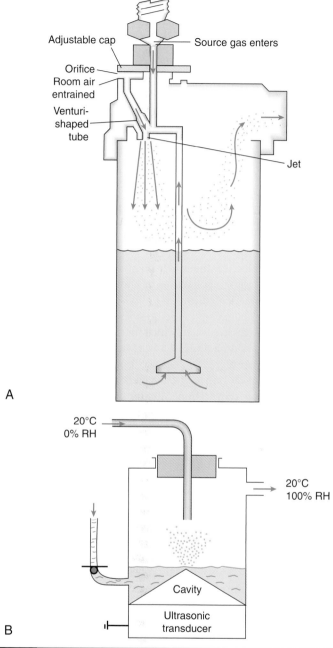

Adjustable cap

Source gas enters

Orifice

Room air entrained

Venturi-shaped tube

Jet

A

20°C
0% RH

20°C
100% RH

Cavity

Ultrasonic transducer

B

FIGURE 4-14

Nebulizers produce aerosols that may be cooled or heated. **A,** Oxygen is forced through a small-lumen cannula in the *jet nebulizer*. This creates subatmospheric pressure at the top of a capillary tube, drawing water upward in the tube. The water is hit by the jet stream and then forced into a baffle, which breaks the aerosol into even finer particles. **B,** The *ultrasonic nebulizer* creates a cavity of high-frequency sound waves that vibrate the solution, creating an aerosol geyser. (*A, Modified from Kacmarek RM, and Stoller JK. Current Respiratory Care. Toronto, BC Decker, 1988. B, Modified from Shelly MP. Inspired gas conditioning. Resp Care 1992; 37:1075.*)

ULTRASONIC NEBULIZER

The ultrasonic nebulizer, which is electrically driven, uses high-frequency sound waves to create an aerosol mist by vibrating the solution. It may be used for continuous therapy but is primarily used for intermittent therapy. Ultrasonic nebulizers are used much less frequently than jet nebulizers, primarily because the latter devices are much simpler and there is less potential for equipment problems.

General Principles: Aerosol Therapy

- The patient's face should be dried periodically as a comfort measure.
- Aerosols may induce bronchoconstriction in patients with hypersensitive airways, such as those with asthma. Consider using a humidification system in these patients.
- Escaped aerosolized toxic medication or microbes exhaled by the patient is a concern for caregivers. Use appropriate protective apparel for airborne respiratory diseases.
- Bacterial contamination of the water may occur. Use strict hand-washing procedures, do not allow condensate in the tubing to drain back into the nebulizer as it is contaminated, and use only sterile water or physiologic saline solution.
- Keep tubing free of excessive water, which increases the delivered F_{IO_2}.
- Overheated water should be drained and replaced because it can cause airway burns. Ensure that the water level does not drop below the indicated level.
- In the pediatric population, long-term continuous administration of bland aerosol may result in overhydration. Monitor fluid balance.

Small-Volume Aerosol Delivery Systems (Nebulizers)

Small-volume aerosol systems are used for the administration of medications. Advantages of the aerosol versus the parenteral route of administration are that smaller doses are required, there is a rapid therapeutic effect because of direct administration of drug into the area in need of treatment, administration techniques are simple, and the use of the aerosol route is associated with fewer systemic side effects. Three types of small-volume aerosol delivery systems are discussed here: small-volume jet nebulizers, metered-dose inhalers (MDIs), and dry powder inhalers (DPIs).

The effectiveness of an aerosol is determined by its ability to deposit a drug in the lung. Factors that determine drug deposition are the size of the aerosol particles and the amount produced, airway characteristics (size, geometry), and the patient's ventilatory pattern. The larger the particle produced by the delivery device, the more proximal the deposition in the airway. The diameter of the airway affects aerosol delivery in that the size of the airway is positively correlated to aerosol deposition. As bronchodilators are administered and the airway dilates, more drug may be deposited with subsequent inhalations. Multiple factors can influence aerosol delivery during mechanical ventilation. Specifically, aerosol drug delivery can be impaired by drug deposition in the ventilator circuit and artificial airway. Only MDIs and nebulizers can be adapted for use during mechanical ventilation. Until recently, the techniques that should be used to optimize aerosol delivery were not well understood and ventilators were not designed to optimize inhaled drug therapy. Technologic improvements and better understanding of aerosol delivery have allowed researchers to overcome the obstacles to efficient aerosol delivery during mechanical ventilation. Humidification increases the loss of aerosol in the ventilator circuit by as much as 40%. Bypassing the humidifier is not recommended for routine inhalation therapy in mechanically ventilated patients and would require breaking the circuit and allowing it to dry. Furthermore, inhaling dry gases can be detrimental to the tracheal mucosa. With careful attention to administration technique the effect of humidity on drug delivery can be overcome by delivering a higher dose. The patient's ventilatory pattern, which enhances drug deposition, is a slow, steady inhalation (occasionally to inspiratory capacity), followed by breath holding at end-inspiration to allow for particle settling. Larger inspiratory volumes result in more aerosol entering the lung; however, this has not been demonstrated to result in greater drug deposition.

SMALL-VOLUME NEBULIZERS

Small-volume nebulizers (SVNs) operate by the same principle as the large-volume jet nebulizer: the Venturi principle and the Bernoulli effect. SVNs are simple devices powered by portable compressors or hospital gas supplies (Fig. 4-15). SVNs are

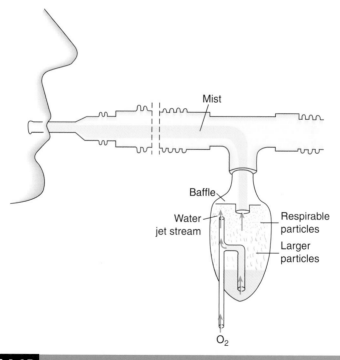

FIGURE 4-15

Typical design of a small-volume jet nebulizer. See text for explanation. *(Modified from Luce JM, Pierson DJ, and Tyler ML. Intensive Respiratory Care. Philadelphia, Saunders, 1993.)*

used in three ways: as handheld devices, incorporated into the breathing circuit of intermittent positive-pressure breathing (IPPB) machines, or placed in the circuitry of a mechanical ventilator. With the advent of disposable respiratory therapy supplies, the incidence of contamination of SVNs has decreased.

After the drug is placed in the nebulizer, it may be diluted to a larger volume with normal saline solution up to a typical fill volume of 3 to 4 mL. Most SVN drugs are available in unit-dose premixed vials. The gas flow rate is set typically at 6 to 8 L/min to achieve maximal drug delivery. As gas flow through the nebulizer increases, particle size decreases. The treatment should continue until no more aerosol can be produced. In all SVN designs, some of the solution remains after the treatment is completed, usually 0.5 to 1.0 mL. This is known as the dead volume and represents the solution that adheres to the inside of the SVN. The amount of dead volume may be diminished by intermittently tapping the sides of the nebulizer throughout the treatment so that the droplets on the walls of the nebulizer fall to the bottom and are renebulized. Devices that allow for control of aerosol only during inspiration or are breath-actuated reduce drug waste from continuous nebulization during both inspiration and expiration. Furthermore, this new generation of handheld nebulizers reduces caregiver exposure to exhaled drug.

The SVN should be placed in the inspiratory limb about 18 inches from the patient's airway because the ventilator circuit then serves as a spacer for aerosol to accumulate between inspirations. The least effective location is between the patient and the Y-connector of the ventilator circuit. If a loss of volume in the circuitry occurs, then the point where the nebulizer is attached should be assessed as the potential cause of a circuit leak. There are significant differences in the output efficiency of different nebulizer brands. A nebulizer can be operated continuously or intermittently. Continuous aerosol generation into the ventilator circuit requires a pressurized gas source, whereas intermittent operation uses a separate line to conduct inspiratory airflow from the ventilator to the nebulizer. Intermittent nebulizer operation is more efficient because it minimizes aerosol waste during exhalation. One factor that may negatively affect intermittent delivery is the driving pressure provided by the ventilator, which is typically lower than a pressurized gas source.

Nebulized drug is deposited both in the artificial airway and in the ventilator circuitry; therefore, the drug doses may need to be increased. Deposition of drug in the artificial airway increases as airway radius becomes smaller. To improve drug deposition to the lower airway, the V$_T$ should be 500 mL or more in adults, which ensures that the dead space is cleared of aerosol. Additional flow from the nebulizer enters the inspiratory circuit; therefore, V$_T$ and pressure limit may need to be adjusted to accommodate this flow. Flow-by, or continuous gas flow, needs to be turned off. Patients who are using pressure support ventilation (PSV) and receiving medication through a continuous-flow SVN must overcome the increased pressure gradient created by the SVN to trigger the ventilator; therefore, the trigger sensitivity should be adjusted appropriately. When the treatment is complete, the SVN should be removed from the circuit, and the ventilator and alarm settings returned to their pretreatment settings. The SVN is rinsed with sterile water and allowed to air dry. To minimize contamination, it is recommended that the SVN be changed every 24 hours or more often if indicated.

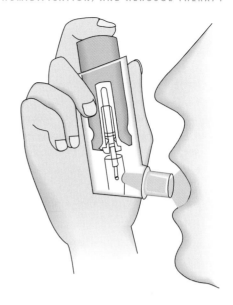

FIGURE 4-16

A metered-dose inhaler. *(Modified from Luce JM, Pierson DJ, and Tyler ML. Intensive Respiratory Care. Philadelphia, Saunders, 1993.)*

METERED-DOSE INHALERS

The MDI consists of a small canister that contains medication and an inert gas propellant. A mouthpiece, or actuator, is attached when the MDI is used by spontaneously breathing patients (Fig. 4-16). It may be used with or without an adjunct known as a spacer (see later). When activated, the MDI delivers a single dose of drug. The canister may contain hundreds of such doses. The gas propellant is typically hydrofluoroalkane (HFA) because chlorofluorocarbons are known to contribute to ozone layer depletion and global warming and therefore were banned worldwide in 2000. MDIs are the most commonly prescribed form of aerosol delivery. They are used to administer bronchodilators, anticholinergics, antiinflammatory agents, and steroids.

The MDI is portable, requires no compressed gas source, is less expensive than the SVN, and is associated with less risk of equipment contamination. In many institutions all patients supported by mechanical ventilation receive their aerosol therapy by MDI unless the drug needed does not come in an MDI. Choice of MDI over SVN in the spontaneously breathing patient depends on the patient's ability to coordinate the timing of activation of the device with proper inhalation. However, the use of a spacer (see later) may eliminate this indication for use of an MDI.

The techniques for MDI administration are outlined in Box 4-3 for the spontaneously breathing patient and in Box 4-4 for the patient undergoing mechanical ventilation. The timing from inhalation to activation of the MDI is crucial to the success of drug delivery to the lungs. After a normal exhalation to functional residual capacity, the MDI should be activated during a slow, deep inhalation, followed by at least a 4-second breath hold. For the mechanically ventilated patient, the MDI should be actuated precisely in synchrony with inspiratory flow ("go with the flow"). The best ventilatory pattern for optimal drug

BOX 4-3	Technique for Administration of Metered-Dose Inhaler (MDI) in Spontaneously Breathing Patients

1. Shake the vial 15 to 20 times after warming it to room temperature.

2. Insert drug canister into actuator and uncap the mouthpiece.

3. When the MDI is new or unused for 24 hours, prime the metering chamber by actuating one puff into the air while holding the MDI upside down.

4. Hold the MDI upright, either between the lips with the mouth open or 4 cm in front of the open mouth. If a spacer is used, hold the MDI between the lips.

5. Exhale normally to resting level (functional residual capacity).

6. Begin to inhale slowly and deeply, and actuate (fire) the MDI. Continue inhaling to total lung capacity.

7. Hold breath for 5 to 10 seconds.

8. Wait a minimum of 30 seconds before repeating steps 4 to 7 for each additional puff ordered.

9. After completion of the treatment, rinse mouth and gargle as necessary to remove drug deposited in the mouth and oropharynx.

BOX 4-4	Technique for Administration of Metered-Dose Inhaler (MDI) During Mechanical Ventilation

1. Assemble MDI spacer and place in ventilator circuitry.

2. Adjust inspiratory flow to minimal rate allowed. Aim for an inspiratory time of over 0.3 of total breath duration.

3. Shake the vial 15 to 20 times after warming it to room temperature.

4. Remove heat and moisture exchanger (HME); do not disconnect humidifier.

5. Place MDI in circuit adapter or spacer and actuate immediately at the start of a ventilator-delivered inspiration. Ensure that the ventilator breath is synchronized with the patient's spontaneous respiratory effort if present.

6. If not contraindicated, apply a 2- to 3-second end-inspiratory pause.

7. Wait 1 minute between puffs and assess the patient for therapeutic and adverse effects.

8. Ensure that all ventilator settings are returned to pretreatment settings and HME is reconnected.

deposition is not known. Lung model studies suggest that aerosol deposition is improved by low inspiratory flows, use of decelerating flow instead of square wave, VT more than 500 mL, and increased inspiratory phase. Furthermore, spontaneous inspiration through the ventilator circuit increased lung deposition as compared to controlled, assist/control, and PSV.

For the spontaneously breathing patient, two types of placement of the mouthpiece at the time of actuation are recommended: (1) between the lips with the mouth open and (2) 4 cm from the open mouth. Consensus as to the optimal method

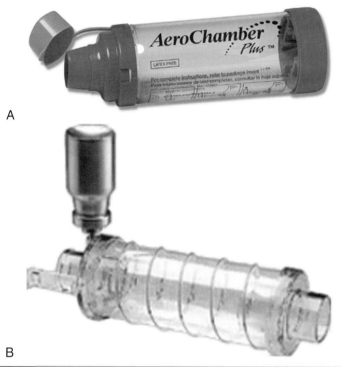

A

B

FIGURE 4-17

Spacers are adjuncts used with the metered-dose inhaler. They are available for (**A**) spontaneously breathing patients or (**B**) as a device that fits into the circuitry of the mechanical ventilator. *(Courtesy of Monaghan Medical Corporation, Plattsburgh, NY.)*

has not been reached. The rationale for placing the mouthpiece at a distance from the lips is that when the lips are closed, the majority of the drug is thought to be deposited in the oropharynx, specifically the tongue.

Spacers

Spacers are adjuncts for use with the MDI to eliminate the need for precise timing of inspiration to activation; they promote steady inspiratory flow and reduce large-particle deposition in the mouth or artificial airway because these particles are deposited in the spacer. In patients using an MDI through their natural airway, the deposition of less drug in the mouth reduces systemic absorption of swallowed drug, oral irritation, and bad taste. The spacer fits between the MDI and the mouth or into the ventilator circuitry (Fig. 4-17). The drug is activated into the spacer, followed by inspiration. Spacers are indicated for individuals unable to time activation and inspiration properly and for all patients undergoing mechanical ventilation. The chamber results in a fourfold to sixfold increase in delivery of aerosol over MDI actuation into an elbow connector (without chamber) attached directly to the ETT. Some commercial spacers used with the natural airway promote slow, steady inspiratory flow by whistling if inspiration is too rapid.

DRY POWDER INHALERS

DPIs are available for a limited number of drugs. The drug is placed in the inhaler in its powder form, sometimes contained within a gelatin capsule. The DPI is breath activated; inspiration draws the powder into the lungs. The device depends on the patient's ability to create turbulent flow to disperse the powder into respirable particles. Advantages of the DPI over the MDI are that problems with exact timing of inspiration are eliminated and a propellant is not required. Disadvantages include a requirement of higher inspiratory flow rates than with the MDI or SVN, an association with heavy oropharyngeal deposition, a limited number of drugs available in DPI form, a limited number of doses provided, clumping of the drugs when they become moist, an association with a greater incidence of bronchospasm (especially in persons with asthma), and their inability to be used in ventilatory circuits. DPIs, however, are as effective as MDIs in drug deposition and response.

RECOMMENDED READINGS

AARC Bronchodilator Administration During Mechanical Ventilation Working Group. AARC clinical practice guidelines: Selection of device, administration of bronchodilator, and evaluation of response to therapy in mechanically ventilated patients. *Respir Care* 1999; 44(1):105–113.

AARC Mechanical Ventilation Guidelines Committee. AARC clinical practice guidelines: Humidification during mechanical ventilation. *Respir Care* 1992; 37(8):887–890.

American Heart Association. Guidelines 2000 for Cardiopulmonary Resuscitation and Emergency Cardiovascular Care. *Circulation* 2000; 102 (Suppl. 1):I95–I104.

Beers MF, Fisher AB. Oxygen toxicity. In RW Carlson, MA Geheb (eds.), *Principles and Practice of Medical Intensive Care* (pp. 949–957). Philadelphia: Saunders, 1993.

Branson RD. Humidification for patients with artificial airways. *Respir Care* 1999; 44(6):630–641.

Dhand R. Basic techniques for aerosol delivery during mechanical ventilation. *Respir Care* 2004; 49(6):611–622.

Fink J. Aerosol drug therapy. In RL Wilkins, JK Stoller, CL Scanlan (eds.), *Egan's Fundamentals of Respiratory Care,* 8th ed. (pp. 761–800). St. Louis: Mosby, 2003.

Hess D, Kallstrom TJ, Mottram CD, et al. AARC evidence-based practice guidelines. Care of the ventilator circuit and its relation to ventilator-associated pneumonia. *Respir Care* 2003; 48(9):869–879.

Kallstrom TJ, and the AARC Clinical Practice Guidelines Committee. AARC clinical practice guidelines: Oxygen therapy for adults in the acute care facility—2002 revision & update. *Respir Care* 2002; 47(6):717–720.

Kallstrom TJ, and the AARC Clinical Practice Guidelines Committee. AARC clinical practice guidelines: Bland aerosol administration—2003 revision & update. *Respir Care* 2003; 48(5):529–533.

Marshak AB. Emergency life support. In RL Wilkins, JK Stoller, CL Scanlan (eds.), *Egan's Fundamentals of Respiratory Care,* 8th ed. (pp. 705–735). St. Louis: Mosby, 2003.

McCabe SM, Smeltzer SC. Comparison of tidal volumes obtained by one-handed and two-handed ventilation techniques. *Am J Crit Care* 1993; 2(6):467–473.

Pruitt WC, Jacobs M. Basics of oxygen therapy. *Nursing* 2003; 33(10):43–45.

Togger DA, Brenner PS. Metered dose inhalers. *Am J Nurs* 2001; 101(10):26–32.

Wissing DR. Humidity and aerosol therapy. In J. Cairo, and S. Pilbeam (eds.), *Mosby's Respiratory Care Equipment,* 7th ed. (pp. 86–129). St. Louis: Mosby, 2004.

CHAPTER 5

Lung Expansion, Positioning, and Secretion Clearance

The provision of supplemental oxygen is often necessary to ensure the adequacy of oxygenation. Oxygen alone should be viewed as only supportive therapy. For the patient to return to an optimal state of oxygenation, without supplemental oxygen, the underlying abnormality must be treated with appropriately chosen bronchial hygiene techniques. The two basic goals of the therapies discussed in this chapter are to expand the lung, thus opening and stabilizing the alveoli and improving lung volume, and to clear the alveoli and airways of secretions.

LUNG EXPANSION THERAPY

Atelectasis

Atelectasis occurs in many hospitalized patients, particularly in the intensive care unit (ICU), where they may not breathe deeply enough or sigh often enough and bed rest may be prolonged. Atelectasis develops because of failure to expand the lung adequately or because of absorption of air distal to congested airways. When the volume of air in the lung is decreased, pulmonary compliance decreases and the work of breathing necessary to expand the lung increases. If the patient is weak and unable to generate the work necessary to expand the lung, the tidal volume decreases, blood gases further deteriorate, and the atelectatic process worsens.

Atelectasis is classified as either microatelectasis or macroatelectasis. The former cannot be seen on x-ray film but is physiologically evident by a widened alveolar-to-arterial oxygen difference (A-a gradient) or a below-normal PaO_2. Macroatelectasis is both radiographically and physiologically evident. The goal of lung expansion therapy, which includes maneuvers that promote larger-than-tidal (closer to inspiratory capacity) inspirations is to prevent, decrease, or correct alveolar collapse and atelectasis.

Deep Breathing

DESCRIPTION

Deep breathing is a simple and yet very effective lung expansion technique. It is indicated for any patient who is at risk of having atelectasis and who can participate in conscious control of ventilation.

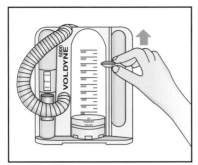
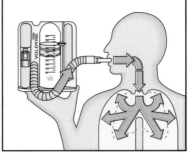

A   B

FIGURE 5-1

The volumetric incentive spirometer provides visual feedback of the inspired volume. **A,** The inspiratory goal is marked by the clinician. **B,** The patient may then independently perform incentive spirometry (IS), working to raise the piston to the prescribed level. *(Courtesy of Hudson RCI, Temecula, Calif.)*

TECHNIQUE

Place the patient in an upright position or, if the patient is in a side-lying position, support the arms, head, and flexed legs with pillows. Instruct the patient to inhale slowly and deeply. To promote diaphragmatic breathing, teach the patient to gently push out the belly during inspiration. For some patients, it is useful to place a hand on their upper abdomen while making a conscious effort to push outward on their hand during inspiration. The deeply inspired breath should be held for several seconds, which may promote collateral ventilation. Exhalation is passive. The patient should be instructed to take 8 to 10 deep breaths per hour while awake and may be motivated to do so if the benefits of this simple respiratory exercise are explained.

Incentive Spirometry

DESCRIPTION

Incentive spirometry (IS) provides patients with a visual cue as to how well they are performing their deep-breathing exercises and therefore may serve as a motivator or provide an "incentive" to their performance. IS is indicated to prevent or correct atelectasis, particularly in the postoperative patient. The visual cue provided to the patient varies according to the type of spirometer. Some spirometers have balls that rise to the top of one or more chambers, whereas others have bellows that contract as the patient inspires. One type of IS allows for the determination of the actual volume that the patient is inspiring. This type is known as a volume spirometer, as opposed to a flow spirometer (Fig. 5-1).

TECHNIQUE

Assist the patient to an upright position. Instruct the patient to exhale fully, insert the mouthpiece firmly between closed lips, and inhale slowly and as deeply as possible (to inspiratory capacity). The breath should be held for 2 to 3 seconds and then the mouthpiece removed from the mouth for exhalation. The patient may rest 30 to

60 seconds between breaths to prevent hyperventilation, respiratory alkalosis, and dizziness. The maneuver should be repeated 6 to 10 times per hour, which mimics the average number of sighs a person usually makes.

If possible, the patient should be coached in the use of the spirometer preoperatively. Preoperative technique and volumes then serve as a reference for comparison of postoperative performance. IS is cost effective because after the staff teaches the patient to use the spirometer and observes a successful demonstration, the patient can perform the exercise independently. Observing the patient performing IS twice daily serves as encouragement and allows for determination of performance, reinforcement of the goal, and further instruction as necessary.

Positioning and Mobilization
ADVERSE EFFECTS OF IMMOBILITY

Regular turning and progressive mobilization are primary therapeutic techniques for lung expansion. It is critical that the nurse, respiratory therapist, physical therapist, and the physician all understand the adverse effects of immobility and the effect of various body positions on lung volume and pulmonary function. Prolonged bed rest is associated with reduction in vascular tone, fluid shifts, regional atelectasis and secretion retention, and musculoskeletal changes including calcium depletion and muscle wasting. Typically the patient is nursed in the supine position, partly for cosmetic benefit but mostly for convenience for delivery of care. The supine position is associated with a tendency for pharyngeal obstruction, retention of airway secretions, reduction in normal sinus drainage and sinus infections, increased reflux and aspiration, and compression of the lungs by the heart and abdomen. Remaining in the supine position for extended periods of time is in dramatic contrast to normal human position and movement. Keane in 1978 explained that even during sleep, human beings change their position approximately every 11.6 minutes, a phenomenon described as the "minimum physiological mobility requirement."

DISTRIBUTION OF VENTILATION-TO-PERFUSION RATIO
IN VARIOUS BODY POSITIONS

Body position affects depth and patterns of ventilation in the lung, perfusion, and lymphatic drainage. Each of these factors affects the ability to effectively keep the lung expanded, clear secretions from the lung, and maintain oxygenation. Areas of the lung in the most dependent regions have the smallest resting volume and thus the greatest tendency to collapse, particularly at reduced inspiratory volumes. The airways are smallest in the dependent regions in all body positions because of the effect of gravitational forces on the lung. Gravity pulls on the lung as it "hangs" in the thorax. Because of this gravitational pull, and because the intrapleural pressure is the most negative, the airways in the uppermost region are expanded to the greatest extent. This is true regardless of body position: supine, upright, lateral decubitus, or prone. Blood flow is also gravity dependent in nature and therefore always greatest in the most dependent regions, tending to compress the alveoli. For a more detailed explanation of the distribution of ventilation and perfusion in the lung, see Chapter 2.

A large volume loss in the lung is associated with the horizontal position. Turning the patient from supine to lateral or prone positively affects the functional residual capacity (FRC). Recall that when the FRC is optimized, so is gas exchange in the lung, specifically oxygenation. Turning the patient affects the distribution of the weight of the mediastinum, lung tissue, and abdominal contents. Lateral positioning mildly improves FRC, whereas more dramatic improvements are associated with head of bed (HOB) elevation, semirecumbency with the feet dependent, and finally upright (standing) positioning (Fig. 5-2). This is not new information. Positive effects of mobility include increased lung volume, secretion mobilization, and maintenance or improvement in the patency of airways. Positioning is beneficial in reducing atelectasis in the bedridden patient. Clearly there is a therapeutic effect of patient positioning.

POSITIONING CRITICALLY ILL PATIENTS

Many factors make it tempting to leave the patient supine for prolonged periods. Concerns about dislodging tubes, monitor leads, and lines; pain with movement; accidental aspiration of ventilator circuit condensate; and simply not enough staff to turn larger patients are all factors that lead to reduced patient mobility. The longer the patient remains supine and motionless, the greater the lung volume reduction, secretion retention, risk of aspiration, and atelectasis formation. Changing the patient's body position may be used prophylactically and therapeutically. Regularly turning and changing of the patient's body position varies the position of the lung and assists in the prevention of atelectasis. For patients who already have atelectasis, placing them in a position with the atelectatic area uppermost may promote reexpansion of the lung.

Traditionally, it is accepted that the patient should be turned minimally every 2 hours. However, as stated previously, more frequent position changes are the human norm. Progressive mobilization from turning to sitting positions or, even better, to ambulation is an excellent lung expansion therapy that is also cost effective. The psychological benefit to the patient of increased mobility, especially getting out of bed, should not be underestimated. Turning and mobilization of patients should be performed with careful planning to avoid complications and monitoring for tolerance throughout and after the position change. Assessment parameters to monitor include oxygen saturation, respiratory frequency, complaints of dyspnea, blood pressure, heart rate, and the patient's overall subjective response.

Head of Bed Elevation

HOB elevation is associated with improved lung volume (Fig. 5-3). Patients may have the HOB elevated by either raising just the HOB or by placing the bed in the reverse Trendelenburg position. The latter position is an ideal way to raise the head when bending the spine is contraindicated. Reverse Trendelenburg also relieves the weight of the abdomen on the diaphragm and lung and therefore results in improved lung volume in all patients, especially those with large abdomens. Drakulovic also demonstrated that HOB to 45 degrees is associated with a statistically significant reduction in ventilator-associated pneumonia (VAP) as compared with supine in mechanically ventilated patients receiving enteral nutrition.

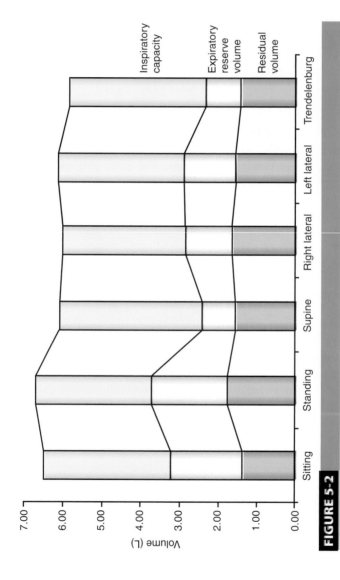

FIGURE 5-2

Changes in lung volume with position changes. Functional residual capacity (residual volume plus expiratory reserve volume) is least in the supine and Trendelenburg positions, increases modestly in the right and left lateral positions, and is best in the sitting and finally standing positions. Inspiratory capacity (*top bar*) follows a similar trend.

(From Fink JB. Clinical Practice of Respiratory Care. Philadelphia: Raven-Lippincott, 1999.)

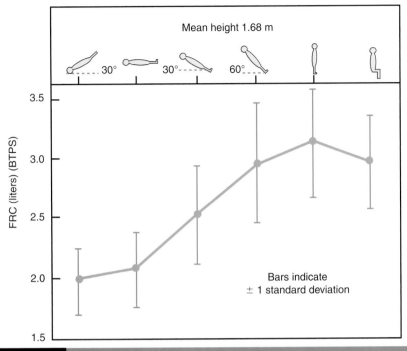

FIGURE 5-3

Changes in the functional residual capacity with changes in head of bed elevation and progression to sitting and standing. A large volume loss is associated with the supine position with dramatic improvements as the patient progresses to upright with the feet dependent. *(From Lumb AB. Nunn's Applied Respiratory Physiology. 6th ed. Philadelphia: Butterworth-Heinemann, 2005.)*

Supine versus Lateral Position in Unilateral Lung Disease

Lateral position is associated with a modest increase in FRC as compared to supine. Therefore, turning the patient from supine to lateral helps expand the lung and reduces the development of atelectasis. Mobilization also reduces the stagnation of secretions and lung water.

Lateral position can be very useful in patients with unilateral lung disease from various causes. Positioning patients in the lateral decubitus position with the good lung down (GLD), results in a higher PaO_2. Perfusion, which is gravity dependent in nature, is greatest to the less diseased lung when that lung is placed in the dependent position. Ventilation, because it is preferentially distributed to areas of best compliance and least resistance, is also best in the dependent lung. Therefore, with the GLD, the matching of ventilation to perfusion in the dependent lung is improved. Investigators demonstrated a decrease in the percentage of shunt when the patient is positioned with the GLD. Therefore, an awareness of the effect of changes in position on pulmonary ventilation and perfusion may permit therapeutic application of patient positioning.

The duration of the immediate effect of body position on gas exchange is unpredictable. A patient with unilateral disease who initially shows enhanced oxygenation with the GLD may demonstrate a gradual fall in oxygenation during a period in which the position is maintained. The mechanism responsible for this deterioration is atelectasis and airway closure by secretions that gradually migrate from the upper lung into the more dependent, and previously relatively less diseased, lung; this leads to a fall in PaO_2.

There are several clinical implications for the use of therapeutic positioning to enhance oxygenation in patients with predominantly unilateral lung disease. First, having the patient lie in a position with the GLD allows ventilation with lower levels of FIO_2 and positive end-expiratory pressure (PEEP). Second, recognition of the phenomenon should help prevent the diagnostic error of overall worsening respiratory status when, in fact, the arterial blood gas was possibly obtained when the patient was positioned in the less favorable lateral position. Third, changing body position without considering its possible ill effects may be life-threatening in patients with severe respiratory insufficiency and unilateral involvement.

In the mechanically ventilated patient, hypoventilation related to three factors may also contribute to a decreasing oxygenation status when the patient is placed in the lateral decubitus position. These three factors are decreased dependent lung motion from mediastinal weight, dependent diaphragm elevation as a result of the weight of the abdominal contents, and relative immobility of the dependent chest wall. Therefore, the use of body position to achieve optimal oxygenation requires careful evaluation of individual patient response over time.

Kinetic Therapy and Continuous Lateral Rotation Therapy

Kinetic therapy (KT) is defined as the continuous turning of a patient slowly along the longitudinal axis to 40 degrees or more onto each side. Continuous lateral rotation therapy (CLRT) is also continuous turning; however, the degree of turn is less than 40 degrees. Rotational surfaces that are firm are referred to as table-based therapy, which can be applied to patients with spinal cord injury and can achieve a turn of 62 degrees. Soft surfaces achieve the turn with alternating inflatable pillows. KT has been shown to significantly decrease the incidence of lobar atelectasis, pneumonia, length of ICU stay, hours intubated, and the need for bronchoscopy. The assumption is that KT improves movement of secretions and prevents stasis of secretions; however, the link between physiologic changes and improved outcomes remains to be determined. The best outcomes are with KT (rotation angle minimally 40 degrees) and rotation occurring at least 18 hours per day.

CLRT data demonstrate a reduction in VAP, infiltrates, atelectasis, and urinary tract infection; however, data are not as robust as KT data. Studies are small, admit to selection bias, or are limited to special patient populations such as liver transplant patients. Multiple clinical, descriptive, process-improvement initiatives reported by hospitals, however, demonstrate favorable results with CLRT. These results include a decrease in hospital and ICU length of stay, ventilator days, readmissions to critical care, and reintubation rate. Results appear to be best when CLRT is applied early (defined as within 24-48 hours of patients' meeting criteria that identify them as being at risk for developing pulmonary problems). As lag time to therapy increases it appears that so do hospital costs, length of stay, incidence of pulmonary problems, and ventilator days. Specialty beds increase the cost of care; therefore, many institutions develop criteria for their use and discontinuation. Common criteria for application of rotational therapy include PaO_2/FIO_2 ratio of 250 or less; chest x-ray evidence of lobar collapse/atelectasis; immobility (spine injury), or the mechanically ventilated patient who is difficult to turn, such as obese patients. When effectively applied and removed, KT may actually save costs because the incidence of VAP is reduced.

An essential part of consistent application and evaluation of therapy is a clinical practice guideline that can be executed by bedside professionals. Application of rotational therapy requires the operator to choose the degree of turn or the percentage of turn, depending on the bed model. A 40-degree turn is the goal, or if degrees are not measurable, then a turn that achieves one lung above the other. Many beds provide an acclimation mode that gradually ramps up the angle of turn, therefore allowing the patient to adjust to the sensation of the bed. Turning is generally tolerated by the patient; however, carefully titrated sedation may improve tolerance. A pause time is also chosen for each position (right, center, and left). Pause times of 10, 5, and 10 result in a 25-minute cycle time to achieve full turning to both sides. The optimal frequency of turning and duration of turn is not known. Cycle times can be made shorter or longer and can be varied for each side. For example, if the patient's right lung is relatively more diseased and desaturation occurs with the right lung down, then the time spent on the right side as well as the degree of angle to that side are adjusted to patient tolerance. Optimal therapeutic benefit occurs when the patient is rotated a minimum of 18 hours/day. All settings, changes in settings, and hours of rotation should be documented.

Evaluation of the therapy includes reviewing the record to determine if therapy was properly applied and patient response to include improvement in daily chest x-ray, PaO_2/FIO_2 ratio, and pulmonary assessment. Average duration of therapy is 5 days. Immediate indications for discontinuing therapy include patient liberation from the ventilator and/or improved patient mobility (frequent self-turning). Many rotational beds also offer the ability to provide percussion therapy. Settings include the intensity and duration of therapy. Little is known about the effectiveness of percussive therapy delivered in this manner.

Prone

Turning the patient prone, called proning, is indicated in patients with severely compromised lungs such as in acute lung injury and acute respiratory distress syndrome (ARDS). No exact level of oxygenation deficit for implementing proning is precisely defined; however, when the following criteria are met, this therapeutic position should be considered: PaO_2/FIO_2 ratio is 200 or less, patient is on 60% or more of oxygen, lung recruitment maneuvers have been tried, and PEEP is 15 cm H_2O or more.

In ARDS, edema and consolidation are greatest in the dependent lung area, which for patients lying in bed is the dorsal region. This observation led researchers to experiment with positioning the patient so that the aerated lung fields (non-dependent lung) became dependent by placing the patient in the prone position. The physiologic effect in patients who respond positively to proning is an improvement in oxygenation. Several mechanisms are thought to result in this improvement. When the patient is prone, a more uniform pleural pressure gradient from the dorsal to ventral body surfaces results, which accounts for a more even distribution and matching of ventilation to perfusion. The prone position eliminates the compressive weight of the heart and great vessels on the lungs because the heart now rests on the sternum. Finally, the airways drain well in the prone position so secretion clearance is enhanced. Ventilator-induced lung injury may also be reduced in the prone position.

Approximately 70% of patients respond to proning. A positive response is defined as a 20% or more increase in PaO_2. As of yet, why some patients respond while others do not is unknown. Of the 70% who respond, approximately 30% to 40% are persistent responders, meaning there is a sustained increase in PaO_2 even when the patient is returned to the supine position. Another equal percentage are nonpersistent responders, meaning when the patient is returned supine, the improvement in PaO_2 is lost. If initial positioning does not result in a positive response, this should not rule out periodic attempts to assess patient response at a later time. There are no criteria for application of proning only during specific stages of ARDS. A positive response should allow for a reduction in FIO_2 and PEEP.

The procedure for moving the patient prone is technically difficult and requires careful planning both to prevent unplanned extubation and malposition or loss of vascular accesses and tubes. Prior to repositioning, the patient should be assessed for the following:

1. Hemodynamic stability (defined as a systolic blood pressure of 90 mm Hg with fluid and vasoactive support) to identify ability to tolerate a position change and to correct imbalances as much as possible before the increase in demand created by the turn
2. Agitation that could lead to safety concerns
3. Size and weight to determine ability to turn within the critical care bed and ability of the caregivers to manage the weight load without injury

Tube feedings should be stopped for 1 hour before the turn. To prevent skin breakdown, eye injury, and accidental extubation, the electrocardiogram leads should be removed from the anterior chest and padding material should be available, eye lubricant applied, and the airway properly secured and suctioned.

A manual turn without any positioning device typically requires four or five personnel: one dedicated to the top of the bed to monitor the airway and the rest on either side of the patient to perform the turn. Use of a positioning device such as the Vollman Prone Positioner reduces the number of needed personnel to three and includes padding/supports for the forehead, chin, upper chest, and pelvis that allows for protrusion of the abdomen to improve diaphragm excursion (Fig. 5-4). As the patient is turned, the person assigned to the airway should be ready to immediately suction the patient's airway. In some patients, large amounts of secretions are immediately mobilized as the patient is turned prone, so much so that it may temporarily be difficult to ventilate the patient. Throughout the turn, tolerance is assessed with pulse oximetry, cardiac monitoring, and end-tidal carbon dioxide monitoring if available to assess position of the airway. Because of the lower chest

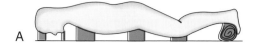

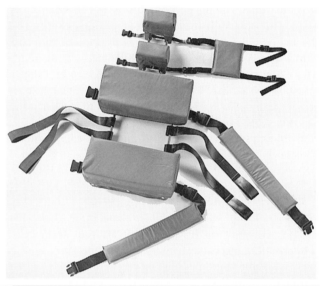

FIGURE 5-4

Proper support and padding are applied when proning to relieve pressure and thus prevent skin breakdown and allow for free abdominal movement. The head is supported at the forehead and chin, relieving pressure and preventing kinking of the airway; thorax and pelvis supports allow for unrestricted abdominal movement; and knee and shin supports prevent breakdown. **A,** Foam blocks or available bedding materials may be used or **B,** padding may be achieved with a commercially available device such as the Vollman Prone Positioner. *(B, Courtesy of Hill-Rom, Batesville, Ind.)*

wall compliance in the prone position, ventilating pressures or volumes may need to be adjusted.

Care of the patient in the prone position should maintain current standards of care and reduce the potential for complications. To avoid skin breakdown, peripheral nerve injury, joint, and eye damage the patient must be maintained with proper support and anatomic alignment. Pillows and supports must be used to prevent overextension or underextension of the cervical spine, bowing of the back in the abdomen-free position, and footdrop. To prevent the latter, supports should be placed to promote slight flexion of the knees and a 90-degree angle of the feet. The patient's head should be repositioned hourly and the eyes lubricated and taped horizontally to ensure they remain closed, thereby preventing corneal abrasions, excessive drying, or contamination with secretions. To prevent brachial plexus injury the arms should be repositioned every 2 hours: one arm up and the other along side the body with the head turned toward the upper arm. Drainage from the nares and mouth may be copious and is suctioned as needed. The patient's family should be informed of the facial edema that will develop and educated that it will resolve when the patient returns supine. Anticipatory planning should be in place for returning the patient to the supine position in the event of an emergency though successful defibrillation is reported with the patient in the prone position.

The length of time to remain in the prone position is unclear. The decision is based on the ability of the patient to sustain an increase in PaO_2 and determination by the health care team of the endpoint for tolerance of remaining in a stationary position. There is no clear direction from the literature on frequency of position change. Prone position should be discontinued prior to attempts to wean the patient. Some authors recommend safe discontinuation of proning when a PaO_2 of 60 mm Hg or more can be sustained by an FIO_2 of 0.4 or less and a PEEP of 8 cm or less H_2O. The effect of proning on survival remains unclear because a well-controlled trial without protocol violations has not been done.

Intermittent Positive-Pressure Breathing

DESCRIPTION

Intermittent positive-pressure breathing (IPPB) is a technique that provides short-term intermittent mechanical ventilation for the purpose of lung expansion, delivering aerosol medications, or assisting ventilation. IPPB augments inflation of the lungs through the application of positive pressure on inspiration. The breaths may be pressure or time limited and pressure, time, or flow cycled. Improvements in the patient with IPPB are short lived (<1 hour), and application is costly because it requires the constant attendance of a respiratory practitioner. Therefore, IPPB may be indicated for the reversal of atelectasis when less expensive therapies, such as deep breathing, IS, coughing therapies, and chest physiotherapy (CPT), are not successful. IPPB promotes lung expansion and improved cough because the patient obtains a larger inspiratory volume than might be taken independently. As the lung is expanded and secretion removal is enhanced, the work of breathing decreases and ventilation/perfusion matching improves. It may be used as short-term ventilatory support; however, devices specifically designed to deliver noninvasive positive-pressure ventilation should be given priority. Hypoxemia, carbon dioxide retention, and acute ventilatory failure should not be viewed as indications for IPPB but, rather, for mechanical ventilation. Perhaps the interpreted success of IPPB in some patients is not because of the treatment itself but due to the fact that pulmonary toileting is receiving concentrated attention.

The most controversial theoretical indication for the use of IPPB is for the delivery of aerosol medication. The effectiveness of aerosol delivery with IPPB is affected by many factors, such as design of the device in terms of flow, volume, and pressure capability; technique such as patient coordination, breathing pattern, selection of inspiratory flow or hold; and the aerosol output and particle size. Only a small percentage of the aerosolized medication deposits optimally in the airway. In fact, as much as a tenfold amount of medication may be needed when administering via IPPB versus a metered-dose inhaler (MDI). Administration of aerosol via IPPB may be considered when other techniques such as MDI with a spacer or holding device or a small-volume nebulizer (SVN) have not proven effective. Patients with neuromuscular disorders or kyphoscoliosis and those who are fatigued or have ventilatory muscle weakness may have improved deposition of the aerosol with the assistance of IPPB. However, based on the available literature, MDI or SVN should be considered the devices of choice for aerosol therapy for chronic obstructive pulmonary disease (COPD) and stable asthma patients. Beneficial effects have not been consistently reproduced in clinical studies, nor have these clinical studies been replicated since aerosol technology has improved. IPPB is more expensive and probably no more effective than handheld nebulizers administered with thorough patient instruction.

The use of IPPB is contraindicated (1) in patients with untreated pneumothorax because the positive pressure may force additional air into the pleural space; (2) in patients who have recently undergone tracheal or pulmonary surgery or pulmonary biopsy because pressure application to the affected area may cause rupture of the site and pneumothorax; (3) in patients who have undergone recent facial, oral, or skull surgery; and (4) in hemodynamically unstable patients because the positive pressure in the thorax may further decrease venous return and impede cardiac output. Hypotension may be particularly pronounced in the patient with hypovolemia. IPPB is also contraindicated in patients who are unable to cooperate because the therapy may be ineffective and gastric distention may occur secondary to air being swallowed or forced into the esophagus.

TECHNIQUE

To initiate the treatment, assist the patient to an upright position. If supplemental oxygen was being administered before IPPB, the same F_{IO_2} should be delivered during the treatment. When the patient is spontaneously breathing, the negative inspiratory effort triggers the IPPB machine to deliver the positive-pressure breath. IPPB may also be time triggered; however, this may result in some dyssynchrony with the patient that would negate a therapeutic effect. Delivery may occur through mouthpiece or mask, or through a tracheostomy with the use of an adapter.

The patient forms a seal around the mouthpiece and inhales, triggering the IPPB machine. The sensitivity should be set at 1 to 2 cm H_2O so the patient will not need to exert excessive negative pressure to trigger a breath. Air and oxygen then flow into the lungs under positive pressure. At the height of inspiration, the patient should hold the breath for 3 to 5 seconds, particularly if medications are being administered, because an inspiratory pause improves their distribution. The patient then exhales passively through the mouthpiece so that exhaled volumes can be registered. The goal of IPPB is to improve lung volume; therefore, the amount of pressure used during the treatment depends on the *volumes exhaled*, which should be 25% larger than the patient's tidal volume (V_T) or larger than pre-IPPB inspiratory capacity. Initial pressures used for IPPB typically range from 10 to 15 cm H_2O; however, the amount of pressure needed is determined by the lung volume goal for each patient. In critical care treatment, frequency ranges from every 1 to 6 hours as tolerated. Each treatment, which typically lasts no longer than 15 to 20 minutes, should provide for 6 to 10 breaths per minute.

Complications from IPPB include the following:

- Hyperventilation when the patient is not properly coached and breathes too rapidly
- Hypotension caused by decreased venous return
- Patient discomfort, emesis, and gastric dilation, which create pressure on the diaphragm and may lead to the development of an ileus
- Nosocomial infection caused by bacterial contamination of poorly managed equipment
- Secretion impaction caused by the positive pressure, especially when IPPB is applied to the patient in the upright position
- Pneumothorax and pneumomediastinum as a result of high volumes and pressure

Positive Airway Pressure Techniques

DESCRIPTION AND PHYSIOLOGIC RATIONALE

Positive airway pressure (PAP) techniques include continuous positive airway pressure (CPAP), positive expiratory pressure (PEP), and expiratory positive airway pressure (EPAP). CPAP provides positive pressure during inspiration to improve lung volume, thereby reversing or preventing atelectasis, and during expiration to splint the lung open. PEP and EPAP, in contrast, provide positive pressure only during expiration to splint open the airway, thereby both improving airflow and promoting secretion clearance. The natural precursor to the development of these therapies is pursed-lipped breathing. Patients with COPD naturally learn the mechanism of breathing against pursed lips, which creates a back pressure in the lungs; splints collapsible, unstable airways during expiration; and relieves air trapping. Positive expiratory pressure, by preventing expiratory collapse, is also thought to improve the distribution of gas in the lungs by promoting gas flow through collateral channels. Expiratory resistance devices mimic this effect.

Cough or other airway clearance techniques must accompany PAP techniques when the therapy is intended to improve secretion clearance. PEP therapy, which may be superior to CPT in promoting clearance of secretions in cystic fibrosis, COPD, and other secretory lung diseases, is less labor intensive. Some devices allow for aerosol medication delivery simultaneous to PAP therapy. A positive outcome from PAP therapies is evident in the following assessment parameters: increased sputum production, improvement in breath sounds and chest x-ray, an improvement in arterial blood gas values or oxygen saturation, and positive subjective response reported by the patient.

INDICATIONS AND CONTRAINDICATIONS

PAP therapies are indicated to reduce air trapping in asthma and COPD, to aid in mobilization of secretions especially in cystic fibrosis and chronic bronchitis, to prevent or reverse atelectasis, and to optimize delivery of bronchodilators in patients receiving bronchial hygiene therapy. There are no absolute contraindications to the application of PAP therapies. Patients should be evaluated for their ability to tolerate the increased work of breathing associated with EPAP or PEP. Additional considerations are discussed later.

CONTINUOUS POSITIVE AIRWAY PRESSURE MASK

Description

The CPAP mask applies a specified amount of positive pressure into the airways in an effort to open the alveoli, improve functional residual capacity, and thereby improve oxygenation. The therapeutic effects of positive pressure occur during exhalation. When the patient expires, it is against the resistance of positive pressure, which creates back pressure in the lungs, promoting alveolar recruitment and improving alveolar stability.

The use of CPAP is indicated for the spontaneously breathing patient with hypoxemia caused by atelectasis. It may be used continuously or applied as a periodic treatment. It is particularly useful when efforts are directed toward avoiding intubation and preventing reintubation in the patient who recently underwent extubation. When CPAP is used intermittently as a treatment, both the duration of the CPAP treatment and the amount of CPAP applied should be documented.

Technique

For application of a CPAP mask, a flow generator is connected to an oxygen source and the flow adjusted to the desired FIO_2 with the use of an oxygen analyzer. A humidification system is connected to the flow generator and tubing. Another piece

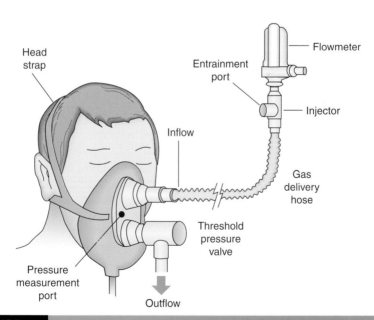

FIGURE 5-5

The continuous positive airway pressure (CPAP) mask fits snugly around the patient's face. Positive pressure, which is applied during expiration, promotes alveolar recruitment and stability, increases the functional residual capacity, and thereby improves oxygenation. See text for further explanation.

of tubing connects the humidification system to the oxygen inlet valve on the CPAP mask. The appropriate PEEP valve is then applied on the bottom port of the mask. The valves generally come in expiratory resistances ranging from 2.5 to 20 cm H_2O, increasing in increments of 2.5 cm H_2O. A head strap is used to attach the system snugly to the patient's face. The flexible head-strap pieces are adjusted by securing the holes in the strap to prongs on the mask (Fig. 5-5). The mask should not be applied until flow is established. The fit of some mask models may be further adjusted by inflation of a cushion seal on the mask.

Advantages of mask CPAP include the application of positive pressure without the use of a ventilator. It may avert the need for intubation and mechanical ventilation, with all the potential complications, and it does not require as much patient effort or cooperation as active deep breathing or incentive spirometry.

Disadvantages and potential complications of mask CPAP include the following:

- Possible gastric insufflation and possible vomiting with aspiration, which may be prevented by using gastric decompression (patient should be told to indicate whether nausea is occurring)
- Discomfort, erythema, and possible skin breakdown around pressure points of the mask (nose, cheeks, chin) (use soft, inflatable seal masks to reduce problem)
- Feeling of being confined or feeling of claustrophobia, particularly when patient's mentation is impaired by hypoxemia
- Decreased cardiac output and hypotension in acute myocardial infarction, untreated pneumothorax, and hypovolemia because the positive pressure in the thorax reduces venous return and thus cardiac output
- Possible carbon dioxide retention because of an increase in dead space if the positive pressure overdistends the normal alveoli
- Possible pneumothorax, with increased risk in patients with bullous lung disease

POSITIVE EXPIRATORY PRESSURE

Description

PEP therapy applies positive airway pressure during expiration. At the start of inspiration, subatmospheric pressures are generated just as with spontaneous breathing. During expiration, positive pressures of 5 to 20 cm H_2O are generated as the patient breathes against a *threshold resistor*. EPAP devices are less complicated than CPAP because a high-flow gas source is not needed. The threshold resistor may take the form of a weighted ball, a flutter valve, a water column, or a spring-loaded valve, to name a few.

PEP therapy is differentiated from EPAP in that the positive expiratory pressure is generated as the patient exhales against a *xed ori ce* resistor (Fig. 5-6). The fixed orifice resistor creates pressure only when expiratory flow is high enough to generate back pressure from the orifice. Think about blowing through a straw at fast versus slow flows, and the concept becomes clear. Pressures of 10 to 20 cm H_2O are generally the goal with PEP therapy.

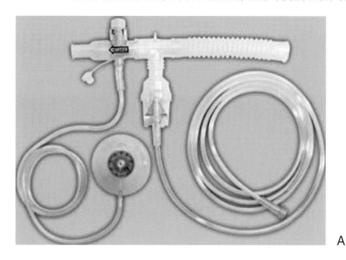

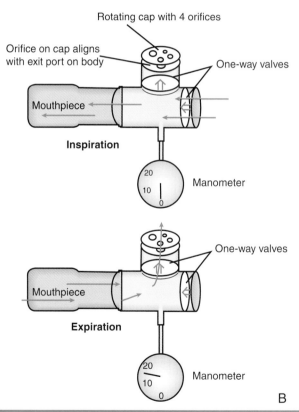

FIGURE 5-6

A, A positive expiratory pressure (PEP) device with variable resistance settings. Along with PEP therapy, aerosol treatments may be administered while monitoring exhaled pressure. **B,** Close-up of the rotating cap with four orifices that allow for variable resistance settings and one-way valves that allow inhalation and exhalation without removing the device from the patient's mouth. *(Courtesy of Mercury Medical, Clearwater, Fla.)*

Technique

After assisting the patient to a comfortable sitting position, the therapy is explained. Cooperation with diaphragmatic breathing and controlled expiratory flow optimizes therapy. If a mask is used, it should be fit comfortably over the nose and mouth. Alternately, a mouthpiece may be used with the lips placed firmly around it if the patient can maintain a seal and not release air through the nose. An inline manometer is placed to measure the expiratory pressure with EPAP and to choose the appropriate-size orifice with PEP. Once the appropriate-size orifice is chosen, the manometer may be removed. The patient is instructed to perform diaphragmatic breathing on inspiration to a volume larger than tidal but not to inspiratory capacity. Expiration is active but not forced. A series of 10 to 20 breaths are performed through the mask or mouthpiece. The patient should then perform several directed coughs and rest briefly. The sequence of therapy, coughing, and rest continues for a therapeutic session lasting approximately 20 minutes, or less if the patient assessment dictates.

Disadvantages and potential problems with EPAP or PEP include potential improper selection of the orifice size, which is key to the PEP technique. Most adults achieve the target 10 to 20 cm H_2O pressure with an orifice size of 2.5 to 4.0 mm.

- Too large an orifice produces a short expiratory phase without achieving the goal expiratory pressure.
- Too small an orifice creates a long expiratory phase, pressures above the target, and an increased work of breathing.

Lung Recruitment Maneuvers

A recruitment maneuver (RM) is the application of a sustained increase in airway pressure. It is advocated to open collapsed alveoli with high opening pressures. The optimal way to perform RMs remains unknown. They can be performed either by maintaining a high (35 to 60 cm H_2O) airway pressure for 20 to 40 seconds (sustained high-pressure RM) or by periodically increasing the inspiratory pressure for a short time and repeating this increase one to three times per minute (periodic high-pressure RM). A common sustained high-pressure RM is the application of CPAP of 35 to 40 cm H_2O for 40 seconds. Other approaches that have been tried include intermittent higher tidal volumes or the use of sighs; intermittent higher PEEP while maintaining tidal ventilation, applied either all at once for several breaths each minutes or in a step-up phase followed by a set-down phase; or pressure control (PC) of 30 above 15 to 20 cm H_2O PEEP for 1 to 2 minutes as tolerated.

Potential problems with recruitment maneuvers include barotrauma secondary to high pressure across the lung and hypotension secondary to increased intrathoracic pressure transmitted to the capillary bed. Hemodynamic compromise seems to be greatest with sustained inflation maneuvers. PEEP may need to be increased after the maneuver to maintain the effects. A number of reports describe improvements in oxygenation with the use of RMs; however, there are no data available that demonstrate they improve outcome.

SECRETION REMOVAL TECHNIQUES

Cough

Coughing is a normal protective pulmonary reflex (see Chapter 1). It is first-line therapy—the most important therapy for the removal of retained secretions. An effective cough requires the development of intraabdominal and intrathoracic pressure, followed by a rapid expiratory flow. The cough maneuver begins with a larger-than-tidal breath. The glottis is then closed, and the thoracic and abdominal muscles contract, building intrapleural and intrapulmonic pressures to maximum levels. As the glottis is suddenly opened, the air in the lungs is rapidly exhaled, moving material in the airways forward to the pharynx, where it can be either expectorated or swallowed.

Ineffective cough may be caused by several factors. The cough reflex may be blunted because of central nervous system abnormalities, or the irritant receptors may lack responsiveness, as may occur with prolonged intubation. The patient may suppress coughing because of pain, particularly after abdominal or thoracic surgery or trauma. The expiratory muscles of the thorax and/or abdomen may be weakened because of disuse or sedation or may be paralyzed by spinal cord injury so that an effective cough cannot be generated. When a patient is intubated, the glottis cannot close; therefore, the development of increased intrathoracic pressure and thus effective forced expiratory flow is impaired. When the patient's cough is ineffective, encouragement and coaching are often necessary. *Directed cough* is any cough that is not reflexive and initiated voluntarily by the patient with or without coaching. Coughing is required only when secretions are present. The effectiveness of the cough may be judged by sputum production and improvement in breath sounds. In addition to cough, airway clearance techniques are used to aid in mucus clearance in a variety of disease states.

COUGH COACHING AND PREPARATION

The patient should be assisted to a position that is conducive to optimal cough. The most effective cough is produced in a sitting position, with the trunk flexed slightly forward so the abdominal muscles can contract and the abdominal contents are pushed up against the diaphragm. The patient who is in bed can achieve optimal muscle contraction either by sitting in the Fowler's position with the knees drawn up or by lying on one side with the knees drawn up. The patient with a surgical incision can also be instructed in methods to splint the incision, such as hugging a pillow or pressing a small blanket against the surgical area. Both maneuvers can help stabilize the thoracic or abdominal wall and lessen the strain placed on the incision line.

An effective method of pain control should be implemented to promote patient cooperation and compliance with coughing. Many methods of pain control are available and should be administered with the goal of controlling the pain while not suppressing the respiratory drive or reflexes. Pain medication may be administered orally, intravenously, epidurally, or in sustained-release topical patches. In many cases, patient-controlled analgesia may be instituted, allowing the patient an active part in the pain control regimen.

COUGH TECHNIQUES

It is a common misperception that if the patient cannot mobilize secretions when instructed to breathe deeply and cough, then more advanced and costly techniques, such as postural drainage and percussion, suctioning, and bronchoscopy, are indicated. However, several cough methods can be tried with the patient to achieve the goal of sputum production.

With all cough techniques, instruct the patient to begin by slowly taking in a deep breath to allow the inspired air to reach the distal airways. The breath should then be held for several seconds, allowing collateral flow to assist in inflating airways that are below functional residual capacity. After coughing, the next breath should be taken through the nose to prevent sucking partially mobilized secretions back down into the airways.

Controlled Cough

The controlled, or voluntary, cough begins with a slow, deep breath held for several seconds. Forceful coughing using the abdominal muscles is then done two or three times in succession during exhalation. Coughing requires effort and can be tiring. Successive coughing may mobilize secretions even in weak patients unable to produce one large, forceful exhalation. The maneuver may be repeated as necessary, with rest between efforts using slow, deep breathing.

Huff Cough

Huffing is similar to the voluntary cough but modified in that the glottis remains open. After taking in a slow, deep breath and holding it for several seconds, the patient holds the glottis open while forcefully exhaling by making the sound *huh*. Because the glottis is held opened, high airway pressures are not produced, and yet secretions are propelled forward in the airways because high linear velocities, or rapid air ow rates, are produced. Less airway collapse occurs in huff coughing because airway pressures are lower. This technique is therefore useful in patients with COPD and in those with reactive airways.

Quad (Assisted) Cough

The quad, or assisted, cough is used in patients with neuromuscular disease that has rendered the abdominal muscles nonfunctional and in patients with diaphragmatic abnormalities. In either case, the patient is unable to generate sufficient expiratory force for effective coughing. After taking a slow, deep breath, the patient is manually assisted to cough during an expiratory effort. The caregiver offering the assistance places the palm of the hand flat on the patient's abdomen, just under the xiphoid process, and pushes inward and upward on the diaphragm just as the patient exhales. Alternatively, if abdominal compression is contraindicated, the caregiver's hands may be placed on the patient's lateral rib cage and quickly pressed inward with each cough (a maneuver called rib springing). For the patient whose respiratory effort also prohibits sufficient inhalation, hyperinflation with a manual resuscitation bag may improve inspiratory volume and thus expiratory flow.

Suctioning

Suctioning of the airway is probably one of the most common respiratory proce-dures performed in the intensive care setting by nurses, respiratory therapists, and appropriately trained technicians. The purpose of suctioning is secretion removal. This goal should be obtained while patient discomfort and adverse hemodynamic effects are minimized and hypoxemia related to suctioning is prevented. Suctioning should be performed when needed, not routinely, because of the potential trauma to the airway and induction of suctioning-related complications. The need for suctioning is determined by auscultation of adventitious breath sounds over the trachea and main-stem bronchi, visual inspection of the airway for the presence of secretions, an increase in peak inspiratory pressure on volume-targeted ventilation, and a decrease in V_T in pressure-targeted modes unexplained by other factors that increase airway resistance, respiratory distress when airway patency is questioned, and suspected aspiration of gastric or upper airway secretions. Although suctioning may be performed nasopharyngeally, this section focuses on the technique of endotracheal suctioning (ETS).

Potential complications of the ETS procedure include cardiac dysrhythmias, hypoxemia, cardiac arrest, vagal stimulation, mucosal trauma, atelectasis, contami-nation of the lower airway and the development of pneumonia, bronchospasm, pulmonary bleeding, and increased intracranial pressure. The cardiac complications may stem from procedure-induced hypoxemia or from tracheal stimulation. Tracheal stimulation may result in tachycardia and hypertension because of increased sympathetic nervous system (SNS) activity. In individuals who have lost SNS control (spinal cord injury above the first thoracic vertebra [T1]), bradycardia may result because vagal activity is unopposed.

It is reasonable that a patient with a marginal oxygenation status tolerates ETS less well than a patient with an optimal baseline PaO_2. Prevention of ETS-induced hypoxemia is paramount; therefore, several techniques targeted toward its elimina-tion are addressed in this section. When intrapulmonary pressure becomes negative because of suction application and the removal of gases from the lung, atelectasis may occur. In patients with increased intracranial pressure (ICP), there is a stepwise increase in ICP with each pass of the suction catheter; therefore the number of passes should be minimal and guided by monitoring of cerebrovascular status. Mucosal trauma is influenced by the vigor with which ETS is performed and also by mucosal invagination into the catheter end or side holes. The result is defoliation of ciliated epithelium from the mucosa, which impairs mucociliary function, causes edema, and possibly results in small hemorrhagic areas, as evidenced by blood streaking in the aspirate. Mechanisms for reducing tracheal trauma are discussed in the sections Suction Catheter Design and Endotracheal Suctioning Technique, later.

SUCTION CATHETER DESIGN

Suction catheters are generally for single use and made of polyvinylchloride. This clear material makes it easier to inspect the aspirated secretions for quantity, color, and character. They are easy to insert into the endotracheal tube (ETT), thereby eliminating the need for lubrication, which would increase catheter manipulation and the opportunity for contamination.

Suction Catheter Size

It is generally recommended that the diameter of the suction catheter should be no greater than approximately half of the diameter of the ETT to allow gases to flow around the catheter during suctioning. Generally, a No. 14 French (range, 12 to 16) suction catheter is used in adults. The No. 14 French catheter has a 4-mm outer diameter and therefore can be used with a tube 8.0 mm or larger. A catheter that is too small makes secretion removal difficult, especially if secretions are thick. The clinician is then tempted to pass the suction catheter more often, which may lead to patient discomfort or procedure-related complications. The catheter should be of sufficient length to extend approximately 2 inches (5 cm) beyond the end of the ETT to enter the main-stem bronchi.

Tip Design

The catheter should have more than one eye at the tip of the catheter for greater contact with secretions during their removal. Catheters with only one eye are associated with increased mucosal trauma from adherence. The quest to develop a catheter that results in reduced mucosal trauma has resulted in the availability of catheters with two eyes, four eyes, beveled tips, blunt tips, and so-called mushroom tips. A more important factor in reducing tracheal injury is probably ETS technique—the intensity with which the procedure is performed, and the onset and duration of the application of negative pressure (see Endotracheal Suctioning Technique, later).

Closed Tracheal Suction Systems

Open suctioning involves disconnecting the patient from the ventilator to insert the suction catheter. A closed tracheal suction system (CTSS) allows the catheter to be advanced into the airway without disconnection from the ventilator. A CTSS consists of a suction catheter housed in a plastic sheath, an adapter that attaches to the ventilator circuitry and allows the system to remain continuously attached, an irrigation port for tracheal lavage solution instillation and for rinsing the catheter after use, and a thumb-activated suction control valve (Fig. 5-7). After insertion of the catheter into the ETT and the performance of suctioning, the catheter is withdrawn back into the plastic sleeve. Advantages of maintaining a closed system include reduction in the potential for contamination to personnel and the environment, maintenance of positive-pressure ventilation, less loss of PEEP and functional residual capacity and therefore less derecruitment and hypoxemia, continuation of oxygen supply, ability to suction safely with one caregiver. Concerns related to use of the CTSS include infection control, effectiveness, creation of excess negative pressure from application of suction in a closed system, and cost.

There clearly is less potential for environmental contamination with the CTSS. This is a distinct advantage, especially in conditions spread by airborne particles, such as tuberculosis. The maintenance of positive-pressure ventilation and PEEP is particularly advantageous in patients who are sensitive to its discontinuation, such as those with apnea or high levels of PEEP. For prevention of suction-related hypoxemia, patients must still undergo hyperoxygenation before, during, and after

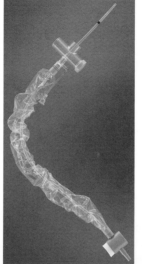

A

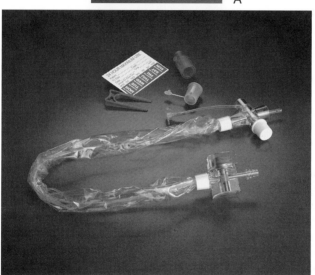

B

FIGURE 5-7

Closed tracheal suction systems. **A,** Ballard Trach Care. **B,** Concord/Portex Steri-Cath. *(A, Courtesy of Kimberly-Clark, Roswell, Ga. B, Courtesy of Smiths Medical, Keene, NH.)*

ETS with a CTSS. The closed system is maintained by performing hyperoxygenation with the ventilator, either by activating the 100% oxygen for suctioning feature, if available, or by adjusting the FiO_2 manually. The addition of hyperinflation further reduces the incidence of hypoxemia.

Studies on the effect of CTSS on the incidence of VAP show conflicting results. Several studies found similar pneumonia rates with closed versus open suction systems. Another study by Combes, however, reported a 3.5 times greater risk of pneumonia in patients randomized to receive open suctioning. The catheter, which becomes contaminated from the ETT or secretions in the patient's lower respiratory tract, must be properly rinsed after each use. Manufacturers of the device recommend that they be changed at regular intervals; however, they do not dictate the time interval. The catheter is an extension of the ventilator circuit. Ventilator circuits do not have to be changed at regular intervals for infection control purposes; therefore, possibly the CTSS does not either. Studies show no difference in pneumonia rates between patients randomized to receive daily changes versus those for whom no routine changes were performed or when the CTSS was changed daily versus weekly. As with ventilator circuits, the maximum duration that CTSS can be used safely is not known; however, they do not have to be changed daily. The current community standard based on comments received on an Internet discussion group appears to be 7 days. Changing the catheter every 7 days also results in considerable cost savings.

Some caregivers believe they cannot remove secretions as effectively with the CTSS because they do not vigorously manually ventilate the patient, which they believe loosens secretions and stimulates cough. Much of this so-called feeling could be the loss of audible feedback that the caregiver receives with open suction and because it is slightly more difficult to visualize secretions through the catheter sleeve. With the CTSS, cough can still be stimulated with the catheter. The purpose of manually ventilating the patient with open suctioning is hyperinflation. With the CTSS, hyperinflation can be performed with the ventilator.

Suction effectiveness is improved by appropriately setting the suction regulator and by *straight* withdrawal of the catheter to prevent kinking at the airway connection or at the suction control valve. Additional practical tips regarding the use of the CTSS are that gloves must always be worn (even though the system is closed) and the catheter must be fully withdrawn until the black mark is visible in the sheath. Partial occlusion of the airway with the catheter, when it is not properly withdrawn into its sheath, results in increased airway resistance and elevated peak airway pressures.

Suctioning in a closed system may result in negative airway pressures when suction flow rates exceed ventilator flow rates. This negative pressure may result in a loss of PEEP, reduction in oxygen supply to the lungs, atelectasis, and hypoxemia. These adverse effects are more likely to occur in the volume assist/control mode of ventilation and at lower tidal volumes. Gas delivery settings that maintain high gas flow in response to closed suction result in the least change in airway pressure. El Masry and colleagues evaluated the effect of closed suctioning on 11 critical care ventilators, during assisted ventilation in pressure and volume modes with two suctioning pressures. They concluded that closed suctioning does not cause ventilator malfunction, that all ventilators maintained gas delivery during suctioning, and that it does result in a decrease in PEEP. However, upon removal of the suction catheter, all ventilators resumed their presuctioning gas delivery within two breaths.

Cost effectiveness is a paramount concern in all health care settings. The CTSS costs more than a single open-system suction catheter set, and therefore if the patient requires only short-term ventilation (e.g., for rapid weaning postoperatively), a CTSS is not warranted. The CTSS is cost effective if the patient requires frequent suctioning. Savings may also be realized in lost charges because of the onetime charge, the saving of personnel time because it is not necessary to gather and set up supplies for each suctioning procedure, and the reduction in infection.

Endotracheal Suctioning Technique

Aseptic technique is imperative during ETS. The hands should be washed both before and after the procedure, and sterile gloves and a sterile suction catheter must be used. It is advisable that eye protection for the clinician be routine. Universal precautions should be adhered to during ETS.

The amount of negative pressure produced by the suction source should be adjusted to 100 to 150 mm Hg, but recommendations in the literature vary. To adjust the suction level, turn the suction source on, occlude the end of the suction tubing, and adjust the vacuum regulator until the dial reads between 100 and 150 mm Hg. As the vacuum regulator is adjusted from 40 to 200 mm Hg, suction flows generally vary from 10 to 30 L/min. Suctioning research has yet to define the ideal suction flow rate for secretion recovery. Furthermore, there is no simple method widely available for measuring suction flow.

Begin the procedure by preoxygenating the patient with 100% oxygen for 30 seconds and performing hyperinflation with three to five breaths. Insert the catheter gently until resistance is met, and then, to prevent the suction catheter from grabbing the mucosa, withdraw the catheter approximately 1 cm before applying suction. The greatest degree of tracheal trauma occurs at the point where the suction catheter meets tissue resistance, especially if suction is applied at this point. No suction is applied during insertion of the catheter into the airway to reduce hypoxemia and atelectasis induced by suctioning. However, Lewis suggested that the application of suction during entry of the catheter may serve the purpose of suctioning out of the airway any biofilm fragments that may be dislodged by the entry of the suction catheter. There is no research to support this practice. The duration of suction application affects the degree of suction-related hypoxemia, presumably because oxygen is also withdrawn from the lungs, along with secretions. Suction application should be limited to 10 seconds and may be continuous or intermittent. Results of research on continuous versus intermittent suction are inconclusive because of the variation in catheters used and the amount of suction applied. Both methods are damaging to the tracheal epithelium. Continuous suction may improve secretion removal but also increases the amount of air drawn from the patient's lungs, especially in a CTSS. Intermittent suction is recommended whenever the catheter may make contact with the mucosa, which occurs to a greater extent in nasopharyngeal suctioning. While the catheter is being removed, it should be twirled between the thumb and fingers so that the eyes of the catheter are exposed to a larger surface area and therefore remove more secretions.

Perform hyperoxygenation and hyperinflation (see later) between passes of the suction catheter. The amount of elapsed time between catheter passes depends on the patient's recovery, as evidenced by cardiopulmonary monitoring, but should minimally be 20 to 30 seconds. The catheter may be cleared of thick secretions with sterile water or normal saline solution between passes of the suction catheter. Most suction catheter kits contain a disposable expandable cup that can be used for this purpose. Clearing the catheter between passes improves suction effectiveness.

After the suctioning procedure is completed, the catheter is rinsed and may then be used to suction the patient's oral cavity and pharynx to remove any excess saliva and oropharyngeal secretions that have pooled on top of the ETT cuff. Care should be taken to avoid oral pharyngeal tissue trauma and gagging during suctioning. Although this practice is generally accepted, it is not known if it introduces microorganisms from the ETT that are not yet present in large numbers to other parts of the airway or whether this creates a reservoir for infection and reinfection of the lower airway. After the suction catheter is disconnected, the suction tubing should also be cleared of secretions with the remaining sterile solution or water. Finally, wrap the catheter around the fingers and pull the glove off inside out, leaving the catheter inside the glove. Dispose of properly.

HYPEROXYGENATION

A universal finding in studies is that hyperoxygenation before and after suctioning is the most critical variable in determining the postsuction PaO_2 and preventing hypoxemia during ETS. Hyperoxygenation may be performed with an MRB or the ventilator; however, no single technique for delivering 100% oxygen is defined as the standard, and further research is needed.

To achieve hyperoxygenation with a manual resuscitator bag (MRB), one must be sure that the bag is capable of delivering 100% oxygen (see Chapter 4). The highest FIO_2 concentrations are delivered in bags with reservoirs when the flow rate is set at 15 L/min and the rate of bag compression is adjusted to allow the reservoir to fill between breaths. Use of an MRB may be sufficient in patients with normal lung function but not in patients with abnormal lung function and dependence on a critical FIO_2 level.

Some ventilators have a 100% oxygen button to aid in the hyperoxygenation of patients before, during, and even after ETS. Factors to be aware of in regard to this ventilator feature are as follows: (1) All ventilators have a washout volume, the internal volume of the ventilator that must be flushed out before the delivered FIO_2 is actually 100%, and (2) the amount of time the ventilator is going to deliver the 100% oxygen varies. These factors must be taken into consideration in determining when to initiate and when to terminate ETS or reactivate the 100% oxygen feature. If the FIO_2 must be turned up *manually*, a time delay occurs before 100% oxygen is delivered to the patient because of the ventilator washout volume. It is critical that the clinician remembers to turn the FIO_2 setting back down to the baseline level after the suctioning procedure is completed.

HYPERINFLATION

Hyperinflation is the delivery of breaths that are larger than tidal volume. It is recommended as an additional mechanism to reduce suction-induced hypoxemia, although hyperoxygenation may be sufficient in many patients. Use of a bag may possibly improve the mobilization of secretions as well as the clinician's feel for the secretions in the airway. Hyperinflation should be used cautiously because of the hazards of overdistention injury. Hyperinflation may be performed with an MRB or the ventilator. When an MRB is used, the patient must be disconnected from the ventilator, which results in the loss of positive-pressure ventilation and PEEP. The volumes delivered with an MRB vary among individuals because of hand size and use of a one- versus two-handed technique. Rarely can an individual actually deliver hyperinflation volumes with an MRB when performing the procedure without an assistant. Use of one hand may result in volumes that are actually smaller than ventilator volumes. Alternating between suctioning and bagging may also result in contamination of the suction catheter. The rate of ventilation may be varied to meet the patient's inspiratory efforts, which may be increased because of the ETS procedure.

Ventilator hyperinflation is performed by activating the sigh feature. The use of a ventilator may be superior because the delivered volume and flow are precisely controlled and PEEP is maintained. The sigh feature should be used cautiously in patients with high peak airway pressures and tracheobronchial disruption, large pleural air leaks, or recent pulmonary surgery.

Hyperinflation is associated with increases in mean arterial pressure and mean airway pressure (possibly caused by technique). Because hyperinflation may have adverse effects in some patient populations, its use should be assessed on a case-by-case basis.

HYPERINFLATION COMBINED WITH HYPEROXYGENATION

In subjects with normal lung function, hyperoxygenation alone for three to five breaths may be sufficient to prevent hypoxemia related to ETS. Hyperinflation without hyperoxygenation is not an acceptable practice with critically ill patients because improved ventilation alone does not prevent suction-related hypoxemia. The combination of hyperinflation and hyperoxygenation with three to five breaths before ETS, between passes of the suction catheter, and after ETS consistently produces the greatest increase in PaO_2 in suctioning studies.

NORMAL SALINE INSTILLATION

The introduction of small amounts of sterile normal saline solution, usually 10 mL or less, is referred to as tracheal instillation or lavage and is a highly controversial practice. Normal saline instillation (NSI) is performed purportedly to dilute or loosen thick secretions and make their passage through the suction catheter easier and to stimulate cough. A controlled clinical trial that assesses the effectiveness of NSI and its adverse effects is needed because many of the studies lack controls and have a small number of subjects. A collaborative effort between nurses and respiratory therapists to perform this research would result in an evidence-based policy and procedure for both disciplines to follow. Surveys asking questions related to NSI with suctioning show that respiratory therapists are twice as likely as nurses to perform NSI with suctioning. Adverse effects of this practice are reported in both nursing and respiratory care literature. However, abandoning this practice is not yet recommended in both literature bases, likely because the practice is a long-held tradition in many settings and there are no definitive reports that demonstrate this can be done without untoward effects (airway obstruction). Conversely, scientific data to support the physiologic benefit of this practice are lacking and risks are identified; therefore, its use as a routine practice should be discontinued. NSI should be strictly reserved for patients with thick secretions until more effective methods of secretion hydration, such as systemic hydration and adequate humidification of inspired gases, can be implemented. Following is a discussion of the proposed benefits and potential hazards of NSI.

Normal Saline Instillation Effect on Secretions

It is known that secretions are not liquefied or diluted by normal saline; in fact, saline and mucus in bulk forms are immiscible. The most effective way to reduce the viscosity of mucus is via systemic hydration. Supplemental humidification of inspired gases also reduces the drying effect of medical gases on the airways and on secretions.

Normal Saline Instillation Effect on Volume of Secretions Removed

Several studies have shown an increase in aspirate volume after NSI; however, the clinical significance is unclear because it is not known whether the increased weight is caused by the recovery of instilled saline or mucus. The aspiration of the lavage fluid itself may lead the practitioner to believe that an increased volume of secretions was removed. In regard to the distribution of NSI, research shows that it does not affect secretions beyond the main-stem bronchi. Normal saline solution that is not removed with the suction catheter may flow deeper into the airways; however, as a lavage technique, NSI is probably very poor. Bronchoalveolar lavage, along with bronchoscopy, is a superior technique (see the Bronchoscopy section, later).

Normal Saline Instillation as a Cough Stimulant

Observations that NSI stimulates cough were reported in the literature for many years. Patients often respond with a vigorous cough that may mobilize secretions to the large airways, where they are subsequently suctioned out. The presence of the catheter in the trachea can induce coughing and may stimulate bronchospasm in patients with reactive airways. Because the suction catheter itself induces cough, NSI is not routinely recommended for this purpose. As a vigorous stimulant of cough, NSI may be deleterious in some patient populations, such as patients with increased ICP. Vigorous coughing could also potentially damage surgical wounds.

Effect of Normal Saline Instillation on Oxygenation

Ackerman reports that saline instillation during suctioning has a statistically significant adverse effect on arterial oxygen situation at 2, 3, 4, and 5 minutes after suctioning in patients with pulmonary infections. The desaturation worsened over time up to the 5-minute measurement, the longest parameter used. The majority of the work on the effect of NSI on oxygenation has focused on oxygen supply. One study by Kinloch assessed mixed venous oxygen saturation ($S\bar{v}O_2$) in a group of postoperative cardiac bypass patients. The $S\bar{v}O_2$ nadir was significantly lower in the NSI group than in the non-NSI group. The $S\bar{v}O_2$ recovery time was also significantly longer, requiring an average of 3.8 minutes longer to return to baseline in the NSI group. Although there were limitations to the study, these results demonstrate the potential harm that NSI can have on critically ill patients. Several other studies showed no significant differences in SaO_2 between the NSI and non-NSI groups. Because NSI is thought to improve secretion removal, there should be evidence of improved oxygenation after suctioning, not the contrary; therefore the findings of these studies do not support a physiologic benefit of NSI on oxygenation. Indeed, instilling a bolus of fluid into the airway may present a potential barrier to gas exchange. Because not all of the normal saline is returned in the aspirate, it is possible that the normal saline solution migrates into the airways and increases intrapulmonary shunt, thereby worsening oxygenation.

Potential of Normal Saline Instillation to Increase Infection

Within hours of intubation, a biofilm composed of white blood cells, bacteria, and polysaccharides forms within the ETT. This bacteria-rich biofilm is highly resistant to antibiotic and host-immune factor penetration. The presence of biofilm is an important consideration in the planning and evaluating care of the intubated patient, especially because prevention of bacterial infection is an important goal of any airway clearance technique. Hagler and Traver demonstrated that passing a suction catheter through the ETT can disrupt the biofilm, releasing up to 60,000 colonies of bacteria into the airway. NSI increased the number of colonies dislodged to 320,000. Washing organisms from the ETT to be aspirated into the lower respiratory tract can result in pneumonia or exacerbation of airway inflammation. Although it is important to look at the short-term effects of an airway clearance technique on pulmonary mechanics, SaO_2, and volume of secretion removed, it is critical that the analysis include the possible effects of increased infection inherent to the technique. The risk of increased infection with NSI is a significant concern.

PATIENT MONITORING DURING ENDOTRACHEAL SUCTIONING

Continuous arterial saturation with a pulse oximeter is the optimal method of assessing the potential for hypoxemia during ETS. In the ICU, all patients have cardiac monitors to allow assessment of heart rate, rhythm, and hemodynamic pressure effects of ETS. When an ICP monitor is present, the effect of the suction procedure on ICP should be closely monitored and used to gauge the timing/continuation of the procedure. Continuous monitoring of $S\bar{v}O_2$ allows assessment of the balance between oxygen supply and demand during ETS. Suctioning stimulates the sympathetic nervous system. Oxygen consumption may increase and $S\bar{v}O_2$ may decrease, despite increases in arterial oxygen saturation (SaO_2), especially in patients with a high oxygen demand or diminished cardiac reserve at baseline. Visual inspection of the patient for color and psychological tolerance should be performed throughout the procedure. The sputum aspirated should be assessed for color, volume, and consistency. After the procedure, the patient should be assessed for suction effectiveness by auscultation of breath sounds, SpO_2, peak airway pressure, and respiratory rate and pattern.

High-Frequency Chest Wall Oscillation

High-frequency oscillation is another method that can be used to facilitate secretion removal. Devices may apply oscillatory forces at the airway or across the chest. When the oscillatory forces are applied across the chest wall, the therapy is called high-frequency chest wall oscillation (HFCWO). The system to deliver HFCWO requires two parts: (1) a nonstretch inflatable vest that covers the patient's entire torso, and (2) an air-pulse generator (Fig. 5-8). Pulses of air fill the vest and can be applied to the chest wall throughout the respiratory cycle or at times chosen by the operator, such as only during the expiratory phase, through a foot pump control. Pulse frequency is adjustable from 5 to 25 Hz. As the Hz are increased, the pressure in the vest ranges from 28 mm Hg at 5 Hz to 39 mm Hg at 25 Hz.

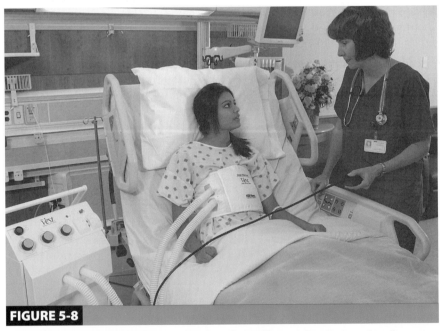

FIGURE 5-8

Therapy vest used for high-frequency chest wall oscillation. Therapeutic system consists of an inflatable vest connected by tubes to an air-pulse generator. *(Courtesy of Hill-Rom, Batesville, Ind.)*

HFCWO techniques were discovered by chance during research on high-frequency ventilation. The volume of the secretions at the upper airway was observed to be increased when high-frequency pulsatile gas flow at 3 to 30 Hz was applied. Enhanced tracheal mucus clearance seen during high-frequency oscillation (HFO) appears to occur as a result of shearing at the air–mucus interface. The changes in airflow with each high-frequency cycle are believed to produce a coughlike force to the mucus layer. Repeatedly applied it mimics ciliary beating, nudging the mucus layer upward toward the larger airways and trachea, where it can be cleared by coughing or suctioning. The majority of studies on HFCWO had patients with cystic fibrosis as the subjects. These studies demonstrated that vest therapy is more effective than postural drainage for secretion clearance. In the acute care setting the therapy is generally well tolerated. With appropriate application HFCWO therapy does not dislodge or disrupt invasive equipment or surgical drains. Vest therapy treats all lobes of the lungs simultaneously and consistently and does not require positioning or breathing techniques. Since less caregiver assistance is required the risk of repetitive motion injury is eliminated.

HFCWO vest devices that are approved for sputum clearance and induction were originally designed for self-administered therapy. As stated earlier, the device consists of a large-volume variable-frequency air-pulse delivery system attached to a nonstretchable inflatable vest that extends over the entire torso down to the iliac crest. The wrap vest used in the acute care setting is disposable and comes in sizes ranging from small to extra large to accommodate patients with chest circumferences ranging from 23 to 67 inches. The vest is placed two finger breadths below the axilla and the Velcro is secured at maximum inspiration. Patients typically are administered 10- to 20-minute therapy sessions at two different oscillatory frequencies, the second setting being 2 Hz higher than the first. Optimal frequencies for clearance by HFCWO are in the range of 10 to 15 Hz. Therefore a patient may start at 10 Hz for 10 minutes and then advance to 12 Hz for another 10 minutes. Between these two frequencies the patient should cough and be suctioned as necessary. In addition to the Hz setting, an oscillatory pressure is set between 1 and 4. Pressure should be set at the highest level that is comfortable for the patient. The sensitivity setting on the ventilator may need to be adjusted to prevent ventilator self-cycling. Opinions vary regarding whether the therapist should remain in attendance throughout the entire treatment. Assessment of patient individual response should dictate the required amount of vigilance. Treatments may be administered one to six times per day depending on assessment of need and clinical response.

Chest Physiotherapy

Chest physiotherapy (CPT) encompasses the techniques of postural drainage, percussion, and vibration. The evidence does not support the use of percussion and vibration independent of active postural drainage. Slow deep breaths, forced expiration, huffing, coughing, or suctioning should also always accompany CPT so that the mobilized secretions can be expelled. CPT may be performed by nurses, respiratory therapists, physical therapists, or other appropriately trained personnel. The purposes of these procedures are to prevent the accumulation of secretions, to mobilize

> **BOX 5-1** Chest Physiotherapy: Therapeutic Considerations
>
> 1. Before chest physiotherapy (CPT) is started, the patient should be positioned comfortably. Support may be provided by pillows, blankets, rolled towels, foam wedges, or other available supplies.
>
> 2. The patient should be maintained on the same amount of supplemental oxygen received before postural drainage. The F_{IO_2} may be increased if a particular position adversely affects oxygenation. If oxygenation remains decreased, the position should be modified or the therapy aborted.
>
> 3. The patient should take slow, deep breaths throughout the therapy.
>
> 4. Premedicate the patient with pain medication as necessary.
>
> 5. Coughing and/or suctioning should be used throughout the treatment as necessary to remove mobilized secretions.
>
> 6. Tube feedings and/or oral intake should be held for 30 minutes to 1 hour before the treatment is initiated.
>
> 7. Appropriate monitoring as determined by the patient's severity of illness and relative stability should be instituted. Monitor the neurologic, cardiovascular, and respiratory systems for evidence of cardiorespiratory compromise.
>
> 8. Examine the secretions produced for color, consistency, texture, odor, and amount.
>
> 9. Evaluate the effectiveness of the CPT through assessment of the following: chest x-ray film, work of breathing, dyspnea, breath sounds, sputum production, lung volumes, Pa_{O_2}, and measures of intrapulmonary shunt.

retained secretions, and to reduce airway obstruction, thereby reducing intrapulmonary shunt and improving oxygenation.

Postural drainage has little or no effect in conditions with scant secretions. Postural drainage, along with the manual techniques of percussion and vibration, is beneficial in disease processes in which sputum production is large or its removal is impeded. In these patients, secretion retention persists despite deep breathing and coughing. Radiologic evidence of obstructive atelectasis caused by mucus plugging of airways (segmental collapse) is another condition that responds to CPT. Specific indications for CPT encompass a number of clinical problems. Patients who are on prolonged bed rest, are paralyzed or unconscious, have neuromuscular disease, have an inhalation injury or multiple-system trauma, or have undergone abdominal or thoracic surgery may be candidates for CPT. Again, CPT is of little or no benefit in patients with minimal secretions but may be indicated when the mucociliary escalator and the cough mechanism have been inadequate in removing pulmonary secretions (Box 5-1).

POSTURAL DRAINAGE

Postural drainage (PD) is the technique of using various body positions to promote the flow of secretions toward the larger airways, where the secretions can then be coughed up or suctioned out. PD takes advantage of the effect of gravity on the flow of mucus. Various body positions, based on an understanding of normal pulmonary anatomy, are used to promote drainage of specific lobar segments (Fig. 5-9 [see pp. 172-173]). The affected area is placed in the most upright position, superior to the carina, in an effort to promote drainage of the lung segment by achieving an optimal gravitational effect on mucus flow. The position to be used with a specific patient is determined by x-ray and auscultatory findings. Positions may need to be modified as indicated by deteriorating neurologic, cardiac, or pulmonary assessment data, by position contraindications secondary to trauma or surgery, or by the presence of tubes or drains. Intermittently the patient should be assisted to cough or suctioned to remove the mobilized secretions. Mobilized secretions can gravitate into nondiseased lung segments, necessitating therapy in these areas as well.

PD requires a sufficient drainage time of 5 to 15 minutes for each position drained and is effective as a technique only if applied with attention to detail. The length of time that a position should be maintained is variable and depends on a balance between achievement of therapeutic effect and patient tolerance. Important to note is that drainage of a position for less than 5 minutes shows no advantage over controls. Therefore, a considerable time investment is required to achieve satisfactory results if multiple segments require drainage. Even if all factors are positively applied, PD has limited benefit in most patients. Two groups appear to benefit from this therapy: patients with cystic fibrosis and those who have difficulty clearing large quantities of sputum.

Evaluation of therapeutic effect should include assessment of volume of sputum production and improvement in breath sounds and chest x-ray. If properly applied PD does not increase sputum production, continuation of its use should be reevaluated. Conversely, if secretion clearance is improved during PD, continued therapy is supported.

PERCUSSION

Percussion is a technique used in conjunction with PD to promote the advancement of secretions toward the larger airways. It can be performed manually with cupped hands or with mechanical devices. Manual percussion is performed by rhythmically and alternately clapping cupped hands (Fig. 5-10) over the relevant area of lung. The cupping of the hands creates a cushion of air, which reduces the force of impact. The action should produce a hollow popping sound, not a slapping one. The shoulders and elbows remain relaxed so that the rhythmic movement is generated from the wrists. Theoretically, the effect of percussion is the transmission of energy waves through the chest, which shakes and vibrates secretions, loosening them, thus aiding in their removal. There is no evidence that percussion alone without positioning is of any value. Clinicians should not interpret an order for CPT to mean percussion without positioning.

Some critical care beds offer the option of a percussion module that allows the practitioner to administer percussion therapy to the patient through the bed itself. With this method, percussion is applied to the dependent lung segments as opposed to the most superior lung segment, which is the principle of CPT. Evidence supporting this application of percussion is lacking. Bed and other forms of percussion often feel good to the patient, which may be a convincing reason to consider applying these techniques.

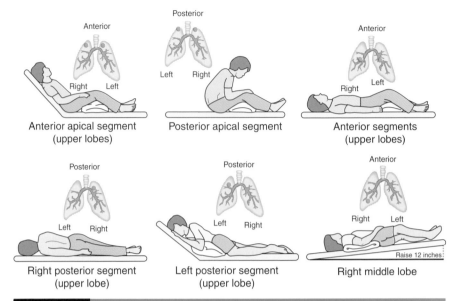

FIGURE 5-9

Body positions used for postural drainage. *Apical segments of right and left upper lobes:* Patient in semi-Fowler's position with the head of bed (HOB) raised 45 degrees. *Posterior apical segment:* Patient sitting upright and leaning forward. *Anterior segments of upper lobes:* Patient supine with the bed flat. *Posterior segment of right upper lobe:* Patient one-quarter turn from prone with the right side up, supported by pillows, HOB flat. *Apical posterior segment of LUL:* Patient one-quarter turn from supine with left side up supported by pillows, with the HOB elevated 30 degrees. *Right middle lobe:* Patient one-quarter turn from supine with right side up and foot of bed (FOB) elevated 12 inches. *(Modified from RL Wilkins, JK Stoller, CL Scanlan (eds.), Egan's Fundamentals of Respiratory Care, 8th ed. St. Louis: Mosby, 2003.)*

The traditional method of delivering percussion with the cupped hand is effective; however, it can be tiring for the person administering the therapy. As a result, several companies have produced various mechanical or electrical devices for delivering therapy. These percussors may operate manually, pneumatically, or electrically. Manual percussors are made of soft vinyl and shaped like a palm to ensure the correct air cushion is applied, therefore minimizing patient discomfort from improper hand position. Pneumatically and electrically powered devices may come with a variety of accessories and offer the ability to vary the force of percussive strokes. Manual methods offer no advantage over mechanical.

Percussion should be performed directly on the chest wall and not over a towel or other covering, as some clinicians advocate. The use of a covering requires that greater force be applied to achieve the same effect, and the air cushion is lost in the covering. Furthermore, anatomic landmarks are not visible, nor is the presence of erythema, petechiae, subcutaneous emphysema, or other indicators that the therapy should be discontinued or altered. Table 5-1 outlines the precautionary factors that need to be considered before the initiation of postural drainage with percussion.

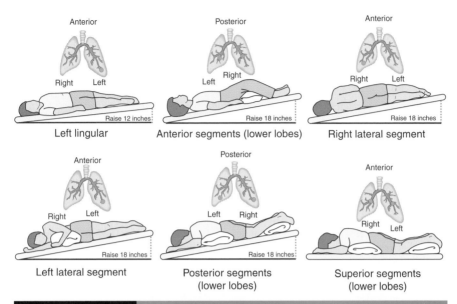

Anterior — Left lingular — Raise 12 inches

Posterior — Anterior segments (lower lobes) — Raise 18 inches

Anterior — Right lateral segment — Raise 18 inches

Anterior — Left lateral segment — Raise 18 inches

Posterior — Posterior segments (lower lobes) — Raise 18 inches

Anterior — Superior segments (lower lobes)

FIGURE 5-9, cont'd

Body positions used for postural drainage, cont'd. *Left lingular*: Patient one-quarter turn from supine with left side up and FOB elevated 12 inches.

Anterior segments of lower lobes: Patient supine with FOB elevated 18 inches.

Right lateral segment: Patient 90 degrees to the left, right side up, and FOB elevated 18 inches.

Left lateral segment: Patient 90 degrees to the right, left side up, and FOB elevated 18 inches.

Posterior segments of lower lobes: Patient prone with FOB elevated 18 inches.

Superior segments of lower lobes: Patient prone with HOB flat and pillow under the abdominal area.

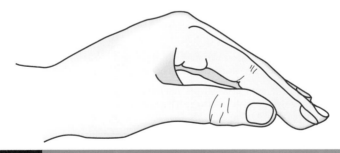

FIGURE 5-10

Cupped position of the hand used for percussion. The thumb and index finger are pinched together; the fingers are then extended, held together, and flexed at a 90-degree angle to the palm of the hand. Incorrect hand position results in a slapping sound, whereas correct hand position results in a hollow, popping sound.

TABLE 5-1 Chest Physiotherapy: Precautionary Factors

Precaution	Rationale
Recent MI and CHF, dysrhythmias	HR and BP may rise, increasing myocardial oxygen demand. Head-down position increases central blood volume, which may not be tolerated in CHF. Restrict to patients who can be monitored closely.
Recent craniotomy or head trauma	Administer CPT (including use of varying degrees of Trendelenburg position) cautiously and only with appropriate monitoring of ICP and CPP. Administer sedation and maintain neck alignment. Restrict to patients with clear benefit and modify therapy as necessary. Head-down position is contraindicated in unrepaired cerebral aneurysm.
Unstable spine injuries or recent spinal surgery	Placing the entire bed in the head-down position while maintaining spinal alignment may be used. Care must be taken not to put stress on recent spinal fusions. Use must be individualized.
Hypoxemia that worsens with body position changes, extreme dyspnea	Monitor patients closely with continuous real-time monitoring (e.g., pulse oximetry). Modify positions as necessary.
Lung abscess	Postural drainage and percussion are therapies of choice. Discontinue if frank hemoptysis occurs. Have suction available to prevent asphyxiation from rapid dislodgment of a large volume of pus. There is risk of spillover of contaminated material into uncontaminated area, with consequent spread of infection.
Pulmonary contusion	May assist in clearing blood and thus reducing this potential bacterial growth medium. Contraindicated in concomitant coagulopathy.
Frank hemoptysis (active or recent)	Percussion and vibration are contraindicated because they may worsen bleeding and dislodge clots. CPT may be given cautiously in conditions in which modest blood streaking is present.
Rib fracture and flail chest, osteoporosis	May be performed by an experienced therapist while monitoring for rib shift or any other motion. When properly performed, percussion may apply less pressure than coughing or lying on the injury. Positive-pressure ventilation may promote internal stabilization of the area.
Subcutaneous emphysema	Monitor for and report any increase in subcutaneous air. When no chest tubes are present, CPT should be held until pneumothorax is ruled out.
Asthma and/or bronchospasm	An inhaled bronchodilator may be given 10 to 20 minutes before CPT.
Chest tubes, vascular lines, artificial airways, incisions	Extreme care must be used not to dislodge lines, drains, or airways. Administer gentle percussion or vibration around incisions and chest tubes.
Tube feedings	Gastric tube feedings should be held for 1 hour before CPT. Small bowel (duodenal/jejunal) feedings may continue if there is no gastric reflux.

BP, Blood pressure; *CHF,* congestive heart failure; *CPP,* cerebral perfusion pressure; *CPT,* chest physiotherapy; *HR,* heart rate; *ICP,* intracranial pressure; *MI,* myocardial infarction.

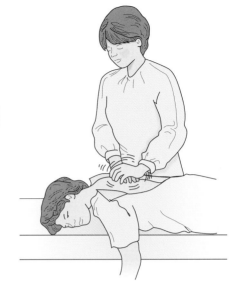

FIGURE 5-11

Chest vibration.

VIBRATION

Chest vibration is used in conjunction with PD. It may be used as an alternative to percussion, particularly around surgical incisions, where it may be more comfortable. It is performed by placing the flat of the hands over the chest wall of the affected lung area and vibrating the hands quickly with a fine tremorous action during the *expiratory* phase of the respiratory cycle (Fig. 5-11). The vibration is superficial and creates an oscillatory movement that is reflected to the deep tissues, thereby assisting in the loosening of mucus and promoting its flow. The procedure should follow a maximal inspiration, which can be facilitated in the patient supported by mechanical ventilation with the delivery of a large breath with a manual resuscitator bag or sighing with the ventilator. If the procedure is performed correctly, the patient has spurts of exhaled air. Mechanical vibrators, which were originally introduced for home care, are available, but they show no clear advantage over manual vibration.

Bronchoscopy

The bronchoscope may be used for therapeutic as well as diagnostic purposes. There are two types of bronchoscopes: rigid and flexible. The use of the rigid bronchoscope is limited to the operating room under general anesthesia. The flexible bronchoscope is used in the ICU setting by the intensivist, surgeon, or pulmonologist because it has many advantages over the rigid scope. This section is limited to discussion of the flexible bronchoscope.

The bronchoscope consists of a rigid hand piece and a flexible extension that averages 55 to 60 cm long. The hand piece contains a viewfinder lens, a thumb lever for flexion and extension of the tip, a finger-activated suction valve, an instrument port, and a site where suction is connected (Fig. 5-12). Visualization of the airways

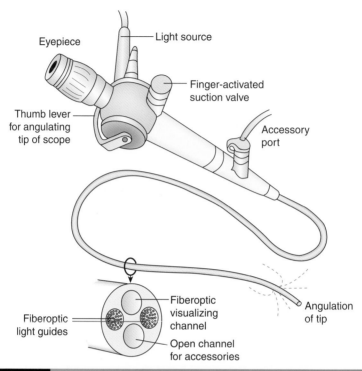

FIGURE 5-12

Component parts of the flexible fiberoptic bronchoscope.

is provided by fiberoptics. The bronchoscope must also be connected to a light source. The bronchoscopy procedure may be performed nasally, orally, or through an endotracheal or tracheostomy tube. The flexible scope provides much greater visualization than the rigid one because it can be advanced to the third or fourth division of the segmental bronchi. The bronchoscope is portable, and the procedure can be easily performed at the patient's bedside, which eliminates the risks inherent in transporting the patient. A portable cart, set up with all the necessary procedural supplies, improves efficiency.

Therapeutic indications for bronchoscopy include removal of aspirated foreign bodies, especially those beyond the reach of a rigid bronchoscope; secretion retention not responsive to less invasive therapies, including CPT, because the bronchoscope can be used to aspirate thick secretions or an abscess; and facilitation of endotracheal intubation. Endotracheal intubation is performed by inserting the bronchoscope through the ETT, advancing the bronchoscope through the glottic opening, and then passing the ETT over the bronchoscope. *Diagnostic indications* for bronchoscopy include acquisition of specimens, biopsy in distal airways, and inspection of the airways, such as in the presence of a mass, a tracheobronchial injury, or hemoptysis.

BRONCHOSCOPY PROCEDURE

During the bronchoscopy procedure, all members of the team should wear a mask, eye protection, and gloves. Protective gowns may also be worn. Prepare the patient who is taking food by mouth by withholding the diet for 6 hours. If the patient is receiving gastric, duodenal, or jejunal tube feedings, hold the feeding for 1 hour and, as an extra precautionary measure, aspirate the stomach contents (if a gastric tube is in place) before initiating the procedure. Instruct the patient on what to expect and how to cooperate with the procedure. Appropriate laboratory studies should be obtained, including coagulation studies, if a biopsy is to be performed.

Prepare for the procedure by gathering all necessary supplies, including medications. Various drugs may be used, including a drying agent such as atropine or topical anesthetics such as 1%, 2%, or 4% lidocaine, cocaine, or Cetacaine, which is a solution of benzocaine and tetracaine used to suppress the gag reflex in non-intubated patients. An analgesic or sedative such as fentanyl, morphine, diazepam, or midazolam is also generally administered. Diazepam and midazolam have the additional benefit of providing the patient with amnesia of the event. Ensure that the patient has a reliable intravenous access for administration of medication or fluids should hypotension occur.

The patient should be monitored throughout and after the procedure to detect any complications early. Minimal monitoring should include pulse oximetry, electrocardiography, and monitoring of the heart rate and blood pressure. The individual performing the bronchoscopy may become absorbed in the procedure; therefore, the assistant is responsible for monitoring the patient and informing the physician of any patient problems. After the procedure, the patient should be monitored for successful recovery. If a biopsy was performed, the presence of increasingly bloody sputum may indicate bleeding.

Patients undergoing mechanical ventilation should receive 100% oxygen throughout the procedure, and in patients supported by PEEP, a bronchoscopy adapter should be used to avoid loss of PEEP. Auto-PEEP may develop because of the resistance to exhalation created by the bronchoscope as it partially occludes the airway. The peak airway pressure alarms may need to be reset to a higher limit because airway pressure rises as the bronchoscope creates an increased resistance to airflow. So that a lower peak airway pressure can be maintained during the procedure, the tidal volume and flow rate may be decreased while the respiratory rate is concurrently increased, thus maintaining a steady minute ventilation. Exhaled tidal volumes and minute ventilation should be monitored for their adequacy, and the tidal volume should be titrated to maintain a sufficient minute ventilation.

SPECIMENS

Various specimens may be obtained during the bronchoscopy procedure. Bronchial washings are the aspirate obtained as the scope is passed through the airways. They may or may not be sent for culture because they may be contaminated with upper airway flora. The physician may prevent contamination by not applying suction until the lower airways are reached.

A double-sheathed brush catheter is used for obtaining sterile bacterial cultures. The brush is enclosed in a sheath as it is advanced through the bronchoscope to the area in question. The brush is then advanced beyond the sheath to obtain the specimen. It is then withdrawn back into the protective sheath, and the whole thing is removed from the bronchoscope.

For bronchoalveolar lavage (BAL), the distal airway is occluded by wedging the bronchoscope tip in the airway and then instilling 20- to 30-mL aliquots of nonbacteriostatic normal saline solution. The fluid is then aspirated into a suction trap. Microbiologic tests are run on the aspirate. BAL is useful for determining the cause of lung infections.

Endobronchial biopsy may also be performed with a variety of needle or forceps appliances.

COMPLICATIONS

When bronchoscopy is performed by a skilled bronchoscopist and with appropriate monitoring, complications are rare. Complications that should be considered include bronchospasm, vasovagal response, postprocedure fever, bleeding, cardiac dysrhythmias, and pneumothorax caused by the development of excessive airway pressures or inadvertent pleural biopsy.

When bronchoscopy is performed on intubated patients, interference with ventilation may occur because the bronchoscope creates resistance to ventilation. A cuffed airway of at least 8.0 mm (inside diameter) may result in less compromise in airflow and tidal volume. Use of a swivel bronchoscope adapter allows mechanical ventilation to continue throughout the procedure. Hypoxemia and cardiac dysrhythmias may occur and may possibly be caused by mechanical obstruction of the airway and/or increased intrapulmonary shunt caused by lavage solutions. Interventions directed toward preventing these complications include increasing the FIO_2, flow rate, or tidal volume; limiting the amount of lavage used; and limiting the duration of suction application.

RECOMMENDED READINGS

Ackerman MH. Instillation of normal saline before suctioning in patients with pulmonary infections: A prospective randomized controlled trial. *Am J Crit Care* 1998; 7(4):261–266.

Ahrens T, Kollef M, Stewart J, et al. Effect of kinetic therapy on pulmonary complications. *Am J Crit Care* 2004; 13:376–383.

Allen JS, Garrity JM, Donahue DM. The utility of high-frequency chest wall oscillation therapy in the post-operative management of thoracic surgical patients. *Chest* 2003; 124(Suppl 4):235SG.

Blackwood B. Normal saline instillation with endotracheal suctioning: *Primum non nocere* (first do not harm). *J Adv Nurs* 1999; 29(4):928–934.

Burns SM, Egloff MB, Ryan B, et al. Effect of body position on spontaneous respiratory rate and tidal volume in patients with obesity, abdominal distention, and ascites. *Am J Crit Care* 1994; 3(2):102–106.

Choi SC, Nelson LD. Kinetic therapy in critically ill patients: Combined results based on meta-analysis. *J Crit Care* 1992; 7(1):57–62.

Chulay M. Suctioning: Endotracheal or tracheostomy tube. In DJ Lynn-Hale Weigand, KK Carlson (eds.), *AACN Procedure Manual for Critical Care*, 5th ed. (pp. 62–70). St. Louis: Saunders, 2002.

Combes P, Fauvage B, Oleyer C. Nosocomial pneumonia in mechanically ventilated patients, a prospective randomised evaluation of the Steri-Cath closed suctioning system. *Intensive Care Med* 2000; 26(7):878–882.

Curley MAQ: Prone positioning of patient with acute respiratory distress syndrome: A systematic review. *Am J Crit Care* 1999; 8:397-405.

Drakulovic MB, Torres A, Baur TT, et al. Supine body position as a risk factor for nosocomial pneumonia in mechanically ventilated patients: A randomized trial. *Lancet* 1999; 354:1851–1858.

El Masry, A, Williams PF, Chipman DW, et al. The impact of closed endotracheal suctioning systems on mechanical ventilator performance. *Respir Care* 2005; 50(3):345–353.

Faling LJ. Chest physical therapy. In GG Burton, JE Hodgkin, JJ Ward (eds.), *Respiratory Care: A Guide to Clinical Practice* (pp. 625–654). Philadelphia: JB Lippincott, 1991.

Fink JB. Positioning versus postural drainage. *Respir Care* 2002; 47(7):769–777.

Fink JB. Positive pressure techniques for airway clearance. *Respir Care* 2002; 47(7):786–796.

Fink JB, Mahlmeister MJ. High-frequency oscillation of the airway and chest wall. *Respir Care* 2002; 47(7):797–807.

Fink MP, Helsmoortel CM, Stein KL, et al. The efficacy of an oscillating bed in the prevention of lower respiratory tract infection in critically ill victims of blunt trauma. *Chest*, 1990; 97:132-137.

Gattinoni L, Gianni T, Pedenti A, et al. Effect of prone positioning on survival of patients with acute respiratory failure. *N Engl J Med* 2001; 345(8):568–573.

Gray JE, MacIntryre NR, Kronenberger WG. The effects of bolus normal saline instillation in conjunction with endotracheal suctioning. *Respir Care* 1990; 35:785–790.

Hagler DA, Traver GA. Endotracheal saline and suction catheters: Sources of lower airway contamination. *Am J Crit Care* 1994; 396:444–447.

Hanley MV, Rudd T, Butler J. What happens to intratracheal saline instillations? [abstract]. *Am Rev Respir Dis* 1978; 117(Suppl.):124.

Hess DR. Managing the artificial airway. *Respir Care* 1999; 44(7):759–772.

Hess DR. The evidence for secretion clearance techniques. *Respir Care* 2001; 46(11):1276–1292.

Hess DR, Bigatello LM. Lung recruitment: The role of recruitment maneuvers. *Respir Care* 2002; 47(3):308–317.

Hess DR, Kallstrom TJ, Mottram CD, et al. Care of the ventilator circuit and its relation to ventilator-associated pneumonia. *Respir Care* 2003; 48(9):869–879.

Kacmarek RM, Dimas S, Mack CW. *The Essentials of Respiratory Care,* 4th ed. St. Louis: Mosby, 2005.

Keane FX. The minimum physiological mobility requirement for man supported on a soft surface. *Paraplegia* 1978–1979; 16:383–389.

Lewis RM. Airway clearance techniques for the patient with an artificial airway. *Respir Care* 2002; 47(7):808–817.

Mackenzie CF, Imle PC, Ciesla N. *Chest Physiotherapy in the Intensive Care Unit.* Baltimore: Williams & Wilkins, 1989.

Mancinelli-Van Atta J, Beck SL. Preventing hypoxemia and hemodynamic compromise related to endotracheal suctioning. *Am J Crit Care* 1992; 1(3):62–79.

McQuillan KA. The effects of the Trendelenburg position for postural drainage on cerebrovascular status in head-injured patients [abstract]. *Heart Lung* 1987; 16(3):327.

Messerole E, Peine P, Wittkopp S, et al. The pragmatics of prone positioning. *Am J Respir Crit Care Med 2002;* 165:1359–1363.

Myslinski MJ, Scanian CL. Bronchial hygiene therapy. In RL Wilkins, JK Stoller, CL Scanlan (eds.), *Egan's Fundamental of Respiratory Care,* 8th ed. (pp. 883–906). St. Louis: Mosby, 2003.

Pelosi P, Brazzi L, Gattinoni L. Prone position in ARDS. *Eur Respir J* 2002; 20:1017–1028.

Raoof S, Chowdhrey N, Raoof S, et al. Effect of combined kinetic therapy and percussion therapy on the resolution of atelectasis in critically ill patients. *Chest* 1999; 115:1658–1666

Richard J-C, Maggiore S, Mercat A. Where are we with recruitment maneuvers in patients with acute lung injury and acute respiratory distress syndrome? *Curr Opin Crit Care* 2003; 9:22–27.

Schwenker D, Ferrin M, Gist AG. A survey of endotracheal suctioning with instillation of normal saline. *Am J Crit Care* 1998; 7(4):255–231.

Sole ML, Byers JF, Ludy JE, et al. A multisite survey of suctioning techniques and airway management practices. *Am J Crit Care* 2003; 12 (3):220–232.

Sorenson HM, Shelledy DC, and the 2003 CPG Steering Committee. AARC clinical practice guideline: Intermittent positive pressure breathing—2003 revision & update. *Respir Care* 2003; 48(5):540–545.

Stoller JK, Orens DK, Fatica C, et al. Weekly versus daily changes of in-line suction catheters: Impact on rates of ventilator-associated pneumonia and associated costs. *Respir Care* 2003; 48(5):494–499.

Vollman KM. Prone positioning in the patient who has acute respiratory distress syndrome: the art and science. *Crit Care Nurs Clin N Am,* 2004; 16:319-336.

Vollman KM. Pronation therapy. In DJ Lynn-Hale Weigand, KK Carlson (eds.), *AACN Procedure Manual for Critical Care,* 5th ed. (pp. 108–120). St. Louis: Saunders, 2005.

CHAPTER 6

Mechanical Ventilation: Indications, Ventilator Performance of the Respiratory Cycle, and Initiation

INDICATIONS FOR MECHANICAL VENTILATION

The primary indication for mechanical ventilation is impending or existing respiratory failure despite maximal treatment. Its use is also indicated after major surgery while the patient is recovering from general anesthesia and in cardiogenic shock to decrease the oxygen cost of breathing at a time of severely reduced cardiac output.

Acute Respiratory Failure

Respiratory failure is the absence of the normal homeostatic state of ventilation as it relates to acid–base status of the blood and the exchange of oxygen and carbon dioxide. Therefore, the candidates for mechanical ventilation are those patients whose lungs can no longer provide an adequate exchange of gases. This inadequacy is reflected in the patient's blood gases. Following is an objective clinical definition of respiratory failure:

A Pa_{O_2} of less than 60 mm Hg on an F_{IO_2} of more than 0.5 (oxygenation)

A Pa_{CO_2} greater than 50 mm Hg, with a pH of 7.25 or less (ventilation)

It is difficult to place a threshold value on a failing oxygenation status because so many factors, such as age and previous history of lung disease, determine the acceptable Pa_{O_2} in any individual patient. It is more helpful to look at the trend of the patient's Pa_{O_2} with time and to determine whether deterioration is signifying respiratory failure. The ventilatory values just listed warn of life-threatening respiratory acidosis and respiratory failure. Clues to the presence of respiratory failure include an increasing respiratory rate, a decreasing tidal volume, an increase in the work of breathing (WOB) as evidenced by an increase in the use of the accessory muscles of ventilation and abnormal breathing patterns, and complaints of dyspnea.

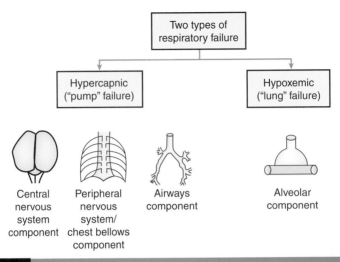

FIGURE 6-1

Acute respiratory failure may be divided into failure to oxygenate (hypoxemic failure) and failure to ventilate (hypercapnic failure). Hypercapnic failure may occur as a result of inability to sustain adequate ventilation by one or more of the three components of ventilation: the central nervous system, the peripheral nervous system innervating the muscles of ventilation, and the airways. Hypoxemic failure results from failure to exchange gases adequately at the alveolar level.

To make appropriate therapeutic decisions, the clinician should differentiate whether the patient has failure to ventilate, failure to oxygenate, or a combination of the two (Fig. 6-1). *Failure to ventilate*, also called ventilatory failure, hypercapnic respiratory failure, or respiratory pump failure, occurs when ventilatory demand exceeds ventilatory supply. Ventilatory demand is the minute ventilation required to maintain a normal or baseline $Paco_2$. Ventilatory supply is the maximal sustainable ventilation that a person can uphold without respiratory muscle fatigue. In disease, not only may ventilatory demand be increased but ventilatory supply may concurrently be markedly decreased, an imbalance that may result in respiratory failure. The primary cause of *failure to oxygenate*, also known as hypoxemic respiratory failure, is physiologic shunt (see Chapter 2). With shunt, the associated hypoxemia stimulates the respiratory drive, but because the ventilated oxygen is not interfacing with the pulmonary capillary, hypoxemia persists. Conservative measures such as the administration of supplemental oxygen may correct the hypoxemia; however, if it is not corrected, then a swift decision to mechanically ventilate must be made to prevent tissue hypoxia. Placing the patient on a ventilator allows for support of an increased ventilatory demand, the application of tidal volumes that will improve functional residual capacity, and the administration of therapies designed to improve oxygenation: high inspired oxygen concentrations and positive end-expiratory pressure (PEEP).

The decision to mechanically ventilate with or without intubation is based on sound clinical decision making after assessment of the patient's oxygenation, ventilation, and WOB. The decision is not an arbitrary one because of the complications associated with artificial airways and positive-pressure ventilation (see Chapter 9). The decision needs to include an evaluation of how invasive support has to be (because sufficient evidence exists to support the initial use of noninvasive positive-pressure ventilation when specific criteria are met) and how aggressive it has to be (i.e., total vs. partial support), and should constantly reevaluate how long the support is really needed.

Apnea and impending respiratory arrest remain general indications for ventilatory support. How impending respiratory arrest is defined involves judgment by the clinical team. Table 6-1 presents a classification of diseases that predispose a patient to respiratory failure. Such a classification is helpful because it offers insight into the pathophysiologic process underlying the failure and suggests suitable therapies. It must be remembered that the application of mechanical ventilation does not correct the underlying disorder. It only provides gas exchange support until the appropriate therapies, such as bronchial hygiene, diuretics, and administration of antibiotics, can be applied to cure the underlying disease.

POSITIVE-PRESSURE VENTILATION

As a comparison of how respiration is altered when a mechanical ventilator is used, review of the mechanics of normal, spontaneous respiration is important. Recall from Chapter 2 that the physiology of spontaneous respiration requires that energy be expended to contract the muscles of respiration. The contraction of the respiratory muscles enlarges the thoracic cavity, creates negative pressure within the chest, and results in the flow of air, at atmospheric pressure, into the lungs. It would be ideal if mechanical ventilators could mimic the mechanics and physiology of spontaneous respiration while achieving the goals of adequate oxygenation and ventilation. Indeed, negative-pressure ventilators attempt to do so. However, ventilators used in inpatient clinical settings are *positive*-pressure ventilators.

The positive-pressure ventilator uses a pneumatic system for delivery of gas into the lungs during inspiration. Expiration occurs passively during positive-pressure ventilation. The patient may exhale to atmospheric pressure or to a set level of PEEP.

In spontaneous breathing, no conscious effort is required to pass through the phases of a respiratory cycle: "inspire, end inspiration, expire, and begin a new inspiration." Imagine how tedious this would be! However, if a machine is to perform the respiratory cycle, it must be told, first, what the component phases of the respiratory cycle are and, second, how to carry out each of the phases as determined by the settings of the phase variables. Every ventilator has four basic phases that it must complete in providing a ventilatory cycle to the patient (Fig. 6-2):
1. Expiratory-inspiratory changeover
2. Inspiration
3. Inspiratory-expiratory changeover
4. Expiration

TABLE 6-1	Categories of Intrapulmonary and Extrapulmonary Disorders Predisposing to Respiratory Failure

Category	Examples
Disorders of the CNS associated with a reduced drive to breathe	Overdose of respiratory depressant drugs such as sedatives and narcotics Cerebrovascular accident Cerebral trauma Subarachnoid hemorrhage
Disorders associated with neuromuscular function*	Guillain-Barré syndrome Multiple sclerosis Poliomyelitis Myasthenia gravis Spinal cord injury Electrolyte disorders (hypophosphatemia, hypomagnesemia)
Disorders associated with musculoskeletal and pleural functions	Kyphoscoliosis Flail chest Pleural effusion Pneumothorax Hemothorax
Disorders of the conducting airways	Upper airway obstruction Epiglottitis Obstructive sleep apnea Postextubation laryngeal edema Asthma Bronchospasm
Disorders of the gas-exchanging units (alveoli and pulmonary capillaries)	Pulmonary contusion Pneumonia Pulmonary edema ARDS Aspiration Interstitial lung disease Near drowning Smoke inhalation

*Function of the peripheral nerves and muscles of ventilation.
ARDS, Adult respiratory distress syndrome; *CNS,* central nervous system.

Phase variables are responsible for each part of the breath and are manipulated by the operator. They provide the ventilator with the necessary information to carry out the phase. The variable that initiates inspiration is the *trigger variable.* The *limit variable* places a maximum value on the parameter chosen to be controlled during inspiration, which could be pressure, volume, flow, or time. The *cycle variable* is the variable causing a breath to end. The *baseline variable* describes what is happening to the breath during expiration. The following is a discussion of each of the four phases of ventilation in a positive-pressure ventilator, the phase variables, and the ventilator settings.

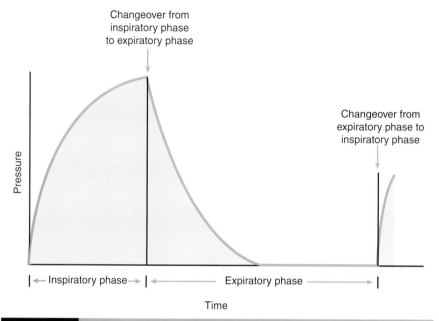

FIGURE 6-2

The four phases of the respiratory cycle on a ventilator. See text for explanation.

Beginning of Inspiration (Expiratory-Inspiratory Changeover): The Trigger Variable

The variable that determines the initiation of a breath is known as the *trigger variable*. Inspiration may be initiated by the patient or by the ventilator. When time is the trigger, the ventilator initiates the breath after a preset time interval. When the patient's spontaneous respiratory effort initiates the breath, pressure, flow, or volume is the trigger variable. The final way in which a ventilator can be triggered into the inspiratory phase is manually. This external cycling mechanism is activated by the clinician, all other cycling mechanisms are overridden, and a controlled breath is delivered.

The most common patient-initiated trigger variables are pressure and flow. When the patient initiates the breath, the ventilator must be able to *sense* the patient's effort and begin inspiration. The *sensitivity*, a ventilator setting controlled by the clinician, is the inspiratory effort that the patient must apply to initiate inspiration.

TIME-TRIGGERING

When time-triggering, the ventilator initiates a breath at a preset time interval. The time interval is determined by the respiratory frequency. When time-triggering is used, the ventilator-initiated breath is called a controlled or mandatory breath.

PRESSURE-TRIGGERING

When pressure is the trigger, a decrease in the pressure within the inspiratory circuit is sensed and inspiration begins. The *sensitivity setting* reflects the amount of

BOX 6-1 Sensitivity Setting

- Also known as triggering effort
- Normal setting: –0.5 to –2 cm H_2O below baseline pressure

Setting too low	Patient must generate more work to trigger the flow of gas. Patient may effectively become "locked out" from initiating gas flow.
Setting too high	Auto-cycling of the ventilator occurs. Patient–ventilator dyssynchrony occurs.

pressure drop below baseline pressure that the patient must develop in the ventilator circuit, on inspiration, to initiate the flow of gas. Sensitivity is also known as *triggering effort*. The sensitivity setting is generally –0.5 to –2 cm H_2O below the baseline pressure. If sensitivity is set at –2 and the PEEP is at 5 cm H_2O, then inspiratory flow begins when pressure in the circuit drops to 3 cm H_2O. If PEEP is not being used, inspiratory flow begins when the patient decreases circuit pressure to –2 cm H_2O. Sensitivity should be set to allow the patient to trigger the ventilator easily. The ventilator's response time is how fast it responds to patient effort. If the patient must use great effort to initiate the flow of gases, or if there is a delay from the time of patient effort to the start of the flow of gases, then the inspiratory muscle work is increased.

A high sensitivity setting, such as –0.5, decreases the amount of patient effort required to trigger the ventilator; that is, the ventilator will be more sensitive to negative inspiratory efforts. If sensitivity is set too high, ventilator self-cycling, or auto-cycling, will occur. In auto-cycling, the machine triggers a breath on its own without patient effort. This could occur regardless of where the patient is in the respiratory cycle. Auto-cycling may occur when there is an air leak, resulting in an inability to maintain the set baseline pressure (PEEP). If the sensitivity setting is too low, so that the ventilator is not sensitive enough to the patient, the patient must generate significant inspiratory effort to initiate the flow of gases; thus, the patient's WOB increases. The patient may demonstrate use of the accessory inspiratory muscles and complain of dyspnea and of being unable to "get enough air." The setting may be so inappropriately low that the patient is effectively locked out from initiating inspiratory flow (Box 6-1).

FLOW-TRIGGERING

Flow-triggering, also known as flow-by (FB), is a mechanism used to eliminate the imposed work of pressure-triggering a breath. With pressure-triggering, the patient works to create the negative pressure in the ventilator circuit and continues this work for a period (measured in milliseconds) known as the *lag time*. The lag time extends from the instant when the patient performs the triggering effort, through the time when the ventilator assist mechanism senses this effort and signals gas flow to begin, until finally the gases travel in the opposite direction to the patient's airway. The patient performs metabolic work during the lag time. With flow-triggering, inspiratory flow is instantly available; therefore, the work associated with patient triggering and lag time is eliminated.

With FB, a predetermined flow of gas, known as the *base flow*, travels through the inspiratory circuit and is continuously and immediately available to the patient, eliminating lag time. The base flow is set in liters per minute, usually 5 to 10 L/min, and is steadily maintained as the microprocessor in the ventilator constantly monitors flow in both the inspiratory and expiratory limbs.

The *flow trigger* is the clinician-chosen setting that represents how much the expiratory flow has to be decreased by the patient to initiate inspiration. It is usually set at 1 to 3 L/min. In the flow-by system, the base expiratory flow is constantly monitored. As the patient inspires, base expiratory flow decreases, signifying flow diversion from the exhalation circuit to the patient's lungs. This change in base flow is sensed by the ventilator and results in an increase in fresh gas flow before base flow is exhausted. Sufficient flow is maintained to meet the patient's immediate demand until the ventilator delivers the type of breath prescribed.

Inspiratory Phase

The *limit variable* for inspiration is a preset target value for pressure, volume, or flow that cannot be exceeded. The limit variable must not be confused with the cycle variable. The limit variable has a maximal setting but does not cycle the ventilator from the inspiratory to the expiratory phase. For example, in the pressure support (PS) mode of ventilation, the breath is pressure limited but flow cycled.

The two most common limit variables are volume and pressure. In a volume-limited breath, volume is preset and the volume waveform does not change from breath to breath. Examples of volume-limited modes are volume assist/control and synchronized intermittent mandatory ventilation (SIMV). Pressure waveform and values change with changes in the patient's compliance and resistance. In a pressure-limited breath, such as in PS or pressure control (PC), the pressure value and waveform do not change from breath to breath. Volume and flow can vary, depending on lung characteristics.

It is during the inspiratory phase that positive pressure is generated to create a pressure gradient that leads to lung inflation. The pressures within the airways, alveoli, and intrapleural spaces all become positive during inspiration, the exact opposite of what occurs during spontaneous inspiration (Fig. 6-3). This positive pressure causes the lungs to inflate and the thoracic cavity to expand. It is this positive pressure that causes most of the complications of mechanical ventilation, such as hemodynamic compromise and barotrauma (see Chapter 9).

Inspiratory-Expiratory Changeover

The phase variable that ends inspiration is called the *cycle variable*. The cycle variable may be pressure, volume, time, or flow. It is important to understand the interrelationships among these four variables during mechanical ventilation of the patient. One factor is controlled, and therefore it functions as the independent variable. The other factors are variable, and the clinician needs to monitor, or appropriately adjust them, on the ventilator (Table 6-2). This essential concept will become clearer with the following explanation of the four mechanisms that cycle the inspiratory-expiratory changeover.

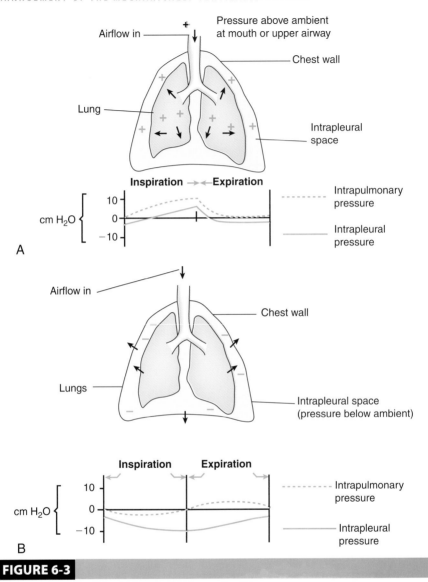

FIGURE 6-3

Comparison of the pressures within the thoracic cavity during positive-pressure ventilation (**A**) versus spontaneous respiration (**B**). *(From Pilbeam SP. Mechanical Ventilation: Physiological and Clinical Applications, 3rd ed. St. Louis: Mosby, 1998.)*

VOLUME-CYCLED VENTILATION

In volume-cycled ventilation, the ventilator cycles to end inspiration and begin expiration when a predetermined volume is delivered into the patient circuit. The time required to deliver the volume, the flow rate, and the pressure developed is variable. Once the predetermined volume and respiratory rate are set on the ventilator, the inspiratory flow rate must be appropriately adjusted so that the tidal volume

TABLE 6-2	Mechanism of Cycling from Inspiration to Expiration on Positive-Pressure Ventilators	
Cycling Mechanism	**Controlled Variable** (*Independent Variable*)	**Variables to Monitor (M) or Adjust (A*)** (*Dependent Variables*)
Volume	Tidal volume	Flow rate (A)
		Inspiratory time (A)
		Airway pressure (M)
Time	Inspiratory time	Flow rate (A)
		Tidal volume (M)†
		Airway pressure (M)
Pressure	Maximal airway pressure	Flow rate (M & A)
		Inspiratory time (M)
		Tidal volume (M)†
Flow	Flow rate	Inspiratory time (M)
		Tidal volume (M)†
		Airway pressure (A)

*Although a variable is adjusted, the implication is that it is also monitored on an ongoing basis so that appropriate adjustments can be made.
†In the use of any ventilatory cycling mechanism in which tidal volume is variable, frequent monitoring of the tidal volume is essential!

is delivered within the desired inspiratory time. The amount of pressure generated to deliver the prescribed tidal volume, the peak inspiratory pressure (PIP), varies depending on compliance and resistance factors, and the clinician must monitor it closely. As compliance decreases or resistance increases, PIP rises because even under these circumstances, the ventilator continues to deliver the committed volume.

TIME-CYCLED VENTILATION

In time-cycled ventilation, inspiration ends and expiration begins after a predetermined time interval is reached. Cycling may be controlled by a simple timing mechanism or by setting the rate and adjusting the inspiratory-to-expiratory (I:E) ratio, or percentage of inspiratory time. Both mechanisms tell the ventilator to cycle from inspiration to expiration after a preset amount of time elapses. When cycling occurs, the airway pressure attained, the inspiratory flow, and the tidal volume may all be variable breath to breath. In time-cycled ventilation, the tidal volume (V_T) is determined by gas flow rate multiplied by inspiratory time (Volume = Flow × Time). Because time is controlled, the flow rate must be adjusted to achieve the desired V_T before the ventilator cycles. Changes in airway resistance and pulmonary compliance vary the airway pressure and may also reduce V_T unless the ventilator is capable of delivering constant flow under varying lung conditions.

PRESSURE-CYCLED VENTILATION

In pressure-cycled ventilation, inspiration ends and expiration begins when a predetermined maximal airway pressure limit is reached. The volume delivered, the flow rate, and the inspiratory time all vary breath to breath. The volume delivered is determined by the set cycling pressure, the flow rate, the patient's lung compliance, airway and circuit resistance to ventilation, and the integrity of the ventilator circuit.

An initial cycling pressure is chosen while the exhaled VT is monitored. Pressure is then adjusted until an acceptable VT is achieved. If the patient's lung characteristics deteriorate, the VT drops and the inspiratory time shortens. Increasing the cycling pressure is the primary mechanism for correcting this problem. Intermittent positive-pressure breathing (IPPB) is an example of pressure-cycled ventilation.

FLOW-CYCLED VENTILATION

In flow-cycled ventilation, inspiration ends and expiration begins when the flow rate decays to a predetermined percentage of its peak value. This critical flow rate in which cycling occurs is called the terminal flow rate. The volume in the lungs and the inspiratory time vary from breath to breath. The volume delivered to the patient's lungs is determined by a chosen generated pressure and by the compliance and resistance of the patient's lungs. At the start of inspiration, the flow rate is maximal, but as the lungs fill with air, pressure within them increases and flow rate decreases. When the terminal flow rate is achieved, the ventilator cycles to the expiratory phase. Flow cycling tends to be more comfortable for the patient than volume cycling because in flow cycling the patient has a greater degree of control over the respiratory cycle. An example of a mode of ventilation that operates by these principles is flow-cycled, pressure-supported ventilation.

Expiration

The variable controlled during the expiratory time on the ventilator is known as the *baseline variable*. In all commonly used ventilators, pressure is the variable controlled during expiration. Exhalation occurs passively because of the elastic recoil of the lung, but the patient passively exhales to a controlled baseline pressure. The end-expiratory pressure when in equilibration with atmospheric pressure is zero. A base-line pressure above atmospheric pressure is known as positive end-expiratory pressure (PEEP) (Fig. 6-4). In the latter case, the patient exhales to a clinician-set amount of positive pressure at the end of exhalation. PEEP improves the functional residual capacity (FRC) by promoting the recruitment and stability of alveoli.

VENTILATOR SETTINGS

Fraction of Inspired Oxygen Concentration

When *initiating* mechanical ventilation for the patient in respiratory failure, it is best to err on the side of caution and use a high fraction of inspired oxygen concentration (FIO_2) (0.7 to 1.0) to ensure adequate tissue oxygenation. After an initial blood gas value is obtained, the FIO_2 may be decreased to achieve the goal of a clinically acceptable partial pressure of oxygen in arterial blood (PaO_2) (>60 mm Hg) with an FIO_2 of 0.5 or less. A PaO_2 of 60 mm Hg or greater achieves an arterial saturation of 90% or greater under conditions of normal body temperature and pH. An FIO_2 of 0.5 or less minimizes oxygen toxicity. If an FIO_2 of more than 0.6 is

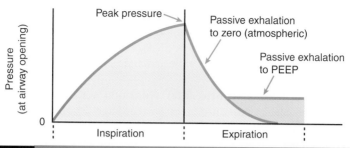

FIGURE 6-4

Expiration on a positive-pressure ventilator occurs passively because of the elastic recoil forces of the lung. Expiration occurs to a controlled *baseline* pressure, which may be zero (atmospheric), or to positive end-expiratory pressure (PEEP).

necessary to maintain oxygenation, the clinician should consider additional strategies that will increase the mean airway pressure, such as the use of PEEP. The persistent use of an FIO_2 more than 0.6 is generally avoided because of the possibility of oxygen toxicity that could damage the lung. However, whenever oxygenation status is in question, the patient is undergoing procedures that increase oxygen demand such as suctioning or bronchoscopy, or during periods of cardiopulmonary instability, an FIO_2 of 1.0 is prudent.

Pulse oximetry should be considered for continuous monitoring of oxygenation and titration of the FIO_2. If blood gas values are used, it is common practice to wait 20 minutes after a ventilator change before obtaining the blood sample. Predictive equations for the selection of a satisfactory FIO_2 exist, but a trial-and-error approach (ideally with the use of a pulse oximeter) is probably just as useful. The reason is that both the patient's underlying disease process and the concurrently administered therapies affect the way individual patients respond to a change in FIO_2.

Use of correct terminology regarding the FIO_2 is to say that the patient is on an FIO_2 of 0.3 or 0.8, which acknowledges that the unit of measure, the FIO_2, is a fraction. Alternatively, one may say that the patient is on 30% or 80% oxygen. It is incorrect to say that the patient is on an FIO_2 of 30% because this terminology mixes two units of measure.

Tidal Volume

The V_T is dictated by the patient's lung characteristics and should be set to ensure that excessive stretch is avoided. The parameter monitored to determine the pressure on the lung is the plateau pressure (Pplat) because it is most reflective of peak alveolar pressure. An acceptable V_T is one that results in a Pplat of 30 cm H_2O or less. A starting point for V_T is 8 to 10 mL/kg ideal body weight. The setting can then be adjusted downward if Pplat is high and pH is acceptable. Conversely, it can be adjusted upward if Pplat is acceptable and the patient's blood gases or comfort would improve by using a larger V_T. In patients with normal lungs or less severe lung injury, larger initial V_T settings might be reasonable to facilitate comfort, to achieve target $Paco_2$ values, and to possibly prevent progressive alveolar collapse. A V_T of 12 mL/kg or more is not usually needed. The goal for V_T setting is that which results in the lowest Pplat possible while maintaining gas exchange and patient comfort goals.

Historically, conventional mechanical ventilation was applied with V_Ts of 10 to 15 mL/kg. Evidence indicates, however, that large V_T ventilation associated with Pplat more than 30 cm H_2O can affect ventilator days and survival. The ARDS Network data published in 2000 showed significantly lower mortality and more ventilator-free days with a V_T of 6 mL/kg titrated to maintain Pplat less than 30 cm H_2O than with 12 mL/kg and a Pplat of 45 to 50 cm H_2O. The strategy advocated as a result of this study is called *low V_T ventilation,* and it is clearly indicated in patients with severe acute lung injury and acute respiratory distress syndrome (ARDS). Indeed, these results demonstrate that high priority should be given to mechanical ventilation strategies that prevent excessive lung stretch. (For more on ventilator-induced lung injury and lung protective strategies, see Chapter 9.)

EXHALED TIDAL VOLUME

Regardless of mode of ventilation, the most accurate measure of the volume received by the patient is the exhaled tidal volume (EV_T). For example, when pressure- or flow-targeted modes of ventilation are used, the generated pressure is set to determine the patient's V_T; however, as previously explained, the actual V_T may vary from breath to breath because of the patient's lung characteristics. Furthermore, when a volume-targeted mode of ventilation is used, the desired V_T is set on the ventilator, but it is misleading to believe that the patient's lungs will always receive this set V_T. Although the desired V_T is predetermined and set on the ventilator control panel, it is not guaranteed to be delivered to the patient. Some volume may be lost because of leaks in the ventilator circuitry, leaks around the airway, or a pleural air leak, or it may be lost as compressible volume in the ventilator circuitry. The volume actually received by the patient, in any mode of ventilation, must be confirmed by monitoring the EV_T on the display panel of the ventilator. When the EV_T deviates from the set tidal volume by 50 mL or more in an adult, the practitioner must troubleshoot the system (see Chapter 9). The EV_T is displayed at variable places on different ventilator models. The bedside practitioner must become familiar with the location of this information so trend monitoring can be carried out properly.

TUBING COMPRESSION AND COMPLIANCE VOLUME

Gas flows not only into the patient when inspiration is initiated but also into the ventilator circuitry. Of course, the gas in the ventilator circuitry, the compressible volume, does not participate in gas exchange. The amount of compressible volume in the circuitry is a function of the space available, the compliance of the ventilator tubing, and the opposing pressure from the patient's lungs. Gases compress when they are under pressure, and flexible ventilator tubing expands. As the patient's pulmonary compliance decreases, a larger percentage of the desired V_T becomes compressible volume because the tubing expands under the greater opposing pressure. More gas is also compressed within the humidifier, connectors, water traps, and internal circuitry of the ventilator. It is important to note that at the end of inspiration, this compressible volume flows out of the expiratory limb, along with the gases from the patient's lungs, and the ventilator interprets it as part of the exhaled V_T.

It is possible to calculate the compressed volume by using the ventilator tubing compliance, or compressibility, factor supplied by the manufacturer. Ventilator tubing compliance is variable, but most tubing has a compliance factor of 1 to 3 mL/cm H_2O. This means that for each centimeter H_2O of airway pressure, 1 to 3 mL of gas are compressed in the circuitry. It becomes clear that when the lungs are noncompliant and airway pressures rise, more volume is compressed in the circuit. Some ventilators automatically measure and calculate the amount of volume lost from tubing compliance and then compensate for it by increasing delivered V_T. Yet on other ventilators, the therapist can enter the tubing compliance into the ventilator, and then the ventilator will compensate for volume compressed in the tubing. Correcting for tubing compliance is especially important in infants and children and when V_T less than 300 mL is used.

The compressible volume in any given patient should remain relatively constant from one breath to the next. Therefore, if the exhaled V_T and minute ventilation that the patient is receiving are sufficient to maintain an appropriate $Paco_2$ and acid–base status, the volume of gas compressed in the ventilator circuitry has little significance. Compressible volume may be reduced by ensuring that the humidifier's water level is kept high and the length of the circuitry is minimal.

Respiratory Rate

The respiratory rate (RR) set on the ventilator should generally be as near physiologic RRs as possible: 10 to 20 breaths/min. Typical initial rate settings are between 8 and 12 breaths/min. Frequent changes in the RR are often required based on observation of the patient's WOB and comfort and on assessment of the $Paco_2$ and pH. Many patients, during initial use of a ventilator, require full ventilatory support. The RR at this time is selected on the basis of the V_T, so the minute ventilation (RR × V_T = Minute ventilation) is sufficient to maintain an acceptable acid–base status. As the patient is capable of participating in the ventilatory work, the ventilator RR should be decreased or the mode changed to allow for more spontaneous breathing.

Slow rates may be useful in patients with obstructive pulmonary disease because, as the rate is decreased, more time is available for exhalation and less air trapping occurs. Fast rates may be useful in patients with noncompliant lungs who require ventilation with smaller V_Ts to prevent barotrauma from increased airway pressures.

Overventilation, which leads to alkalosis, is a common problem in the patient supported by mechanical ventilation. Respiratory alkalosis should be avoided because it is associated with hypokalemia, hypocalcemia, decreased cerebral blood flow, and decreased oxygen unloading from hemoglobin at the tissue level. (In patients with acute intracranial hypertension, mild hyperventilation and subsequent respiratory alkalosis may be indicated.) It is therefore desirable for patients to set their own RR by using a mode of ventilation that allows patient-initiated breaths. Depending on the patient's ability to partially support ventilation, a guaranteed number of breaths may be supplied while the patient is allowed to breathe over this rate. The patient then adjusts the RR and $PaCO_2$ levels and thus maintains a more normal acid–base status (eucapnia). In some modes of ventilation (PS and CPAP), when both the patient's respiratory drive and the ability to work are sufficient, no RR is set on the ventilator.

Flow Rate

Flow rate is the speed with which the V_T is delivered; it is measured in liters per minute. Generally, an initial flow rate of 40 to 100 L/min satisfies the patient's inspiratory demands and achieves a desirable I:E ratio. The inspiratory flow rate is the chief determinant of inspiratory time and thus of the I:E ratio. Therefore, the flow rate must be adjusted for each patient on the basis of the desired I:E ratio, the V_T, and the RR (see Relationships Among V_T, Flow Rate, RR, and I:E Ratio, later). The V_T must be delivered within an appropriate, comfortable time, and flow must meet or exceed the patient's inspiratory flow demand; if not, the patient experiences so-called air hunger, the WOB is increased, and patient–ventilator dyssynchrony results.

Higher flow rates (>60 L/min) shorten inspiratory time, thereby lengthening expiratory time (decreased I:E ratio), and they may be desirable in patients with chronic obstructive pulmonary disease (COPD) and air trapping. Increasing the flow rate may have the negative consequences of increasing the PIP and adversely affecting the distribution of gases because flow becomes more turbulent. Slower inspiratory flow rates (20 to 50 L/min) prolong inspiratory time, improve the distribution of gases, and reduce PIP as a result of a more laminar flow. Most ventilators are capable of delivering flow rates up to a range of 120 to 180 L/min, which should meet the needs of any condition in which the minute ventilatory demands are high or when the lungs are noncompliant and high RR/low V_T ventilation is needed (Box 6-2).

With pressure ventilation, flow is variable and determined by the pressure level and the algorithm used by the ventilator to achieve the pressure target. The ventilator provides sufficient flow to achieve the pressure target in the time allowed by the ventilator's logic. Some ventilators allow adjustment of peak inspiratory flow rate during pressure support ventilation (PSV). This setting is known as the *rise time* and represents the amount of time it takes for the set pressure to be reached from the beginning of inspiration. Rise time should be set to enhance patient comfort by

BOX 6-2 Flow Rate	
Definition	Speed with which the tidal volume is delivered.
Average setting	40–60 L/min
High flow rates	Decrease inspiratory time.
	Increase PIP (peak inspiratory pressure) (more turbulent flow).
	May lead to maldistribution of gas.
	Required for high minute ventilation demands.
Low flow rates	Increase inspiratory time.
	Decrease PIP (more laminar flow).
	May improve distribution of gases.

satisfying peak inspiratory demand. During PS ventilation, the pressure time scalar assists the clinician in setting rise time. An initial overshoot in pressure above the PS level indicates that the rise time is too short, whereas a concave rise in initial airway pressure curve usually indicates the rise time is too long and flows are less than patient demand.

FLOW-WAVE PATTERNS

The flow of gases may be delivered in variable configurations known as flow-wave patterns (Table 6-3). There are four main categories of waveforms: rectangular (sometimes referred to as square); sinusoidal; accelerating (ascending ramp); and decelerating (descending ramp). In pressure-targeted modes of ventilation, the ventilator is committed to the delivery of gases in a descending ramp pattern.

TABLE 6-3 Standard Mechanical Ventilator Flow-Wave Patterns

Label	Flow-Wave Pattern	Description
Rectangular (square)		Peak flow rate is delivered immediately at the onset of inspiration, maintained throughout the inspiratory phase, and abruptly terminated at the onset of expiration.
		Common default pattern with volume-targeted modes.
Sinusoidal		Inspiratory flow rate gradually accelerates to peak flow and then tapers off.
		Believed to mimic spontaneous inspiratory patterns.
		May increase PIP (peak inspiratory pressure).
Accelerating (ascending ramp)		Flow gradually accelerates in a linear fashion to the set peak flow rate.
Decelerating (descending ramp)		Flow is at peak at onset of inspiration and gradually decelerates throughout inspiratory phase.
		Flow ceases and ventilator cycles to expiratory phase when flow decays to a percentage of peak flow, usually 25% but varies by ventilator model. Terminal flow criteria may be adjustable in some newer ventilators.
		Rapid initial flow raises mean airway pressure and may assist in alveolar recruitment.
		May improve the distribution of gases when there is inhomogeneity of alveolar ventilation.
		Decreases dead space, increases arterial oxygen tension, and reduces PIP.

Little research validates the advantages of one waveform over another. Some evidence shows that the use of the decelerating waveform improves the distribution of gas in patients who have a diffuse, nonhomogeneous disease process in which adjacent alveoli require differing inspiratory times for adequate filling. (These are known as alveoli with varying time constants; see Chapter 2.) Both pressure and volume assist/control ventilation with a decelerating flow waveform provided better oxygenation at a lower PIP and higher mean airway pressure (Paw) than volume assist/control ventilation with a rectangular flow waveform. When the decelerating flow waveform is used for both modes, there is no significant difference between VC ventilation and PC ventilation in terms of airway pressures, gas exchange, and hemodynamic values.

Optimal flow pattern is not an exact science. A flow pattern is chosen on the basis of the patient's disease process and the pattern's ability to promote optimal gas distribution and affect inspiratory pressures. Higher inspiratory flows lead to an increase in the PIP; adjusting the flow-wave pattern (i.e., switching from the rectangular to the descending ramp pattern) may reduce the PIP. Modification of the flow-wave pattern should be done while the caregiver remains at the bedside to evaluate the effect of any change in patient comfort and the desired parameters (i.e., PIP) and with awareness that changes in flow pattern can affect peak inspiratory flow rate as well as inspiratory and expiratory times.

Inspiratory-to-Expiratory Ratio

The I:E ratio is the duration of inspiration in comparison with expiration. Inspiratory time during mechanical ventilation is an important consideration, and in most adults a time of 1 second (0.8 to 1.2 seconds) is a good initial setting. Generally, the I:E ratio is set at 1:2; that is, 33% of the respiratory cycle is spent in inspiration and 66% in the expiratory phase. This setting is believed to mimic spontaneous respiration when lung function is normal. It is also generally used because (1) shorter inspiratory times contribute to dead-space ventilation by overexpanding the most compliant alveoli, and (2) longer inspiratory times increase the mean airway pressure, which while promoting improved oxygenation, may also lead to hemodynamic instability. An I:E ratio of 1:3 or 1:4 or longer may be necessary to ventilate the lungs of an individual with COPD and air trapping because the longer expiratory time promotes more complete exhalation, and air trapping is reduced.

The I:E ratio is a function of inspiratory flow rate, inspiratory time, and frequency. Ventilators use several approaches to adjust the I:E ratio. For ventilators with inspiratory time or percentage inspiratory time, rate, and VT control, the set inspiratory time and tidal volume determine the flow rate. In these ventilators when the I:E ratio is manipulated directly, by adjusting the inspiratory time, inspiratory flow rate adjusts appropriately. For example, if the patient's RR is 12 breaths per minute, 60 is divided by 12 to ascertain that a period of 5 seconds is devoted to each respiratory cycle. If the desired I:E ratio is 1:2, then multiplying 5 by 0.33 (the percentage of time allowed for inspiration) determines the inspiratory time of 1.7 seconds. This time, or the percentage inspiratory time, is entered directly into the ventilator. In other ventilators the I:E ratio is set by adjusting the peak inspiratory flow rate while taking into consideration the patient's RR and the need to deliver the

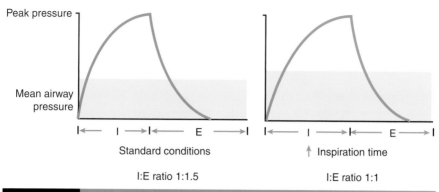

Peak pressure

Mean airway
pressure

|← I →|← E →| |← I →|← E →|

Standard conditions   ↑ Inspiration time

I:E ratio 1:1.5   I:E ratio 1:1

FIGURE 6-5

The effect of altering the inspiratory-to-expiratory (I:E) ratio on mean airway pressure (*shaded area*). As inspiratory time is lengthened, so is the amount of time that positive pressure is applied to the thorax; therefore, the mean airway pressure rises.

VT in a comfortable time. A higher inspiratory flow rate shortens inspiratory time and allows more time for exhalation. To lengthen the inspiratory time, the flow rate is decreased. For example, if the patient's I:E ratio is 1:3 and the desired I:E ratio is 1:2, the flow rate is decreased.

Consideration of the I:E ratio is important because the longer the inspiratory phase, the higher the mean airway pressure (mPaw) (Fig. 6-5). As the mPaw increases, so does the potential for hemodynamic compromise. Positive-pressure ventilation may reduce cardiac output by three mechanisms: decreasing venous return, increasing right ventricular (RV) afterload, and reducing, as a result, RV systolic emptying and left ventricular compliance (because the interventricular septum is displaced by the increased RV end-systolic volume).

INVERSE I:E RATIOS

I:E ratios of 1:1, 2:1, 3:1, and 4:1 are called inverse I:E ratios. An inverse I:E ratio may be employed when conventional strategies to improve oxygenation fail, which may occur in noncompliant lung conditions in which the disease process exhibits a nonhomogeneous distribution. An inverse I:E ratio is used to improve oxygenation. In noncompliant lungs, the short inspiratory time of a normal I:E ratio allows unstable alveoli to collapse during the relatively longer expiratory phase. The inspiratory effect of an inverse I:E ratio is to allow unstable lung units more time to fill and an equilibration of volume between the alveoli as a result of collateral ventilation. The longer inspiratory time provides a longer so-called dwell time for gas mixing and alveolar recruitment to occur. Dead-space ventilation and the percentage of shunt both decrease because gas is more evenly distributed in the lung. The relatively compliant alveoli are not overdistended by gases that preferentially flow to them, as may occur during an inflation period of standard duration. The simultaneous shortening of the expiratory phase prevents unstable alveoli from collapsing because the next inspiration begins before they reach closing volume (Fig. 6-6).

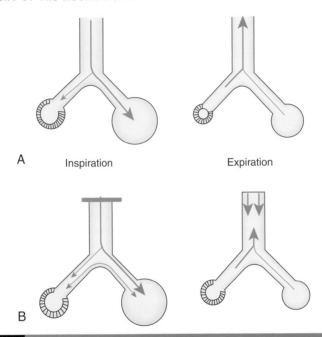

A   Inspiration   Expiration

B

FIGURE 6-6

Inspiratory and *expiratory* effects of standard ventilation (**A**) and inverse-ratio ventilation (**B**) on the distribution of gases in lung units with varying time constants. *Shaded area* represents alveolus with decreased compliance (i.e., a longer time constant). **A,** With a short inspiratory and longer expiratory time, noncompliant alveoli do not have time to fill during inspiration (shunt), whereas adjacent compliant alveoli may become overdistended (dead space). On expiration, unstable alveoli collapse as they reach closing volume before the end of the expiratory phase. **B,** Prolonging the inspiratory time allows noncompliant alveoli more time to fill and equilibration of gases between lung units of varying time constants. Reinflation after a shortened expiration causes gases to be trapped in the lung, which creates a PEEP-like effect promoting alveolar recruitment and stability.

Inverse I:E ratio ventilation increases mPaw because of the prolonged inspiratory time, as shown in Figure 6-5. mPaw is the average airway pressure over the entire respiratory cycle and a key determinant of oxygenation. An increase in mPaw results in an increase in alveolar stability and recruitment. An increase in the functional residual capacity ensues, and thus oxygenation improves. A higher mPaw has the negative effect of creating more positive pressure in the thorax, which may lead to hemodynamic compromise by the mechanisms described earlier (see the Inspiratory-to-Expiratory Ratio section and Chapter 9, Complications of Mechanical Ventilation). Little overall improvement in the patient will be appreciated if arterial oxygenation improves but tissue oxygen delivery falls. Therefore, the clinician must monitor tissue oxygen delivery (DO_2) closely, optimize all aspects of DO_2, and find the ideal I:E ratio for any given patient that improves *overall* oxygenation.

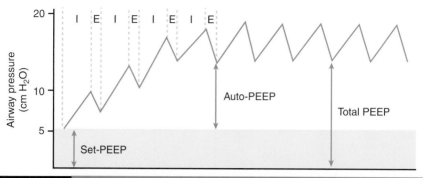

FIGURE 6-7

Phenomenon of auto-PEEP, caused by inversion of the I:E ratio. Insufficient expiratory time permits the trapping of gases in the lung. This trapped gas creates pressure, which is known as auto-PEEP.

A phenomenon known as intrinsic PEEP, or auto-PEEP, may develop when expiratory time impinges on inspiratory time. Because the expiratory phase is shortened, the alveoli may not have sufficient time to empty completely during expiration, and gas becomes trapped in the lung. This trapped gas creates pressure in the alveoli known as auto-PEEP (Fig. 6-7). Auto-PEEP prevents end-expiratory alveolar collapse and adds a cumulative PEEP effect to the operator-chosen, or set-PEEP. The auto-PEEP plus the set-PEEP equals the total PEEP. Measurement of auto-PEEP requires the implementation of an end-expiratory pause (see Intrinsic PEEP section, later). Air trapping does not always occur with use of an inverse I:E ratio, but its development must be monitored.

Inverse I:E ratios are generally most safely applied with the use of PC ventilation, but they may also be applied in the volume control mode by using an end-inspiratory pause or a slow inspiratory flow rate (Marcy and Marini, 1991). Because the respiratory pattern is unusual, it may result in patient discomfort, and because it is important to prevent the patient from breathing out of synchrony with the altered I:E ratio, sedation is usually required. A new approach to address this concern is to allow unrestricted spontaneous breathing throughout the respiratory cycle. This requires an active exhalation valve and is possible with a variety of modes that have different names depending on ventilator manufacturer but function similarly (e.g., airway pressure release ventilation, bilevel ventilation, or biphasic ventilation).

Although prolonged inspiratory time ventilation may improve oxygenation, its use has not been subjected to well-designed large-outcome studies. It cannot be concluded that simply improving oxygenation with a mechanical ventilator will improve survival. In the ARDS Network trial, the patients in the low VT group who showed improved survival had lower Pao_2-to-Fio_2 ratios than the high VT group. There are many factors related to how the ventilator is set that may affect patient outcome.

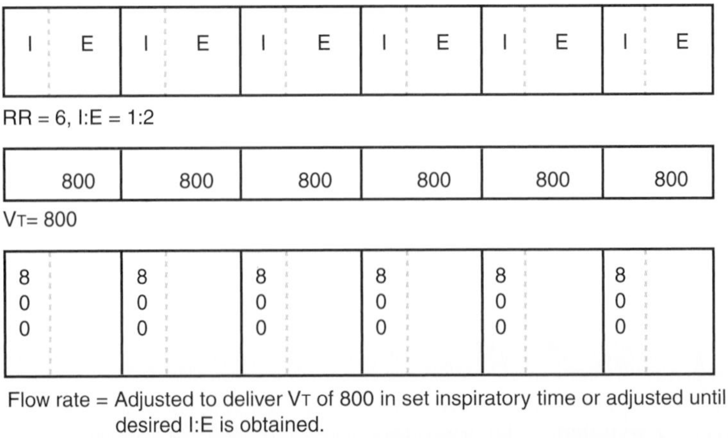

I	E	I	E	I	E	I	E	I	E	I	E

RR = 6, I:E = 1:2

800	800	800	800	800	800

VT= 800

8 0 0	8 0 0	8 0 0	8 0 0	8 0 0	8 0 0

Flow rate = Adjusted to deliver VT of 800 in set inspiratory time or adjusted until desired I:E is obtained.

FIGURE 6-8

Relationships among tidal volume (VT), flow rate, respiratory rate (RR), and the inspiratory-to-expiratory (I:E) ratio.

Relationships Among VT, Flow Rate, RR, and I:E Ratio

After an appreciation of the variables of VT, flow rate, RR, and the I:E ratio is gained, it becomes evident that they are interrelated. For example, increasing the RR affects the I:E ratio if the flow rate is not adjusted appropriately. To enhance understanding further, Figure 6-8 depicts the relationships among these variables graphically.

End-Inspiratory Pause

An end-inspiratory pause takes place when the lungs are held in an inflated state at a set pressure or volume, for a specified period (usually <2 seconds) at the end of inspiration. This maneuver is called an inflation hold, inspiratory plateau, or end-inspiratory pause. In the past, this maneuver was recommended to allow for improved distribution of inhaled gases by increasing the mPaw and lung recruitment and thereby improving oxygenation. The use of a longer inspiratory pause is advocated in acute lung injury and ARDS as a lung recruitment maneuver (see Chapter 5). An end-inspiratory pause maneuver is most commonly used to obtain a reading of Pplat and determination of resistance and static compliance. The pause is instituted at the peak of inspiration. The airway pressure dial then drops to the Pplat. The Pplat reflects pressure within the alveoli. The difference between peak and plateau pressures is caused by resistance to gas flow in the airways. As discussed in Chapter 2, the Pplat reading is also used to calculate static pulmonary compliance, where $C_{ST} = EV_T/Pplat - PEEP$.

Sigh

All human beings sigh approximately 10 times per hour. The purpose of the sigh is to counteract small airway closure, which can occur when VTs are monotonous.

| **TABLE 6-4** | Initial Ventilator Settings: Guidelines |

Parameter	Initial Setting
Fraction of inspired O_2 (F_{IO_2})	0.7–1.0 (Err on side of caution; wean to 0.5 or less to prevent O_2 toxicity.)
Tidal volume (V_T)	8–12 mL/kg; adjust to ensure Pplat ≤30 cm H_2O; may need 4–6 mL/kg in ARDS
Respiratory rate (RR)	10–20 breaths per minute
Flow rate	40–80 L/min (Adjust to deliver tidal volume in desired inspiratory time, appropriate rise time in PS.)
Inspiratory time	1.0 second (0.8–2.0 seconds)
Inspiratory-to-expiratory (I:E) ratio	1:2–1:3
Sensitivity	Pressure trigger: –0.5 to –1.5 below baseline Flow trigger: 1–3 L/min
Positive end-expiratory pressure (PEEP)	3–5 cm H_2O

ARDS, Acute respiratory distress syndrome; *F_{IO_2},* fraction of oxygen in inspired gas; *I:E ratio,* inspiratory-to-expiratory ratio; *PEEP,* positive end-expiratory pressure; *Pplat,* plateau pressure; *PS,* pressure support; *RR,* respiratory rate; *V_T,* tidal volume.

Sigh breaths delivered by the ventilator are usually set at 1.5 times the V_T of machine-cycled breaths. A single sigh may be delivered, or sigh breaths may be given in multiples. Sighs should not be used when supraphysiologic tidal volumes (10 to 15 mL/kg) are being used. Some believe that sighs are not necessary when PEEP is used. Under either of these conditions, the addition of a sigh may cause excessive peak airway pressures and possible barotrauma to the lungs. Table 6-4 lists guidelines for initial ventilator settings.

POSITIVE END-EXPIRATORY PRESSURE

PEEP is the application of a constant, positive pressure in the airways so that, at end-expiration, the pressure is never allowed to return to atmospheric pressure. PEEP is measured in centimeters of H_2O. Typical settings for PEEP range from 5 to 20 cm H_2O. The positive pressure is actually applied throughout the ventilatory cycle (the baseline pressure is raised), but it is used for its physiologic effects at end-expiration. By exerting positive pressure at end-expiration, PEEP recruits atelectatic alveoli, internally splints and distends already patent alveoli, counteracts alveolar and small-airway closure during expiration, and redistributes lung water. PEEP redistributes extravascular lung water from alveoli to the perivascular space, where the effect of excess lung water on gas exchange is decreased. Through these mechanisms, PEEP decreases intrapulmonary shunting, increases the FRC, improves compliance, decreases the diffusion distance for oxygen, and *improves oxygenation.*

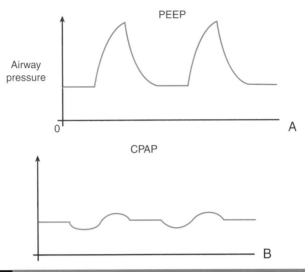

FIGURE 6-9

A, *Positive end-expiratory pressure* (PEEP) is the correct term when positive end-expiratory pressure is applied with any other form of ventilatory support. **B,** Continuous positive airway pressure (CPAP) is positive pressure applied to the spontaneously breathing patient (with or without use of the ventilator) who is receiving no other ventilatory assistance.

PEEP versus Continuous Positive Airway Pressure

PEEP and continuous positive airway pressure (CPAP) are identical in their mechanism, but the terms are not interchangeable. The use of one term rather than the other provides a description of the amount of ventilatory support the patient is receiving. Positive pressure applied at the end of expiration may be administered to patients who are either spontaneously breathing or undergoing mechanical ventilation. *PEEP* is the correct term when patients are receiving positive end-expiratory pressure along with any other mechanical ventilatory assistance, such as PS or assist/control ventilation (Fig. 6-9). CPAP is the correct term when positive pressure is being used with the spontaneously breathing patient who is receiving no other ventilatory assistance. CPAP is measured in centimeters of H_2O pressure and may be administered through a ventilator or with a CPAP mask. See Chapter 7 for further information about indications for CPAP use and patient monitoring.

Indications and Relative Contraindications for Use of PEEP

In patients whose PaO_2 is 60 mm Hg or less (SaO_2 ≤90%) on an FIO_2 of 0.5 or greater, PEEP is therapeutically indicated to improve oxygenation. With the addition of PEEP, it may be possible to provide oxygenation with a lower FIO_2, thus reducing the chance of pulmonary oxygen toxicity. Simultaneous to the addition of PEEP, therapies designed to treat the underlying condition and improve oxygenation (e.g., diuresis, postural drainage, chest physiotherapy, antibiotics, and body positioning) should be applied. PEEP does not correct underlying disorders such as congestive heart failure, fluid overload, and pneumonia. It only supports oxygenation until the underlying condition is corrected.

Clinical indications for PEEP are to prevent atelectasis both postoperatively and in the bedridden patient and to reverse established atelectasis. PEEP may also be used to provide internal stabilization of the chest wall and minimize paradoxical chest wall movement in flail chest if oxygenation is unsatisfactory. Some caregivers consider a small amount of PEEP, 3 to 5 cm H_2O, "physiologic" when it is applied to intubated patients, purporting that it mimics the amount of PEEP usually created by the glottic apparatus, which is interrupted by the artificial airway. This latter point is a controversial one. However, 5 cm H_2O PEEP may be applied to preserve a more normal FRC, which is decreased when an artificial airway is inserted and in the supine position, a position assumed the majority of the time by the critically ill patient supported by mechanical ventilation. PEEP is advocated when auto-PEEP is present because of expiratory airflow obstruction, also known as dynamic airway closure (see Intrinsic PEEP section, later). In cardiogenic pulmonary edema, PEEP levels of 5 to 10 improve oxygenation. The application of PEEP increases intrathoracic pressure and reduces preload and afterload. These effects improve left ventricular end-diastolic pressure and volume and cardiac output. Finally, PEEP is indicated for patients with ARDS in whom the goal is to improve lung volume and prevent unstable alveoli from closing at end-expiration. PEEP levels of 10 to 20 cm H_2O may be needed in ARDS.

Relative contraindications to the use of PEEP include unilateral lung disease because the application of PEEP may result in alveolar overdistention in the healthy lung, which both increases dead space and redistributes perfusion to the bad lung. This redistribution of perfusion to the relatively less ventilated lung results in an increase in intrapulmonary shunt. Under these conditions, independent lung ventilation may be indicated (see Chapter 12). In lung disease resulting in hyperinflation (emphysema), patients already have an increased FRC because of air trapping. PEEP may not improve oxygenation in these patients and may even worsen gas exchange by mechanisms similar to those in unilateral lung disease (overdistention and shunting of blood to less ventilated alveoli), while subjecting the patient to the possibilities of pulmonary barotrauma and decreased cardiac output. In patients with an increased intracranial pressure (ICP), the application of PEEP may result in a reduction of venous return and a further increase in ICP. A careful balance of measures to reduce ICP and improve oxygenation must be maintained. Other relative contraindications are hypovolemia because of the cardiac effects of PEEP and bronchopleural fistula because PEEP may worsen airflow through the defect. One contraindication to PEEP is untreated pneumothorax because the positive pressure forces more air into the chest cavity, leading to a more rapid decline. The clinical significance of these relative contraindications is that one needs to be aware of the effect of PEEP on these conditions so the risk/benefit ratio can be weighed properly and preventive measures, such as volume loading, can be readied.

Adverse Effects

It is important to be aware of the adverse effects of PEEP and how they are prevented or managed. Problems related to the use of PEEP lie in the possibly precipitous reduction in cardiac output (CO), and thus in tissue oxygen delivery, that can occur as a result of the increase in intrathoracic pressure. Three primary factors result in a decrease in CO. First, much of the reduction in CO is attributable to a decrease in venous return, which occurs because of an increase in right atrial transmural pressure. Second, pulmonary vascular resistance is increased because of referred positive pressure from the alveoli. This increases RV afterload, impairing RV emptying. Third, as RV end-systolic volume increases, the interventricular septum shifts, impairing diastolic filling of the left ventricle and further depressing CO.

Management of the adverse hemodynamic effects of PEEP begins by ensuring that the patient has adequate intravascular volume. After optimal preload is achieved, inotropic and afterloading agents are added in the appropriate setting. These agents may be necessary to maintain adequate tissue oxygen delivery, the ultimate goal. Use of a pulmonary artery catheter for monitoring CO and calculation of tissue oxygenation should be considered when 10 cm H_2O or more PEEP is applied.

Barotrauma may also occur with the application of PEEP and is primarily the result of overdistention and an increase in peak inspiratory pressure. The lowest level of PEEP to achieve improved oxygenation and careful monitoring of peak pressure is indicated. Overdistention with the application of PEEP is more likely to occur when lung disease is heterogeneous, especially as in unilateral lung disease.

Institution and Withdrawal of PEEP

When PEEP is indicated, the initial setting is generally 5 cm H_2O. PEEP may then be increased in increments of 3 to 5 cm H_2O until satisfactory oxygenation is obtained. The response to each change should be evaluated, either with the use of pulse oximetry or with assessment of arterial blood gas (ABG) values and the patient's condition. As a general guideline, ABG values should be obtained 20 minutes after the change in PEEP. In ARDS, ideally PEEP should be set just above the lower inflection point of the pressure-volume curve. However, graphing the pressure-volume curve requires paralysis of the patient and a time-consuming process of applying varying Vts and measuring the Pplat, then graphing and interpreting the curve. High PEEP may be applied after a recruitment maneuver or large Vt was applied and then slowly titrated down while monitoring oxygen saturation. Pragmatically, in all patients for whom PEEP is indicated, the goal is to find the best PEEP, which is the least amount of PEEP required to obtain an oxygen saturation of 92% or more, a Pao_2 of 60 mm Hg or more, on an Fio_2 ideally less than 0.6 that does not impair delivery of oxygen to the tissues. If PEEP decreases CO in an uncorrectable fashion, then the preservation of tissue oxygenation will require the PEEP to be lowered and the Fio_2 increased, if necessary, and additional strategies to improve oxygenation such as inverse I:E ratio or prone positioning may be indicated. Excess PEEP overdistends the alveoli, causing compression of the adjacent pulmonary capillaries and thus creating dead space and its attendant hypercapnia (Fig. 6-10).

Once the Fio_2 is reduced to 0.5 or less, and assessment indicates that the reduction in ventilatory support is appropriate, withdrawal of PEEP may begin. PEEP should be decreased in increments of 2 to 5 cm H_2O, with the adequacy of oxygenation evaluated after each change. The patient's condition should be allowed to stabilize for 4 to 6 hours after each 5 cm H_2O decrease in PEEP, or for 6 to 12 hours

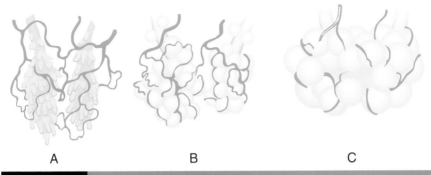

FIGURE 6-10

Effect of the application of PEEP on the alveoli. **A,** Atelectatic alveoli before PEEP application. **B,** Optimal PEEP application has reinflated alveoli to normal volume. **C,** Excessive PEEP application overdistends the alveoli and compresses adjacent pulmonary capillaries, creating dead space with its attendant hypercapnia.

if the underlying disease process affecting oxygenation has been prolonged. Abrupt withdrawal of PEEP may rapidly result in hypoxemia because of airway closure and the need to reinstate PEEP at possibly higher levels than were previously required. For this reason, an inline suction catheter should be used for patients receiving high levels of PEEP. Furthermore, if the ventilator circuit is disrupted, manual ventilation with a bag-valve-mask (BVM) device, with an appropriately set PEEP valve, should be instituted.

Interpretation of Vascular Pressures During PEEP

Positive pressure applied to the lungs is referred throughout the thoracic cavity and therefore to the vascular structures. Formulas were developed to determine the effect of positive pressure applied to the lungs on the vascular pressure readings, specifically the pulmonary artery occlusion pressure (PAOP). These formulas provide the so-called corrected PAOP by subtracting a percentage of the PEEP from the PAOP. The use of these calculations is misleading, however, because the compliance of the lungs (which is not a variable in the equation) affects the amount of pressure referred beyond the lungs into the thoracic cavity and vascular structures. Another method used in some clinical settings is to subtract the amount of PEEP being used from the PAOP to obtain a corrected PAOP. This method has no scientific basis either. Saying that 5 cm H_2O PEEP adds 5 mm Hg pressure to the PAOP is incorrect simply because the units of measure are not equal. Finally, removing the patient from the ventilator to eliminate the effect of PEEP on the vascular pressure is fraught with potential hazards because of the wide fluctuations in oxygenation that could occur. For consistency, vascular pressures should be measured while the patient–ventilator system remains intact.

No magic formula can determine the effect of PEEP on the vascular pressures; however, the amount of PEEP (set and auto) must be documented and taken into consideration as the vascular pressures are interpreted. For example, if the patient's vascular pressure readings rise concurrently with an increase in PEEP, making this connection will assist in ruling out new-onset heart failure or hypervolemia as a cause of the elevation.

Intrinsic PEEP

Intrinsic PEEP (auto-PEEP), by definition, is the spontaneous development of PEEP as a result of insufficient expiratory time. Causes of auto-PEEP formation include rapid respiratory rate, high minute ventilatory demand, airflow obstruction, and inverse I:E ratio ventilation. Expiratory time is inadequate when the lung does not reach its resting expiratory volume before the next inspiration begins. Inadequate expiratory time causes gases to become trapped in the lung. These trapped gases create positive pressure in the thorax. Auto-PEEP continues to develop until the elastic recoil forces in the lung overcome the tendency to trap further gases, as shown in Figure 6-7. Auto-PEEP is also known as pulmonary gas trapping, endogenous PEEP, occult PEEP, intrinsic PEEP, dynamic hyperinflation, or inadvertent PEEP when it occurs unwittingly.

Extrinsic PEEP is the amount of PEEP that the clinician sets on the ventilator. It is the PEEP you know about that can readily be read on the pressure manometer on the ventilator display panel at end-expiration. Auto-PEEP (intrinsic PEEP) is the PEEP you may not know about and cannot detect on the ventilator pressure manometer without performing a special maneuver. When auto-PEEP forms, the end-expiratory pressure is above the ambient level but is not read by the ventilator pressure manometer because the manometer is open to the atmosphere during exhalation and reads only the set-PEEP. For measurement of auto-PEEP, the exhalation valve must be occluded just before the next breath would begin (similarly to performing the end-inspiratory hold maneuver when static compliance is being measured). An end-expiratory hold should be performed as quickly as possible to prevent discomfort from interrupting the respiratory cycle and pattern. Occluding the exhalation port for several seconds allows the ventilator pressure manometer to read both the circuit pressure (set-PEEP) and the airway pressure (auto-PEEP) (Fig. 6-11). The airway-pressure manometer reading therefore reflects *total* PEEP. For determination of the auto-PEEP value, the following calculation is then performed:

$$\text{Auto-PEEP} = \text{Total PEEP} - \text{Set-PEEP}$$

The effective PEEP is the total PEEP—that is, both set-PEEP and auto-PEEP function physiologically in the same manner.

The detection and monitoring of auto-PEEP are important because of its physiologic effects. If auto-PEEP is being used therapeutically, it should be monitored and adjusted like all other ventilator settings. If it is unintentional, then the clinician who is unaware of its presence is unable to manage its potentially adverse effects on the patient. Just as with set-PEEP, auto-PEEP places the patient at risk for barotrauma and hemodynamic compromise. Not being aware of the presence of auto-PEEP may also lead to the misinterpretation of vascular pressures. Auto-PEEP

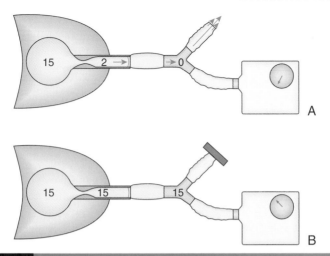

FIGURE 6-11

Measurement of auto-PEEP. **A,** Auto-PEEP is not constantly read by the ventilator pressure manometer because the manometer is open to atmosphere during exhalation and reads only the set-PEEP. **B,** For determination of auto-PEEP, the exhalation port is occluded just before the beginning of the subsequent breath. Circuit and airway pressure equilibrate, allowing for the measurement of total PEEP. The following calculation is used to determine auto-PEEP: Auto-PEEP = Total PEEP − Set-PEEP. *Shaded area* represents an area of airway obstruction. For additional causes of formation of auto-PEEP, see the text.

may subject the patient to an increased WOB to trigger the inspiratory flow of gases. When auto-PEEP is present, the patient must draw back through both the auto-PEEP and the set sensitivity level (usually −2 cm H_2O) to initiate inspiratory flow. A final problem that may occur when the presence of auto-PEEP is unknown is the miscalculation of compliance. In measurements of both static and dynamic compliance, the total PEEP value must be used or errors will result (see Chapter 2).

Correction of unwanted auto-PEEP requires making ventilator adjustments that provide for a longer expiratory time to allow the lungs to return to their resting volume before the next breath. Such ventilator adjustments include decreasing the RR or V_T or increasing the peak inspiratory flow rate so the desired volume is given in a shorter inspiratory time. Another mechanism is removal of any set-PEEP so that the total PEEP is reduced. Bronchodilators may also be used as a method of reducing obstruction to expiratory flow.

Clues to the presence of auto-PEEP are excessive negative inspiratory effort by the patient to trigger the ventilator, rapid respiratory rates (RRs) and high minute ventilation. Auto-PEEP should also be suspected when causes of flow obstruction, such as wheezing, are present, which may indicate high expiratory resistance or a history of COPD.

In patients with airway obstruction, applied PEEP is advocated to counteract auto-PEEP. In this setting, auto-PEEP is measured and then set-PEEP is applied at 50% to 80% of this value. The effect of PEEP is to maintain stability in the airway during expiration and release trapped gases. Auto-PEEP should be measured again to ensure it has been reduced.

VENTILATORY ADJUNCTS

Automatic Tube Compensation

Automatic tube compensation (ATC) is a new ventilatory adjunct that compensates for the flow-dependent pressure decrease across an endotracheal tube (ETT) during inspiration and expiration. The resistance of the tube can increase the ventilatory work. Because the ETT is not present after extubation, it is widely accepted that the intubated patient should be compensated for the increased WOB related to the ETT by using PS. PS provides a constant support level and therefore can lead to undercompensation during the inspiration start phase (high gas flow) and over-compensation during the last part of the inspiration (low gas flow). In contrast, ATC compensates continuously during inspiration and expiration according to the actual gas flow. When ATC is applied, the pressure assist is adjusted continuously during the ventilatory cycle to the change in flow rate and therefore to the change in flow-dependent pressure decrease across the ETT.

The variable entered into the ventilator is the tube size. The ventilator then performs continuous measurement of gas flow rate and airway pressure (proximal to the tube) and rapid calculation of the pressure decrease across the ETT, whereby the ventilator then provides immediate adjustments in support using sophisticated technology. In endotracheally intubated patients, ATC is associated with reduced WOB, a more physiologic breathing pattern, and improved synchronization between patient and ventilator. ATC has also been referred to as electronic extubation because the practitioner can evaluate the patient's breathing by using ATC alone without any additional ventilatory support. This evaluation might provide a useful predictor of successful extubation; however, this has not been clinically tested. ATC, a very new adjunct, is not available on all ventilators, nor can it be expected to perform identically on those ventilators that provide this option.

CORRECTING OXYGENATION AND VENTILATION PROBLEMS

Once the initial ventilator settings are applied, the analysis of ABGs should be performed, generally 20 minutes later. The ABG values allow assessment of the adequacy of oxygenation and ventilation and determination of the correlation between the pulse oximeter saturation of hemoglobin with oxygen in arterial blood (SaO_2) value and the laboratory-quantified SaO_2 value. Ventilator adjustments, if necessary, may then be made to correct problems with oxygenation and ventilation (Table 6-5). Chapters 7 and 9 further explore the adjustment of ventilator settings.

TABLE 6-5	Correction of Oxygenation and Ventilation Problems Through Adjustment of the Ventilator Settings

Problem	ABG Findings	Ventilator Setting Adjustments
Excessive oxygenation	Pao_2 >100 mm Hg Sao_2 100%	Decrease Fio_2 Return I:E ratio to 1:2 if prolonged I:E was applied Decrease PEEP
Inadequate oxygenation	Pao_2 <60 mm Hg Sao_2 <90%	Increase Fio_2 Increase PEEP Prolong inspiratory time to increase mPaw
Respiratory acidosis	$Paco_2$ >45 mm Hg pH ≤7.35	Increase V_T while maintaining PIP ≤40 cm H_2O Increase RR
Respiratory alkalosis	$Paco_2$ <35 mm Hg pH ≥7.45	Decrease V_T Decrease RR

ABG, Arterial blood gas; *Fio₂,* fraction of oxygen in inspired gas; *I:E ratio,* inspiratory-to-expiratory ratio; *Paco₂,* partial pressure of carbon dioxide in arterial blood; *Pao₂,* partial pressure of oxygen in arterial blood; *mPaw,* mean airway pressure; *PEEP,* positive end-expiratory pressure; *PIP,* peak inspiratory pressure; *RR,* respiratory rate; *Sao₂,* saturation of hemoglobin with oxygen in arterial blood; *V₸,* tidal volume.

RECOMMENDED READINGS

Amato MBP, Barbas CSV, Medeiros DM, et al. Effect of a protective-ventilation strategy on mortality in the acute respiratory distress syndrome. *N Engl J Med* 1998; 338:347–354.

Bone RC. Acute respiratory failure: Definition and overview. In RC Bone (ed.), *Pulmonary and Critical Care Medicine* (pp. 1–7). St. Louis: Mosby, 1993.

Branson RD. Flow-triggering systems. *Respir Care* 1994; 39(2):138–144.

Brower RG, Matthay MA, Morris A, et al. Ventilation with lower tidal volumes as compared with traditional tidal volumes for acute lung injury and the acute respiratory distress syndrome. *N Engl J Med* 2000; 342(18):1301–1309.

Burns SM. Auto-PEEP calculation. In DJ Lynn-McHale, KK Carlson (eds.), *AACN Procedure Manual*, 4th ed. (pp. 158–160). Philadelphia: Saunders, 2001.

Dupuis Y. Flow-by. In Y Dupuis (ed.), *Ventilators: Theory and Clinical Application* (pp. 230–235). St. Louis: Mosby, 1992.

Eisner MD, Thompson T, Hudson LD, et al. Efficacy of low tidal volume ventilation in patients with different clinical risk factors for acute lung injury and the acute respiratory distress syndrome. *Am J Resp Crit Care Med* 2001; 164:231–236.

Elsasser S, Guttman J, Stocker R, et al. Accuracy of automatic tube compensation in new-generation mechanical ventilators. *Crit Care Med* 2003; 31(11):2619–2626.

Haberthur C, Elsasser S, Eberhard L, et al. Total versus tube-related additional work of breathing in ventilator dependent patients. *Acta Anaesthesiol Scan* 2000; 44:749–757.

Hess DR, Kacmarek RM. *Essentials of Mechanical Ventilation.* New York: McGraw-Hill, 2002.

MacIntyre NR. Setting the frequency-tidal volume pattern. *Respir Care* 2002; 47(3): 266–274.

Marcy TW, Marini JJ. Inverse ratio ventilation in ARDS: Rationale and implementation. *Chest* 1991; 100(2):494–504.

Nellcor Puritan Bennett, Inc. *The ABC's of Smarter Breath Delivery: Understanding and Controlling Distinct Elements of Pressure-Based Breaths.* Pleasanton, Calif: Nellcor Puritan Bennett, Inc., 2002.

Oakes DF, Shortall SP. *Oakes' Ventilator Management: A Bedside Reference Guide.* Orono, Me: Respiratory Books, 2002.

Pierson DJ. Indications for mechanical ventilation in adults with acute respiratory failure. *Respir Care* 2002; 47(3):249–265.

Pilbeam SP. *Mechanical Ventilation: Physiological and Clinical Applications,* 3rd ed. St. Louis: Mosby, 1998.

Sassoon CSH. Mechanical ventilator design and function: The trigger variable. *Respir Care* 1992; 37(9):1056–1069.

Sassoon CSH, Lodia R, Rheeman CH, et al. Inspiratory muscle work of breathing during flow-by, demand-flow, and continuous-flow systems in patients with chronic obstructive lung disease. *Am Rev Respir Dis* 1992; 145:1219-1222.

Saura P, Blanch L. How to set positive end-expiratory pressure. *Respir Care* 2002; 47(3):279–295.

Shelledy DC, Peters JI. Initiating and adjusting ventilatory support. In RL Wilkins, JK Stoller, CL Scanlan (eds.), *Egan's Fundamental of Respiratory Care,* 8th ed. (pp. 1003–1053). St. Louis: Mosby, 2003.

Zavala E, Ferrer M, Polese G, et al. Effect of inverse I:E ratio ventilation on pulmonary gas exchange in acute respiratory distress syndrome. *Anesthesiology* 1998; 88:35–42.

CHAPTER 7

Modes of Mechanical Ventilation

There are many methods by which the patient and ventilator interact to perform the ventilatory cycle. These variable techniques are called *modes* of mechanical ventilation. The number of modes continues to increase in the effort to improve the efficiency of mechanical ventilation. As each new mode emerges, so do pro and con arguments about its use and about its advantages and disadvantages over previously described modes. That there are so many modes could be viewed as advantageous in the approach to the complex indications for mechanical ventilation. Confusion about differing modes, however, is compounded by manufacturers using different terms to describe the same mode. Companies do this as an attempt to differentiate their ventilator from all the others. There is no one best mode for management of the patient requiring ventilatory support, and limited clinical studies are available to prove the effectiveness of newer modes. Therefore, there is no exact science to the application of the various modes. Experience and skill rank very high in the success of a mode's application.

This chapter describes the modes of mechanical ventilation, their indications, their advantages and disadvantages, and the focus areas of patient monitoring. The focus areas of patient monitoring are key areas of total assessment that may have greater variability when the mode under discussion is used and therefore need to be monitored closely. It is assumed that a complete assessment is performed on each patient and includes physical examination, laboratory and radiograph findings, ventilator settings, and patient data such as the peak inspiratory pressure (PIP), exhaled tidal volume (EVT), and minute ventilation ($\dot{V}E$).

BREATH TYPES

The naming of breath types is very important to understanding ventilator modes. There are four different breath types that a patient on a ventilator may demonstrate clinically (Table 7-1). Breath types are classified by whether the patient or the ventilator triggers, limits, and cycles the breath. Recall from Chapter 6 that *cycling* is the changeover from the inspiratory to the expiratory phase. Machine-cycled breaths may be mandatory or assisted, and patient-cycled breaths may be supported or spontaneous.

In controlled ventilation, the ventilator initiates the breath and performs all the work of breathing (WOB). In assisted ventilation, the patient initiates and terminates

TABLE 7-1 Mechanical Ventilation Breath Types

Breath Type	Description
MACHINE-CYCLED	
Mandatory breath	A breath that is triggered, limited, and cycled by the ventilator. Ventilator performs all of the work of breathing throughout the phases of ventilation
Assisted breath	A breath that is triggered by the patient, then limited and cycled by the ventilator.
PATIENT-CYCLED	
Supported breath	A breath that is triggered by the patient, limited by the ventilator, and cycled by the patient. A spontaneous breath with an inspiratory pressure greater than baseline.
Spontaneous breath	A breath that is triggered, limited, and cycled by the patient. The patient performs all of the work of ventilation.

all or some of the breaths, with the ventilator giving variable amounts of support throughout the respiratory cycle. Hence the modes of ventilation vary in degree of patient versus ventilator effort. The mode chosen for a particular patient depends on how much of the WOB the patient can perform—that is, on how much work it is appropriate for the patient to perform, considering the patient's pathologic condition.

FULL VERSUS PARTIAL VENTILATORY SUPPORT

The question of which mode is the so-called right mode of ventilation for respiratory failure of a particular cause has no simple answer because there are many therapeutic options. Ventilatory support can be classified according to two general approaches: full ventilatory support (FVS) and partial ventilatory support (PVS). FVS constitutes mechanical ventilation in which the ventilator performs all of the WOB without any contribution from the patient. The ventilator alone provides the minute volume of gases required to satisfy the patient's respiratory needs. PVS occurs when both the ventilator and the patient contribute toward the WOB and meeting the minute volume of gases required to satisfy respiratory needs.

FVS may be the initial application of mechanical ventilation required by patients with acute respiratory failure (ARF). Common modes for providing FVS are volume or pressure continuous mandatory ventilation (CMV). FVS may be necessary to relieve the patient of the WOB, allow the diaphragm and ventilatory muscles to recuperate from fatigue, and allow time for the underlying pulmonary abnormality to begin to resolve. FVS is also indicated in patients with apnea; patients who are heavily sedated or paralyzed; patients with depressed neurologic status, drug overdose, or stroke; and when negative respiratory effort is contraindicated, such as in severe flail chest. The term *FVS* should not be construed to mean that the ventilator has complete control of ventilatory processes; instead, it means that the ventilator provides all of the patient's ventilatory needs.

The advantages of PVS include allowing the patient to respond to increases in carbon dioxide by increasing $\dot{V}_E$ and promoting use of the respiratory muscles, thereby preventing disuse atrophy. Allowing some degree of spontaneous breathing during mechanical ventilation improves ventilation/perfusion matching and may help prevent adverse effects of mechanical ventilation such as hemodynamic compromise, atelectasis formation, and need for sedation. PVS can be provided by most currently available modes through titration of the amount of support offered. The proliferation of new modes designed to provide PVS is partly because of the known benefits of spontaneous breathing and partly because of tremendous progress in microprocessor technology over the past 10 years. As a result, patient-ventilator interactions are more complex during these spontaneous breathing modes as compared to controlled mechanical ventilation. Therefore, the principal purpose of the new PVS modes is to enhance coordination between the patient's spontaneous breathing and mechanical assistance at all phases of the respiratory cycle. The principal purpose of a new controlled mode is to improve oxygenation without further damaging the lung.

As pulmonary mechanics and compliance improve during PVS and the patient is able to generate more of the WOB, ventilator assistance should be reduced accordingly. The workload must be balanced between the patient and the ventilator in a way that prevents ventilatory muscle atrophy or fatigue. To apply this principle objectively, one must appreciate all the components of the patient's WOB: normal physiologic WOB, the WOB imposed by the airway and ventilator circuitry, and the physiologic WOB imposed by the disease process. Thorough assessment of the patient's condition and an understanding of how each mode operates and therefore interacts with the patient to perform the WOB are essential. In titrating PVS, clinical judgment plays a key role.

PRESSURE CONTROL VERSUS VOLUME CONTROL

Modes of positive-pressure ventilation may be classified as volume controlled, pressure controlled, or dual control. This classification stems from the limit variable—the target value—set for inspiration. The limit variable is the variable that the ventilator maintains at a preset value during inspiration. It is the maximum value a variable can attain. The limit variable (pressure, volume, or both in dual control) is manipulated to control the breath but does not cause inspiration to end. The variable that ends the inspiratory phase is the cycle variable. For example, a patient could be ventilated using a pressure-limited mode set at a pressure of 12 cm H_2O. If this pressure-limited mode is pressure support (PS), then inspiration will end when a preset flow is attained. Therefore, the breaths are pressure limited and flow cycled. The pressure is limited, or controlled, but reaching the pressure does not end inspiration; flow does.

The breath delivery type (pressure or volume) is used as a prefix in the nomenclature for identifying the mode of ventilation. Throughout this chapter, pressure and/or flow waveforms are used to depict the typical ventilation pattern resulting from the use of a mode. Figure 7-1, a graph of spontaneous ventilation, serves as an example of these waveforms.

213

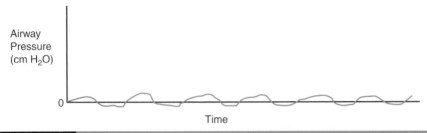

FIGURE 7-1

Spontaneous ventilation. Pressure, in centimeters of H_2O, is graphed on vertical axis against time on horizontal axis. Negative deflections represent patient inspiratory effort. Spontaneous respirations are sinusoidal in shape. *(Modified from Pilbeam SP. Mechanical Ventilation: Physiological and Clinical Applications, 3rd ed. St. Louis: Mosby, 1998.)*

VOLUME CONTROL VENTILATION

A delivered breath is volume controlled when volume is constant for every breath. The ventilator maintains the volume waveform in a specific pattern for every breath. The pressure waveform varies because pressure is variable and depends on the patient's lung, chest wall, and breathing circuit mechanics. The mode name is preceded by a V, indicating it is volume controlled.

Continuous Mandatory Ventilation

DEFINITION AND DESCRIPTION

With volume continuous mandatory ventilation (V-CMV), the patient receives a preset number of breaths per minute of a preset tidal volume (VT). Patient effort does not trigger a mechanical breath. The ventilator performs all the WOB. The breaths are machine triggered, limited, and cycled (Fig. 7-2). On many ventilators, the CMV mode differs from the volume assist/control (V-A/C) mode only when the sensitivity

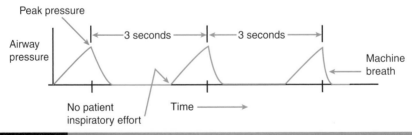

FIGURE 7-2

Controlled mechanical ventilation (CMV). Patient receives a preset number of breaths of a preset tidal volume, delivered at equal time intervals. Patient effort will not trigger either a spontaneous or mechanical breath. *(Modified from Pilbeam SP. Mechanical Ventilation: Physiological and Clinical Applications, 3rd ed. St. Louis: Mosby, 1998.)*

is set so the ventilator will not respond to the patient's inspiratory efforts. Some manufacturers use the term *CMV* to refer to the A/C mode, which leads to confusion between these two modes. The rationale for their use of the term *CMV* involves redefining it to mean controlled *mandatory* ventilation, in which every breath is of a mandatory VT. However, nomenclature varies by manufacturer.

INDICATIONS
1. For patients with no respiratory effort because of dysfunction of the central nervous system (e.g., Guillain-Barré syndrome, high-level spinal cord lesions).
2. To provide a fail-safe method of ventilating the patient's lungs under conditions such as anesthesia or as a backup to assisted ventilation.

ADVANTAGES AND DISADVANTAGES
V-CMV was used widely before the advent of A/C ventilation. Because the patient cannot achieve a spontaneous breath, attempts to breathe result in patient effort with no flow delivered. This can lead to sensations of air hunger and significantly increase the WOB. This disadvantage has relegated the use of CMV to the indications just listed.

This mode is inefficient if the patient attempts to breathe because breathing will cause patient-ventilator asynchrony. Evidence that the patient is attempting to initiate a breath may include contractions of the inspiratory accessory muscles and sternal retractions. Accordingly, patients who can generate spontaneous respiratory efforts should be ventilated with a more appropriate mode. If the patient splints the chest wall or exhales during inspiration, the peak airway pressure limit set on the ventilator may be reached. This causes the remainder of the inspiratory volume to be dumped from the ventilator into the atmosphere, commonly called *bucking the ventilator.*

With CMV, alveolar ventilation and the respiratory contribution to acid-base balance are completely controlled by the clinician. Acid-base balance must be closely monitored and ventilator settings adjusted with changing physiologic scenarios, such as fever, change in nutritional intake, and stress.

Respiratory muscle weakness and atrophy may result from disuse if CMV is used for an extended period, making it harder to wean the patient from the ventilator. Adverse hemodynamic effects may occur with use of this mode because every breath is delivered under positive pressure.

FOCUS AREAS OF PATIENT MONITORING
1. PIP because it is variable and adjusts according to changes in compliance and resistance.
2. EVT because even though the clinician presets the VT, delivery is not guaranteed. If EVT deviates from the set VT by 50 mL or greater in adults, look for a source of the loss of VT (e.g., leaks in system or circuit, patient chest tubes, etc.) (see Chapter 9).
3. Acid-base balance because the clinician controls the respiratory component.
4. Patient-ventilator asynchrony that may be caused by flow rate or respiratory rate (RR) settings that are inadequate to meet the patient's ventilatory needs.
5. Adequate sedation to suppress spontaneous respirations.

Volume Assist/Control Mode

DEFINITION AND DESCRIPTION

The V-A/C mode is a method of ventilation in which the ventilator delivers a preset number of breaths of a preset V_T. Between time-triggered, machine-initiated breaths, the patient may trigger spontaneous breaths. When the ventilator senses the patient's spontaneous respiratory effort, it delivers an assisted breath of the preset V_T. The patient cannot vary the volume of spontaneously initiated breaths (Fig. 7-3). The difference between A/C and CMV is that with the A/C mode, the ventilator is sensitive and responds to the patient's spontaneous respiratory efforts. The work that the patient must perform is the negative inspiratory effort required to trigger the vent on the patient-initiated breaths. The ventilator performs the bulk of the work if the flow rate and sensitivity are set correctly. Many manufacturers use the term *CMV* to mean A/C. Their rationale involves redefining CMV to mean controlled *mandatory* ventilation, in which every breath is of a mandatory V_T. Other manufacturers' terms for this mode include volume control.

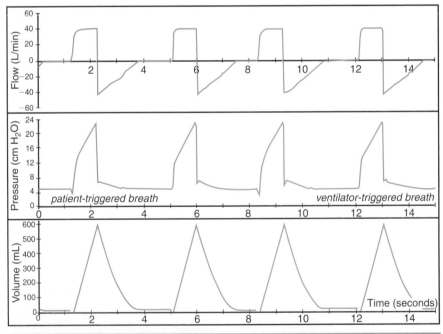

FIGURE 7-3

Volume assist/control (V-A/C) mode of ventilation. Patient receives a preset number of control breaths of a preset tidal volume. The patient may trigger additional breaths. These machine-assisted breaths will be of the preset tidal volume. An assisted breath is evident by the negative pressure deflection created by the patient when triggering the ventilator. A control breath shows no negative deflection. *(Modified from Hess DR, Kacmarek RM. Essentials of Mechanical Ventilation, 2nd ed. New York: McGraw-Hill, 2002, p 38.)*

INDICATIONS

1. Normal respiratory drive, but respiratory muscles are too weak to perform the WOB (e.g., when a patient is emerging from anesthesia).
2. Normal respiratory drive, but respiratory muscles are unable to perform the WOB because it is increased (e.g., in pulmonary abnormalities in which lung compliance is decreased).
3. When it is desirable to allow patients to set their own rate and thereby assist in maintaining a normal partial pressure of carbon dioxide in arterial blood ($Paco_2$). Patient cannot control volume or duration of breath.

ADVANTAGES AND DISADVANTAGES

The A/C mode allows the patient to control the rate of breathing, and yet it guarantees the delivery of a minimal preset rate and volume. The A/C mode also allows some work to be performed by the respiratory muscles, although it is minimal if the flow rate and sensitivity are set appropriately. It is indicated when it is desirable for the ventilator to perform the bulk of the ventilatory work.

Disadvantages include respiratory alkalosis that may ensue because of patients' tendency to hyperventilate related to anxiety, pain, or neurologic factors. Significant alkalosis suppresses ventilatory drive and is detrimental to many metabolic functions. Hyperventilation may also lead to the formation of intrinsic positive end-expiratory pressure, also known as auto-PEEP, because of a shortened expiratory time. Variability in the patient's hemodynamic status may occur with the A/C mode because every breath is delivered under positive pressure. The patient may ride the ventilator, become lazy, and not participate in breathing.

FOCUS AREAS OF PATIENT MONITORING

1. PIP because it is variable in this volume-cycled mode of ventilation and will adjust in relationship to changes in compliance and resistance.
2. EVT because although VT is preset on the ventilator control panel, delivery is not guaranteed. If EVT deviates from the set VT by 50 mL or greater in adults, look for a source of the loss of VT (see Chapter 9).
3. Evaluation of patient's sense of comfort. Monitor airway pressure manometer during patient's spontaneous respiratory effort and adjust sensitivity to allow for minimal triggering effort. Adjust flow rate to meet patient's inspiratory demands by monitoring the pressure-time curve. Pressure should rise smoothly during inspiration. If the curve is concave, the patient is actively inspiring because his or her demands are not met. Increase the flow until the curve becomes convex. The trigger sensitivity and the flow rate are the chief variables affecting the patient's WOB when the A/C mode is used.
4. Close monitoring of acid-base status. If the patient is hyperventilating, consider sedation or changing to a mode in which the patient has greater control (i.e., IMV [intermittent mandatory ventilation], synchronized IMV, or PSV).

Volume-Intermittent Mandatory Ventilation and Synchronized Intermittent Mandatory Ventilation

DEFINITION AND DESCRIPTION

Volume intermittent mandatory ventilation (V-IMV) and volume synchronized intermittent mandatory ventilation (V-SIMV) are modes of ventilation in which the patient receives a set number of breaths of a set V_T. Between these mandatory breaths, the patient may initiate spontaneous breaths. The volume of the spontaneous breaths depends on the muscular respiratory effort that the patient is able to generate. The difference between IMV and SIMV is that, in the latter, the mandatory breaths are synchronized to the patient's spontaneous respiratory efforts. With IMV the mandatory breaths are delivered at a precise time, regardless of where the patient is in the ventilatory cycle, whereas with SIMV the ventilator synchronizes the delivery of the mandatory breath when it senses the patient's inspiratory effort. This is achieved in SIMV by the ventilator's monitoring for the patient's spontaneous inspiratory effort within a window of time (assist window) and then delivering the mandatory breath in synchrony with the patient's inspiratory effort if it occurs within this timing window (Fig. 7-4). If the patient does not make an inspiratory effort within the timing window, the mandatory breath is delivered at the scheduled time. The ventilator then resets to respond to the next spontaneous inspiratory effort.

The main difference between the IMV and A/C modes is the volume of the *patient-initiated* breaths. Patient-initiated breaths in the A/C mode result in the patient's receiving a guaranteed V_T, whereas in SIMV spontaneous breath V_T is variable because it depends on patient effort and lung characteristics. IMV was originally developed in an effort to create a mode in which the patient could interact with the ventilator, using the respiratory muscles; thus, it is useful for weaning patients from ventilatory support. As the IMV rate is lowered, the patient initiates more spontaneous breaths, therefore assuming a greater portion of the ventilatory work. As the patient demonstrates the ability to generate more work, the mandatory breath rate is decreased accordingly.

INDICATIONS

1. Normal respiratory drive but respiratory muscles unable to perform all WOB.
2. In situations in which it is desirable to allow patients to set their own RR and thus assist in maintaining a normal Pa_{CO_2}.
3. Weaning from mechanical ventilation, however, compared to other weaning modalities SIMV is associated with the longest weaning and the lowest success rates.

ADVANTAGES AND DISADVANTAGES

The patient is guaranteed a minimum $\dot{V}_E$ and a guaranteed volume with each mandatory breath. Respiratory alkalosis is less of a problem in this mode than in the A/C mode because the patient can modify rate and volume of the spontaneous breaths. Less atrophy of the respiratory muscles may occur because the patient may participate more in ventilation, using the ventilatory muscles to a greater degree than

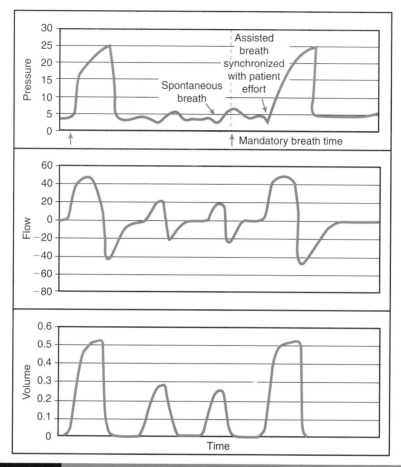

FIGURE 7-4

Synchronized intermittent mandatory ventilation (SIMV). Mandatory breaths are volume controlled and delivered in synchrony with spontaneous breaths if they fall within the mandatory breath-timing window. The up arrow represents the clock time where a mandatory breath is due based on the set respiratory rate. First breath is a mandatory (time-triggered) breath. At the second up arrow the patient is in the expiratory phase of a spontaneous breath. The SIMV timing-window algorithm allows the patient to complete this breath and synchronizes the next mandatory breath with the patient's inspiratory effort. *(Modified from Hess DR, Kacmarek RM. Essentials of Mechanical Ventilation, 2nd ed. New York: McGraw-Hill, 2002, p 63.)*

when CMV or A/C is used. The hemodynamic effects of positive-pressure ventilation may be less with IMV than CMV or A/C because ventilation occurs at a lower mean airway pressure (mPaw) when spontaneous breaths are taken; therefore, the average mean airway pressure over time is less. Also, the distribution of gas within the lung is better during spontaneous breathing.

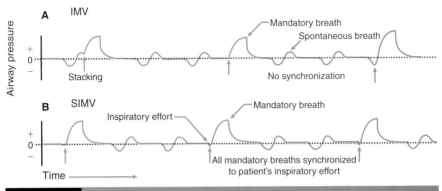

FIGURE 7-5

Intermittent mandatory ventilation (IMV) and synchronized intermittent mandatory ventilation (SIMV). Pressure waveform shows essential differences between IMV and SIMV. Mandatory breaths are marked with vertical arrows. In IMV (**A**), mandatory breaths are given at equal time intervals regardless of where the patient is in the ventilatory cycle. This can result in breath stacking. In SIMV (**B**), mandatory breaths are delivered in synchrony with the patient's negative inspiratory effort. *(Modified from Dupuis YG. Ventilators: Theory and Clinical Application, 2nd ed. St. Louis: Mosby, 1992.)*

IMV fails to monitor the patient's spontaneous respiratory efforts and may deliver a mandatory breath during the patient's own ventilatory cycle (Fig. 7-5). This may lead to breath stacking, in which a mechanical breath falls during or at the end of the patient's breath. This creates patient-ventilator dyssynchrony, discomfort, inadequate ventilation, and potentially barotrauma. If breath stacking leads to pressure limiting on inspiration, then the ventilator vents the rest of the V_T to the atmosphere. Synchronizing mandatory breaths with the patient's readiness to breathe improves patient comfort, reduces competition between ventilator and patient, and prevents breath stacking and its potential problems, such as barotrauma and loss of V_T as a result of pressure limiting.

Spontaneous breaths in an SIMV system may be provided through a continuous-flow system or through a demand valve. The opening of the demand valve occurs in response to a drop in circuit pressure created by the patient's inspiratory effort. When this drop in pressure is sensed, the flow of fresh gas is initiated to meet the patient's respiratory needs. Demand flow systems vary considerably in circuit resistance and the amount of negative effort the patient must generate to initiate the flow of gases. The WOB associated with the demand valve system comes from several sources: from the amount of work required to open the valve; from the ongoing ventilatory muscle work performed during the lag time, which begins at the onset of the flow of gases and ends when the patient actually receives the gas; and from flow rates that are insufficient to meet the patient's ventilatory demand. The realization that some demand valve systems impose significant work has led in the newer generation of ventilators to the development of demand flow systems that require less work to activate. Flow-triggering is designed to provide continuous flow and eliminate the lag time from onset of breath to delivery of gas (see Chapter 6). The WOB associated with triggering spontaneous breaths is reduced by the operator, ensuring the flow rate is set adequately to meet the patient's inspiratory demands. Finally, the WOB imposed by the ventilator circuit and the artificial airway may be eliminated with the use of PS, which provides inspiratory ventilatory assistance.

FOCUS AREAS OF PATIENT MONITORING

1. The patient's RR. If the RR increases, then the VT of the spontaneous breaths should be assessed. Ideal VT of the spontaneous breaths should be 5 to 7 mL/kg. If the patient is beginning to fatigue, a more shallow and rapid respiratory pattern may develop. This ventilatory pattern will lead to atelectasis, a reduction in compliance, further increase in the WOB, and the need for greater ventilatory support.

2. PIP because it is variable in this volume mode of ventilation and will change in relationship to changes in compliance and resistance.

3. EVT of mandatory breaths because even though a VT is set, delivery is not guaranteed. If EVT deviates from set VT, look for a source of the loss of VT (see Chapter 9).

4. EVT of spontaneous breaths. Volume should be 5 to 7 mL/kg. Volumes less than 5 mL/kg promote the development of atelectasis and indicate that the patient does not have sufficient respiratory muscle strength to generate an adequate VT.

5. Patient comfort and patient-ventilator synchrony. If the patient complains of feeling unable to get enough air, ensure that the sensitivity and flow rates are adjusted appropriately. If patient-ventilator dyssynchrony is a problem, especially during weaning trials, assess that ventilatory demands are being met. If so, talk with the patient calmly and reassuringly, coaching him or her to work with the ventilator, that is, to relax and allow the ventilator to deliver the mandatory breaths. Provide sedation and anxiolytic medications as necessary in doses that will not suppress the respiratory drive. If patient discomfort remains a problem and weaning is the goal, consider a mode that allows the patient more control over the breathing pattern, such as PS.

Mandatory Minute Ventilation

DEFINITION AND DESCRIPTION

Mandatory minute ventilation (MMV) is a mode where the patient breathes spontaneously, yet a constant minute ventilation ($\dot{V}_E$) is guaranteed. If the patient's spontaneous ventilation does not match the target $\dot{V}_E$, the ventilator provides whatever part of the $\dot{V}_E$ the patient does not achieve. The method of delivering the deficit in $\dot{V}_E$ depends on ventilator model. In volume mandatory minute ventilation (V-MMV), if the patient's $\dot{V}_E$ falls below the prescribed level, the ventilator responds by delivering mandatory volume breaths (increasing the breath rate). Therefore, both spontaneous and mandatory breaths are provided as in IMV. The assisted breaths are patient triggered, machine (volume) limited, and machine (volume) cycled. The mandatory breaths are volume controlled, machine (time) triggered, machine (volume) limited, and machine (volume) cycled.

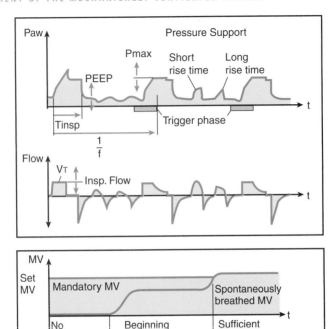

FIGURE 7-6

Mandatory minute ventilation. The patient can breathe spontaneously and therefore contribute to reaching the target minute ventilation. The first half of the figure demonstrates V-MMV; the second, P-MMV. This mode is intended for weaning patients by incrementally reducing the mandatory portion of overall minute volume. *(Courtesy Draeger Medical, Inc., Telford, Pa.)*

In pressure mandatory minute ventilation (P-MMV), the ventilator increases the level of PS when the target $\dot{V}E$ is not met. Essentially, the patient is receiving variable PS. Therefore, P-MMV is classified as pressure-controlled, patient-triggered, pressure-limited, patient-cycled ventilation. There are no mandatory breaths with P-MMV, and if the target $\dot{V}E$ is met, there are no PS adjustments (Fig. 7-6).

Sophisticated algorithms typically monitor a moving time-averaged $\dot{V}E$ and vary the rate or level of inspiratory pressure as necessary. The $\dot{V}E$ set as the target varies according to indication for using MMV. If used to ensure adequate ventilation in patients with a fluctuating ventilatory drive, the target $\dot{V}E$ should be one that results in an acceptable $Paco_2$. If used as a weaning mode, $\dot{V}E$ should be set to ensure a $Paco_2$ necessary to stimulate spontaneous breathing. A $\dot{V}E$ that is 80% to 90% of the patient's $\dot{V}E$ requirements is usually acceptable.

MMV was originally designed to address the problems encountered with weaning with IMV. This mode ensures a safe level of ventilation if during IMV weaning the patient's ability to breathe spontaneously is inadequate or declines. The ventilator simply increases the amount of mechanical support provided to ensure adequate ventilation. Likewise, as the patient's ventilatory function improves, the ventilator gradually delivers less and less support. The designers of MMV developed a system that required less user interface while ensuring a constant, safe level of ventilation. Indeed, MMV is the first closed-loop mode of ventilation. Closed loop means that the ventilator changes its output based on a measured input variable.

Manufacturers use a variety of terms to describe the modes available on their ventilators that provide MMV. These modes include minimum mandatory ventilation, augmented minute volume (AMV), and extended mandatory minute ventilation (EMMV). The patient may be breathing spontaneously or under controlled conditions, depending on the mode that is operating under the principles of MMV.

INDICATIONS

1. As a weaning tool, MMV may enhance the weaning process by promoting muscle strength while preventing fatigue.
2. When there is a desire for spontaneous breathing but the patient has an unstable ventilatory drive, MMV may be used to smooth transitions in the patient's ventilatory support needs, especially when there are fluctuations in ventilatory drive or effort.

ADVANTAGES AND DISADVANTAGES

MMV prevents hypoventilation and possible resultant hypercapnia and respiratory acidosis. The possibility of hypoventilation related to administration of sedative narcotics for the treatment of agitation or pain or during procedures is eliminated. Patients can breathe spontaneously while a safety net is always provided. Whether MMV provides a smoother transition from mechanically ventilatory support to spontaneous ventilation is not known. Maintenance of a stable $\dot{V}_E$ may result in fewer arterial blood gas (ABG) measurements and fewer manual ventilator adjustments, and it therefore may reduce the cost of ventilator weaning. However, MMV certainly does not eliminate the need for the bedside practitioner to assimilate all the data and then to guide the ventilator's settings and monitor its function.

The primary disadvantage of MMV is that MMV systems do not monitor the quality of the spontaneous breaths; thus, the patient with a rapid, shallow breathing pattern can achieve the target $\dot{V}_E$ without alveolar ventilation being adequate. This defeats the basic premise of the system. Atelectasis may then develop. If the patient's $\dot{V}_E$ demand increases because of fever, activity, etc. and the target $\dot{V}_E$ is not adjusted, the patient's needs will not be met. Another concern regarding MMV is that patient care may be adversely affected by the purported reduction in required patient assessment and intervention. The caregiver may be lulled into a false sense of security that the ventilator is managing the patient's ventilatory needs, and a less thorough assessment may ensue.

FOCUS AREAS OF PATIENT MONITORING

1. RR because patient can have a rapid, shallow breathing pattern and meet the $\dot{V}_E$ target. Alveolar ventilation will become increasingly inadequate while dead-space ventilation increases. In fact, alveolar ventilation could become negligible if the patient's V_T nears physiologic dead space. A high RR alarm must be set.
2. Monitor PIP in V-MMV because it will be variable.

PRESSURE CONTROL VENTILATION

A delivered breath is pressure controlled when pressure is constant for every breath. The ventilator maintains the pressure waveform in a specific pattern for every breath. The volume waveform varies because volume is variable and depends on the patient's lung, chest wall, and breathing circuit mechanics. The mode name is preceded by a P, indicating it is pressure controlled.

Continuous Positive Airway Pressure

DEFINITION AND DESCRIPTION

Continuous positive airway pressure (CPAP) is positive pressure applied throughout the respiratory cycle to the spontaneously breathing patient (Fig. 7-7). The patient must have a reliable ventilatory drive and an adequate VT because no mandatory breaths or other ventilatory assistance is given the patient. Furthermore, the patient performs all the WOB.

CPAP provides positive pressure at end-exhalation, thus preventing alveolar collapse, improving the functional residual capacity (FRC), and enhancing oxygenation. CPAP can also help splint the airways open, thus reducing airway resistance and flow limitation. When flow limitation results in trapped gases in the lung causing auto-PEEP, CPAP can equalize the pressure at the mouth and the alveoli and reduce the WOB.

As discussed previously (Chapter 6), CPAP is identical to PEEP in its physiologic effects. *CPAP* is the correct term when the baseline pressure is elevated in the *spontaneously* breathing patient both when the ventilator is used and when it is not. *PEEP* is the term used when the baseline pressure is elevated and the patient is receiving some form of additional respiratory support (e.g., A/C, SIMV, PS).

INDICATIONS

1. During spontaneous breathing trials when weaning from mechanical ventilation. CPAP is used to promote alveolar stability and improve the FRC, in comparison with breathing on T-piece or trach mask without CPAP.
2. Adequate ventilation but incompetent oxygenation because of conditions that decrease the FRC, such as atelectasis or secretion retention.
3. Obstructive sleep apnea.
4. Dynamic hyperinflation and auto-PEEP to reduce the WOB.

ADVANTAGES AND DISADVANTAGES

The primary advantage of CPAP is that it increases the FRC and reduces intrapulmonary shunt. CPAP also maintains and promotes respiratory muscle strength because the patient is given no other ventilatory assistance and therefore performs all the WOB. CPAP is often incorporated into a weaning plan as a mechanism to build respiratory muscle strength. For example, CPAP periods may be alternated with periods of full ventilatory support. The time spent in the CPAP trial should be increased as the patient's respiratory muscle function improves.

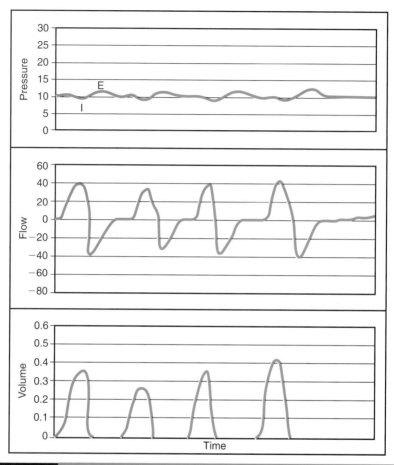

FIGURE 7-7

Continuous positive airway pressure (CPAP). Patient is breathing spontaneously, with positive pressure applied throughout ventilatory cycle. Therefore, both inspiratory positive airway pressure (IPAP) and expiratory positive airway pressure (EPAP) are present. The baseline is always positive at the level of CPAP set, never returning to ambient pressure. Note that the waveform of spontaneous respiration is sinusoidal. *I,* Inspiration; *E,* expiration. *(Modified from MacIntyre NR, Branson RD. Mechanical Ventilation. Philadelphia: Saunders, 2001.)*

Because the patient is still connected to the ventilator, when using CPAP as a weaning mode the practitioner benefits from low EV_T and apnea alarms and the delivery of mandatory breaths as a backup in the event of apnea. None of these options are present when weaning is accomplished with a T-piece or trach mask trial. Furthermore, the adequacy of the V_T can be readily monitored on the display panel of the ventilator. For further information on the use of CPAP as a weaning mode, see Chapter 11, Weaning from Mechanical Ventilation.

The application of positive pressure may cause decreased cardiac output, increased intracranial pressure, and pulmonary barotrauma. Levels of positive pressure generally used with CPAP are 5 to 10 cm H_2O. These levels are unlikely to cause serious adverse effects unless significant hypovolemia or cardiac dysfunction is present. If the latter is present, then a mode that requires the patient to perform less WOB is indicated.

FOCUS AREAS OF PATIENT MONITORING

1. The patient's RR. If the RR increases, the EVT should be assessed. If the patient is becoming fatigued, a more shallow and rapid respiratory pattern may develop. This pattern will lead to atelectasis and a reduction in compliance, further increasing the WOB and the need for greater ventilatory assistance.

2. The EVT, which should be 5 to 7 mL/kg. Volumes less than 5 mL/kg promote the development of atelectasis and indicate that the patient does not have sufficient respiratory muscle strength to generate an adequate VT. The mode of ventilation may need to be switched to one that provides additional assistance, such as PS, V-SIMV, P-SIMV, or A/C. If the patient is in a weaning trial and the RR is increasing and VT decreasing, these are signs of fatigue, and the chosen resting mode should be reinstated.

3. Patient comfort. If the patient complains of feeling unable to get enough air, ensure that the flow rate is adjusted appropriately. If the patient is anxious, especially during weaning trials, talk with the patient in a calm and reassuring manner and stay at the bedside until both you and the patient are confident that ventilation is adequate. Provide sedation and/or anxiolytic medications as necessary in doses that will not suppress respiration.

Pressure Support

DEFINITION AND DESCRIPTION

PS is a mode of ventilation in which the patient's spontaneous respiratory activity is augmented by the delivery of a preset amount of inspiratory positive pressure. When the patient triggers the onset of inspiration, the preselected amount of PS is delivered and then held constant throughout inspiration, thereby promoting the flow of gas into the lungs (Fig. 7-8). With PS there is no set VT. The VT is variable, determined by patient effort, the amount of applied PS, and the compliance and resistance of the system (patient and ventilator). Gas flow is delivered with the decelerating flow-wave pattern, in which the flow rate naturally decays as the patient's lungs fill with air on inspiration. The patient can vary the inspiratory flow on demand. Inspiration ends (the breath cycles) when the inspiratory flow rate decreases to a set terminal flow or a percentage of the initial inspiratory flow, i.e., 25% of peak flow, depending on ventilator model. PS is therefore a flow-cycled mode of ventilation. Because inspiration ends on the basis of a flow criterion (not pressure, time, or volume), the patient retains control over respiratory frequency, inspiratory time, and volume.

Other important components of the PS breath are the *trigger* and the *rise time*. Breaths may be triggered by detection of either a change in pressure or flow (Fig. 7-9).

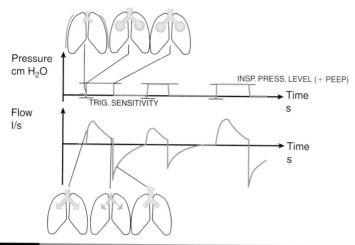

FIGURE 7-8

Pressure support (PS) ventilation. In PS ventilation, the patient's spontaneous respiratory effort is provided inspiratory pressure augmentation to promote the flow of gas into the lungs. The applied PS level is held constant throughout the inspiratory phase. *(Courtesy MAQUET, Inc., Bridgewater, NJ.)*

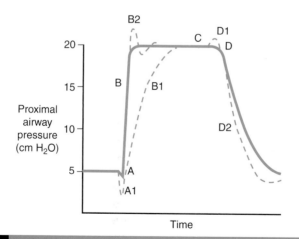

FIGURE 7-9

Important components of a PS breath. *A,* Trigger; *B,* rise time; *C,* pressure limit; *D,* cycle. The PS breath, if delivered, ideally appears as the solid line. Patient effort and manner of ventilator operation can affect the breath. *A1,* Incorrect sensitivity setting or slow response time; *B1,* slow rise time relative to patient demand, which can cause an increased work of breathing; *B2,* rise time too fast, causing overshoot; *D1,* pressure spike caused by patient actively exhaling because inspiratory time too long; *D2,* breath cycles too early because of B2 or early cycle criteria. *(Modified from MacIntyre NR, Branson RD. Mechanical Ventilation. Philadelphia: Saunders, 2001.)*

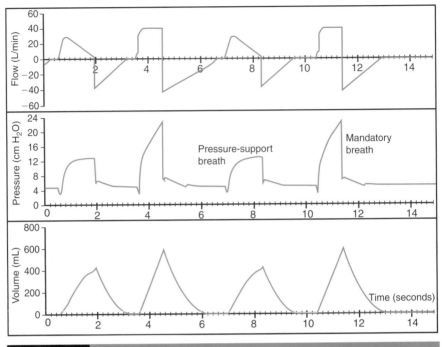

FIGURE 7-10

Synchronized intermittent mandatory ventilation (SIMV) with pressure support (PS) ventilation. In SIMV and PS, mandatory breaths of a preset tidal volume are administered in the fashion of SIMV. In this figure the square waveform is applied to the mandatory breaths. Only spontaneous breaths are pressure supported, not the mandatory breaths. *(Modified from Kacmarek RM, Dimas S, Mack CW. The Essentials of Respiratory Care. St. Louis: Mosby, 2005.)*

It is important that the trigger sensitivity be set to result in minimal work to initiate the flow of gas (see Chapter 6).

The rise time is the amount of time it takes for the set pressure to be reached. It should be set to meet the patient's peak inspiratory demand. An initial overshoot in pressure above the set PS level indicates the rise time is too rapid. Conversely, a concave wave on the initial airway pressure indicates that the rise time is too slow, which results in an increased WOB. As rise time is shortened, peak flow increases. As peak flow increases there is greater flow to meet inspiratory demand, and breath cycling may occur more rapidly. Therefore, pressure, rise time, and flow termination criteria are interrelated. If one is adjusted, the others should be evaluated. The best method to evaluate appropriateness of settings is to monitor the airway pressure graphics.

The PS mode may be used alone or in conjunction with SIMV (Fig. 7-10). Straight PS should only be used in patients who display a reliable respiratory drive because all breaths are patient initiated. When PS is used with SIMV, only the spontaneous breaths are pressure supported. One advantage of using SIMV and PS concurrently is that in the event of apnea, the patient is assured of a preset backup number of mandatory breaths.

PS may be delivered at either a high level or a low level. In high-level PS (PSV_{max}), the amount of PS is increased until the patient achieves full ventilatory support. When PS is used in this manner, no additional volume-cycled breaths are required as long as the patient has a consistent respiratory drive. In low-level PS, the amount of support is adjusted until the patient achieves a V_T that is acceptable for spontaneous breathing: 5 to 7 mL/kg. Low-level PS may be used alone; however, it is often used with an SIMV backup rate to ensure minimal alveolar ventilation. With either high- or low-level PS, the amount of support given to the patient is decreased as respiratory muscle strength increases and as the respiratory system mechanics improve, as evidenced by an improving V_T.

It is incorrect to say the patient is on PS and CPAP because CPAP is a mode in and of itself. Confusion arises about this latter point because of the terms used by ventilator manufacturers. If the PIP increases as a result of such events as splinting, coughing, or kinking of the ventilator circuit or airway, then the high-pressure-limit alarm parameter set by the operator will be reached, causing the ventilator to cycle into expiration. Recall that in PS the pressure limit is not the mechanism that routinely causes the ventilator to cycle from inspiration to expiration. PS is a flow-cycled, pressure-limited mode of ventilation.

INDICATIONS
1. Weaning from mechanical ventilation. The quality and quantity of work applied to the respiratory muscles can be tightly controlled by varying the level of PS. PS is used as for spontaneous breathing trials.
2. PS, by augmenting inspiratory flow, reduces the WOB associated with the artificial airway and the ventilator circuitry.
3. Noninvasive ventilation to augment spontaneous inspiratory volumes.

ADVANTAGES AND DISADVANTAGES
PS may be used to overcome the resistance work associated with moving inspiratory flow through an artificial airway and the ventilatory circuitry. If the WOB is decreased, so is the oxygen consumption in relation to ventilation. Decreasing the WOB also increases the likelihood that the patient will better tolerate weaning. PS improves patient-ventilator synchrony and patient comfort because the patient has control over the process of ventilation. The patient determines when to initiate a breath, the timing of inspiration and expiration, and the ventilatory pattern. Therefore, the patient also maintains greater control over the $Paco_2$ and acid-base balance.

PS allows the operator to augment inadequate spontaneous V_T to any desired degree and to set the PIP. The amount of assistance afforded the patient and the quality and quantity of work applied to respiratory muscles for reconditioning are more "titratable" than with the volume-cycled modes of ventilation. With PS, every spontaneous breath is assisted and the amount of assistance can be reduced in increments as small as 2 cm H_2O, thereby gradually titrating the amount of work being relinquished to the patient. In comparison, when the number of mandatory breaths is reduced in SIMV, all WOB previously done by the ventilator to achieve those breaths is handed over to the patient. The kind of work (high volume/low pressure) performed by the respiratory muscles during PS promotes endurance, as opposed to strength (see Chapter 11, Weaning from Mechanical Ventilation). Finally, a lower mean airway pressure is achieved because the PIP is generally lower than with volume-cycled ventilation.

The main disadvantage of PS is that the V_T is variable and therefore the alveolar ventilation is not guaranteed. If compliance decreases or resistance increases, because of either patient or ventilator circuitry factors, then V_T decreases. PS should be used with great caution in patients who exhibit extremely variable respiratory system impedance, such as those with bronchospasm or significant secretions.

The ventilator may fail to cycle to expiration if an extensive air leak occurs, either around the airway, through bronchopleural fistulae, or in the circuit, because the flow rate that terminates inspiratory PS will not be reached. This will result in a prolonged inspiratory cycle and application of positive pressure. Most ventilators, for safety, provide for a time criteria for the termination of inspiration, usually 3 seconds. This prevents prolonged inspiration under the conditions of flow-cycling and an air leak.

Finally, the use of an inline nebulizer should be limited with PS ventilation because the increased flow created by the nebulizer may be erroneously sensed by the ventilator as the patient's minute ventilation. This may result in failure to detect apnea. Medications should be administered with metered-dose inhalers (MDIs) to avoid this potential complication.

FOCUS AREAS OF PATIENT MONITORING

1. Exhaled V_T. When PS is used for full ventilatory assistance, the V_T should be sufficient to meet the patient's minute ventilation demands with a comfortable RR. Partial ventilatory assistance V_Ts should be 5 to 7 mL/kg. The cause of low EV_T needs to be rapidly investigated because volumes less than the goal for the patient promote the development of atelectasis. Assess systematically the patient-related versus ventilator circuitry–related causes of decreased exhaled V_T (Table 7-2). V_T is increased by increasing the amount of PS. If the patient is in a weaning trial and the RR is increasing and EV_T is decreasing, these are signs of fatigue. The patient should be provided more ventilatory support: Increase the PS level, increase the number of mandatory breaths, or return the patient to the chosen resting mode.

2. Airway cuff leaks because the ventilator will not reach the PS level and may persist in the inspiratory phase of respiratory cycle.

3. The patient's RR, which should remain at less than 25 breaths/min. If the RR increases, the V_T should be assessed. If the patient is becoming fatigued, a shallower and more rapid respiratory pattern may develop. This ventilatory pattern will lead to atelectasis, a reduction in compliance, further increase in the WOB, and the need for greater ventilatory assistance.

4. Hemodynamic effects of positive-pressure ventilation, especially when PS_{max} is being used.

TABLE 7-2	Troubleshooting Potential Causes of Low Exhaled Tidal Volume with a Pressure Mode of Ventilation

PATIENT RELATED

Reduction in compliance: for example, pleural space disease, infiltrative process

Increase in resistance: airway narrowing, as in bronchospasm, secretions in airway

Insufficient respiratory muscle strength to meet ventilatory demands

Loss of tidal volume through pleural air leak

VENTILATOR CIRCUIT RELATED

Increase in resistance to gas flow: kinking of endotracheal tube, patient biting on airway, circuit tubing compressed between bed rail and mattress or patient lying on it, closed suction catheter not fully withdrawn from airway, water in tubing

Loose connection in exhaled gas limb of circuitry, allowing gases to escape

Loss of tidal volume from around artificial airway cuff

Pressure Assist Control

DEFINITION AND DESCRIPTION

Pressure control continuous mandatory ventilation (PC-CMV), also known as pressure assist control (P-AC), is a mode of ventilation in which there is a preset RR and every breath is augmented by a preset amount of inspiratory pressure (Fig. 7-11). With PC there is no set V_T. The V_T that the patient receives with each breath is

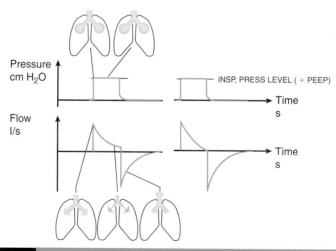

FIGURE 7-11

Pressure control (PC) ventilation. A preset number of breaths per minute are delivered, every breath being augmented by a preset amount of inspiratory pressure. Flow is delivered with the use of the decelerating flow-wave curve. Tidal volume is variable. Inspiratory/expiratory changeover is time cycled. (*Courtesy MAQUET, Inc., Bridgewater, NJ.*)

variable and determined by the set inspiratory pressure, the inspiratory time, pulmonary compliance, and airway and circuit resistance.

In PC, mandatory breaths are machine (time) triggered at the set rate, machine (pressure) limited, and machine (time) cycled. The ventilator responds to the patient, allowing additional breaths to be triggered. After the patient triggers the breath, it is augmented by the preset amount of pressure. These additional assisted breaths are patient triggered, machine (pressure) limited, and machine (time) cycled.

The onset of inspiration is determined primarily by the timing mechanism. Once triggered, the inspiratory flow of gas is augmented by the preselected amount of pressure, that is, the PC level. This amount of pressure is held constant throughout inspiration. Flow is delivered with the decelerating flow-wave pattern, as opposed to the square or sinusoidal-wave patterns primarily used with volume-cycled modes of ventilation. With the decelerating flow-wave pattern, flow rate naturally decays as the patient's lungs fill with air on inspiration. Unlike PS, which is a flow-cycled mode of ventilation that gives the patient control over the ventilatory pattern, PC is time cycled to end inspiration and begin expiration. The patient has no control over the ventilatory pattern.

INDICATIONS

PC may be used as a method of providing full ventilatory support in patients with noncompliant lungs who exhibit high airway pressures and poor oxygenation while supported by volume-cycled ventilation. PC can be utilized to get the airway pressure under the control of the clinician, who uses only the amount of inspiratory pressure necessary to achieve the desired VT. In comparison with volume ventilation, in the same noncompliant lung conditions, the PIP may be reduced, thereby reducing the potential for pulmonary barotrauma. Concurrently, the mean airway pressure is increased, which improves oxygenation.

ADVANTAGES AND DISADVANTAGES

During P-AC, the ventilator provides constant pressure of air to the patient throughout inspiration. The ventilator also produces appropriate flow at the onset of the breath to quickly achieve and maintain the set inspiratory pressure. PC ventilation is more proficient than other modes in maintaining open airways and improving gas distribution. Greater proportions of average flow, pressure, and volume are delivered earlier in inspiration than when volume ventilation with a square wave pattern is used. The rapid initial pressure possibly assists in opening collapsed alveoli at the beginning of inspiration. Pressure is then sustained throughout the inspiratory phase, splinting the airways and allowing for improved gas distribution. In volume-cycled ventilation, in contrast, flow is constant while airway pressure gradually rises to a maximum, possibly reaching the critical opening pressure of noncompliant alveoli at the peak of inspiration. However, at that point the flow stops and expiration begins, preventing noncompliant lung units from filling adequately.

Under the conditions where the lungs are very noncompliant and the disease process is diffuse, the delivery of volume-cycled ventilation with a square wave pattern may result in a high PIP and maldistribution of gases. The high PIP generated is associated with pulmonary barotrauma. That is not to say that the higher the PIP, the

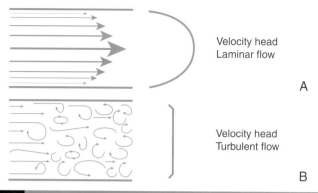

FIGURE 7-12

Velocity profile of gas particles moving along the airways during (**A**) laminar flow and (**B**) turbulent flow. The decelerating flow-wave pattern used with pressure support (PS) and pressure control (PC) ventilation promotes laminar flow. Laminar flow creates less airway trauma and promotes a more even distribution of gas. *(Modified from Dupuis YG. Ventilators: Theory and Clinical Application, 2nd ed. St. Louis: Mosby, 1992.)*

more barotrauma. Pulmonary barotrauma occurs when the PIP is high and there is uneven expansion of the lung and uneven pressure gradients between the alveoli. These conditions, which exist in nonuniform disease processes, lead to shear forces and injury in the lung. Reducing the PIP may reduce pulmonary barotrauma.

PC ventilation is postulated to reduce pulmonary barotrauma associated with high ventilating pressures and uneven gas distribution. Reduced airway pressures are promoted by limiting the application of inspiratory pressure to that which achieves the desired VT. This pressure is typically much lower than that which is generated with volume-cycled ventilation and a square flow-wave pattern. Because the pressure is limited, more normal areas of the lung may be spared from overdistention during inspiration. When the lungs are stiff and gases are delivered with "bulk flow," as with a square wave pattern, flow in the lung is turbulent, causing increases in lateral pressure and airway trauma. The decelerating flow-wave pattern used with PC ventilation changes the nature of the flow pattern in the lung and promotes laminar flow, which is more ideal because it leads to a more even distribution of gas (Fig. 7-12). Laminar flow waves wedge their way into airways and alveoli, creating less airway trauma and a more uniform gas distribution. The decelerating flow-wave pattern is associated with a significant reduction in total resistance, improved pulmonary compliance, a decrease in dead-space ventilation, and an increase in oxygenation. V-A/C may also be administered using the decelerating flow-wave pattern, and many of the same benefits may be achieved.

When a pressure mode of ventilation is used, the mean airway pressure, which is the mean pressure in the airway throughout the ventilatory cycle, increases. Mean airway pressure increases in pressure ventilation because airway pressure rapidly rises and is sustained at the PIP throughout inspiration. Mean airway pressure is a key determinant of lung volume and therefore oxygenation. Manipulation of the mean airway pressure contributes to achieving the goal of restoring lung volume through the recruitment of collapsed alveoli and the redistribution of lung water, thereby improving oxygenation. Increases in mean airway pressure may be unfavorable in that they are also associated with reductions in cardiac output because of lung distention, which reduces preload and increases right ventricular afterload. Appropriate monitoring should be implemented when a pressure mode of ventilation is applied, so that a reduction in cardiac output can be detected rapidly and managed as necessary with preload augmentation and inotropic agents. The patient will not benefit from an improved PaO_2 if overall tissue oxygen delivery is compromised.

FOCUS AREAS OF PATIENT MONITORING

1. Be thoroughly familiar with all ventilator settings, including the inspiratory pressure level—for example, PC of 34 cm H_2O, RR of 20 breaths/min, 15 cm H_2O PEEP, and FIO_2 0.6. In this example, PC of 34 cm H_2O refers to an inspiratory pressure level of 34, not 34 breaths/min. A common error is to believe that the PC level is the set RR. The likely reason is that an A/C or SIMV of 8 means 8 breaths/min.

2. With the P-A/C mode, rapid RRs may result in respiratory alkalosis, air trapping, the formation of auto-PEEP, and hemodynamic compromise. Sedate the patient as necessary or consider switching to a mode that allows more spontaneous breathing (P-SIMV).

3. Monitor exhaled V_T and minute ventilation closely because any factor that reduces compliance or increases airway resistance will adversely affect V_T. Conversely, if the PC level is not decreased commensurately with improvement in the patient's lung characteristics, the increase in V_T may result in overdistention and excessive ventilation. Key safety features are the setting of high and low V_T and $\dot{V}_E$ alarms.

4. Understand what constitutes the PIP. On some ventilators, the PIP equals the PC level plus any level of applied PEEP, whereas on others, the PIP is the true PC level.

5. Monitor hemodynamics closely, anticipating possible compromise as a result of increases in mean airway pressure.

6. Monitor and prevent airway cuff leaks because the ventilator may not reach PC level and may persist in the inspiratory phase of the respiratory cycle. Set inspiratory cycle time limits.

7. See the later discussion of PC inverse inspiratory-to-expiratory (I:E) ratio ventilation to learn how to make ventilator setting changes for optimal gas exchange.

Pressure Control: Synchronized Intermittent Mandatory Ventilation

DEFINITION AND DESCRIPTION

Pressure control synchronized intermittent mandatory ventilation (PC-SIMV) is a combination of P-AC and spontaneous breathing. The patient receives a preset number of mandatory P-A/C breaths by the ventilator. Between the mandatory breaths, the patient may trigger additional breaths. These spontaneous breaths are typically supported by a set amount of inspiratory PS (Fig. 7-13). If the patient

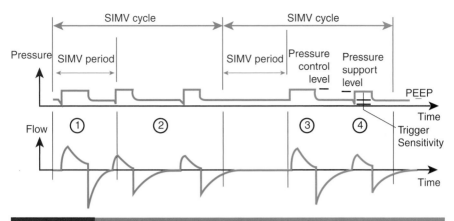

FIGURE 7-13

PC-SIMV where spontaneous breaths are pressure supported. **1,** When the patient triggers a breath within the SIMV period, a PC breath is delivered. **2,** Patient-triggered assisted breath delivered with PS at the preset PS level. **3,** If an SIMV period passes without any spontaneous breathing effort, a mandatory PC breath is given. **4,** Breaths are triggered when the sensitivity level is reached.
(Courtesy MAQUET, Inc., Bridgewater, NJ.)

initiates a breath within the timing window where the ventilator is scheduled to deliver a mandatory breath, then a full machine-assisted breath is delivered in synchrony with patient effort. The mandatory breaths are machine (time) triggered, machine (pressure) limited, and machine (time) cycled. The spontaneous breaths, when PS is used, are patient (flow or pressure) triggered, pressure limited, and patient (flow) cycled.

INDICATIONS

- Normal respiratory drive but respiratory muscles unable to perform all of the work.
- When it is desirable to progress the patient from full ventilatory support and have the patient begin to breathe spontaneously, assume a portion of the WOB, and retain some respiratory muscle strength.
- When a guaranteed backup rate of ventilation is required.

ADVANTAGES AND DISADVANTAGES

The patient is guaranteed a minimum $\dot{V}_E$ and a guaranteed volume with each mandatory breath. Respiratory alkalosis is less of a problem in this mode than in the P-A/C mode because the patient can modify rate and volume of the spontaneous breaths. Less atrophy of the respiratory muscles occurs because the patient participates more in ventilation, using the ventilatory muscles to a greater degree than when P-A/C is used. The hemodynamic effects of positive-pressure ventilation may be less with P-SIMV than P-A/C because ventilation occurs at a lower mean airway pressure when spontaneous breaths are taken; therefore, the average over time is less. Also, the distribution of gas within the lung is better during spontaneous breathing.

FOCUS AREAS OF PATIENT MONITORING

1. The patient's RR. If the RR increases, then the V_T of the spontaneous breaths should be assessed. The V_T of the spontaneous breaths should be 5 to 7 mL/kg. If the patient is beginning to fatigue, a more shallow and rapid respiratory pattern may develop. This ventilatory pattern will lead to atelectasis, a reduction in compliance, further increase in the WOB, and the need for greater ventilatory support.

2. EV_Ts of mandatory breaths and spontaneous breaths because they are variable in this pressure mode of ventilation and will decrease with changes in compliance and resistance. Key safety features are the setting of high and low V_T and $\dot{V}_E$ alarms.

3. Understanding what constitutes the PIP. On some ventilators, the PIP equals the PC or PS level plus any level of applied PEEP, whereas on others, the PIP is the true PC or PS level.

4. Monitoring hemodynamics closely, anticipating possible compromise as a result of increases in mean airway pressure.

5. Monitoring and preventing airway cuff leaks because the ventilator may not reach PC level and may persist in the inspiratory phase of the respiratory cycle. Set inspiratory cycle time limits.

Pressure Control with Inverse Inspiratory-to-Expiratory Ratio Ventilation

DEFINITION AND DESCRIPTION

PC, as previously discussed, is a mode of ventilation in which there is a preset RR and every breath is augmented by a preset amount of inspiratory pressure. Inversion of the I:E ratio is an additional strategy used with this mode of ventilation when further efforts to improve oxygenation are needed. The I:E ratio is inverted—1:1, 2:1, 3:1—in such a way that inspiratory time equals or exceeds expiratory time. This is done to improve gas distribution in the lung and increase the mean airway pressure for improvement of oxygenation.

In addition to changing the inspiratory and expiratory times, the RR may be set rapidly enough so that the patient does not exhale completely before the initiation of the next breath. A shortened expiratory time results in gas trapping in the lung (auto-PEEP), which keeps the critical closing volume above the point of alveolar collapse (Fig. 7-14). Continuous monitoring of a terminal flow curve assists in the appropriate rate selection. Because the ventilatory pattern is altered, sedation is necessary and possibly medical paralysis to maintain patient-ventilator synchrony. Inversion of the I:E ratio, use of a sufficient inspiratory pressure to overcome the opening pressure of the lung, and use of a critical rate to promote the formation of auto-PEEP are strategies to improve oxygenation that build on the previously described benefits of PC ventilation. Read the earlier section on PC ventilation as a foundation for understanding PC with inverse I:E ratio ventilation. In addition, see the sections in Chapter 6 on inverse I:E ratios and auto-PEEP for a thorough discussion of these critical topics. The I:E ratio may be inverted with volume control ventilation; however, the development of auto-PEEP with a volume mode of ventilation is dangerous because of the associated increase in PIP.

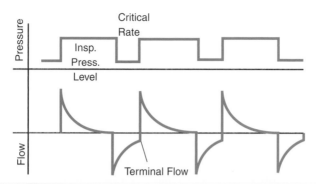

FIGURE 7-14

Pressure control (PC) with inverse inspiratory-to-expiratory (I:E) ratio ventilation. A critical pressure achieves the desired tidal volume and splints the alveoli throughout inspiration. The critical rate is determined by setting each new breath to begin just before terminal flow of the previous breath returns to zero. Appropriate rate and I:E ratio settings result in the desired formation of auto-PEEP.

INDICATIONS

Pressure control inverse I:E ratio ventilation (PC-IRV) may be used as a means of providing full ventilatory support in patients with noncompliant lungs who exhibit high airway pressures and poor oxygenation when volume-cycled ventilation is used. PC ventilation can be used to get the airway pressure under the control of the clinician, with only the necessary amount of inspiratory pressure used to achieve the desired VT. In comparison with volume ventilation, in the same noncompliant lung conditions, the PIP may be reduced, thereby reducing the potential for pulmonary barotrauma. Concurrently, inversion of the I:E ratio further increases mean airway pressure, which promotes optimal gas distribution to lung units with longer time constants and improves oxygenation.

ADVANTAGES AND DISADVANTAGES

In surfactant-deficient lung disease such as acute respiratory disease syndrome (ARDS), the pattern of pulmonary abnormality is diffuse and nonuniform through-out the lung. Lung units with varying resistances and compliances exist in adjacent areas of the lung. Alveoli with relatively more disease have longer time constants and require more time to fill. In conventional ratio ventilation, alveoli with long time constants may not have adequate time to fill and may remain in a collapsed state, resulting in persistent intrapulmonary shunt and hypoxemia. Inverting the I:E ratio increases the inspiratory time and thereby allows the alveoli with long time constants adequate time to fill, which improves overall gas distribution in the lung. Inspiratory time is prolonged to the point where it encroaches on expiratory time. On exhalation, the alveoli then do not have time to empty to their resting volume, and gas is trapped in the lung (dynamic hyperinflation). This trapped gas creates pressure in the lung known as auto-PEEP. Auto-PEEP splints the unstable alveoli at end-expiration. After this shortened expiratory phase, the lungs are rapidly reinflated before the alveoli reach their closing volume; therefore, fewer lung units collapse.

PC-IRV results in an increase in the FRC, a reduction in intrapulmonary shunt, improved oxygenation, and a reduction in dead-space ventilation. The primary disadvantage of this mode of ventilation is that hemodynamic embarrassment may occur as a result of increases in both the mean airway pressure and the level of total PEEP.

INSTITUTION OF PRESSURE CONTROL WITH INVERSE I:E RATIO VENTILATION

The typical patient for whom inverse I:E ratio ventilation should be considered has progressively worsening radiographic infiltrates, increasing PIP, worsening oxygenation despite a high FIO_2 and a high level of PEEP, and a high minute ventilation. Table 7-3 outlines guidelines for initial ventilator settings.

The following important patient management and monitoring principles apply to the patient who is to receive support with PC inverse I:E ratio ventilation:

■ Before implementing PC-IRV, ensure that appropriate patient monitoring is implemented. Monitoring equipment should include a pulse oximeter, electrocardiograph, arterial line, and, ideally, an end-tidal carbon dioxide monitor. A pulmonary artery catheter may also be indicated for the assessment of hemodynamic and advanced oxygenation indices. The clinician should be prepared to stay with the patient on implementation of this mode to monitor

TABLE 7-3	Pressure Control with Inverse I:E Ratio Ventilation: Guidelines for Initial Ventilator Setting
Parameter	**Initial Setting**
FIO_2	1.0
I:E ratio	1:1
Inspiratory pressure (pressure control level)	Adjust to achieve VT of 8 mL/kg, usually accomplished at Pplat patient had on volume ventilation; use lowest pressure that achieves best VT, minute ventilation, and $PaCO_2$ (in disease processes resulting in severely noncompliant lungs, smaller VTs, 6 mL/kg, may be desirable and permissive hypercapnia necessary)
Respiratory rate	To prevent complete exhalation and allow auto-PEEP formation: Adjust at sufficiently rapid rate so that before exhalation is completed, subsequent breath begins—usually approximately 20 to 25 breaths per minute; use terminal flow curve.
	To prevent dynamic hyperinflation, set RR to allow for terminal flow curve to reach zero before next breath.
Set-PEEP	Approximately 5 cm H_2O; remember that auto-PEEP forms because of rapid rate and incomplete exhalation.
	If dynamic hyperinflation is not allowed, set PEEP high enough to prevent alveolar closure at end-exhalation.

FIO_2, Fraction of oxygen in inspired gas; *I:E ratio,* inspiratory-to-expiratory ratio; *$PaCO_2$,* partial pressure of carbon dioxide in arterial blood; *PEEP,* positive end-expiratory pressure; *Pplat,* plateau pressure; *VT,* tidal volume.

cardiac and pulmonary response and to manage hemodynamic alterations. All supplies should be in the room, including intravenous fluid for volume resuscitation and an inotropic agent, to be initiated and titrated especially if the patient has questionable cardiac reserve. All components of oxygen delivery should be optimized.

- The patient must be deeply sedated and possibly paralyzed. This ensures patient comfort and prevents the patient from breathing out of phase with the ventilator. Patient interruption of the I:E ratio will result in a loss of PEEP, a reduction in the FRC, and hypoxemia.

- A closed system should be used for suctioning the patient. This type of system eliminates the need to break the patient-ventilator circuit, with a resultant loss of PEEP. Suction as indicated by chest assessment and provide hyperoxygenation before each pass of the suction catheter.

VENTILATOR SETTING ADJUSTMENTS

As pulse oximetry and end-tidal carbon dioxide monitoring are performed and ABG values are obtained, the ventilator must be adjusted appropriately to achieve optimal gas exchange. It is important to introduce a key concept before oxygenation and ventilation are discussed as separate issues. When the PEEP is changed, the clinician must appreciate that *any increase in the baseline pressure will decrease the* V_T because the change in pressure from baseline to PIP is a primary determinant of inspired volume (Fig. 7-15). Consequently, when adjustments are being made in the

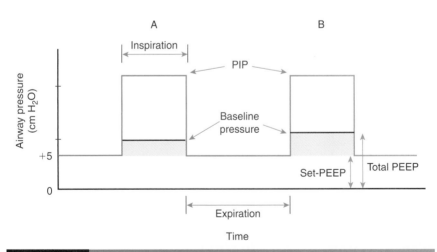

FIGURE 7-15

Pressure control (PC) and PC inverse inspiratory-to-expiratory (I:E) ratio ventilation. Any change in the baseline pressure that is not associated with a concurrent change in the applied inspiratory pressure will affect tidal volume (V_T). The important concept here is that the change in pressure from baseline (total PEEP) to peak inspiratory pressure (PIP) is a key determinant of V_T. In this example, both breaths A and B have 5 cm H_2O set-PEEP applied to them. Hashed area represents auto-PEEP, which is greater in breath B. Breath A will therefore have a larger change in pressure from baseline (total PEEP) to PIP than breath B and consequently a larger V_T.

PEEP to affect oxygenation, ventilation may also be affected. The clinician must develop an understanding of this concept, which requires new thought processes regarding how to make ventilator setting changes and differs from the effect of these parameters on each other during use of volume-controlled modes.

Strategies to Improve Oxygenation (Pao$_2$)

- Increase the Fio$_2$, trying to keep it in a nontoxic range (<0.6).
- Increase the auto-PEEP by adjusting either the RR or the I:E ratio. Increasing the respiratory frequency shortens the duty cycle, shortening expiratory time and promoting gas trapping and auto-PEEP formation. The RR should be increased in increments of 3 to 5 breaths/min. Utilization of a terminal flow curve provides visual guidance for the changes. Progressively altering the I:E ratio from 1:1 to 2:1 to 3:1 will also increase auto-PEEP formation as expiratory time is shortened. The clinician must be prepared because this setting is the most difficult to change because of hemodynamic instability. Perform the adjustment of the I:E ratio beyond 2:1 after the preceding maneuvers have been used to their fullest extent.

Strategies to Improve Ventilation (Paco$_2$)

- If the patient has respiratory acidosis, then the suitable response is to increase the minute ventilation. This may be achieved by increasing the inspiratory pressure level or increasing the RR.
- Make increases in the inspiratory pressure level in increments of 3 to 5 cm H$_2$O to a maximum PIP of 40 cm H$_2$O while EVt is monitored to assess patient response. An increase in the EVt is the desired response. If there is no change in the EVt and the Paco$_2$ is worsening, then the pressure is exceeding the distensibility of the pulmonary tissue. Go back to the prior inspiratory pressure level and tolerate an elevated Paco$_2$ (permissive hypercapnia; see Chapter 9).
- Increase the RR. After reaching a rate at which subsequent breaths encroach on the prior breath, further rate increases may raise the auto-PEEP, worsening the Vt and carbon dioxide excretion. Be cautious regarding hemodynamic instability resulting from increased auto-PEEP.
- Conversely, if the patient presents with a respiratory alkalosis, decrease the minute ventilation by decreasing either the RR or the inspiratory pressure level. When the RR is decreased, auto-PEEP may decrease, affecting oxygenation.

WEANING FROM PRESSURE CONTROL WITH INVERSE I:E RATIO VENTILATION

When the patient is weaned from PC, the mean airway pressure should be maintained with the PC level and the total PEEP until the Fio$_2$ can be reduced to 0.5 or less while an oxygen saturation of 90% or more is maintained. When the patient demonstrates stability, the I:E ratio is the next setting to change. The inspiratory time is decreased cautiously because the response can be unpredictable. The mean airway pressure may drop significantly, especially on the initial change, allowing alveolar units to collapse, reducing the FRC, and leading to deterioration in oxygenation. No less than a 6-hour period of stability should elapse before another change is made. Once the I:E ratio is at 1:2, and if a set-PEEP greater than 10 cm H_2O is still necessary, the PEEP should be reduced before further weaning from ventilatory support.

FOCUS AREAS OF PATIENT MONITORING

1. Be familiar with all the ventilator settings and where to find both ventilator settings and patient data on the ventilator's control and display panels.
2. Monitor EVTS because any factor that reduces pulmonary compliance or increases airway and circuit resistance will decrease the EVT.
3. Monitor the level of auto-PEEP by performing an end-expiratory pause maneuver for 2 to 4 seconds (see Chapter 6). The reading on the pressure manometer will be total PEEP:

$$Auto\text{-}PEEP = Total\ PEEP - Set\text{-}PEEP$$

4. Monitor the PIP, which should equal the inspiratory pressure level plus the level of set-PEEP.
5. Document data clearly and completely, ensuring that all caregivers are using the same terminology, particularly when referring to the various forms of PEEP.
6. Monitor the patient's hemodynamic status closely because the hemodynamic effects of this mode of ventilation can be profound. Optimize all aspects of tissue oxygen delivery.
7. Ensure sedation to a level that suppresses the patient's respiratory drive. Institute paralysis as necessary. See Box 7-1 for a PC inverse I:E ventilation case study.

Airway Pressure Release Ventilation

DEFINITION AND DESCRIPTION

Airway pressure release ventilation (APRV) is a mode of ventilation specific to the Drager Evita ventilator. Similar variations are available on newer generation ventilators. APRV provides two levels of CPAP while allowing unrestricted spontaneous breathing at any point during the respiratory cycle. APRV starts at an elevated pressure—the CPAP level or pressure high (PHIGH or P1)—followed by a release pressure—pressure low (PLOW) (Fig. 7-16). After the airway pressure release, the CPAP level is restored. The time spent at PHIGH is known as time high (THIGH) or time 1 (T1). It is followed by the release phase, which is a brief period at the lower pressure (PLOW or P2) known as time low (TLOW) or time 2 (T2). Each pressure level is machine (time) triggered, machine (pressure) limited, and machine (time) cycled.

The time spent at PHIGH is generally prolonged, 4 to 6 seconds, whereas TLOW is set very short, generally 0.5 to 1.1 seconds in adults. Therefore, when observing the pressure waveform, APRV is similar to PC-IRV. However, unlike the PC-IRV, APRV offers the patient unrestricted spontaneous breathing at an elevated CPAP level because the exhalation valve is "active" or "floating." What this means is that any time during PC ventilation if the set PIP is exceeded, the exhalation valve opens. The expiratory time is also much shorter in APRV.

BOX 7-1 Pressure Control Inverse I:E Ventilation: Case Study

Male, 52 years of age, who suffered multiple-system trauma including bilateral hemopneumothoraces. The patient had multiple hypotensive episodes that necessitated massive volume resuscitation. Two days after injury:

1. *Ventilator settings:* A/C 22, patient's rate 29, FIO_2 1.0, VT 650, PEEP 18 cm H_2O, PIP 58 cm H_2O

2. *ABG values:* pH 7.29; PaO_2 45.5; $PaCO_2$ 47.5; HCO_3^- 22.9; BE −3.7/87% saturation

PC inverse I:E ratio ventilation was initiated:

Ventilator Settings	Patient Data	ABG
PC 28	PIP 36 cm H_2O	PaO_2 43
RR 28	EVT 560	$PaCO_2$ 55
FIO_2 1.0	$\dot{V}E$ 15.7	pH 7.25
PEEP (set/total) 8/12		Saturation 83%
I:E ratio 2:1		HCO_3^-/BE 24.5/−3.0

The primary goal—to improve oxygenation—was achieved by increasing the RR to increase the auto-PEEP formation. This made it possible to reduce the FIO_2. To reduce the degree of respiratory acidosis, minute ventilation was increased by increasing the inspiratory pressure level to the maximum allowable PIP of 40. Recall that any increase in the baseline pressure will decrease the EVT if there is not an associated increase in the PC level. In this example, despite the increase in the PC level, the EVT decreased with the increase in total PEEP. This is likely explained by the concurrent markedly shortened expiratory time. These ventilator changes were guided by pulse oximetry and end-tidal CO_2 monitoring and validated with ABG determinations.

Ventilator Settings	Patient Data	ABG
PC 32 ↑	PIP 40 cm H_2O	PaO_2 110
RR 36 ↑	EVT 520	$PaCO_2$ 32
FIO_2 0.5 ↓	$\dot{V}E$ 18.7	pH 7.47
PEEP (set/total) 8/18 ↑		Saturation 96%
I:E ratio 2:1		HCO_3^-/BE 23.4/+1.5

Six hours later:

Ventilator Settings	Patient Data	ABG
PC 32	PIP 40 cm H_2O	PaO_2 173 ↑
RR 36	EVT 580	$PaCO_2$ 28 ↓
FIO_2 0.5	$\dot{V}E$ 20.1	pH 7.50 ↑
PEEP (set/total) 8/20		Saturation 97%
I:E ratio 2:1		HCO_3^-/BE 20/0.0

The PC level was decreased to reduce the minute ventilation and correct the respiratory alkalosis:

Ventilator Settings	Patient Data	ABG
PC 28 ↓	PIP 36 cm H_2O	PaO_2 152
RR 36	EVT 500	$PaCO_2$ 34 ↑
FIO_2 0.5	$\dot{V}E$ 18.0	pH 7.46
PEEP (set/total) 8/20		Saturation 97%
I:E ratio 2:1		HCO_3^-/BE 21/−0.3

ABG, Arterial blood gas; *BE,* base excess; *EVT,* exhaled tidal volume; *FIO₂,* fraction of oxygen in inspired gas; *I:E ratio,* inspiratory-to-expiratory ratio; *PaCO₂,* partial pressure of carbon dioxide in arterial blood; *PaO₂,* partial pressure of oxygen in arterial blood; *PC,* pressure control; *PEEP,* positive end-expiratory pressure; *PIP,* peak inspiratory pressure; *RR,* respiratory rate; *V̇E,* minute ventilation.

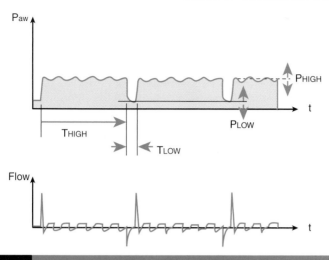

FIGURE 7-16

Airway pressure release ventilation (APRV). Free spontaneous breathing is allowed throughout the ventilatory cycle. An elevated CPAP pressure level (P$_{HIGH}$) is followed by a brief period of low pressure (P$_{LOW}$) called the pressure release. Additional ventilator settings include the time at the high pressure (T$_{HIGH}$) and the time at the low pressure (T$_{LOW}$). *(Courtesy of Drager Medical, Inc., Telford, Pa.)*

During APRV, FRC is maintained at the upper CPAP level. During the release phase, gases are allowed to leave the lung passively. Passive lung deflation during airway pressure release augments alveolar ventilation and promotes carbon dioxide elimination. Synchronous airway pressure release occurs during spontaneous expiration, whereas synchronous restoration of CPAP occurs during spontaneous inspiration.

APRV is distinguished from other modes of ventilation in that as opposed to increasing airway pressure to generate a V$_T$, the pressure is released, generating a release volume. The rationale for a brief expiratory phase, T$_{LOW}$, is that it limits closure of unstable alveoli, therefore maintaining recruitment. Exhalation and carbon dioxide removal, however, are not limited to the release phase because ventilation is allowed throughout the respiratory cycle. See Table 7-4 and Figure 7-17 for recommendations for initial ventilator settings in patients with severe lung injury. The clinician should be aware that, just as with PC-IRV, it may take several hours for positive results to be realized, especially if the patient has significant lung injury. Maximal beneficial effect on oxygenation may take up to 8 hours.

INDICATIONS

1. Acute lung injury, resulting in a decrease in lung compliance and the FRC. APRV recruits alveoli and prevents derecruitment.
2. Chronic obstructive pulmonary disease (COPD) because the rapid expiratory flow rates with APRV reduce expiratory flow limitation.

TABLE 7-4	Airway Pressure Release Ventilation: Guidelines for Initial Ventilator Settings in Acute Lung Injury
Parameter	**Initial Setting**
P$_{HIGH}$ or P1	P$_{HIGH}$ equal to Pplat in conventional volume ventilation or peak pressure in pressure ventilation (maximum value: 35-40 cm H$_2$O). New intubated patient set at 25-35 cm H$_2$O and titrate.
P$_{LOW}$ or P2	Set at 0-3 cm H$_2$O to reduce expiratory resistance and maximize expiratory flow rate.
T$_{HIGH}$ or T1	Set 4-6 sec (shorter time decreases Paw and oxygenation). Make as long as possible to promote gas diffusion and reduce number of cyclical opening and closing of airways.
T$_{LOW}$ or T2	Optimal release provides adequate ventilation while minimizing lung volume loss. Set between 0.5 and 1.0 sec (generally 0.8 sec in adults as a starting point). Monitor expiratory flow waveform for truncation and end release when expiratory flow is 25%-50% of peak expiratory flow rate.

mPaw, Mean airway pressure; *Pplat,* plateau pressure.

ADVANTAGES AND DISADVANTAGES

APRV increases the mean airway pressure, which results in recruitment of non-compliant, unstable alveoli; reduction in intrapulmonary shunt; and an improvement in oxygenation. APRV has been shown to result in better gas exchange than V-CMV in acute lung injury. The hazards associated with high peak airway pressures are minimized in this pressure control mode of ventilation because the PIP does not exceed the high CPAP level, thus reducing barotrauma and circulatory compromise. Because the patient is allowed to breathe spontaneously, patient-ventilator dyssynchrony is reduced, decreasing sedation requirements; distribution of gas is enhanced; and cardiac performance may be improved.

Disadvantages include that V$_T$ is variable and depends on compliance and resistance factors in the patient-ventilator system. It is difficult to auscultate breath sounds because of the very short release interval when bulk flow is occurring. Study of a large number of patients is still needed to determine the applications of APRV, how it compares with other modes, and its effect on patient outcome.

Strategies to Improve Oxygenation (Pao$_2$)
- Increase the F$_{IO_2}$, trying to keep it in a nontoxic range (<0.6).
- Adjust the mean airway pressure by increasing the area under the pressure-volume curve as follows:
  - Increase P$_{HIGH}$.
  - Lengthen T$_{HIGH}$ with awareness that this will decrease the respiratory frequency (number of releases) and may cause an increase in Paco$_2$.
  - Shorten T$_{LOW}$ to increase air trapping.

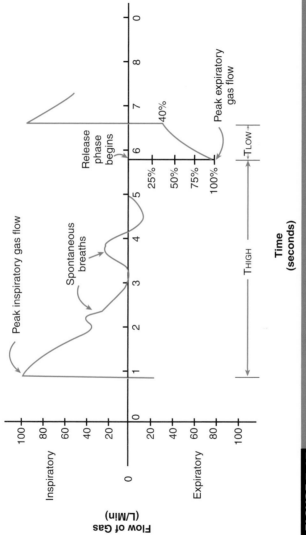

FIGURE 7-17

Flow of gas during inspiration and expiration with APRV. The expiratory portion of the flow curve is used to adjust the release time. When expiratory flows falls to approximately 25% to 50% of peak expiratory flow, the release should end, allowing airway pressure to return to P_HIGH. *(Modified from Frawley PM, Habashi NM. Airway pressure release ventilation: theory and practice. AACN Clin Issues 2001; 12:234–246.)*

Strategies to Improve Ventilation (PaCO_2)

■ If the patient has respiratory acidosis, the suitable response is to increase the alveolar ventilation. This may be achieved by increasing the pressure change between P1 and P2.

■ Increase PHIGH while EVT is monitored. An increase in the EVT is the desired response. If there is no change in the EVT and the PaCO_2 is worsening, the pressure is exceeding the distensibility of the pulmonary tissue and dead-space ventilation is being created. Go back to the prior inspiratory pressure level and tolerate an elevated PaCO_2 (permissive hypercapnia; see Chapter 9).

■ Decrease PLOW.

■ Conversely, if the patient presents with a respiratory alkalosis, the minute ventilation should be reduced by decreasing PHIGH, increasing P2, or decreasing the number of releases by lengthening T1. Decreasing P1 may adversely effect oxygenation.

WEANING FROM AIRWAY PRESSURE RELEASE VENTILATION

When the patient is ready to be weaned from APRV, support is reduced through manipulation of PHIGH and THIGH. PHIGH is lowered in increments of 2 to 3 cm H_2O; THIGH is lengthened in 0.5- to 2.0-second increments, depending on patient tolerance. This strategy, called the "drop and stretch" approach, was developed by Dr. Habashi. The drop and stretch method allows for reshaping of mean airway pressure and inducement of increasing spontaneous breathing. As these changes are made, the mean airway pressure is reduced; therefore, the effect on oxygenation should be monitored closely. Similarly, exhaled V_T and $\dot{V}_E$ are tracked in conjunction with PaCO_2. The goal is to arrive at straight CPAP, at which point the CPAP could be weaned further or the patient extubated. Patients with more severe forms of acute lung injury need to be weaned from APRV gradually and cautiously as with any other mode of mechanical ventilation.

FOCUS AREAS OF PATIENT MONITORING

■ Minute ventilation, spontaneous VT, and release volumes because all can be variable with this pressure-controlled mode of ventilation.

■ Total RR. Respirations should be counted for a full minute and recorded. The patient's spontaneous breaths may be small if the lungs are already being held at the FRC. Very high respiratory frequency may indicate the patient has increased minute ventilation demands, the cause of which should be evaluated (could be pain, anxiety, sepsis, etc.).

■ Expiratory gas flow to prevent derecruitment by allowing expiratory flow to return to zero. However, patients with COPD, asthma, and airway edema, as in thermal injuries requiring longer expiratory times, may develop significant air trapping that may not be hemodynamically tolerated. T2 should be adjusted accordingly.

BiLevel

DEFINITION AND DESCRIPTION

BiLevel is a mode of mechanical ventilation specific to the Puritan Bennett 840 ventilator. BiLevel is a form of augmented pressure ventilation like APRV that allows for unrestricted spontaneous breathing at any time during the ventilatory cycle. Settings include a high CPAP level ($PEEP_H$) and a low CPAP level ($PEEP_L$). The operator also sets a time for the two levels that determines the mandatory breath rate. Mandatory and spontaneous breaths are therefore combined.

BiLevel is not restricted to any specific T_{HIGH} to T_{LOW} (I:E) ratio. However, BiLevel with prolonged I:E ratio is identical to APRV. During BiLevel, if the time spent at the upper and lower PEEP is long enough to allow spontaneous breathing at both levels, this mode is commonly referred to as BiPhasic. During BiLevel, patient-initiated breaths at both PEEP levels can be pressure supported (patient triggered, pressure limited, flow cycled), and transitions between PEEP levels are synchronized with patient breathing. All patient-initiated breaths are supported with at least 1.5 cm H_2O PS (Fig. 7-18). Additional PS, if desired, is above $PEEP_L$, which means the PIP is the PS level + $PEEP_L$. Spontaneous breaths are supported as follows: PS is applied to spontaneous breaths at $PEEP_L$ provided there is sufficient time; it is applied to spontaneous breaths at $PEEP_H$ if the PS level is higher than $PEEP_H$. If the patient does not initiate any spontaneous breaths, this mode functions like P-A/C with mandatory breaths that are machine (time) triggered, machine (pressure) limited, and machine (time) cycled.

When BiLevel is initiated as APRV, it has all of the advantages and disadvantages outlined earlier. The difference between the Drager and the Puritan Bennett form of APRV is that on the Drager, no PS is applied to patient-initiated breaths. An adjunct called automatic tube compensation (ATC) can be applied on the Drager, however. BiLevel can transition from PC to P-SIMV to all levels of PS ventilation and therefore may be useful across the entire course of mechanical ventilation. Both the Puritan Bennett 840 and the Drager Evita monitor mandatory minute volume and rate

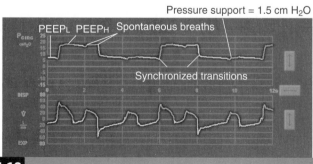

FIGURE 7-18

BiLevel. Spontaneous breathing is allowed throughout. *(Courtesy of Puritan Bennett, Pleasanton, Calif.)*

separately. This provides a clear picture of the patient's spontaneous ventilation contribution to total ventilation.

To begin BiLevel as APRV, the settings are initiated as suggested earlier. If the patient had no history of mechanical ventilation and inverse I:E ratio is not desired, the BiLevel settings are as in P-A/C; the low pressure level is adjusted to the desired PEEP, and the high pressure is set to achieve the desired exhaled V_T based on the compliance of the lung and a PIP limit of 40 cm H_2O. Because no scientific evaluations of BiLevel are available, experience and careful monitoring guide the approach. Suggestions for weaning include a reduction in $PEEP_H$ followed by subsequent lengthening of the duration of the low pressure period to achieve a breath frequency of 4 breaths/min. The last step is to switch to CPAP at a level corresponding to the mean airway pressure of the last BiLevel setting.

DUAL CONTROL MODES

Dual control modes are able to control volume or pressure. However, these modes cannot control both volume and pressure at the same time, only one or the other. The logic behind how these modes function is the closed-loop feedback system where the control of one output variable is based on the measurement of an input variable. Dual control modes are classified as either dual control within a breath or dual control from breath to breath.

A dual control within a breath mode is capable of switching from pressure control to volume control in the middle of a single breath. Dual control breath-to-breath modes function by adjusting the pressure level of a pressure breath based on a clinician-selected target value for V_T and/or $\dot{V}_E$. The result is pressure ventilation with a volume guarantee.

Dual Control Within a Breath

Pressure augmentation (PA) and volume-assured pressure support (VAPS) are two names for dual control within a breath ventilation. The breath may be either patient or ventilator triggered and is delivered as a pressure-limited breath. The ventilator continuously compares the volume delivered to the desired V_T set as the target by the operator. If it appears that the target V_T is not going to be reached, the ventilator continues inspiration at peak flow until the target V_T is reached. Therefore, the ventilator has switched within the breath from pressure-limited to volume-limited ventilation. Because the feedback control occurs within a single breath, the ventilator must monitor the V_T being delivered, not the exhaled V_T. Two types of breaths can be delivered. The first type is pressure-controlled, patient- or time-triggered, pressure-limited, flow-cycled breath. The second type is volume-controlled, patient- or time-triggered, flow-limited, and volume-cycled breath (Fig. 7-19).

The input variable is a minimal set value of the inspired V_T. Ventilator output is variable based on the relationship between the volume delivered and the minimum set V_T.

If the delivered and the set V_T are equal, then the breath is a pressure-supported or pressure-controlled breath.

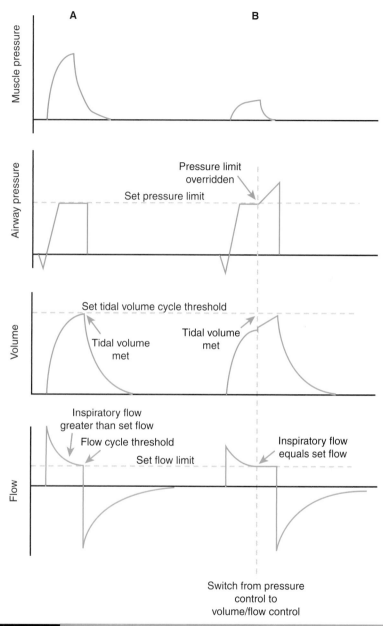

Muscle pressure

A   B

Airway pressure

Pressure limit
overridden

Set pressure limit

Volume

Set tidal volume cycle threshold

Tidal volume
met

Tidal volume
met

Flow

Inspiratory flow
greater than set flow

Flow cycle threshold

Set flow limit

Inspiratory flow
equals set flow

Switch from pressure
control to
volume/flow control

FIGURE 7-19

Dual control within breath ventilation. **A,** Patient-triggered, pressure-limited, flow-cycled breath. Target V$_T$ was reached before flow decayed to the set flow limit; therefore, breath continues as a pressure-limited breath until the flow-cycle value is reached. **B,** Breath switches from pressure to volume because flow decayed to the set flow limit *before* the target V$_T$ was reached. This occurred because of a smaller patient effort. Inspiration continues at the set flow and pressure rises. *(Modified from Wilkins RL, Stoller JK, Scanlan CL, et al. [eds.]: Egan's Fundamentals of Respiratory Care, 8th ed. St. Louis: Mosby, 2003.)*

If the ventilator reaches a set peak flow value and it is determined that the delivered VT will not match the target VT, the breath changes from a pressure-limited to a volume-limited breath. Flow remains constant, increasing the inspiratory time until the target VT is delivered. Airway pressure can rise, during this volume portion of the breath, above the set PS level. This scenario occurs when patient's inspiratory effort is diminished. Important safety features during this type of breath are the setting of a maximum inspiratory time of 3 seconds, after which the breath will be time cycled, and a high-pressure alarm will sound.

The third manner of ventilator response is that if the delivered VT is larger than the target VT, the ventilator allows this and makes no adjustments. The breath remains a PS or pressure controlled flow-cycled breath. This response is important to allow for normal variations in VT with sighing, increased effort, and activity.

Dual Control Breath to Breath: Pressure-Limited, Flow-Cycled Ventilation

Volume support (VS) and variable pressure support (VPS) are two dual control breath-to-breath, pressure-limited, flow-cycled modes. These modes are PS, closed-loop ventilation with VT or V̇E as the input variable. They provide the positive features of PS ventilation with the security of a V̇E and VT as in V-A/C. As lung mechanics improve or patient effort increases, the ventilator will automatically make adjustments to reduce the level of PS. Description of these modes is provided here by an in-depth discussion of VS as currently available on the Servo 300. VS, also available on the Puritan Bennett 840, operates slightly differently.

DEFINITION AND DESCRIPTION

VS is a mode of ventilation that pressure supports every breath to a level that guarantees a preset VT. The patient triggers every breath. Initial ventilator settings include a value for the expected spontaneous RR and minimum VT/V̇E.

Initially, and after any patient disconnection from the ventilator, the machine gives a sequence of four test breaths. The initial test breath is given at a pressure level of 10 cm H_2O above the PEEP setting, and the delivered volume at this pressure is measured. The ventilator then determines the pressure needed to achieve the target VT by performing a calculation involving the pressure used for the previous breath (dynamic compliance), the target VT, and the actual VT of the previous breath. The next breath in the test breath sequence is delivered at 75% of the calculated pressure needed to deliver the target VT. This process continues for the final two breaths of the test breath sequence. The inspiratory pressure with each subsequent breath can change up to plus or minus 3 cm H_2O, being regulated to a value based on the compliance calculation for the previous breath compared to the preset target VT/V̇E. If the patient breathes above the preset VT, the ventilator lowers the PS in a stepwise fashion until the target VT is achieved. Breaths may be flow cycled or time cycled (Fig. 7-20).

The ventilator responds to a decrease in the patient's RR that is less than the expected spontaneous rate by calculating a new target VT based on the preset minimum V̇E and the measured RR. The ventilator uses the new calculated target VT as the reference to regulate inspiratory pressure. The new calculated target VT is

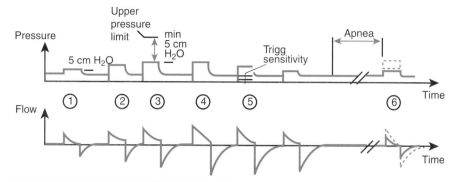

FIGURE 7-20

Volume support. **1,** Patient trigger initiates a test breath. **2,** If target tidal volume (VT) not achieved, pressure support (PS) is added stepwise. **3,** Maximum PS is 5 cm H_2O below preset upper pressure limit. **4,** If PS results in larger VT than the target, then PS is lowered stepwise. **5,** Every breath is patient triggered, and spontaneous breathing is allowed. **6,** Apnea condition results in switch to pressure-regulated volume control. *(Courtesy MAQUET, Inc., Bridgewater, NJ.)*

compared to the preset VT, and if the new VT exceeds the preset VT by 50%, the increase in inspiratory pressure is stopped at the level required to achieve a volume that is 150% of the set VT. The patient is guaranteed the minimum minute volume up to the point where the delivered VT reaches 150% of the initial VT. If the patient's RR drops below the apnea alarm threshold during VS, the ventilator automatically switches to PRVC and remains in this mode until the alarm is reset by the clinician. The ventilator switches back to VS after the apnea alarm is reset.

INDICATIONS

VS is suitable for spontaneous breathing patients who do not have sufficient respiratory muscle strength to consistently guarantee an adequate VT. Evidence is lacking that dual control of pressure-support breaths performs any function other than a volume guarantee.

ADVANTAGES AND DISADVANTAGES

VS may be viewed as refined PS and, therefore, has all of the advantages of PS ventilation. In addition, the ventilator strives to use the lowest required pressure. Unlike PS, however, VT is guaranteed, and the pressure varies depending on the compliance of the lungs and on ventilator circuit and airway resistance factors. Unlike MMV modes, the patient cannot achieve the set V̇E using a rapid, shallow breathing pattern. Patients may be more comfortable because they have control over RR and inspiratory time.

Asynchrony and VT instability were reported by Sottiaux in three patients ventilated with VS using the Siemens Servo 300 ventilator. In patients with expiratory obstruction and auto-PEEP formation, the target VT might not be achieved because auto-PEEP limits the pressure change from end-expiratory pressure to the PS level.

The ventilator will respond by increasing the PS level. This response further aggravates auto-PEEP formation. When auto-PEEP is present, the patient may not be able to trigger the ventilator although effort is made. Ventilator dyssynchrony is present as missed efforts.

There are additional disadvantages. Because ventilator support decreases when it is sensed that the patient is meeting the $\dot{V}E$ target, the ventilator could erroneously respond to the patient with an increased $\dot{V}E$ demand, by decreasing ventilatory support. If the minimum set $\dot{V}E$ is too high, the patient will remain on too much ventilatory support.

FOCUS AREAS OF PATIENT MONITORING

1. Monitor the exhaled V_T to ensure that the patient is receiving the target minimum $V_T/\dot{V}E$. Patients may receive V_Ts as large as 150% of the target V_T in the event their RR decreases.
2. Monitor the peak inspiratory pressure to determine the amount of pressure required to achieve the desired V_T. Set the upper pressure limit 10 to 15 cm H_2O above the average required inspiratory pressure. When the peak inspiratory pressure reaches 5 cm H_2O below the upper pressure limit, inspiration will continue. If this occurs for three consecutive breaths, the upper pressure limit alarm sounds, and the display reads "limited pressure." If the actual upper pressure limit is reached, inspiration is terminated.
3. Ensure that all parameters used in PRVC are preset for apnea ventilation.
4. Monitor the patient's RR. If the patient's RR increases to more than 25 breaths/min and the $\dot{V}E$ demands are increasing, assess the patient's ability to continue to manage the WOB associated with a spontaneous breathing mode. The patient's $\dot{V}E$ may exceed the set value because the set value indicates minimum acceptable $\dot{V}E$.
5. Set appropriate alarms for $\dot{V}E$, high pressure, and RR, which are critically important to the safe use of VS.

Dual Control Breath to Breath: Pressure-Limited, Time-Cycled Ventilation

This technique is essentially PC closed-loop ventilation with a guaranteed V_T and $\dot{V}E$. The input variable is V_T, and the pressure limit automatically reduces as lung mechanics improve or patient effort increases. Breaths are time or patient triggered, pressure limited, and time cycled. Modes that function in this manner include pressure-regulated volume control (PRVC), adaptive pressure ventilation (APV), auto-flow, variable pressure control (VPC), and volume control plus (VC+). Description of these modes is provided here with an in-depth discussion of one of them, PRVC, which is currently available on the Servo 300, because how each ventilator performs the mode is fairly consistent.

DEFINITION AND DESCRIPTION

PRVC is a control mode of ventilation in which the patient receives a preset number of breaths of a preset V_T that is given in the form of a pressure breath. Initial

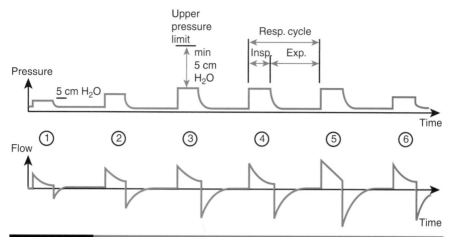

FIGURE 7-21

Pressure-regulated volume control. **1,** First breath is a machine-triggered test breath. **2,** Pressure control (PC) level changes breath to breath until target tidal volume (VT) is reached. **3,** Maximum PC level is 5 cm H_2O below preset upper pressure limit. **4,** Breaths are delivered with preset minute volume, respiratory frequency, and inspiration time. **5,** When measured VT equals target value, PC level remains constant. **6,** If measured VT exceeds target value, PC level decreases in stepwise increments. *(Courtesy MAQUET, Inc., Bridgewater, NJ.)*

ventilator settings include RR, inspiratory time, and the target $V_T/\dot{V}_E$. The ventilator strives to achieve the target V_T using the lowest possible pressure.

Initially, and after any patient disconnection from the ventilator, the machine gives a sequence of four test breaths. The initial "test breath" is given at a defined pressure level above the PEEP setting, and the delivered volume at this pressure is measured. The ventilator then determines the pressure needed to achieve the target V_T by performing a calculation involving the pressure used for the previous breath, the target V_T, and the actual V_T of the previous breath. The next breath in the test breath sequence is delivered at 75% of the calculated pressure needed to deliver the target V_T. This process continues for the final two breaths of the test breath sequence. The inspiratory pressure with each subsequent breath can then change up to plus or minus 3 cm H_2O, being regulated to a value based on the volume/pressure calculation for the previous breath compared to the preset target $V_T/\dot{V}_E$ (Fig. 7-21).

The ventilator always goes to the lowest pressure possible to achieve the desired V_T. Thus, if the measured V_T is too large, the pressure decreases in the same manner as just stated until the preset and measured volumes are equal. The maximum pressure control level allowed is 5 cm H_2O below the set upper pressure limit. For patient safety, the upper pressure limit should be set as low as possible.

INDICATIONS

PRVC is suitable for patients for whom PC ventilation is appropriate who do not have a reliable respiratory drive either because of underlying pathologic changes or because of sedation or other agents. It is useful for patients who demonstrate non-compliant lungs caused by disease processes that result in lung units with varying time constants. Some research has been done on these modes comparing them to VC that found lower PIP. This finding was likely because of the decelerating waveform versus the constant flow waveform used with VC as opposed to the closed-loop function of PRVC. No research has been done comparing consistency of VT delivery between these modes and conventional therapist-adjusted PC ventilation. Theoretically, this mode would be beneficial in patients with potentially changing compliance and resistance and limited respiratory care resources.

ADVANTAGES AND DISADVANTAGES

PRVC combines the advantages of pressure and volume-controlled ventilation: The patient can be ventilated with low pressure while the VT is guaranteed. A decelerating flow pattern is delivered that promotes more even distribution of gas in nonuniform disease processes. The ventilator automatically regulates inspiratory pressure as compliance, and resistance factors affect the volume/pressure relation. A hazard of PRVC is that in the event of a large air leak, the vent may continue to raise the pressure control level in a stepwise fashion, chasing the volume lost through the leak, and possibly aggravating air loss through the defect.

FOCUS AREAS OF PATIENT MONITORING

1. Monitor the patient's exhaled VT and V̇E to ensure the set parameters are being achieved.
2. Monitor the inspiratory pressure to determine the amount of pressure required to achieve the desired VT. Set the upper pressure limit 10 to 15 cm H_2O above the average required inspiratory pressure. When the peak inspiratory pressure reaches 5 cm H_2O below the upper pressure limit, inspiration will continue. If this occurs for three consecutive breaths, the upper pressure limit alarm sounds and the display reads "limited pressure." If the actual upper pressure limit is reached, inspiration is terminated.

Dual Control Breath to Breath: Combined Time- and Flow-Cycled Ventilation

This technique allows for the automatic switching between dual control breath-to-breath time-cycled breaths and dual control breath-to-breath flow-cycled breaths. The variable that provides the feedback to determine which breath type will be delivered is patient effort. Two modes are partnered with each other to provide the two levels of support (e.g., PRVC and VS). If the patient makes triggering efforts, the ventilator switches to the support mode. If the patient becomes apneic for a set period of time, the ventilator switches back to the controlled mode.

Modes that function with this option include *automode* (Siemens 300a) and *volume ventilation plus* (VV+; Puritan Bennett 840). The proposed potential benefit is that the ventilator will adapt to the patient's breathing effort and therefore not provide either too little or too much ventilatory support. Patients whose ventilatory effort is widely variable, therefore, may benefit from this technique. One potential concern is that decreases in mean airway pressure that occur during switches from time-cycled to flow-cycled modes could adversely effect oxygenation.

Adaptive support ventilation (ASV) is another mode that combines dual control breath-to-breath time-cycled and flow-cycled breaths. This mode is interestingly based on the work of Otis done in 1950 describing the mechanics of human breathing. This work states that patients optimize their breathing pattern (VT and rate) based on the compliance and resistance of the lung, which results in the lowest WOB while maintaining oxygenation and acid-base balance. The equation of minimal work is incorporated into the ASV algorithm along with the patient's ideal body weight (IBW), which is entered by the clinician. The ventilator continuously monitors resistance and compliance and adjusts frequency, VT, pressure limit, and I:E ratio for the mandatory breaths. It also calculates the expiratory time constant and adjusts I:E ratio to prevent auto-PEEP formation.

NONINVASIVE POSITIVE-PRESSURE VENTILATION

Definition and Description

Noninvasive positive-pressure ventilation (NPPV) is the provision of any form of ventilatory support applied without the use of an endotracheal tube (ETT). It is usually applied with either a nasal or oral face mask. NPPV may also be known as bilevel positive airway pressure ventilation or noninvasive ventilation. Use of NPPV ventilation in the intensive care unit (ICU) has increased in recent years as a result of successful application in multiple patient populations and improved equipment (Fig. 7-22).

Noninvasive ventilation may provide adequate ventilatory support without the need to perform endotracheal intubation, eliminating its associated complications. Sedation needs are less and the incidence of health-care-acquired pneumonia is reduced. Patients can eat and speak, and they are free from the discomfort of an artificial airway.

Contraindications to NPPV include apnea, cardiovascular instability (hypotension, uncontrolled dysrhythmias, and myocardial ischemia), claustrophobia, somnolence, high aspiration risk, viscous/copious secretions, inability to clear secretions, recent facial or gastroesophageal surgery, craniofacial trauma or burns, and fixed nasopharyngeal abnormality.

Indications/Patient Selection

1. COPD patients with acute exacerbation, as an early intervention to prevent deterioration to the point of requiring endotracheal intubation. Use when at least two are present: moderate to severe dyspnea with use of accessory muscles and paradoxical abdominal motion; moderate to severe acidosis (pH 7.30 to 7.35); and hypercapnia ($PaCO_2$ 45 to 60 mm Hg) or respiratory frequency more than 25 breaths/min. If patient is alert, NPPV should be the therapy of first choice unless exclusion criteria are present. NPPV has been investigated extensively in COPD patients with hypercapnic ARF. It is highly effective in improving gas-exchange abnormalities, decreasing the need for intubation, reducing length of hospital stay, and lowering mortality.

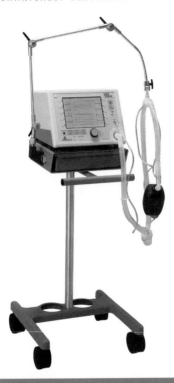

FIGURE 7-22

Noninvasive positive pressure ventilation (NPPV), also known as bi-level positive airway pressure, may be administered through a mask with the BiPAP Vision ventilatory support system (BiPAP; Respironics, Murrysville, Pa.). This system is capable of operating in four modes. In the spontaneous *(S)* mode, the unit synchronizes with the patient's respiratory pattern, cycling from inspiratory to expiratory positive airway pressure (IPAP to EPAP). This is pressure support (PS) ventilation. In the spontaneous/timed *(S/T)* mode, the mode delivered is PS, but in the event of apnea, pressure control (PC) breaths are given on the basis of a clinician-set breaths-per-minute setting. In the timed *(T)* mode, the unit cycles between IPAP and EPAP levels according to set respiratory rate (RR) and percentage IPAP time controls. This is PC ventilation. The continuous positive airway pressure (CPAP) mode allows the system to be used for the delivery of CPAP. *(Photo courtesy of Respironics, Inc., Murrysville, Pa.)*

2. Patients with hypoxemic respiratory failure who are hemodynamically stable, without severely impaired mental status, and not in need of an artificial airway for secretion management or aspiration protection. Conditions could include pneumonia, atelectasis, trauma, aspiration, and postoperative respiratory failure. NPPV can improve gas exchange, reduce the need for intubation, prevent reintubation, and reduce ICU length of stay in patients with acute hypoxemic respiratory failure. Mask ventilation can be used to administer PEEP and recruit underventilated alveoli, increase the FRC, and thus improve oxygenation. NPPV is associated with fewer serious complications such as sinusitis and pneumonia.

The wide variety of diagnoses in this category makes it difficult to apply results to individual diagnostic groups. Patients must have a patent natural airway, a spontaneous drive to breathe, and be able to assist in the management of their secretions because the lack of artificial airway access reduces control of the airway for suctioning secretions or protecting from aspiration. NPPV should be used with caution in patients with basilar skull fracture. A case of pneumocephalus was reported in a trauma patient with unrecognized basilar skull fracture.

3. Patients who fail planned or unplanned extubation to avoid reintubation and thereby the associated complications. Noninvasive ventilation may provide an adequate level of support for respiratory distress with a lower level of complications. There is a trend toward lower success rates in unplanned as opposed to planned extubation. Carefully select patients and closely monitor them until stabilized.

4. Immunocompromised patients with early acute hypoxemic respiratory failure to avoid intubation. Early use of NPPV results in improved oxygenation, lower intubation rates, and lower mortality. Patients experience less serious complications.

5. Patients with acute cardiogenic pulmonary edema in the absence of myocardial infarction (MI). CPAP rapidly improves oxygenation by reexpanding fluid-filled alveoli, increasing the FRC, and therefore improving lung compliance. These effects reduce the WOB and improve RR. Favorable effect is also demonstrated in reduced need for intubation, reduced ICU length of stay, and improved hospital mortality. Exercise caution in the use of CPAP in patients with good ventricular performance and low filling pressures because venous return may be reduced, resulting in a decreased cardiac output.

6. Patients for whom intubation and mechanical ventilation are undesirable. For example, do-not-intubate patients, patients with late-stage disease or terminal conditions, or patients in whom the respiratory failure is caused by an acute condition that could be reversed during brief mechanical ventilatory support. Patients who decline intubation could possibly benefit from noninvasive support administered concurrently with therapies to treat an acute respiratory process. In patients with poor prognoses, noninvasive ventilatory support may allow time to make resuscitate/do-not-resuscitate decisions and to address life-closure tasks. Ethical concern arises regarding possible use of noninvasive ventilation when further intervention is futile.

7. Patients with acute on chronic respiratory disorders who are unable to meet extubation criteria but are otherwise good candidates for NPPV. When the respiratory muscles are unable to manage the workload independently, NPPV provides effective ventilator assistance without the risks of prolonged intubation and with improved patient comfort. This approach shortens duration of invasive mechanical ventilation. Results are inconsistent for reducing ICU and hospital length of stay, need for tracheostomy, and pneumonia. Be cautious when selecting patients for early extubation. Ensure that the patient is a good candidate for NPPV (i.e., proven applications of NPPV such as COPD and cardiogenic pulmonary edema). The clinician should be very experienced in application of NPPV. Outside of these groups the use of noninvasive ventilation to support extubation is not proven.

8. Nocturnal ventilatory support in patients with obstructive sleep apnea, cystic fibrosis, obesity hypoventilation syndrome, etc. NPPV was originally developed for the relief of obstructive sleep apnea, the inspiratory positive airway pressure (IPAP) creating an adequate VT and expiratory positive airway pressure (EPAP) stenting the airway.

Application

MASK TYPE

Selection of the proper mask interface and assurance of a proper fit is necessary to success. Oronasal (full-face) masks deliver higher ventilation pressures with less leak and may lower carbon dioxide more effectively (providing dead space is not increased); require less patient cooperation; and may benefit mouth breathers. But they may generate feelings of claustrophobia, making patients unable to tolerate NPPV; may be harder to fit and therefore generate leaks; place a barrier to communication; and limit oral intake. Nasal masks add less dead space; allow for speech, expectoration, and oral intake without mask removal; and are sensed as more comfortable by the patient. When a nasal mask is applied, patients must have patent nasal passages and breathe solely through the nares with the mouth closed.

Masks come in a variety of sizes and materials (Fig. 7-23). Most are clear and made of soft materials with either an air or soft silicone open cushion seal. As pressure increases in the mask, the cushion pushes against the face, promoting a good seal. Some are made with a swivel adapter. A mask with a transparent dome is preferable because it allows visualization of the airway and secretions. The mask should be carefully sized as per the manufacturer's instructions, to ensure proper fit and patient comfort.

Masks are secured to the head with adjustable straps or head caps that attach to prongs on the mask. The nasal or oronasal masks used to administer noninvasive ventilation must have a tight seal to ensure the patient receives the full benefit of ventilatory support. However, fastening too tight does not ensure a better seal and causes patient discomfort. The straps should be adjusted so that one finger can still pass between the strap and face. Straps come with cushions, called forehead spacers, which improve comfort and can reduce pressure injury (Fig. 7-24).

Nasal bridge skin erythema or breakdown is the most common complication of NPPV. Compliance with therapy diminishes when patient discomfort increases. In addition to using minimum strap tension to achieve a seal, mask position should be altered to prevent areas of pressure and skin breakdown. At the first sign of pressure and before skin breakdown occurs, apply a patch of wound care dressing to prevent further problems.

VENTILATORS, MODES, AND SETTINGS

NPPV can be delivered with critical care ventilators or bilevel ventilators that were first designed for sleep apnea and are now specifically designed for the application of this technique. Because critical care ventilators have oxygen blenders, they may be superior for patients with hypoxemia. They also have separate inspiratory and expiratory circuits that limit rebreathing. The biggest disadvantage of a critical care

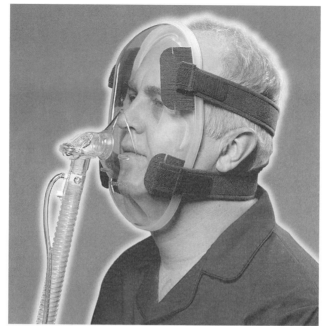

A

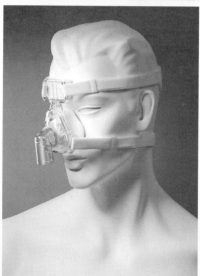

B

FIGURE 7-23

Noninvasive positive-pressure ventilation (NPPV) masks. **A,** Total face mask for patient who cannot tolerate nasal mask or full-face mask. The fast, effective seal, one size, and no fitting make this mask useful for patients in need of immediate ventilation. **B,** Nasal mask. The top of the nasal mask should rest a third of the way down from the bridge of the nose, which is approximately just above the junction of the cartilaginous nostrils and the nasal bone. A mask resting too high may result in leaks in the eye area. The bottom of the nasal mask should be just above the upper lip. *(Courtesy of Respironics, Murrysville, Pa.)*

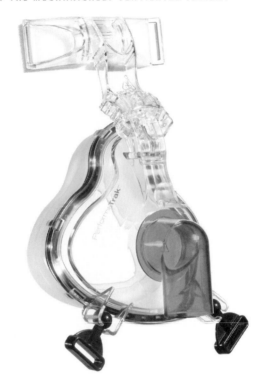

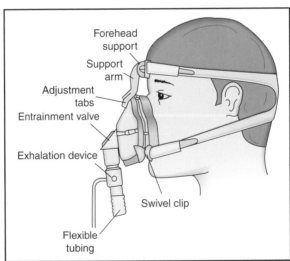

FIGURE 7-24

Full-face mask for noninvasive positive-pressure ventilation (NPPV). The top of the oronasal, or full-face, mask is fit just like the nasal mask (one third of the way down from the bridge of the nose); however, the bottom of the mask should rest just below the lower lip. Forehead support minimizes mask force on the bridge of the nose while maintaining an effective seal. *(Courtesy Respironics, Murrysville, Pa.)*

ventilator is its inability to deal with leaks with leak compensation. The newest model ICU ventilators are capable of software upgrades with features needed to provide mask ventilation.

Ventilators designed to provide NPPV are more leak tolerant in that they have leak compensation. It may be difficult to create a perfect seal, so a system that detects leaks around the mask and compensates for them by increasing flow is ideal. The BiPAP Vision operates under such a principle and does so without affecting the sensitivity of the flow-triggering mechanism. Because flow-triggering is used, as opposed to pressure-triggering, the WOB associated with triggering the ventilator is eliminated.

NPPV systems are typically single-hose systems without a true exhalation valve. Expired gases leave through a fixed leak in the system. One concern is the potential for carbon dioxide rebreathing, which may occur in single-tube systems when two levels of airway pressure are used. This side effect of the technique could prevent $PaCO_2$ from dropping in hypercapnic patients. Setting PEEP 4 to 6 cm H_2O can resolve the rebreathing problem.

Disadvantages in NPPV systems include the limitation in the amount of support that the ventilator can offer to the patient. The intent, however, of the portable NPPV machine is to assist the patient's respiratory efforts, not to override them. When resources for ventilator purchase are limited, the purchase of a separate system for the delivery of NPPV may be prohibitive. These costs must be weighed against potential savings from ventilator days and reduction in complications of mechanical ventilation.

Modes used when applying NPPV can be pressure or volume. Pressure modes are preferred because they are better tolerated. The use of a pressure-targeted mode enables the peak pressure in the mask to be limited, which may reduce leaks and gastric insufflation and improve synchrony, especially in the presence of leaks. Deliver NPPV using a combination of low-level PEEP to improve FRC and oxygenation and to offset auto-PEEP in COPD (which significantly reduces inspiratory workload) and inspiratory positive pressure. PS is adjusted to achieve the desired exhaled V_T, to correct gas-exchange abnormalities, and to unload the respiratory muscles sufficiently as evidenced by patient comfort. Set inspiratory pressure low and titrate up to avoid discomfort caused by air pressure and flow. Typical PS levels are 10 to 20 cm H_2O. Typical PEEP values are 5 to 10 cm H_2O.

Pressure assist control and CPAP are other commonly used modes. Controlled modes reduce inspiratory workload better than PSV and may be better in more severe disease and unstable ventilatory drive. CPAP is highly beneficial in cardiogenic pulmonary edema in the absence of hemodynamic instability. Choice of mode should be based on the same indications and rationale outlined previously for each of the modes while taking into account local expertise.

CAREGIVERS

The initiation of NPPV is time consuming. Achieving the right interface, coaching the patient, titrating the degree of support to patient comfort and synchrony, and monitoring for leaks are some of the tasks that must be performed frequently. The nurse, respiratory therapist, and physician on the team must all be committed to the success of NPPV. Each brings expertise to ensure the patient meets selection criteria, the ventilator is managed optimally, and problems such as poor mask fit and skin breakdown are minimized. The patient being placed on NPPV requires a high intensity of monitoring. It is highly likely that some of the positive outcomes experienced with NPPV can be attributed to this caregiver vigilance. Likewise, because the airway is not protected, the converse could result if team members are not readily available. It is not recommended that NPPV be implemented in the general care areas. However, it may be used in the emergency department before transporting the patient to a unit where ventilator care is the routine.

FOCUS AREAS OF MONITORING

1. Exhaled V_T (EV_T), which will be variable in this pressure mode of ventilation. The EV_T should be at least 5 to 8 mL/kg. Prevent all factors that will increase resistance to ventilation and decrease V_T. If the EV_T is less than the goal, atelectasis may develop, resulting in the need for increased ventilatory assistance.
2. Assess for air leaks and preferably use a system that detects air leaks and compensates for them by increasing flow. This increases the assurance that patient will receive adequate V_T. When an air leak occurs, check to see if exhaled V_T is compromised, reposition the mask, apply wound care dressing to seal leaks, increase the amount of PEEP as tolerated, or try another mask.
3. The PIP. Determine whether altering the EPAP level also changes the IPAP level in the system being used to deliver noninvasive pressure support ventilation (NIPSV).
4. Mouth breathing. Consider the use of a chin strap if the patient tends to breathe through the mouth.
5. Pressure areas, particularly over the bridge of the nose, caused by the mask. Comfort between the interface of patient's skin and the mask is probably one of the most important areas of patient compliance. At the first sign of pressure, the application of a patch of wound care dressing may prevent further problems.
6. Monitor for gastric distention because when administering positive-pressure ventilation with a face mask, air may be swallowed or forced down the esophagus. To reduce the possibility of gastric insufflation, adjust inflation pressures if possible and use peak mask pressures of 30 cm H_2O or less. Place a gastric tube for decompression as indicated, although it is usually not necessary. If a gastric tube is placed, it may be more difficult to seal a mask, which creates another point of concern for pressure necrosis and creates a resistance to gas flow through the nares with nasal ventilation.
7. Monitor patient's nasal passages and upper airways for excessive drying. Mucous membranes of the nose may become dry from inspiration of high-volume dry gases. It is not necessary to heat the inspired gases because the upper airways that normally heat inspired gases are not bypassed. Nasal dryness may respond to normal saline nasal spray or drops. If dryness fails to respond to these measures, a humidification system is an option (nonheated pass-over humidifier) and should be added on the basis of patient comfort and assessment of the secretions and upper airways.

8. Leakage of gases around the nasal portion of the mask may dry the eyes, leading to conjunctivitis. Use artificial tears to moisten the eyes and a humidification system for the inspired gases.

SUMMARY

The various modes of ventilation give the clinician the opportunity to change the therapeutic option when the patient's condition changes. A thorough understanding of what is known to date about each mode's mechanism of action will contribute to sound clinical judgment regarding their use. Much is still to be learned about the appropriate choice of ventilator mode for the various conditions for which mechanical ventilation may be required. Limited research is available on newer modes, which continue to proliferate partly as a result of ventilator manufacturers competing to offer a so-called better mode. Dual control modes function using the principles of a closed feedback system and strive to respond to changing patient conditions. A dramatic expansion in the use of noninvasive ventilation has occurred and will likely continue to rise as patients can be ventilated without the hazards of an artificial airway. A solid understanding of how a mode operates will result in accurate settings, appropriate safety limits, detection of problems, and knowledgeable adjustment of the parameters to ensure optimal patient-ventilator interaction. New knowledge continues to bring about change in the way we perceive and use the current modes. What remains the same is the clinical outcome goal: to support gas exchange, without compromise of pulmonary or systemic perfusion, while preventing complications of applied therapy.

RECOMMENDED READINGS

Abraham E, Yoshihara G. Cardiorespiratory effects of pressure controlled ventilation in severe respiratory failure. *Chest* 1990; 98(6):1445–1449.

Al-Saady N, Bennett ED. Decelerating inspiratory flow waveform improves lung mechanics and gas exchange in patients on intermittent positive-pressure ventilation. *Intensive Care Med* 1985; 11:68–75.

Antonelli M, Conti G, Rocco M, et al. A comparison of noninvasive positive-pressure ventilation and conventional mechanical ventilation in patients with acute respiratory failure. *N Engl J Med* 1998; 339(7):429–456.

Branson RD. Understanding and implementing advances in ventilator capabilities. *Curr Opin Crit Care* 2004; 1:23–32.

Branson RD, Campbell RS. Modes of ventilator operation. In NR MacIntyre, RD Branson (eds.), *Mechanical Ventilation* (pp. 51–84). Philadelphia: Saunders, 2001.

Branson RD, Johannigman JA. What is the evidence base for the new ventilation modes? *Respir Care* 2004; 49(7):742–760.

Branson RD, Johannigman JA, Campbell RS, et al. Closed loop mechanical ventilation. *Respir Care* 2002; 47(4):427–451.

Calzia E, Pradermacher P. Airway pressure release ventilation and biphasic positive airway pressure. A 10-year literature review. *Clin Intensive Care* 1997; 8:296–301.

Campbell RS, Davis BR. Pressure-controlled versus volume-controlled ventilation: Does it matter? *Respir Care* 2002; 47(4):416–424.

Chatburn RL, Primiano FP. A new system for understanding modes of mechanical ventilation. *Respir Care* 2001; 46(6):604–621.

Davis K, Branson RD, Campbell RS, et al. Comparison of volume control and pressure control ventilation: Is flow waveform the difference? *J Trauma* 1996; 41:808–814.

Esteban A, Frutos-Viva F, Ferguson ND, et al. Noninvasive positive-pressure ventilation for respiratory failure after extubation. *N Engl J Med* 2004; 350(24):2452–2461.

Ferrer M, Esquinas A, Arancibia F, et al. Noninvasive ventilation during persistent weaning failure: A randomized controlled trial. *Am J Respir Crit Care Med* 2003; 168:70–76.

Frawley PM, Cowan J. Airway pressure release ventilation: The future of trauma ventilatory support? [case study]. *J Trauma Nurs* 2002; 9(3):75–78.

Frawley PM, Habashi NM. Airway pressure release ventilation: Theory and practice. *AACN Clin Issues* 2001; 12(2):234–246.

Habashi, NM. Other approaches to open-lung ventilation: Airway pressure release ventilation. *Crit Care Med* 2005; 33[Suppl.]:S228–S240.

Hess DR, Kacmarek RM. *Essentials of Mechanical Ventilation,* 2nd ed. New York: McGraw-Hill, 2002.

Hill N. *Noninvasive Positive Pressure Ventilation: Principles and Applications.* Armonk, NY: Futura, 2001.

International Consensus Conference in Intensive Care Medicine. Noninvasive positive pressure ventilation in acute respiratory failure. *Am J Respir Crit Care Med* 2001; 163(1):283–291.

Jaber S, Delay JM, Matecki S. Volume-guaranteed pressure-support ventilation facing acute changes in ventilatory demand. *Int Care Med* 2005; 31:1181–1188.

Kuhlen R, Rossaint R. The role of spontaneous breathing during mechanical ventilation. *Respir Care* 2002; 47(3):296–303.

Liesching T, Kwok H, Hill NS. Acute applications of noninvasive positive pressure ventilation. *Chest* 2003; 124:699–713.

MacIntyre NR, McConnell R, Cheng KG, et al. Patient-ventilator flow dyssynchrony: Flow-limited versus pressure-limited breaths. *Crit Care Med* 1997; 25:1671–1677.

Marcy TW, Marini JJ. Inverse ratio ventilation in ARDS: Rationale and implementation. *Chest* 1991; 100(2):494–504.

Marini JJ, Ravenscraft SA. Mean airway pressure: Physiologic determinants and clinical importance. Part 2. Clinical implications. *Crit Care Med* 1992; 20(11):1604–1616.

Oakes DF, Shortall SP. *Oakes' Ventilator Management: A Bedside Reference Guide.* Orono, Me: Respiratory Books, a division of Health Educator Publications, Inc., 2002.

Otis AB, Fenn WO, Rahn H. Mechanics of breathing in man. *J Appl Physiol* 1950; 2:592–607.

Pilbeam SP. *Mechanical Ventilation: Physiological and Clinical Applications,* 3rd ed. St. Louis: Mosby, 1998.

Poelaert JI, Vogelaers DP, Colardyn FA. Evaluation of the hemodynamic and respiratory effects of inverse ratio ventilation with a right ventricular ejection fraction catheter. *Chest* 1991; 99(6):1444–1450.

Putensen C, Jutz NJ, Putensen-Himmer G, et al. Spontaneous breathing during ventilatory support improves ventilation-perfusion distribution in patients with acute respiratory distress syndrome. *Am J Respir Crit Care Med* 1999; 159:1241–1248.

Putensen C, Zech S, Wrigge H, et al. Long-term effects of spontaneous breathing during ventilatory support in patients with acute lung injury. *Am J Respir Crit Care Med* 2001; 164:43–49.

Schonhofer B, Sortor-Leger S. Equipment needs for noninvasive mechanical ventilation. *Eur Respir J* 2002; 20:1029–1036.

Sottiaux TM. Patient-ventilator interactions during volume support ventilation: Asynchrony and tidal volume instability—A report of three cases. *Respir Care* 2001; 46(3):255–262

Stock MC, Downs JB. Airway pressure release ventilation: A new approach to ventilatory support during acute lung injury. *Respir Care* 1987; 32(7):517–524.

Wysocki M, Tric L, Wolff MA, et al. Noninvasive pressure support ventilation in patients with acute respiratory failure: A randomized comparison with conventional therapy. *Chest* 1995; 107:761–768.

Ventilator Graphics and Waveform Analysis

Sean P. Shortall and Linda A. Perkins

The availability of ventilator graphics has had a tremendous impact on the science of mechanical ventilation. Through the analysis of these pressure, volume, and flow waveforms, critical care clinicians can now more accurately assess not only the current state of lung function but the status of patient-ventilator interaction as well. Considering the emphasis placed on employing lung protective strategies and the judicious use of sedation and other chemical agents, knowledgeable practitioners will find understanding ventilator graphics a valuable adjunct to their clinical expertise.

This chapter provides descriptions of scalar and loop waveforms, the significance of each, and graphic representations of normal and abnormal waveforms. It can be used as a basic guide for the beginner or as a reference for the experienced clinician. Unless otherwise designated, the ventilator graphics displayed are of volume ventilation.

SCALARS

A waveform is a graphic display of patient ventilation data. The three most important parameters reflective of ventilation status are pressure, flow, and volume. Scalar waveforms are representations of each of these variables plotted against time. Typically, the horizontal, or *x*, axis depicts time, and the vertical, or *y*, axis depicts the designated parameter. Each type of scalar provides a view of lung mechanics, ventilator function, or the patient's response to ventilation. Scalars are also known as curves. Figure 8-1 depicts normal pressure-time, flow-time, and volume-time scalars for three different breath types.

The *pressure-time scalar* depicts airway pressure (Paw), measured in cm H_2O, on the *y* (vertical) axis, and time, measured in seconds, on the *x* (horizontal) axis. Reflecting positive pressure, the waveforms rise above the baseline (0 cm H_2O) and remain positive. If positive end-expiratory pressure (PEEP) is set on the ventilator, the waveforms will begin at that set point (5 cm H_2O PEEP lifts the baseline to 5 cm H_2O). Note that the flow and volume of both breaths A and B are identical: a characteristic of volume assist/control ventilation. The gradual rise in pressure while the volume is being delivered resembles a shark's fin. The pressure required to reach

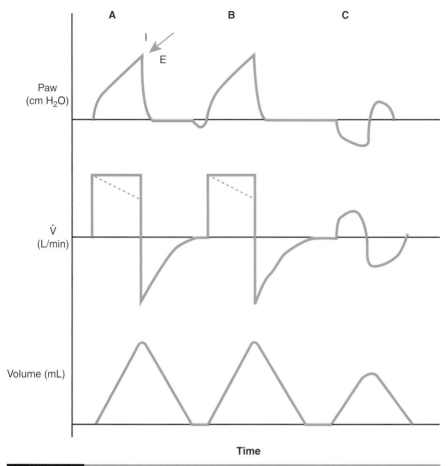

FIGURE 8-1

Normal pressure-time, flow-time, and volume-time scalars. Breath A is a mandatory, volume-control, time-triggered breath. Breath B is a volume-control, patient-triggered breath. Breath C is a sponta- neous breath. Note on the flow curve that breaths A and B are delivered with a square flow-wave pattern. The dashed line represents the appearance of a decelerating flow-wave pattern. Breath C is a sine wave, which is characteristic of spontaneous ventilation. *I*, Inspiration; *E*, expiration.

the set volume is variable and depends on the patient's lung mechanics. The slight negative deflection immediately before the waveform in breath B depicts the patient's inspiratory effort. The depth of the deflection and the period of time below the baseline reflect the degree of patient effort necessary to trigger the ventilator. An increase in patient effort reflects an increased work of breathing (WOB) and may be caused, for example, by auto-PEEP, pneumothorax, or fluid overload.

Pressure-time scalars can be used to determine the following:

- Breath type delivered (volume or pressure control)
- Patient versus machine triggering

- Work required to trigger the breath
- Breath timing: inspiratory (I) versus expiratory (E)
- Adequacy of inspiratory flow
- Airway pressure

Detecting if a breath is patient-triggered versus machine-triggered is important in determining the effectiveness of neuromuscular blocking drugs. In the chemically paralyzed patient, so-called breakthrough breathing may be present despite reaching the desired train-of-four muscle twitch response with a peripheral nerve stimulator (PNS). The train-of-four muscle twitch response is the most common method for assessing level of paralysis; however, it may be difficult to obtain or may not reflect the degree of paralysis accurately. The pressure-time scalar is an objective, real-time measure that can be used to titrate the paralytic to elimination of patient-initiated breaths.

Another important function of the pressure waveform is the identification of end-expiration, a significant factor in accurately interpreting hemodynamic waveforms such as pulmonary artery occlusion pressure and cardiac output. Some newer bedside monitors designate a channel for airway pressure waveforms to be continuously visualized along with pulmonary artery catheter data. When this function is not readily available, a technique known as continuous airway pressure monitoring (CAPM) can be applied to any monitor with an unused channel and a transducing system. CAPM allows waveform visualization along with the pressure measured in the ventilator circuit. This procedure provides clinicians access to pressure waveforms and can be implemented regardless of the simplicity of the bedside monitor or the availability of graphics on the ventilator.

The *flow-time scalar* shows flow (V), in liters per minute, on the vertical axis, and time, in seconds, on the horizontal axis (see Fig. 8-1). Flow depicted above the zero flow line is inspiratory, and flow below the zero flow line is expiratory. The set inspiratory flow can be constant (square waveform) or decelerating, as depicted by the dashed lines, and it is not affected by the patient's lung mechanics.

Flow-time scalars can be used to evaluate the following:

- Inspiratory and expiratory flow rates
- Type of breath (volume or pressure control)
- Type of inspiratory flow pattern (in volume ventilation)
- Adequacy of inspiratory time (in pressure control [PC] ventilation)
- Presence of auto-PEEP
- Expiratory resistance and response to bronchodilators
- Presence and degree of continuous air leaks

The *volume-time scalar* plots volume of gas in milliliters on the vertical axis against time in seconds on the horizontal axis (see Fig. 8-1). Inspiratory volume is depicted by the up slope of the waveform; the down slope represents the expiratory volume. Expiration begins when the set tidal volume (VT) is reached (volume cycled). These curves may be used to detect air trapping or leaks in the patient circuit.

Spontaneous ventilation is depicted in Figure 8-1 breath C. Note that the flow, pressure, and volume are generally lower than ventilator breaths. The breath is patient triggered and patient cycled. The flow above the baseline is inspiratory and

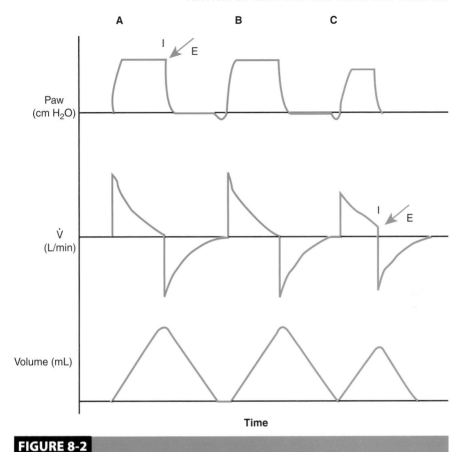

FIGURE 8-2

Normal pressure ventilation scalars. **Breath A,** Pressure control, time triggered. **Breath B,** Pressure control, patient triggered. **Breath C,** Pressure supported, patient triggered.

below the baseline is expiratory. Inspiratory pressure is negative (below the baseline) and rises to positive (above the baseline) with expiration. The volume may vary with each breath because of patient effort and lung mechanics. If continuous positive airway pressure (CPAP) is set on the ventilator, the pressure waveform reflects that pressure as the baseline.

Figure 8-2 represents the square pressure waveform and the descending flow waveform of PC ventilation. Breath A is a mandatory time-triggered breath. Breath B is patient triggered, as noted by the initial negative deflection on the pressure waveform. Although the pressure graphics remain the same breath to breath, the flow and the volume vary depending on the airway resistance and the lung compliance. Both breath A and B are time cycled, meaning expiration begins when the set inspiratory time has elapsed. The inspiratory time, once set by the clinician, remains constant.

The pressure support (PS) waveform in Figure 8-2 breath C is similar to the PC scalars shown in breaths A and B. The following important differences should be noted by the clinician:

- All PS breaths are patient triggered, as depicted by an initial negative deflection on the pressure-time scalar waveform.
- Inspiration ends and expiratory cycling begins when the machine flow decreases to a set terminal flow criterion, which is typically 25% of peak inspiratory flow. Consequently, the descending flow waveform never reaches the zero baseline. This expiratory parameter may be less depending on the ventilator model and may be adjustable on some newer ventilators. This adjustable parameter is called expiratory sensitivity.
- The delivered volume is typically less than a PC breath and varies, depending on the amount of PS and patient effort, compliance, and resistance.

LOOPS

Graphic loops display two of the three ventilator variables plotted against one another. A *volume-pressure (V-P) loop* usually displays pressure on the *x* (horizontal) axis and volume on the *y* (vertical) axis (Fig. 8-3). The lower curve of the loop depicts inspiratory pressure and volume; the upper curve depicts expiratory parameters. The slope of the loop is defined by the angle of the inspiratory and expiratory curves. The degree of slope depicts lung and chest wall compliance.

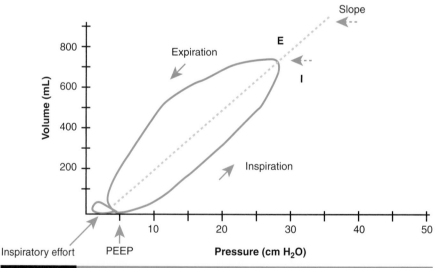

FIGURE 8-3

Volume-pressure loop depicting volume-control ventilation. Note the trigger-tail, representing degree of patient effort to trigger the breath.

V-P loops are used to assess the following:

- Changes in resistance and compliance
- Adequacy of peak inspiratory flow rates (in volume ventilation)
- Work required to trigger a breath
- Lung overdistention

On the V-P loop, positive-pressure breaths are plotted counterclockwise. The starting point is at the intersection of zero on the volume axis and zero, or the set-PEEP, on the pressure axis. A patient-initiated breath forms a small "trigger-tail" to the left of the vertical axis. Analysis of this indicator of patient effort provides the clinician with information on patient triggering and WOB. The larger the trigger-tail, the greater the patient effort and therefore work. To the right of the vertical axis, the loop follows an elliptical tract plotting a simultaneous rise in pressure and volume until peak inspiratory pressure and set VT are reached. Then expiration begins, and the loop falls in an elliptical path to the baseline values. The slope of the loop provides information regarding lung compliance. The steeper the slope of the V-P loop, the better the lung compliance. This concept is discussed in greater detail later.

The V-P loop of a pressure-control ventilation breath is also plotted in a *counterclockwise* direction and assumes a more rectangular shape than a volume-control breath. The set pressure on the horizontal axis is reached quickly before the volume, on the vertical axis, rises (Fig. 8-4, *A*). At the end of inspiration, the volume

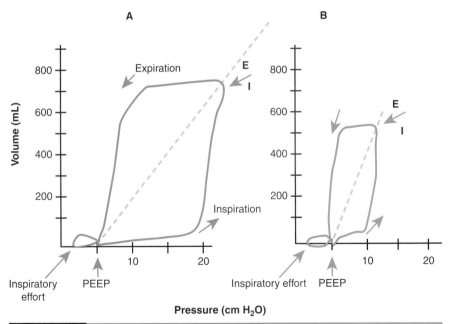

FIGURE 8-4

Normal pressure ventilation volume-pressure loop. **Breath A,** Pressure control, patient triggered. **Breath B,** Pressure support.

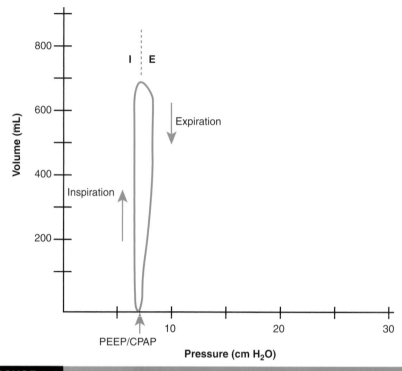

FIGURE 8-5

Normal spontaneous ventilation volume-pressure loop.

is held steady while the pressure returns toward the baseline. Only then does the volume returns to zero. A patient-triggered breath is noted by a trigger-tail to the left of the vertical axis.

PS ventilation depicted in Figure 8-4 breath B resembles pressure control ventilation with the following exceptions:

- Each breath is patient triggered.
- Pressure and volume are usually less than pressure control ventilation.

A spontaneous breath V-P loop is plotted in a *clockwise* fashion. The loop begins with the negative inspiratory force plotted to the left of the patient's baseline pressure (zero or CPAP) and increases to maximum volume (Fig. 8-5). The positive expiratory loop is plotted to the right of the pressure baseline and returns to baseline as the volume returns to zero. Pressure and volume values are typically lower than with positive-pressure ventilation.

A *flow-volume loop* displays flow on the *vertical* axis and volume on the *horizontal* axis (Fig. 8-6). In most cases, inspiratory flow is above the horizontal axis and expiratory flow is below, depending on the configuration of the particular ventilator. The shape of the inspiratory loop is determined by the flow setting on the ventilator (e.g., constant or descending). The shape of the expiratory portion of the

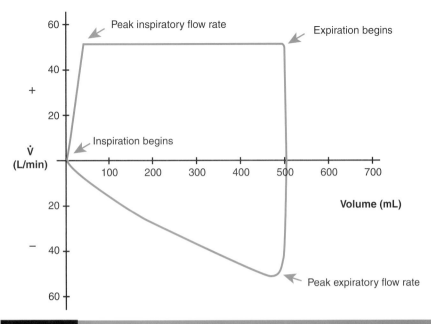

FIGURE 8-6

Normal volume ventilation flow-volume loop, volume-control ventilation. Peak inspiratory flow is achieved at the beginning of inspiration and maintained during the entire inspiratory phase, resulting in the square wave pattern. Expiration begins after the set tidal volume is reached and then flow drops to below baseline to a value known as the peak expiratory flow rate. Flow and volume decrease simultaneously until zero flow and zero volume are reached.

flow-volume loop is determined by the patient's lung characteristics. This loop is used primarily to assess the effect of bronchodilator therapy but may also demonstrate other changes in airway resistance. Flow-volume loops may also be used to detect auto-PEEP and volume leaks.

The flow-volume loop of PC ventilation is plotted in a clockwise fashion as in volume-control ventilation (Fig. 8-7). The peak inspiratory flow rate is achieved quickly and then decelerates throughout the inspiratory phase. PS ventilation resembles PC ventilation with the following differences:

- The amount of flow and volume are usually less.
- The inspiratory phase is terminated when the inspiratory flow decreases to a set ventilator flow parameter (usually 25% but depends on the configuration of the ventilator model). Hence, expiration begins above the point of zero flow.

The flow-volume loop plotted during spontaneous ventilation starts at the intersection of flow and volume and proceeds in a clockwise loop. Just as with mechanical ventilation breaths, flow above the zero baseline is inspiratory and flow below the baseline is expiratory. Flow and volume values are lower than ventilator breath values.

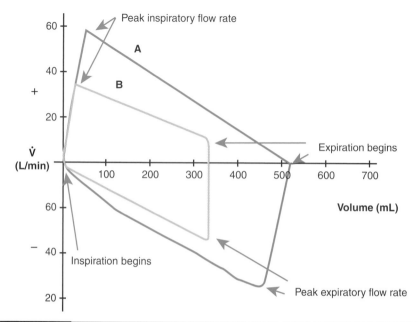

FIGURE 8-7

Normal pressure ventilation flow-volume loops. **Breath A,** Pressure control. **Breath B,** Pressure support. Pressure support (PS) breaths are typically lower volume and pressure than pressure control (PC) breaths. Breath cycling from inspiration to expiration results from different criteria in a PC versus a PS breath. See text for explanation.

ABNORMAL GRAPHIC WAVEFORMS

It is important that the clinician gain comfort with rapid recognition of normal scalars, volume-pressure loops, and flow-volume loops. This will allow greater confidence at detecting abnormal conditions and using the waveforms to evaluate response to therapeutic interventions.

Air Leaks

Air leaks may occur during inspiration or expiration. Inspiratory leaks are ventilator related, such as loose connections, a faulty flow sensor, or ventilator malfunction. In volume ventilation, the set volume is not reached. In pressure ventilation, the set pressure may not be reached. Expiratory leaks are more common and primarily patient related, and they may be caused by a leak around the endotracheal/tracheostomy tube cuff, air loss through a chest tube, or a gastric tube placed inappropriately in the trachea. It is easiest to detect air leaks on ventilator graphics by looking at the waveforms that represent volume (Fig. 8-8). An inspiratory leak is represented by a smaller VT on the volume scalar and a decreased peak inspiratory pressure on the pressure waveform. Expiratory leaks are demonstrated by an

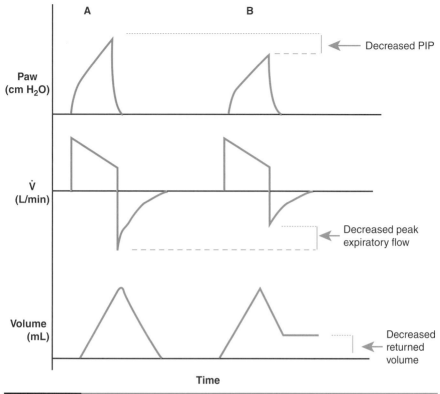

FIGURE 8-8

Abnormal scalars depicting air leak in breath B on each of the three curves during volume-control ventilation. Expiratory leak results in a decreased expiratory tidal volume (V_T) and a decreased peak expiratory flow. An inspiratory leak is represented by a smaller V_T on the volume scalar (not shown) and a decreased peak inspiratory pressure on the pressure waveform as shown in *B*.

expiratory V_T smaller than the set (inspiratory) V_T. If a leak is suspected, the volume curve will show quantitatively how much volume is being lost. When a leak is present, the peak expiratory flow will also be decreased relative to the breaths where no leak was present.

It is also possible to detect and quantify an air leak on the V-P loop (Fig. 8-9). On the V-P loop when all of the volume fails to return, the result is an incomplete loop. Figure 8-10 depicts a flow-volume loop with an air leak. On the flow-volume loop when an expiratory leak is present, the expiratory portion of the curve returns to a value greater than zero.

Auto-PEEP

Auto-PEEP, or intrinsic PEEP ($PEEP_I$), refers to the presence of positive pressure in the lungs at the end of exhalation (air trapping). This is depicted by expiratory

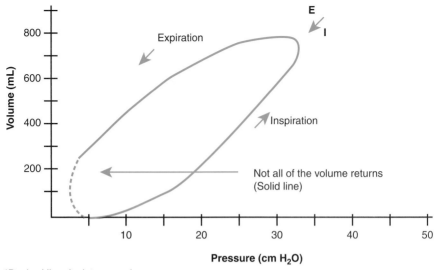

*Dashed line depicts normal

FIGURE 8-9

Volume-pressure loop demonstrating an air leak. Approximately 200 mL of volume is lost even though the pressure returns to its baseline value of 5 cm H_2O.

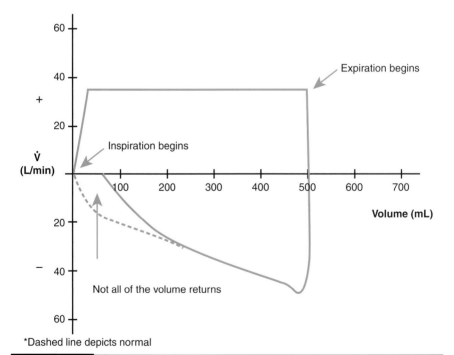

*Dashed line depicts normal

FIGURE 8-10

Flow-volume loop during volume-control ventilation demonstrating an expiratory air leak. Flow returns to baseline (zero) but approximately 75 mL of volume is lost.

flow that does not return to baseline before the next inspiration. Most often, auto-PEEP is the result of insufficient expiratory time, but it also can be related to conditions with increased airway resistance (Raw) as in asthma and chronic obstructive pulmonary disease (COPD). Bronchospasm and early collapse of unstable alveoli during exhalation reduce expiratory outflow.

The consequences of intrinsic PEEP are as follows:

- Hemodynamic compromise
- Increased WOB related to decreased lung compliance from hyperinflation
- Interference with ventilator triggering
- Decreased returned volume in pressure ventilation

In Figure 8-11, auto-PEEP is readily recognized on the expiratory portion of the flow scalar. Expiratory flow does not return to the baseline as a result of increased

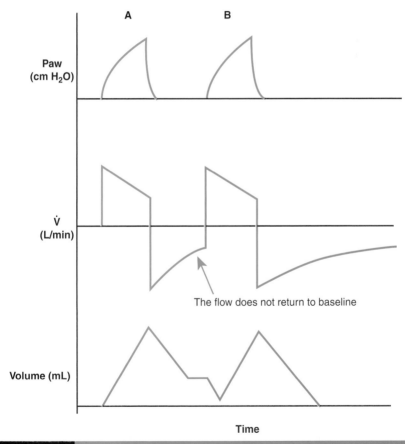

FIGURE 8-11

Detection of auto-PEEP on scalars. **Breath A,** Auto-PEEP is evident on the flow curve as expiratory flow that does not return to the baseline. On the volume curve (also breath A), auto-PEEP presents as a loss of expiratory volume.

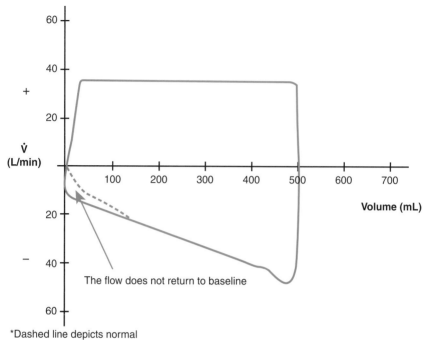

*Dashed line depicts normal

FIGURE 8-12

Flow-volume loop where flow does not return to baseline. Retained expiratory flow provides evidence of auto-PEEP.

resistance and/or an expiratory time that is too short for complete exhalation. Auto-PEEP may also be evident by a loss of expiratory volume on the volume scalar. When the respiratory rate is high, auto-PEEP on the volume-time scalar may mimic a leak. The flow-volume loop depicted in Figure 8-12 also demonstrates retained expiratory flow, which should alert the clinician to evaluate further for the presence of auto-PEEP.

Auto-PEEP can be reduced by increasing flow to shorten inspiratory time or by decreasing respiratory rate; both are means of increasing expiratory time. Bronchodilators may also assist with reducing expiratory airway resistance. Adding moderate amounts of extrinsic PEEP ($PEEP_E$) offsets the intrinsic PEEP ($PEEP_I$) by stenting open collapsed airways, therefore improving expiratory flow. The $PEEP_E$ should be no more than 85% of the $PEEP_I$. Normal ventilator pressure-triggering depends on a drop in intrathoracic pressure to –1 to –2 cm H_2O depending on the sensitivity set on the ventilator. A patient with auto-PEEP has to generate a negative inspiratory pressure equal to the auto-PEEP plus the –1 to –2 cm H_2O to trigger the ventilator flow; this situation increases the WOB dramatically. Reducing or eliminating auto-PEEP improves patient triggering and reduces the patient's WOB.

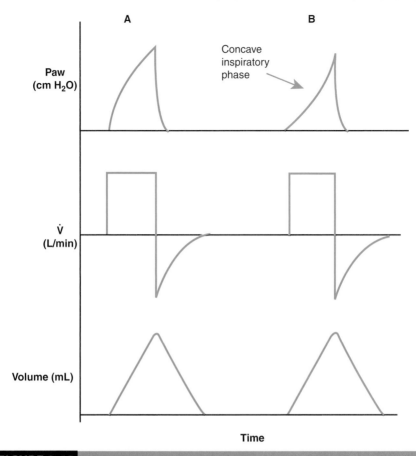

FIGURE 8-13

Scalars graphing volume-control ventilation. **Breath A,** Normal convex, shark's fin configuration of the pressure curve; no evidence of flow dyssynchrony. **Breath B,** Pressure scalar: Flow starvation is evident by the concave shape of the inspiratory limb.

Auto-PEEP can be measured on the ventilator by employing an expiratory hold maneuver. At end-expiration, the ventilator circuit is closed. In this static environment, the amount of pressure trapped in the alveoli can be measured. This maneuver is accurate only if the circuit is closed long enough for the pressure to equilibrate, typically 2 to 3 seconds, and if the patient does not attempt to initiate a breath during the hold.

Flow Starvation (Flow Dyssynchrony)

Active patient effort after the initiation of a ventilator breath indicates the patient is not receiving enough flow, which is referred to as flow starvation. Flow starvation is represented on the pressure-time scalar (Fig. 8-13) and on the V-P loop (Fig. 8-14).

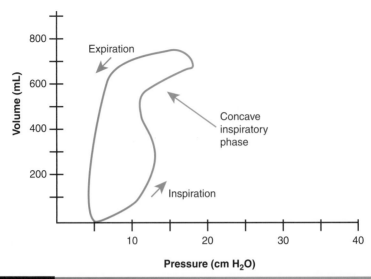

FIGURE 8-14

Volume-pressure loop demonstrating flow starvation or flow dyssynchrony. The patient's negative inspiratory effort is evident during inspiration.

On the pressure scalar, the result of the patient's demand for more flow is a concave appearance of the inspiratory limb of the curve. This is a result of the patient creating negative pressure during inspiration in an effort to draw in more gas. The flow dyssynchrony may look more pronounced in the V-P loop. Again, the inspiratory limb is sucked in as a result of the patient's attempt to pull more flow than the ventilator is delivering. This active patient effort increases the WOB. Increasing the flow will satisfy the patient's demand. Another option is to switch from volume ventilation to pressure ventilation, which provides a variable flow.

Cycling Dyssynchrony

Cycling is the transition of the ventilator from the inspiratory to the expiratory phase. Cycling dyssynchrony occurs when the patient's inspiratory time, known as the neural time ($T_I$neural), is not synchronized with the set inspiratory time on the ventilator, known as mechanical time ($T_I$mech). If the $T_I$mech is set too short, the patient's inspiratory needs are not met. This could cause the patient to trigger the ventilator during the expiratory phase, resulting in a double triggering effect. Conversely, if the $T_I$mech is set too long, the patient wants to exhale during the inspiratory phase. Both of these situations cause dyssynchrony and increased WOB.

During PS ventilation when the cycling criterion is set too low for the patient, the $T_I$mech is too long. The patient wants inspiration to end before the ventilator cycles it to end. This will be evident on the pressure-time scalar as a spike at the end

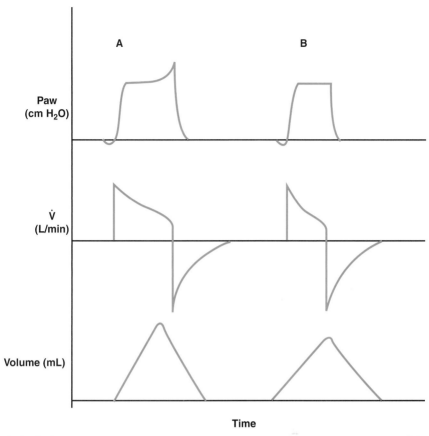

FIGURE 8-15

Pressure-supported breath with cycling criteria is set too low, resulting in cycle dyssynchrony. The pressure scalar in breath A shows a pressure spike at the end of inhalation. The inspiratory cycling criterion is increased in breath B, lowering the threshold for exhalation (shortening mechanical time [$T_I$mech]).

of inspiration (Fig. 8-15). Increasing the cycling criterion shortens $T_I$mech and enables the $T_I$neural and the $T_I$mech to match, resulting in patient-ventilator synchrony. If the ventilator does not have adjustable cycling criteria for the pressure-supported breaths, it may be difficult to achieve synchrony in some patients.

Trigger Dyssynchrony

Trigger dyssynchrony may occur as a result of an inappropriate sensitivity setting or as the effect of auto-PEEP. On the pressure-time scalar, an attempt to initiate breaths that are not sensed by the ventilator appears as negative deflections that are

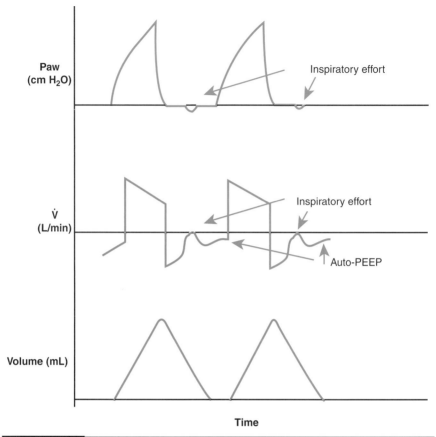

FIGURE 8-16

Scalars showing trigger dyssynchrony. On the pressure scalar, the attempt to initiate breaths (negative deflections) is not sensed by the ventilator and therefore it is not followed by a breath. Because of lack of patient triggering, a time-triggered machine breath occurs. On the flow scalar, the expiratory flow is interrupted by an inadequate patient inspiratory effort, followed by a time-triggered machine breath. The presence of auto-PEEP is evident by expiratory flow not returning to baseline.

not followed by a positive-pressure breath. On the flow-time scalar, expiratory flow is interrupted by small positive inspiratory flow attempts, representing inadequate patient inspiratory effort (Fig. 8-16).

Auto-PEEP increases the WOB as the patient takes a breath and is a cause of trigger dyssynchrony. To trigger a breath when auto-PEEP is present requires the patient to create negative pressure sufficient to draw back through the auto-PEEP and continue this negative pressure until the trigger sensitivity is reached. Trigger dyssynchrony can lead to increased patient WOB and may lead to increased oxygen requirements.

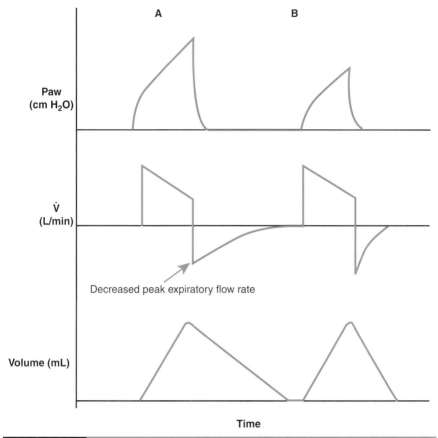

A   B

Paw
(cm H$_2$O)

$\dot{V}$
(L/min)

Decreased peak expiratory flow rate

Volume (mL)

Time

FIGURE 8-17

Scalars representing resistance changes. Breath B is a normal breath for comparison purposes. Breath A changes because of increased resistance include increased peak inspiratory pressure on the pressure waveform, decreased peak expiratory flow and a prolonged expiratory phase on the flow waveform, and a prolonged expiratory phase on the volume waveform.

Even in the absence of auto-PEEP, an inappropriately low sensitivity setting hinders triggering because a greater inspiratory effort is needed to initiate a breath. If the sensitivity is set too high, triggering may result from very little effort, causing auto-cycling. The ventilator triggers breath after breath rapidly, disregarding the patient's own respiratory pattern.

Resistance Changes

Changes in Raw may be related to a disease state such as asthma or COPD or related to the endotracheal tube (ETT) or ventilator circuit. Airway resistance may be increased and expiratory flow decreased in bronchospasm, when an expiratory filter or heat and moisture exchanger (HME) is blocked, or when the ETT is partially obstructed, kinked, or too small. Figure 8-17 provides scalar waveform evidence of

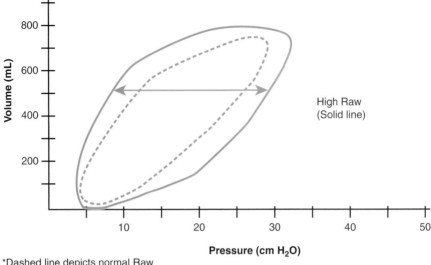

*Dashed line depicts normal Raw

FIGURE 8-18

Volume-pressure loop representing resistance changes. The inner loop (*dashed lines*) represents a normal volume-pressure loop. The outer loop demonstrates the higher pressures required to deliver the volume (inspiratory resistance) and the prolonged expiratory phase (expiratory resistance). *Raw*, Airway resistance.

increased airway resistance and decrease in expiratory flow. The following changes in expiratory flow are depicted on the scalars:

■ On the flow waveform, peak expiratory flow is decreased and the expiratory phase is prolonged.
■ On the pressure waveform, peak inspiratory pressure is increased, and
■ On the volume waveform, the expiratory phase is prolonged.

The V-P loop in Figure 8-18 displays the changes that occur with increased resistance. When resistance is increased, a higher pressure results on inspiration and the expiratory phase is increased. Airway resistance changes can also be detected on the flow-volume loop (Fig. 8-19). These waveforms are helpful not only in detecting resistance problems but also in evaluating the effect of bronchodilator or other therapies on improving airflow.

Compliance Changes

As lung compliance changes, the V-P loop's slope changes (Fig. 8-20). If lung compliance decreases, as in acute respiratory distress syndrome (ARDS), the slope of the loop shifts downward toward the pressure axis. This represents an increase in pressure required to deliver the set volume. If the lung compliance is high as in COPD,

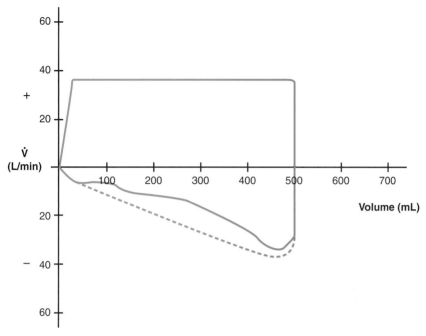

*Dashed line depicts normal expiratory flow

FIGURE 8-19

Flow-volume loop representing resistance changes. Increased expiratory resistance is depicted as decreased peak expiratory flow and a concave shape to the expiratory limb. The dashed lines represent normal flow or an improvement in flow after intervention.

the slope of the loop shifts upward toward the volume axis. This demonstrates that less pressure is required to achieve the set volume, a characteristic of decreased elasticity of the lung. These conditions normally occur over time. It is helpful to record and save a loop to compare with a real-time loop later in the patient's stay in the intensive care unit (ICU). Not all ventilator graphic packages have a recording feature.

Overdistention

Overdistention occurs when an increase in pressure yields little or no volume increase. This could be the result of too much volume in volume ventilation or too much pressure in pressure ventilation. In Figure 8-21, the so-called beaking at the top of the inspiratory limb depicts the overdistention. Overdistention could cause barotrauma and volutrauma that result in ventilator-induced lung injury. The pressure or volume needs to be decreased to avoid lung injury.

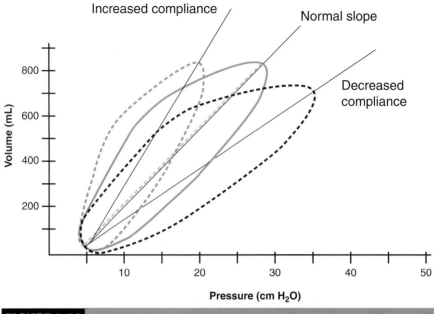

FIGURE 8-20

Volume-pressure loop representing compliance changes.

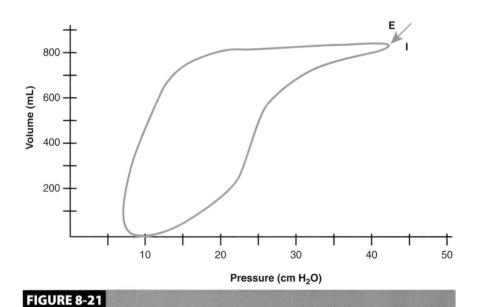

FIGURE 8-21

Volume-pressure loops representing overdistention. See text for description.

SUMMARY

For clinicians just learning ventilator graphic waveforms, the process may seem overwhelming at first. The authors suggest isolating one abnormal waveform at a time and identifying it on the ventilator screen. When one abnormality is easily recognized in daily practice, the clinician is encouraged to progress to another.

All those managing mechanical ventilators should have a solid understanding of these waveforms. Clinicians who familiarize themselves with ventilator graphics will have a more precise image of lung physiology as it relates to the constant changes occurring during mechanical ventilation. This will enable improved care because the clinician will more readily identify problems and then track patient progress as interventions are performed.

RECOMMENDED READINGS

Branson RD, Davis K Jr, Campbell RS. Monitoring graphic displays of pressure, volume and flow: The usefulness of ventilator waveforms. *World Federation J Crit Care* 2004; 1(1):8–12.

Burns SM. Working with respiratory waveforms: How to use bedside graphics. *AACN Clin Issues* 2003; 14(2):133–144.

Burns SM. Continuous airway pressure monitoring. *Crit Care Nurse* 2004; 24(6):70–74.

Dennison F. Basic ventilator waveform analysis. In DW Chang (ed.), *Clinical Application of Mechanical Ventilation,* 2nd ed. (pp. 264–324). Clifton Park, NY: Delmar Learning, 2000.

Hess DR, Kacmarek RM. *Essentials of Mechanical Ventilation,* 2nd ed. (pp. 264–283). New York: McGraw-Hill, 2002.

MacIntyre NR. Patient-ventilator interactions. In NR MacIntyre, RD Branson (eds.), *Mechanical Ventilation* (pp. 189–203). Philadelphia: Saunders, 2001.

MacIntyre NR. Respiratory system mechanics. In NR MacIntyre, RD Branson (eds.), *Mechanical Ventilation* (pp. 146–160). Philadelphia: Saunders, 2001.

MacIntyre NR. Ventilator monitors, displays, and alarms. In NR MacIntyre, RD Branson (eds.), *Mechanical Ventilation* (pp. 131–144). Philadelphia: Saunders, 2001.

Oakes DA, Shortall SP. *Ventilator Management: A Bedside Reference Guide* (pp. 8-1–8-46). Orono, Me: Health Educator Publications, 2002.

Pruitt WC. Ventilator graphics made easy. *Respir Ther* 2002; 15(1):23–24, 50.

Waugh JB, Deshpande VM, Harwood RJ. *Rapid Interpretation of Ventilator Waveforms.* Upper Saddle River, NJ: Prentice-Hall, 1999.

CHAPTER 9

Complications of Mechanical Ventilation and Troubleshooting the Patient-Ventilator System

It is indisputable that in many circumstances, mechanical ventilation is a life-saving therapy. However, the introduction of a machine to any clinical setting presents the need for the mastery of skills associated with a highly technical therapy and its potential complications. It is imperative that the clinician appreciate the problems associated with the use of mechanical ventilators, understand how to perform a respiratory assessment of the ventilated patient, and understand the proper function and troubleshooting of the patient-ventilator system.

COMPLICATIONS OF MECHANICAL VENTILATION

Problems Related to Positive Pressure

Recall from Chapter 2 that the pressure within the thoracic cavity during spontaneous ventilation is negative. This negative pressure in the chest promotes venous return to the heart and even distribution of gas in the lung. When we place a patient on a positive-pressure ventilator, the lungs fill with gas through the application of positive pressure. Although positive-pressure ventilation (PPV) provides the benefit of adequate ventilation to the patient, it is also responsible for many of the complications. These complications are related to increases in thoracic pressure in general and, more specifically, to increases in mean and plateau airway pressures.

VENTILATOR-INDUCED LUNG INJURY

Over the last 10 years, it has become clear that the inappropriate application of mechanical ventilation can result in injury to the lung that is indistinguishable from acute respiratory distress syndrome (ARDS). There is a debate regarding whether the lung is injured because of volumes that are too large or pressures that are too high. It is generally believed that there is a safe alveolar pressure where the lung will not be damaged regardless of tidal volume (V_T) as long as the pressure is maintained below this level. This is believed because high-peak alveolar pressure is associated with alveolar overdistention and injury. Therefore, in the clinical setting, the alveolar pressure is monitored and maintained at 30 cm H_2O or less as a prudent mechanism for reducing lung injury. To be most accurate, alveolar pressure should be measured as end-inspiratory static pressure, also known as end-inspiratory plateau pressure (Pplat). Pplat should be measured at regular intervals, after any change in ventilatory support that results in a higher inspiratory flow or VT, and with any change in patient condition that could result in a reduction in compliance or increase in resistance.

Because the peak inspiratory pressure (PIP) is more easily monitored clinically on a continuous basis, it may be chosen as the trend variable and should be kept at 40 cm or less H_2O pressure. The PIP, however, is only a trend variable because it reflects more than alveolar pressure. It is affected by changes in airway resistance, which can vary significantly in the clinical setting. If PIP is trended, then controllable factors affecting resistance, such as the inspiratory flow rate and pattern, must be kept constant or taken under consideration when trending the PIP. Furthermore, the relationship between PIP and Pplat must be intermittently measured and reevaluated.

Lung trauma occurs to a greater extent when gases are unevenly distributed in the lung. Gas flow is more turbulent under these conditions, creating greater shear forces and uneven distention of the alveoli. Because there is no practical mechanism for monitoring regional overdistention, airway pressures are closely monitored. Predisposing factors for lung injury include high ventilating pressures and volumes, a high mean airway pressure (mPaw), and preexisting lung disease. The types of injuries to the lung that can occur as a result of mechanical ventilation include barotrauma, volutrauma, atelectrauma, oxygen toxicity, and biotrauma.

Barotrauma

Barotrauma, or pressure trauma, historically was the injury to the lung most associated with mechanical ventilation. In barotrauma, alveolar injury or rupture occurs as a result of excessive pressure, excessive peak inflating volume (volutrauma), or both. The alveoli rupture, or tear, so that air escapes. Forms of pulmonary barotrauma include pulmonary interstitial emphysema, pneumothorax, pneumomediastinum, pneumopericardium, pneumoperitoneum, pneumoretroperitoneum, and subcutaneous emphysema.

When an overdistended alveolus ruptures, the escaped gas follows the path of least resistance. It moves centrally along perivascular sheaths toward the mediastinum, where it may rupture into the mediastinum or travel through pleural reflections of the great vessels into the pericardium. Alternatively, the air may dissect along fascial planes into the neck and torso, forming subcutaneous emphysema. Subcutaneous emphysema or pneumomediastinum is not likely to cause the patient a serious problem. However, the clinician should head these warnings that more serious complications are likely to occur if ventilatory management is not altered. Air in the pleural cavity (pneumothorax), however, causes varying degrees of lung collapse, adversely affecting ventilation. Progression to a tension pneumothorax may result in rapid cardiovascular decompensation. A pneumothorax must therefore be identified in a timely fashion and pleural decompression achieved through chest tube insertion (see Appendix III, Chest Drainage Systems).

Volutrauma

Lung parenchymal injury induced by end-inspiratory overdistention is called volutrauma. The term *volutrauma* is used because it is believed that localized or regional overdistending volume causes the damage. The lung damage is similar to early ARDS and probably the result of local stress and strain on the alveolar-capillary (A-C) membrane. It is manifested by an increase in the permeability of the A-C membrane, pulmonary edema, the accumulation of neutrophils and protein in the interstitial and alveolar spaces, and reduction in surfactant production. Because local overdistention is not easily assessed at the bedside, pressure is used as a surrogate for volume and maintained at the levels stated earlier to reduce volutrauma.

Atelectrauma

Atelectrauma is ventilator induced lung injury (VILI) related to unstable, or atelectatic, alveolar units opening on inspiration and then closing at end-expiration. This repetitive opening upon application of sufficient positive pressure and closing on expiration occurs with each breath. Atelectrauma is postulated to be sheer, or stress, injury at the junctions where open and closed alveoli interface. The mechanism to prevent atelectrauma is to recruit the unstable alveolar units and then maintain their opened state (prevent derecruitment) with the application of sufficient positive end-expiration pressure (PEEP).

Biotrauma

The activation of inflammatory mediators secondary to damage to the lung from injurious ventilatory patterns is called biotrauma. It results from alveolar overdistention (volutrauma) and repetitive opening and closing of lung units (atelectrauma). Proinflammatory mediators such as cytokines and chemokines are activated and are the cellular response to mechanical stress. These mediators increase edema formation and migration of neutrophils, and they promote relaxation of vascular smooth muscle. When PEEP is applied and results in sustained lung recruitment, the level of inflammatory mediators is reduced. Opportunities for pharmacologic interventions may be identified as the biotrauma cellular response is further identified.

Because VILI can also result in stress fractures in the pulmonary capillaries, these inflammatory mediators can gain access into the systemic circulation. Translocation of pro-inflammatory mediators and bacteria may cause tissue injury and impaired oxygen delivery to distal organs (Fig. 9-1). The lung ventilated with injurious patterns, therefore, may be the source of the inflammatory cascade that results in multiple organ dysfunction syndrome (MODS).

Oxygen Toxicity

The exposure of the pulmonary tissues to a high oxygen tension can lead to pathologic parenchymal changes. The degree of injury is related to the duration of exposure and to the oxygen tension of the inspired air, not to the partial pressure of oxygen in arterial blood (PaO_2). Generally, a fraction of oxygen in inspired gas (FIO_2) of more than 0.5 is considered toxic. The first signs of oxygen toxicity are caused by the irritant effect of oxygen and reflect an acute tracheobronchitis. After only a few hours of breathing 100% oxygen, mucociliary function is depressed and clearance of

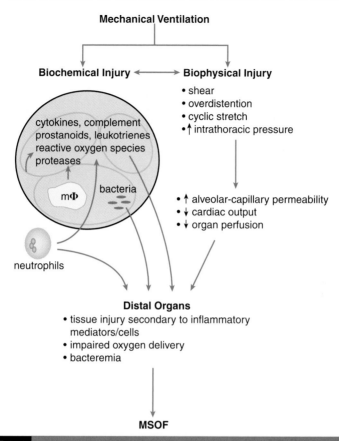

Mechanical Ventilation

Biochemical Injury ←→ **Biophysical Injury**

cytokines, complement
prostanoids, leukotrienes
reactive oxygen species
proteases

mΦ   bacteria

neutrophils

• shear
• overdistention
• cyclic stretch
• ↑ intrathoracic pressure

• ↑ alveolar-capillary permeability
• ↓ cardiac output
• ↓ organ perfusion

Distal Organs
• tissue injury secondary to inflammatory
  mediators/cells
• impaired oxygen delivery
• bacteremia

MSOF

FIGURE 9-1

Mechanisms whereby inappropriately applied mechanical ventilation results in biochemical and biophysical injury to the lung and possibly contributes to the development of multiple organ dysfunction syndrome (MODS). *(Modified from Slutsky AS, Trembly L. Pulmonary perspective. Am J Crit Care Med 1998; 157:1721–1725.)*

mucus is impaired. More prolonged exposure to high oxygen tension may lead to changes in the lung that mimic ARDS. The tissue injury in the lung caused by hyperoxia results from the production of biochemically reactive, oxygen-derived free radicals that overwhelm the body's antioxidant defenses. Disruption of the endothelial lining of the pulmonary microcirculation results in leakage of proteinaceous fluid. An exudate consisting of edema, hemorrhage, and white blood cells forms in the lung. The damage to the lung may progress to cell death. The function of the pulmonary macrophage is also depressed, rendering the patient more susceptible to infection. Termination of exposure to toxic levels of oxygen allows cellular repair to begin; however, the repair may also result in varying degrees of pulmonary fibrosis.

Lung-Protective Mechanical Ventilatory Strategies

Recognition that the application of mechanical ventilation can lead to VILI has led to the development of lung protective ventilatory strategies. This strategy focuses on avoiding overdistention and repetitive opening and closing of unstable lung units. The turning point for recognition of the value of this strategy was the ARDS Network study that demonstrated that mechanical ventilation of patients with acute lung injury and ARDS with lower V_T ventilation (lung protective strategy) as compared to traditional ventilation resulted in a 25% reduction in mortality. In fact, the study was stopped early because mortality was lower in the treatment group. Traditional ventilation involved an initial V_T of 12 mL/kg and a plateau pressure of 50 cm H_2O or less, whereas lower V_T ventilation involved an initial V_T of 6 mL/kg or less and a Pplat of 30 cm H_2O or less. The first primary outcome was death prior to discharge and breathing without assistance; the second primary outcome was number of ventilator-free days between days 1 and 28. Other outcomes were number of days without organ or system failure and the occurrence of barotrauma. Patients who met study criteria were randomly assigned to receive mechanical ventilation involving either traditional V_Ts or lower V_Ts. The volume assist/control mode was used for all patients. In the group treated with traditional V_T, the initial V_T was 12 mL/kg. This was subsequently reduced or increased in stepwise increments to maintain the Pplat 45 to 50 cm H_2O. In the group treated with lower V_T, the V_T was reduced by 6 mL/kg. V_T was adjusted in stepwise increments to maintain Pplat 25 to 30 cm H_2O. Data were collected at baseline, and on days 1, 2, 3, 4, 7, 14, 21, and 28. Mortality was lower in the group treated with lower V_Ts than in the group treated with traditional V_Ts (31.0% vs. 39.8%, $P = 0.007$), and the number of vent days was also lower in the treatment group ($P = 0.007$). The mean V_Ts on days 1 through 3 were 6.2+/−0.8 and 11.8+/−0.8 mL/kg of predicted body weight ($P < 0.001$), respectively, and the mean Pplats were 25+/−6 and 33+/−8 cm H_2O ($P < 0.001$), respectively. There was no significant difference in duration of mechanical ventilation between the two groups. The number of days without nonpulmonary organ or system failure was significantly higher in the low V_T group ($P = 0.006$). The incidence of barotrauma was similar in the two groups.

A lung protective strategy should always be used for patients with acute lung injury (ALI) and ARDS. ARDS affects lung function in a nonhomogeneous distribution. Less involved areas of the lung receive a disproportionate share of the V_T. Conventional ventilatory strategies that use high V_T, FiO_2, and levels of PEEP may result in high peak inspiratory and alveolar pressures and regional alveolar overdistention. Patients with acute respiratory failure (ARF) with asthma and chronic obstructive airway disease also benefit from lung protective strategies because ARF in asthma and chronic airway disease is associated with significant expiratory obstruction and hyperinflation of the lung. The increased expiratory lung volume causes an increased pressure in the lung that can cause volutrauma and barotrauma. A lung protective strategy incorporates the following key points, described further in Table 9-1:

- ■ Maintain stable alveoli (i.e., prevent derecruitment) by applying adequate PEEP.
- ■ Limit the Pplat to ≤30 cm H_2O.

- Minimize exposure to toxic level of F_{IO_2} if possible.
- Use low V_T ventilation to achieve target Pplat, and if necessary allow permissive hypercapnia.

PERMISSIVE HYPERCAPNIA. Permissive hypercapnia (PHC) is an inherent element in a ventilatory strategy designed to reduce barotrauma caused by high inspiratory airway pressures. In fact, no data have evaluated the efficacy of hypercapnia independent of a lung protective strategy. In PHC, airway pressures are reduced by using small V_Ts. To achieve the target airway pressure, a V_T as small as 4 to 6 mL/kg may be needed. Smaller volumes are permitted because ventilatory requirements are reduced by allowing the partial pressure of carbon dioxide in arterial blood ($Paco_2$) to rise gradually to 50 to 100 mm Hg or greater. Staged, deliberate limitation of ventilatory support results in a gradual increase in $Paco_2$ that is generally tolerable, possibly because intracellular pH levels change gradually, and partial to complete metabolic compensation may occur.

The systemic hemodynamic effects of hypercapnic acidosis are relatively benign, even as the pH falls to 7.15 when the $Paco_2$ is allowed to increase gradually as determined by tolerance of respiratory acidosis. Patients typically experience no change or small increases in cardiac output and blood pressure. However, rapid induction of hypercapnic acidosis over a 2-hour period has resulted in significant hemodynamic alterations. Potentially adverse effects of increased $Paco_2$, which should be monitored for, include cardiac depression, neurologic depression, and increased pulmonary vascular resistance. Both children and adults have survived exposure to extreme levels of acidosis applied in a controlled manner. Hypercapnia is contraindicated, however, in the presence of increased intracranial pressure (ICP) and may be poorly tolerated by patients with a preexisting metabolic acidosis, which is an indicator of existing cellular stress.

Buffering the acidosis induced by PHC is a common but controversial clinical practice. Buffering with sodium bicarbonate was permitted in the ARDS Network study. Concern about the use of bicarbonate to correct an acidosis has resulted in the removal of bicarbonate therapy from routine use in cardiac arrest algorithms. To be an effective buffer, the ability to excrete carbon dioxide should be intact. Bicarbonate may further raise systemic carbon dioxide levels under conditions of reduced alveolar ventilation. It may actually worsen intracellular acidosis because the carbon dioxide produced when bicarbonate reacts with metabolic acids readily diffuses across cell membranes, whereas bicarbonate cannot. A positive feature of bicarbonate infusion is that it provides an osmolar load and may improve retention of intravascular volume and augment cardiac output. There are no outcome data to support the use of bicarbonate to buffer hypercapnic acidosis. Its use should be accompanied by a clear rationale, such as to reduce identified side effects of acidosis, and must be evaluated on a case-by-case basis.

The $Paco_2$ is gradually increased to avoid an acute, intolerable reduction in the pH and to make the infusion of bicarbonate solutions unnecessary. During the escalation phase, an increase in the ventilatory drive, in response to an increased $Paco_2$, accompanied by an unacceptable increase in the work of breathing (WOB), may be blunted with the use of deep sedation and/or chemical paralysis. As the

TABLE 9-1 Lung Protective Ventilation

Strategy	Rationale	Comments
Maintain stable alveolar units by applying an adequate level of PEEP to recruit alveoli, increase the functional residual capacity, and keep recruited alveoli open throughout the respiratory cycle.	Excessive PEEP stretches alveoli and leads to injury. Too little PEEP allows recruited alveoli to collapse during exhalation requiring the next positive-pressure breath to "snap open" the alveolus before it can fill. Repetitive alveolar collapsing and opening contributes to parenchymal injury (shear stress) during positive-pressure breathing. Providing enough PEEP to prevent repeated small airway and alveolar opening and closing reduces alveolar injury. This is known as the "open lung" strategy.	Determining the amount of PEEP to recruit and maintain alveoli above the opening pressure of the lung is a challenge. Some authors suggest developing a pressure volume (PV) curve of the lung and adjusting PEEP to levels above the lower inflection point on the curve, which correlates to the opening pressure of the lung. However, others say that alveolar recruitment occurs along the entire inspiratory limb of the PV curve. Titrate PEEP by monitoring oxygenation and hemodynamics. An estimated 10-20 cm H_2O PEEP may be required. As possible, titrate $F_{I}O_2$ down to 0.5 while ensuring SpO_2 of ≥90%. Then incrementally decrease PEEP to lowest level while maintaining SpO_2 of 90%-95%.
Limit peak plateau (alveolar) pressure to 30 cm H_2O.	Pplat is used as a surrogate to monitor for alveolar overdistention because regional overdistention is not easily monitored. Lung damage may be minimized by preventing overdistention of alveolar units.	The mode of ventilation may vary; however, many believe that pressure controlled modes are an attractive option for a lung protective strategy because the peak pressure cannot rise above the preset value.

To accomplish the goal of limiting Pplat, ventilate the patient with V_T 6 mL/kg ideal body weight. If plateau pressure remains ≥30 cm H_2O, reduce the V_T further, and permit the $Paco_2$ to rise (permissive hypercapnia) unless the presence, or risk, of raised ICP or other contraindication exists that would demand a more normal CO_2. Avoid rapid rises in $Paco_2$. Slow reduction of V_T may allow renal compensation of the respiratory acidosis. Minimize Fio_2 to ≤0.6 while maintaining arterial oxygen saturation of ≥90%.	To limit plateau pressure in the lung to protect the lung from further injury, maintenance of a normal CO_2 may be sacrificed. Control elevation in the $Paco_2$ to prevent complications related to rapid induction of respiratory acidosis.	Potential harmful effects of low V_T ventilation include progressive atelectasis and derecruitment. Although high V_T (12 mL/kg) should be avoided, intermediate ventilation (8-10 mL/kg) could be considered if plateau pressure remains in the safe range.
	Exposure to a high Fio_2 increases alveolar Po_2 (Pao_2). High Pao_2 increases microvascular permeability to protein, can lead to absorption atelectasis and surfactant inactivation, and may impede tracheal mucus flow because of ciliary abnormalities and goblet cell hyperplasia. Hyperoxia can also lead to excess oxidant production, lipid peroxidation, protein oxidant damage, and cell death.	Concerns of oxygen toxicity should never supersede appropriate administration of oxygen to prevent tissue hypoxia.
Determine the recruitment potential through periodic applications of high sustained airway pressure (i.e., recruiting maneuvers).	Opening of collapsed alveoli may be achieved through a recruitment maneuver. A variety of approaches have been tried, such as the application of CPAP of 35-40 cm H_2O for 40 seconds, intermittent higher tidal volumes, intermittent higher PEEP, extended sigh, or PC of 30 above 15-20 cm H_2O PEEP for 1-2 minutes as tolerated. The actual opening pressure of the alveoli is determined by the transpulmonary pressure, which varies depending on patient characteristics and stage of ARDS.	Potential problems with recruitment maneuvers include barotrauma secondary to high pressure across the lung and hypotension secondary to increased intrathoracic pressure transmitted to the capillary bed. PEEP may need to be increased after the maneuver to maintain the effects. The optimal way to perform recruitment maneuvers remains unknown and no data are available that demonstrate they improve outcome.

ARDS, Acute respiratory distress syndrome; *CPAP,* continuous positive airway pressure; *Fio₂,* fraction of oxygen in inspired gas; *ICP,* intracranial pressure; *Paco₂,* partial pressure of carbon dioxide in arterial blood; *PC,* pressure control; *PEEP,* positive end-expiratory pressure; *Po₂,* partial pressure of oxygen; *Pplat,* plateau pressure; *PV,* pressure volume; *Spo₂,* saturation of hemoglobin with oxygen in arterial blood measured with pulse oximetry.

airway pressure is reduced during PHC initiation, the mPaw may decrease, resulting in a decrease in oxygenation. Strategies to improve a deteriorating oxygenation status include the addition of PEEP or an extension of the inspiratory time.

As the underlying disease process resolves and the patient's clinical status improves, the $PaCO_2$ should gradually be brought back to the patient's baseline. Rapid reversal of PHC should be avoided because it will result in metabolic alkalosis, whose magnitude depends on the degree of metabolic compensation that occurred during the therapy.

REDUCTION IN CARDIAC OUTPUT AND OXYGEN DELIVERY

PPV may result in hypotension and decreased cardiac output (CO). These complications are more pronounced when the lungs are compliant or when the chest wall is noncompliant because, under both conditions, more positive pressure is transmitted to the mediastinal structures. The hemodynamic effects of PPV are also more prevalent in the patient with hypovolemia, in the patient with poor cardiac reserve, and when PEEP is applied. Patients with high inflating pressures and on PEEP of 10 cm H_2O or greater should have CO and tissue oxygenation monitored through the use of a pulmonary artery catheter.

Three mechanisms are involved in the development of decreased CO under the condition of PPV:

1. Positive pressure increases lung volume, alveolar pressure, and pleural pressure. In the spontaneously breathing individual, venous blood return to the right side of the heart is promoted by negative pressure in the thorax on inspiration. With PPV, thoracic pressure rises above atmospheric pressure, resulting in decreased venous return to the right side of the heart (Fig. 9-2).
2. Pulmonary vascular resistance is increased as the increase in lung volume results in referred pressure to and possible compression of adjacent pulmonary capillaries. The right ventricular (RV) afterload is therefore increased, impeding the ability of this low-pressure, thin-walled chamber of the heart to eject its volume into the pulmonary vasculature and over to the left side of the heart.
3. Increased RV afterload may result in increased RV end-systolic volume, causing the interventricular septum to bulge into the left ventricle. This decreases the size, volume, compliance, and output of the left ventricle (Fig. 9-3).

Management of hypotension and decreased CO primarily involves the use of adequate volume to increase preload, followed by use of an inotropic agent as needed. Reduction of the mPaw is also beneficial and may be achieved by using modes that allow more spontaneous breathing or lower peak inspiratory pressures.

Just as the application of positive thoracic pressure decreases venous return, its removal promotes return of fluid to the central veins. This may precipitate cardiac decompensation in patients with minimal cardiac reserve. Such an event could occur, for example, when a patient supported by ventilation in the assist/control (A/C) mode is disconnected from the ventilator for a T-piece spontaneous breathing trial.

ALTERATION IN RENAL FUNCTION AND POSITIVE FLUID BALANCE

Under the conditions of PPV, renal blood flow may be decreased as a result of a reduction in CO. Furthermore, renal vein pressure may rise, shifting blood flow from

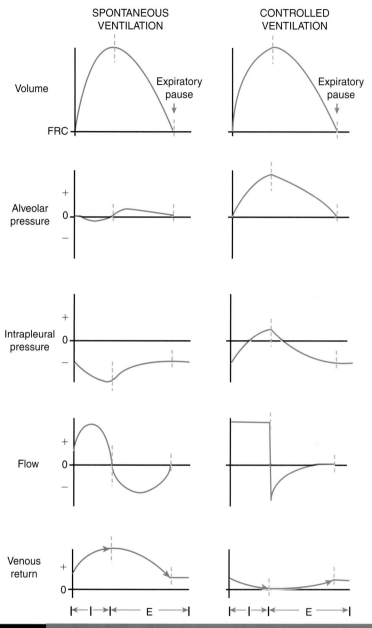

FIGURE 9-2

Physiologic differences in thoracic pressures under conditions of spontaneous versus positive-pressure ventilation. *(Modified from Dupuis YG. Ventilators: Theory and Clinical Application, 2nd ed. St. Louis: Mosby, 1992.)*

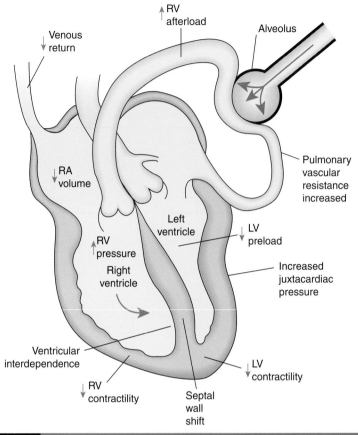

FIGURE 9-3

Factors responsible for a reduction of cardiac output during mechanical ventilation and PEEP. See text for details.

cortical to medullary areas, enhancing sodium reabsorption and decreasing filtration rate and therefore urine output. A decrease in renal perfusion, caused by a decrease in CO, fools the kidneys into thinking there is an overall fluid deficit, with the result that the renin-angiotensin-aldosterone system is stimulated to retain additional sodium and water.

Fluid retention also results from a series of reactions that increase antidiuretic hormone (ADH) and decrease atrial natriuretic peptide (ANP). ADH promotes a decrease in urine output through fluid retention. ADH production by the posterior pituitary gland is stimulated by vagal receptors in the right atrium that sense the decreased venous return and interpret it as hypovolemia. ANP is a natural diuretic that also inhibits secretion of aldosterone and renin. When right atrial pressure rises with PPV (because pressure is referred back from the pulmonary circulation to the right side of the heart), secretion of ANP decreases. This results in less circulating natural diuretic and more aldosterone, and therefore sodium and water retention. Positive fluid balance is therefore primarily caused by the kidneys' precipitating the conservation of salt and water through several mechanisms. Water can also be absorbed in the lung, and insensible losses through the respiratory tract are reduced because the inspired gases are humidified.

The patient's weight should be monitored frequently to allow fluid status trends to be determined. Diuretics should be administered as indicated. When peripheral edema is excessive, skin care must be performed meticulously.

IMPAIRED HEPATIC FUNCTION

Many factors may contribute to hepatic dysfunction in critically ill patients, prolonged application of positive pressure being only one of them. In the patient supported by mechanical ventilation, the downward movement of the diaphragm and impaired venous return to the right side of the heart may lead to an increase in portal vein pressure, followed by decreased portal venous blood flow to the liver and impairment of bile and hepatic vein flow. It is difficult, however, to discern adverse effects of PPV on hepatic function from manifestations of an underlying disease process.

INCREASED INTRACRANIAL PRESSURE

Persons who have had craniocerebral trauma, have cerebral tumors or vascular malformations, or have undergone neurosurgical procedures are at risk of having an increase in ICP and/or a decrease in cerebral perfusion pressure (CPP) when PPV and PEEP are applied. Increases in superior vena cava and jugular vein pressure diminish cerebral venous outflow and as a result may increase the ICP. The CPP may be decreased if the CO and mean arterial pressure (mPaw) fall, as a result of increased intrathoracic pressures, when PPV is employed. Furthermore, the infusion of large amounts of volume to restore normal hemodynamics after the institution of PPV and PEEP should be avoided in patients with cerebral edema and increased ICP. Overall, high mean intrathoracic pressure should be avoided in the patient supported by mechanical ventilation who has an altered cerebrovascular status because ICP may increase or CPP decrease. PPV has no adverse effects on ICP in individuals with normal cerebrovascular hemodynamics.

VENTILATION/PERFUSION MISMATCH

Ventilation/perfusion ($\dot{V}/\dot{Q}$) mismatch may occur as a result of alveolar overdistention caused by elevated airway pressure, large Vts, and use of excessive PEEP. Alveolar overdistention results in compression of the adjacent pulmonary capillaries and regional hypoperfusion. This increase in dead-space ventilation decreases carbon dioxide elimination. Overdistention of some units may also result in redistribution of pulmonary blood flow to unventilated regions. This increase in capillary shunt results in hypoxemia.

Mechanical ventilation strategies should achieve optimal $\dot{V}/\dot{Q}$ matching, not worsen it. In nonuniform disease processes in which the Vt is maldistributed, alveoli are especially vulnerable to overdistention. Strategies to reduce alveolar overdistention and iatrogenic $\dot{V}/\dot{Q}$ mismatch should be employed. In unilateral lung disease, independent lung ventilation may be indicated (see Chapter 12).

Problems Related to the Artificial Airway

To manage the patient-ventilator system successfully, one must pay detailed attention to the artificial airway. Complications related to artificial airways and the principles of airway management are outlined in Chapter 3.

Infection (Ventilator-Associated Pneumonia)

Placement of an artificial airway provides a conduit for contamination of the lower airway. Contamination may lead to pneumonia, especially in the presence of impaired host resistance. Critically ill patients who are intubated for more than 24 hours are at 6 to 21 times the risk of developing ventilator-associated pneumonia (VAP). The risk increases 1% to 3% per day of mechanical ventilation. Additional risk factors for VAP include events or factors that can lead to aspiration, such as decreases in level of consciousness, gastric distention or presence of gastric or small intestine tubes, supine positioning, and factors that influence changes in the gastrointestinal (GI) environment such as gastric ulcer prophylaxis with agents that decrease the pH of the stomach. Surgical patients undergoing upper abdominal or thoracic procedures, patients with chronic lung disease, and those requiring reintubation are also at risk. Attributable mortality associated with VAP, defined as the percentage of deaths occurring in excess of that expected because of the underlying disease process, is calculated at 27%.

Factors contributing to infection in the patient supported by mechanical ventilation include poor oral hygiene; aspiration; contaminated respiratory therapy equipment; poor hand washing by caregivers; breach of aseptic technique during suctioning or handling of respiratory equipment; impairment of the mucociliary system because of oxygen toxicity, inadequate hydration, suboptimal humidification, trauma during suctioning, or poor nutrition; and the decreased ability of the patient to produce an effective cough and remove secretions or diminished airway reflexes.

The principal mechanism for development of nosocomial pneumonia appears to be aspiration of gastric and oropharyngeal organisms, primarily colonized gram-negative bacteria, into the tracheobronchial tree. When these organisms overwhelm the patient's antibacterial defenses, pneumonia develops. Gram-negative colonization of the mouth is known to occur within 48 hours of admission to the intensive care unit (ICU). Furthermore, gram-negative colonization is promoted by the presence of a nasogastric tube, enteral nutrition, patient position, and manipulation of the gastric pH with antacids or H_2-receptor blocking agents as approaches to stress ulcer prophylaxis. The following strategies are aimed at reducing gram-negative colonization and nosocomial pneumonia:

- Elevate head of bed (HOB) 30 to 45 degrees, if not medically contraindicated, to prevent reflux and aspiration of gastric contents. HOB elevation is associated with a 26% absolute risk reduction in pneumonia.
- Do not routinely change, on the basis of duration of use, the ventilator circuit. Only change when visibly soiled or malfunctioning.
- Prevent inoculation of the airway with condensate that collects in the tubing of the ventilator. Circuit condensate should be viewed as infectious waste. It should

always be emptied from the tubing and *never* drained back into the humidifier because this action contaminates the entire water reservoir.

■ Use only sterile fluid for humidification or nebulization.

■ Practice proper hand hygiene before and after patient contact or contact with any respiratory device used on the patient.

■ Wear gloves for handling respiratory secretions or objects contaminated with respiratory secretions.

■ Use an endotracheal tube (ETT) with a dorsal lumen above the endotracheal cuff if feasible. This tube provides continuous or intermittent aspiration of secretions that pool above the cuff in the subglottic area (see Chapter 3, Airway Maintenance).

■ Ensure secretions are cleared above the cuff before cuff deflation or tube removal.

■ Use the oral route preferentially to the nasal route for the insertion of the artificial airway and gastric tubes to reduce incidence of sinusitis.

■ Exercise meticulous oral care using a well-defined comprehensive oral hygiene program. The goal is to reduce bacterial burden in the oral cavity. Chlorhexidine oral rinse twice a day has been shown to reduce pneumonia in cardiac surgery patients; however, its routine use cannot be recommended for all critically ill patients. Other strategies to reduce bacteria in the oral cavity include a mechanism to remove dental plaque mechanically, such as brushing the teeth with a solution containing an antibacterial agent (peroxide) at least twice a day. Moisturize the mouth to prevent xerostomia (excess drying) and potential cracking of the mucosa, and in the absence of an airway with subglottic suction, frequent suctioning of pooled oral secretions is recommended. The required frequency of these aspects of oral care is not yet known and the significance of each of these measures is not clear. Further controlled, prospective research is needed in this important area of pulmonary care.

■ Use noninvasive ventilation whenever feasible.

Aids to infection management and early detection include monitoring of vital signs and breath sounds, chest x-ray examination, observation of the character of the sputum, sputum culture and sensitivity, and leukocyte count. Prevention of all other contributing factors just listed should be attempted. Finally, the role of adequate nutrition in maintaining host defenses must not be minimized.

Patient Anxiety and Stress

The patient and family may demonstrate anxiety related to the disease process, diagnostic tests and procedures, and mechanical ventilation therapy. Some individuals may fear a grave prognosis associated with the use of what they call an "artificial respirator." They may have misconceptions as a result of viewing television programs or reading books that are not factual. They may have strong perceptions because of the increased discussions in the media and even upon admission into the hospital regarding advance directives, end-of-life decisions, and withdrawal of ventilatory and other life support measures. Some individuals may lose hope as the need for continued therapy becomes prolonged or if reintubation is required. Alarms are also frightening to those who do not understand their function.

Patients have many reasons to be stressed and anxious. After all, they have lost autonomy over a vital body function: breathing. Their ability to communicate is also impaired. Disruption of sleep-wake cycles by procedures is common, and noise in the ICU compounds sleep loss. The patient may be unable to determine day from night, the date, or the time. Position changes are limited by being attached to a ventilator, and physical restraint may be necessary to prevent self-extubation. Imposed immobility may create physical discomfort and frustration. The patient may experience pain from the ETT, from suctioning procedures, or from the tugging of the ventilator tubing on the airway.

The clinician should reduce anxiety by providing sufficient, which often means repetitive, realistic information relevant to the patient's and family's level of under-standing. Periods of uninterrupted sleep should be arranged, and meaningless noise and stimulation eliminated. A clock and a calendar should be placed within the patient's view. Frequent position changes are imperative, and the patient should be advanced to sitting in the chair or ambulating as tolerated. Whenever the patient is moved, the ventilator tubing should be supported to minimize discomfort and potential injury from tugging on the airway.

SEDATION AND ANALGESIA

Intubated and mechanically ventilated patients often receive opioids and sedatives for discomfort and anxiety. The administration of these agents should be directed by a goal that is objective and communicated using terminology common to all members of the team. For example, pain medication is titrated to a pain score of 4 or less on a scale of 1 to 10, and sedation is targeted to a specific level on a valid and reliable sedation scale such as the Ramsey scale or the Riker Sedation-Agitation scale (SAS). It is very important that the nurse, respiratory therapist, and physician are all using the same objective sedation and analgesia scoring system to promote unambiguous communication.

Duration of mechanical ventilation and sedation practices are related. Continuous infusion of sedatives is associated with a prolonged duration of mechanical ventilation. Depth of sedation is also increasingly recognized as contributing to delayed weaning from mechanical ventilation and associated ICU complications. Prolonging the duration of mechanical ventilation may predispose the patient to an increased risk of VAP, lung injury, and other complications related to the presence of an artificial airway. The association among sedation, duration of mechanical ventilation, and the patient's ability to participate in weaning has spawned discussion about the best method of ensuring the patient is maintained on the lowest dose and lightest level sedation possible. As a result of these concerns, concepts such as the "daily interruption" or "sedation vacation" and continuous titration to lowest dose are becoming more formalized. Just as excessive sedation may affect outcomes, insufficient sedation may precipitate ventilator dyssynchrony and associated physiologic alterations in thoracic pressures and gas exchange. Inadequate sedation is also associated with unplanned extubation. Optimal sedation of the mechanically ventilated patient is present when the patient resides at a state where patient-ventilator harmony exists and the patient remains capable of taking spontaneous breaths in readiness for weaning, when appropriate.

COMMUNICATION

Studies of the experiences of ICU patients show significant relationships between the inability to talk and feelings of panic and insecurity, sleep disturbances, and stress level. A means of communication should be established. Gestures are identified as the most frequently used method of nonvocal communication among intubated ICU patients, but they are often inhibited by wrist restraints. Gestural communication and lip reading can convey some basic needs; however, augmentative communication devices may facilitate even better communication. Pencil and paper is difficult for seriously ill patients to use because they are often too weak or poorly positioned to write or lack the concentration to spell. A board with pictures improved communication in postcardiothoracic surgical patients and was preferred by a small group of critical care survivors who were interviewed about augmentative communication methods. A picture board with icons representing basic needs and possibly the alphabet that can be easily cleaned between patients should be available in every ICU. Both nurses and patients report that family members can serve as a communication link between the patient and the care providers. It is important to reassure the patient that the loss of the voice is temporary and that speech will again be possible after the tube is removed.

Gastric Distress

ABDOMINAL DISTENTION

Gastric distention may occur as air is swallowed or forced down into the stomach during use of a resuscitation bag and mask before insertion of an artificial airway. The stomach may become quite enlarged, and a gastric bubble may be evident on x-ray examination. A nasogastric tube should be inserted to decompress the stomach. Stool softeners should be administered as necessary because immobility and the inability to close the glottis may make defecation difficult.

STRESS MANIFESTATIONS: ULCERS AND GASTRITIS

Stress, anxiety, and critical illness may precipitate the formation of gastritis or gastric ulcers. GI bleeding is related to the use of mechanical ventilation and to the severity of illness. Its incidence increases the longer mechanical ventilation continues and in severe respiratory disease such as ARDS.

Randomized trials of stress ulcer prophylaxis versus no prophylaxis suggest that using some form of prophylaxis rather than none is important in reducing the risk for upper GI bleeding. However, elevation of the gastric pH is also associated with a higher incidence of gram-negative colonization of the stomach. Gastric organisms may be transmitted into the tracheobronchial tree, resulting in nosocomial pneumonia. The use of prophylaxis other than antacids or H_2 blockers lessens the incidence of gastric colonization and nosocomial pneumonia.

Gastric mucosal blood flow may be compromised if splanchnic blood flow is reduced during a hypotensive episode. This may result in gastric mucosal ischemia, tissue sloughing, and GI bleeding. The patient with inadequate perfusion pressure is therefore at higher risk of having GI bleeding.

The patient should be monitored for gross blood in the gastric aspirate and stools. GI prophylaxis should be implemented early, and the gut should be used for feeding as soon as possible. The clinician should attempt to identify patient stressors and reduce them as much as possible, communicate with the patient in a calm and reassuring manner, and administer anxiolytic and/or sedative agents as necessary.

Complications Attributed to Operation or Operator of the Ventilator

Complications related to the operation or operator of the ventilator stem primarily from miscommunication of patient condition or treatment plan, carelessness, or lack of knowledge of the ventilator's functioning. Examples of such errors are inaccurate settings, incompatible settings, incorrect assembly, and failure to set and activate all alarm systems correctly. The patient-ventilator system must be checked a minimum of every 4 hours, but ideally every 2 hours, as described later in this chapter, and all alarm conditions must be investigated rapidly. Electrical, pneumatic, or microprocessor malfunction can also result in failure to provide ventilation for the patient. A manual resuscitation bag with an oxygen flowmeter should be readily available at the bedside of each mechanically ventilated patient so that manual ventilation can be provided in the event of mechanical failure.

Accidental disconnection from breathing systems is a significant problem. The most common site of disconnection is the patient-machine interface. Disconnection from this site occurs more frequently in patients with a tracheostomy tube than in those with a nasotracheal or orotracheal tube. The likely explanation for the higher occurrence in patients with a tracheostomy is that the connection is made more gently at this site to minimize patient discomfort during manipulation. Other common disconnection sites include the exhalation line connection, the nebulizer connections, and the connections between the circuit tubing and the humidifier. Preventive measures include heightened awareness, consistent full use of alarm systems, rapid response to all alarm conditions, reduction of the weight and tension of the circuit tubing on the airway, and twisting of the component connections together, as opposed to pushing them together (twisting provides a stronger connection).

MONITORING THE PATIENT-VENTILATOR SYSTEM

The primary goals of continuous monitoring and frequent assessment of the patient and ventilator are to prevent complications and detect problems early, when they are easier to correct. The most efficient assessment is performed using a systematic approach. The patient-ventilator system should be checked (1) to evaluate the patient's response to the current level of ventilatory support, (2) to determine accuracy and appropriateness of the current ventilator settings, and (3) to ensure the presence and proper functioning of the necessary equipment at the bedside.

Monitoring the Patient

An understanding of the patient's medical history, current diagnosis, and clinical course is imperative in formulating a database that leads to sound clinical reasoning and decision making. Key components of monitoring the patient undergoing mechanical ventilation are identified later. The patient should be assessed at least every 2 hours and with any setting change, with the use of whatever portions of the examination are appropriate. The traditional techniques of the examination—inspection, palpation, percussion, and auscultation—are all performed. However, modifications of the traditional physical examination of the chest are required when the patient is undergoing mechanical ventilation. All findings should be described with terminology common to all caregivers. Furthermore, when the location of findings is described, the imaginary lines of the thorax are used (Fig. 9-4).

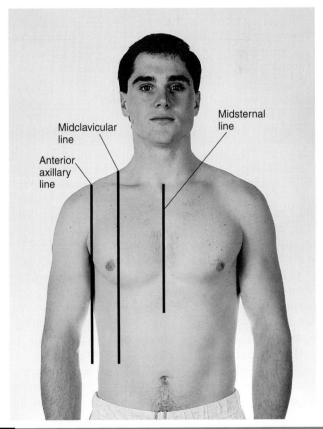

Midsternal line

Midclavicular line

Anterior axillary line

A

FIGURE 9-4

Imaginary lines of the thorax used to describe location of findings from physical examination techniques of observation, palpation, percussion, and auscultation. **A,** Imaginary lines of the anterior chest. *(From Jarvis C. Physical Examination & Health Assessment, 4th ed. St. Louis: Mosby, 2004.)*

Continued

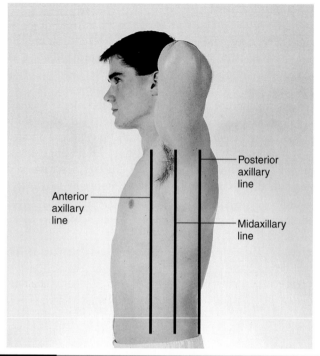

Anterior axillary line

Posterior axillary line

Midaxillary line

B

FIGURE 9-4, cont'd

Imaginary lines of the thorax used to describe location of findings from physical examination techniques of observation, palpation, percussion, and auscultation. **B,** Imaginary lines of the lateral chest. *(From Jarvis C. Physical Examination & Health Assessment, 4th ed. St. Louis: Mosby, 2004.)*

In the mechanically ventilated, versus the spontaneously breathing, patient, *observation* of the ventilatory rate and pattern may not provide the same degree of information regarding disease severity. The reason is that varying amounts of ventilatory control are achieved by the ventilator, depending on the mode of ventilation used. Generally speaking, the more spontaneous breathing the patient is performing, the more useful are the rate and pattern indicators. Observation of the equality of chest excursion is best performed by observing the rise and fall of the exposed chest from the foot of the bed. Unequal chest excursion may be caused by disorders or interventions resulting in unequal air distribution, such as right main-stem intubation, pleural effusion, atelectasis, consolidation, lobectomy, pneumothorax, and pneumonectomy. Paradoxical chest wall motion is the sucking in of a portion of the chest wall on inspiration and its protrusion on expiration (the opposite of normal chest wall movement). This phenomenon is caused by flail chest, in which several adjacent ribs have been broken in more than one location, creating a free-floating section of the chest wall.

TABLE 9-2	Percussion Sounds over the Lung Fields	
Sound	**Description**	**Clinical Significance**
Resonance	Drumlike, hollow, low-pitched sound	Normal air-filled lungs
Hyperresonance	Louder and lower pitched than resonant sound; somewhat musical or booming	Increased air in thorax, as in emphysema or pneumothorax
Flatness	Soft, higher pitched, dull sound heard over very dense, almost airless tissue	Conditions replacing air with fluid or mucus: pneumonia, atelectasis, consolidation, pulmonary edema
Dullness	Soft, short, muffled thud like sound heard over airless tissue	Lung tumor, pleural effusion; also heard over liver
Tympany	Loud, high-pitched sound heard over completely air-filled organ	Normally heard over stomach; large pneumothorax or herniated bowel

Palpation is useful in identifying the presence of subcutaneous emphysema or crepitus, which may indicate bony instability. The intubated patient is unable to perform the necessary maneuvers for eliciting tactile vocal fremitus or vocal resonance because the artificial airway courses through the glottis. Furthermore, in such a patient, palpation of the tracheal position rarely elicits tracheal deviation because the ETT tends to splint the trachea. If the pathologic condition is severe, however, as in tension pneumothorax, the trachea may deviate, thus providing useful clinical information.

Percussion is limited by the ability to position the patient as needed and by the presence of wound and intravenous line dressings, incisions, electrocardiograph leads, and possibly braces or slings. Percussion may be used to gain further assessment data in a suspect area. Table 9-2 identifies the terms used to describe percussion notes and commonly associated pulmonary findings.

Auscultation is most often performed anteriorly and laterally in the mechanically ventilated patient, particularly in the critical care setting. Every opportunity to listen posteriorly should be seized. A systematic sequence should be used during auscultation, with sounds from one side of the chest wall compared with those from the other (Fig. 9-5). The clearest sounds, free of artifact, are appreciated when all water is drained from the circuitry and when the artificial airway cuff is appropriately inflated. An air leak around a cuff may be misinterpreted as wheezing. The examiner should listen over the tracheal area for such a leak and correct it before completing the auscultatory portion of the examination. The stethoscope tubing should not touch the ventilator circuitry because air and water sounds in the circuitry will transmit to the examiner's ears. This artifact may be misinterpreted as adventitious sounds. Auscultation should not be performed over clothing because breath sounds, both normal and adventitious (Tables 9-3 and 9-4), will be more difficult to hear. The crackling sound of chest hair may be misinterpreted as adventitious sounds. Wetting the hair may reduce the amount of artifactual sound created.

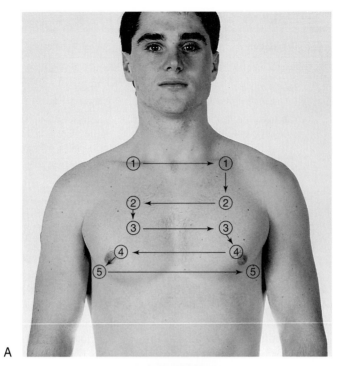

A

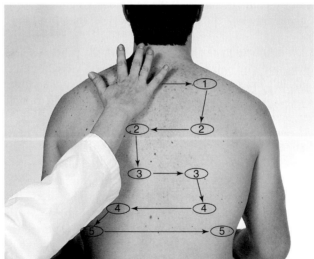

B

FIGURE 9-5

Sequence of systematic movements for auscultation, percussion, and palpation of the anterior (**A**) and posterior (**B**) chest. Comparison of the right and left sides of the chest should be performed by moving from side to side, beginning proximally and moving distally down the chest wall. *(From Jarvis C. Physical Examination & Health Assessment, 4th ed. St. Louis: Mosby, 2004.)*

TABLE 9-3 Normal Breath Sounds

Sound/Description	Location	Cause	Clinical Significance
Bronchial—tubular, hollow, loud intensity, high pitched	Larynx, trachea	Turbulent flow of air through large airways	None unless heard over peripheral lung fields, which indicates consolidation.
			Normally, air-filled alveoli filter these sounds from reaching periphery.
			Consolidation creates denser lung tissue, which transmits bronchial sounds to periphery.
Bronchovesicular	Main-stem bronchi; anteriorly at 1-2 ICS; posteriorly between scapulas	Turbulent flow in central airways; less intense and lower pitched than bronchial because of filtering of sound by chest wall tissue	None unless heard peripherally, which indicates consolidation.
Vesicular—soft, breezy, low pitched	Periphery of lung	Air movement through smaller airways	When diminished or absent, indicates decreased sound *production* (shallow breathing) or decreased sound *transmission* (less dense lung tissue, as in hyperinflation or partial physical obstruction such as with mucus).
			Absent vesicular sounds indicate that transmission is blocked, as in pleural effusion, pneumothorax.

ICS, Intercostal space.

Monitoring the Patient Undergoing Mechanical Ventilation: Key Components

VITAL SIGNS AND HEMODYNAMICS

Monitor blood pressure, heart rate and rhythm, temperature, and respirations, including patient and ventilator rates, pattern, and depth. Monitor volume status: pulmonary artery catheter readings, urinary output, intake and output, and weight. Monitor cardiac output. Finally, monitor the effect of the respiratory cycle on interpretation of hemodynamic parameters.

TABLE 9-4 Adventitious Breath Sounds

Sound/Description	Cause	Clinical Significance	Additional Descriptors/Comments
Crackles—discontinuous, explosive, bubbling sounds of short duration	Air bubbling through fluid or mucus, or alveoli popping opening on inspiration	Atelectasis, fluid retention in small airways (pulmonary edema), retention of mucus (bronchitis, pneumonia), interstitial fibrosis	Fine: soft, short duration. Coarse: loud, longer duration. Wet or dry. Other common (older) term: rales.
Rhonchi—coarse, continuous, low-pitched, sonorous, or rattling sound	Air movement through excess mucus, fluid, or inflamed airways	Diseases resulting in airway inflammation and excess mucus (e.g., pneumonia, bronchitis, or excess fluid, as in pulmonary edema)	Inspiratory and/or expiratory; may clear or diminish with coughing.
Wheezes—high- or low-pitched whistling, musical sound heard during inspiration and/or expiration	Air movement though narrowed airway, which causes airway wall to oscillate or flutter	Bronchospasm, as in asthma, partial airway obstruction by tumor, foreign body or secretions, inflammation, or stenosis	High or low pitched; inspiratory and/or expiratory.
Pleural friction rub—coarse, grating, squeaking, or scratching sound, as when two pieces of leather rub together	Inflamed pleura rubbing against each other	Pleural inflammation, as in pleuritis, pneumonia, tuberculosis, chest tube insertion, pulmonary infarction	Pleural rub occurs during breathing cycle and is eliminated by breath holding. Need to discern from pericardial friction rub, which continues despite breath holding.
Stridor—high-pitched, continuous sound heard over upper airway; a crowing sound	Air flowing through constricted larynx or trachea	Partial obstruction of upper airway, as in laryngeal edema, obstruction by foreign body, epiglottitis	Potentially life-threatening.

PHYSICAL EXAMINATION

Include in the physical examination patient comfort and WOB, use of accessory muscles, retractions, synchrony with the ventilator, and symmetry of chest wall excursion. Also observe skin color, temperature and moisture, and the presence or absence of crepitus or subcutaneous emphysema. Determine the presence and quality of pulses. Note the type, position, and stability of the artificial airway. Breath sounds are noted, including their presence and character and the presence of air leak around the cuff of the artificial airway. Monitor for air leak through the chest tube; the color, character, and amount of chest tube drainage; the color, amount, and character of secretions; the airway reflexes (cough, gag, and swallow); the presence of gastric distention; and the location, functioning, and patency of gastric decompression and feeding tubes. Finally, determine nutrition status.

LABORATORY AND X-RAY FINDINGS

Monitor arterial blood gases (ABGs): oxygenation, ventilation, and acid-base status. Determine serum potassium, sodium, magnesium, and phosphorus concentrations. Determine end-tidal CO_2 value. Determine when the most recent chest x-ray film was done and its findings, the hemoglobin level, results of sputum cultures, and the leukocyte count. If resources are available, perform a more advanced assessment by determining the central venous oxygen saturation ($S\textsc{c}\textsc{v}O_2$), the mixed venous oxygen saturation ($S\bar{\textsc{v}}O_2$), the arterial-venous oxygen content difference ($AV\textsc{d}O_2$), oxygen consumption ($\dot{\textsc{v}}O_2$), oxygen extraction, alveolar-arterial oxygen tension difference ($A\text{-a}\textsc{d}O_2$), percentage of shunt ($\dot{Q}s/\dot{Q}t$), and dead space/tidal volume ratio ($V\textsc{d}/V\textsc{t}$).

BEHAVIORS AND COMPLAINTS

Observe level of consciousness. Monitor for anxiety, fear, restlessness, agitation, confusion, disorientation, inappropriate behavior, delirium, somnolence, obtundation, dyspnea, degree of relaxation, level of sedation, pain, twitching and/or tetany, and psychological wellness.

SAFETY

Provide appropriate (least restrictive) application of restraints, secure airway safely, have spare airway of correct size readily available, and keep manual resuscitation bag and a mask at the bedside.

Monitoring the Ventilator: Key Components

The ventilator should be checked systematically on a scheduled, institution-specific basis, no less often than every 4 hours, and usually every 2 hours. A check should also be performed before ABG values or bedside pulmonary function data are obtained, after any change in ventilator settings, as soon as possible after an event of patient deterioration, and at any time when the function of the ventilator is questionable. When caring for the patient, tune into the normal sounds of the ventilator and the patient's respiratory pattern as a means of providing constant patient monitoring.

SETTINGS

Check for correctness to prescribed order. Monitor information found on front panel: FiO_2; set rate; V_T; mode; level of PEEP; level of pressure support or pressure control; peak inspiratory flow rate and waveform; inspiratory-to-expiratory (I:E) ratio or percentage of inspiratory and expiratory times; sensitivity; and sigh volume, interval, and multiples.

PATIENT DATA

Monitor the following information found on the display panel: peak, mean, and plateau airway pressures; PEEP; respiratory rate (RR) (ventilator and patient); exhaled V_T (mandatory and spontaneous breaths); minute ventilation ($\dot{V}E$) and contour of pressure, volume, and flow waveforms. Measure compliance, resistance, vital capacity, and negative inspiratory force as indicated. Measure total PEEP as indicated to determine presence and amount of auto-PEEP formation. Monitor cuff pressure.

ALARMS

Ensure that all alarms are activated and appropriate alarm limits are set.

TECHNICAL CONSIDERATIONS

Secure all connections. Check system temperature and function of humidifier. Ensure patency of tubing and that water in tubing is properly drained by means of universal precautions.

TOUR OF ALARMS AND ALARM PARAMETERS AND THEIR TROUBLESHOOTING

Alarms warn of technical or patient events that require the attention or action of the caregiver. They may provide audible and/or visual warnings depending on the severity of the condition but should never be viewed as fail-safe. Although alarm systems on ventilators are becoming increasingly sophisticated, especially on microprocessor ventilators, they serve a purpose only if set properly. Furthermore, alarms are intended only as a backup to close patient observation.

In the ICU, there are many alarms. A ventilator alarm, however, may be the one with the highest priority. When it sounds, it may indicate a problem with the patient's airway or breathing, the two highest priorities in the ABCs (airway, breathing, and circulation). When any ventilator alarm sounds, the first thing to do is look at the patient. If the patient is disconnected from the ventilator, reconnect the patient to the machine. If the patient is connected to the ventilator and is in distress and you cannot readily identify the cause, disconnect the patient from the machine and provide manual ventilation while calling for help in troubleshooting the problem. Finally, if an alarm sounds and the patient is not in respiratory distress, determine which alarm is sounding and proceed with problem solving.

For rapid problem solving, clinicians must be familiar with the status messages and front panel indicators on the ventilator with which they are working. In general, ventilator panels or screens are divided into fields of information with a common theme. A field or panel contains touch pads or dials that are grouped according to function. A field may be categorized further into an area of either display or control. The *control panel* is where ventilator settings and alarm parameters are established. The *display panel* provides patient information such as exhaled VT, minute ventilation, and peak inspiratory pressure; or status messages such as messages related to alarm indicators or battery function. Figures 9-6 *A* through *D* show the control and display panels of several ventilators. The monitoring of the patient's ventilator in most settings is a collaborative function between the respiratory therapist/practitioner and the nurse. The respiratory therapist can also play an instrumental role in teaching the nurse how to quickly read the ventilator's messages.

Refer to Chapter 8 to learn the respiratory waveforms, which provide additional objective information useful in troubleshooting a variety of conditions such as air leak, patient-ventilator dyssynchrony, auto-PEEP formation, and so on.

Oxygen

Set oxygen above and below prescribed FIO_2. Alarm will sound if delivered FIO_2 deviates from the prescribed setting.

Cause	Assessment and Management
Set FIO_2 inadvertently changed	Return oxygen setting to prescribed value.
Intentional change in FIO_2 for delivery of 100% oxygen during suctioning	
Oxygen analyzer error	Calibrate analyzer.
Oxygen source failure	Correct failure (see low oxygen pressure, later).

Pressure Alarms

HIGH-PRESSURE LIMIT

The high-pressure limit is usually set 10 cm H_2O above the patient's average PIP. The alarm will sound if pressure increases anywhere in the circuit. When this alarm is activated, the ventilator terminates the inspiratory phase. Airway pressures are observed on a gauge on the ventilator display panel. The pressure gauge reflects, on a breath-to-breath basis, the peak inspiratory and end-expiratory airway pressures (Fig. 9-7). Normal PIP for a patient ventilated with a volume control mode is between 20 and 30 cm H_2O. An increase in the PIP is caused by changes in pulmonary compliance or airway resistance (see Chapter 2 for a detailed discussion of these essential physiologic principles). In general, airway pressure will rise more gradually if it is a problem with pulmonary compliance, the exception being the development of a tension pneumothorax. Changes in resistance to gas flow may cause the airway pressure to rise more suddenly. Compliance and resistance can be quantifiably measured, as explained in Chapter 2. Serial measurements may therefore be a part of troubleshooting the cause of high PIP and evaluating the effects of interventions designed to reduce the high pressure.

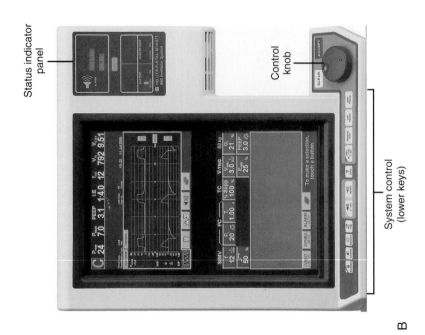

Status indicator panel

Control knob

System control (lower keys)

B

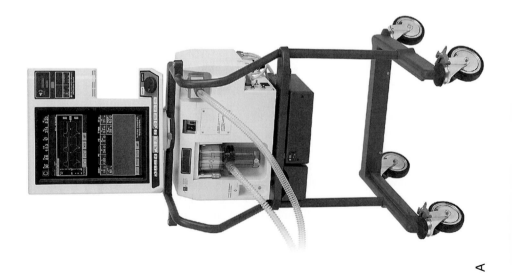

A

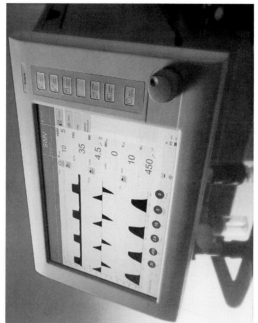

D

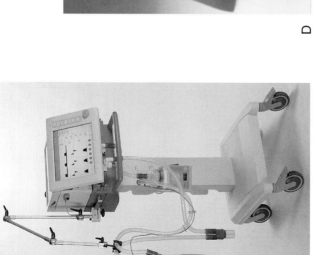

C

FIGURE 9-6

Rapid problem solving requires familiarization with the display, control panels, and screens of the ventilator in use. Several models are shown in parts A through D. **A,** Puritan Bennett model 840 ventilator (*top*). **B,** The PB 840 graphic interface unit, status panel indicator (visual messages regarding alarm conditions), and lower row of system control keys (control panel). **C,** Drager Evita XL. **D,** The basic screen of the Evita XL is configurable and displays ventilator graphics and a trend. Controls and values related to mode or function are logically grouped according to function and directly accessible on the main page. Additional screens are readily available. (*A and B, Courtesy of Puritan Bennett Corporation, Pleasanton, Calif.; C and D, courtesy of Drager Corp, Telford, Pa.*)

315

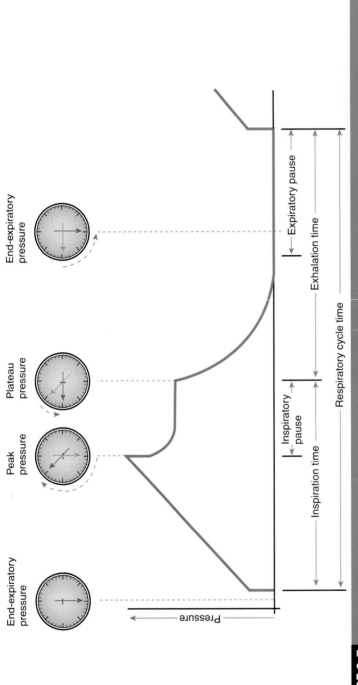

FIGURE 9-7

Peak airway pressure is a function of pressure created as a result of pulmonary compliance and airway resistance. When the PIP rises, a quick measurement of plateau pressure (Pplat) may assist in troubleshooting the cause of the elevation. The Pplat reflects alveolar pressure and therefore pulmonary compliance. The difference between the PIP and the Pplat, which is generally approximately 10 cm H_2O, reflects the pressure caused by airway resistance. If the difference is greater than 10 cm H_2O, the cause of high PIP is an increase in resistance to gas flow, that is, rising PIP with no change in the Pplat. If the PIP increases and the difference between peak and plateau pressures remains approximately 10 cm H_2O, then the cause of the elevated PIP is generally a reduction in compliance. (*Modified from Dupuis YG. Ventilators: Theory and Clinical Application, 2nd ed. St. Louis: Mosby, 1992.*)

Cause	Assessment and Management
Increase in resistance to gas flow	Possible causes of airflow obstruction (increased resistance) include kinks or water in tubing, biting of tube by patient, secretions in airway, closed suction catheter not fully retracted into sheath, migration of airway into right main-stem bronchus, herniation of cuff over end of tube, and bronchospasm. Straighten airway and other tubing to eliminate kinks, drain water, place bite-block or sedate patient, auscultate breath sounds for wheezes, and administer bronchodilator. Evaluate airway for change in placement; reposition if necessary. If unable to pass suction catheter or significant resistance is met during attempt to pass catheter, suspect cuff herniation. Deflate cuff and replace tube.
Decrease in pulmonary compliance	Pathologic conditions that cause the lungs to be stiffer, such as atelectasis, pneumonia, ARDS, pulmonary edema, pulmonary fibrosis, and pneumothorax, and hemothorax.
	Auscultate lungs for diagnostic clues such as crackles indicating edema, decreased breath sounds indicating atelectasis or infiltrate, and absent breath sounds indicating pleural space disease or consolidation.
	Assess chest x-ray film.
	Treat underlying pathologic condition with appropriate therapies: PEEP; mobilization of secretions with chest physiotherapy and suctioning; use of techniques that enhance ventilation such as turn, cough, deep breathing, and positioning; administration of diuretic for edema; evacuation of pleural effusion; pneumothorax or hemothorax.
	Assessment findings accompanying a tension pneumothorax including a sudden increase in PIP, decreased to absent breath sounds, and hyperresonance on the affected side. The pulmonary artery and central venous pressures rise and acute cardiovascular decompensation occurs as a result of mediastinal shifting and kinking of the great vessels. Correct tension pneumothorax with needle thoracentesis, followed by chest tube insertion. Maintain chest tube drainage system.
	Correct causes of reduction in chest wall compliance: If patient is splinting respirations, then control pain, perform escharotomies on circumferential chest wall burns, and determine cause of patient's breathing out of synchrony with ventilator (see section, Patient Fighting Ventilator or Breathing Out of Synchrony with Ventilator, later).
	Determine trend of serial measurements of static compliance. Adjust ventilator settings: decrease flow rate or V_T if possible, change flow pattern, or use pressure control mode.
Patient received sigh	Adjust pressure limit for sigh volumes.

Cause	Assessment and Management
Patient gagging, coughing, or attempting to talk	Determine what is causing gagging. For example, patient may be attempting to "tongue out" tube, tube may have been accidentally jarred or pulled, or patient may be vomiting. Correct problem, and reassure and calm patient. Suction as necessary. Explain to patient why he or she is unable to vocalize and that vocalization should be avoided. Develop alternative form of communication.
Patient fighting ventilator	See section, Patient Fighting Ventilator or Breathing Out of Synchrony with Ventilator, later.

LOW INSPIRATORY PRESSURE

The low inspiratory pressure alarm is usually set 5 to 10 cm H_2O pressure below the patient's average PIP. Alarm will be activated if pressure in system falls and is not reaching the level generally required for adequate ventilation in a particular patient.

Cause	Assessment and Management
Patient-ventilator disconnection or leak in system	Determine cause of leak: patient-ventilator disconnection, loose connection in circuitry, site of inline thermometer, or leak around cuff of airway. Correct cause of leak.

LOW OXYGEN PRESSURE

The low oxygen pressure alarm warns of inadequate pressure in the oxygen lines supplying the ventilator.

Cause	Assessment and Management
Loss of oxygen source or loss of adequate pressure within oxygen source	May be caused by accidental disconnection of O_2 line from O_2 outlet or to an array of problems generally handled by engineering department: for example, main oxygen line may have been interrupted because of construction occurring in another part of the facility. Check O_2 hose assembly for proper connection and reconnect if necessary. If main O_2 source is the problem, quickly apply manual resuscitation bag to *portable* oxygen source and provide manual ventilation to patient.

LOW AIR PRESSURE

The low air pressure alarm warns of inadequate pressure in the air lines supplying the ventilator. If the air source is lost, most ventilators provide 100% oxygen in an attempt to maintain an adequate source of fresh gas to the patient.

Cause	Assessment and Management
Loss of air source or loss of adequate pressure within air source	Check to see whether air hose assembly is properly connected. If ventilator becomes nonfunctional because its performance relies on high-pressure gas, then disconnect patient and provide manual ventilation until problem is corrected.

LOW PEEP/CPAP

The low PEEP/CPAP (continuous positive airway pressure) alarm parameter is usually set 3 to 5 cm H_2O below the set PEEP/CPAP level. The alarm is activated if the PEEP/CPAP level is not being maintained.

Cause	Assessment and Management
Usually a leak in the circuit	Evaluate the circuitry systematically for source of leak, and make correction. Patient-related sources of leaks are around the artificial airway or through a pleural chest tube (e.g., because of a bronchopleural fistula).

Volume Alarms

LOW EXHALED TIDAL VOLUME OR MINUTE VENTILATION

Volume alarm parameters are usually set 10% below the set V_T and the patient's average minute ventilation ($\dot{V}_E$). The low exhaled tidal volume (EV_T) alarm generally is set 100 mL less than the prescribed V_T. Some microprocessor ventilators automatically set these alarms on the basis of measured parameters. These alarms are valuable for ensuring adequate alveolar ventilation, particularly in the patient whose respiratory status is frequently changing.

Cause	Assessment and Management
Patient disconnected, or possible air leak somewhere in the patient-ventilator system	Audible leak may come from mouth or circuitry connection. Patient may be able to phonate and may exhibit signs and symptoms of hypoxemia and hypercapnia.
	Assess patient and circuit systematically for source of air leak, and correct it. Common sites for a leak are at the patient airway and circuit connection, connections in the circuitry such as at the humidifier, and at sites of inline thermometers.
	Air may need to be added to the cuff to reinstate seal (see Chapter 3 for technique). Leak may also be caused by malposition of artificial airway.
	If leak is not immediately correctable, such as a large pleural air leak, reset alarm parameters and adjust set V_T to compensate for volume loss.

Cause	Assessment and Management
Patient undergoing ventilation with pressure controlled mode of ventilation and a decrease in compliance, increase in resistance, or patient fatigue occurs	Assess for and treat cause of decreased pulmonary compliance or increased airway resistance (see High-Pressure Limit, under Pressure Alarms, earlier). Assess patient for other signs and symptoms of respiratory muscle fatigue: increased RR, irregular breathing pattern, use of accessory muscles. Provide additional ventilatory assistance by increasing inspiratory pressure assistance to achieve adequate V_T, providing an increased number of mandatory breaths, or placing patient on a volume controlled mode of ventilation.
High-pressure alarm limit reached, causing ventilator to dump rest of V_T	Troubleshoot cause of high peak inspiratory pressure (see High-Pressure Limit, under Pressure Alarms, earlier).
Insufficient gas flow	Patient complains of not being able to "get enough air." Assessment findings include a prolonged inspiratory time in modes in which patient has control over I:E ratio or an abnormal inspiratory flow-wave form. Correct by increasing the flow rate.

HIGH EXHALED TIDAL VOLUME OR MINUTE VENTILATION

Alarm parameters for high EV_T or $\dot{V}_E$ are set 10% to 15% above the desired V_T and $\dot{V}_E$. The alarm is activated when volumes of gas larger than the set alarm parameters are passing the flow sensor.

Cause	Assessment and Management
Increase in RR or V_T	Determine the reason that patient has increased $\dot{V}_E$: anxiety, pain, hypoxemia, or metabolic acidosis caused by decreased tissue perfusion, fever, or loss of bicarbonate base through an abdominal drain, for example. Determine cause of anxiety, reassure patient, and administer anxiolytic agents as necessary. Control pain. Determine cause of hypoxemia (see Low Pao_2, later), and correct. If patient has craniocerebral abnormality, the cause of hyperventilation may have a central neurogenic origin. Manage resulting respiratory alkalosis (see Respiratory Alkalosis, later).
Inappropriate or incompatible ventilator settings	Too high V_T, $\dot{V}_E$, or RR set on the ventilator, or alarm parameter not set appropriately for prescribed settings of V_T, RR, or $\dot{V}_E$.

Cause	Assessment and Management
Ventilator self-cycling because of incorrectly set sensitivity	Assist light is illuminated in the absence of patient inspiratory effort. Decrease sensitivity setting.
Excessive noise (water in tubing) as possible cause of false readings	Drain and discard appropriately all water from ventilator tubing.

Apnea

Alarm is activated when no exhalation is detected for an operator-selected period, usually set at approximately 20 seconds. Some ventilators automatically default to a safety mode of ventilation whenever apnea is detected. A message appears on the ventilator stating that this function was called into play.

Cause	Assessment and Management
No detectable spontaneous respiratory effort from the patient	Assess patient for respiratory excursion. If no spontaneous effort occurs, determine cause: lethargy, heavy sedation, respiratory arrest. Physically stimulate lethargic patient and instruct patient to take a breath. You may need to use a mode that provides more support until patient is less lethargic. Weaning may have to be discontinued if apneic periods are frequent. Consider giving agents such as naloxone to reverse effects of narcotics.
	If patient is in respiratory arrest, remove from ventilator and provide ventilation manually with a manual resuscitation bag. If patient is pulseless, call for assistance and perform cardiopulmonary resuscitation.
Loose connection to exhalation flow sensor	Secure the connection.

Inspiratory-to-Expiratory Ratio

The alarm for the I:E ratio alerts caregiver when the I:E ratio exceeds 1:3 or is less than 1:1.5 (generally). Parameters may be altered when I:E ratios other than 1:2 are in use.

Cause	Assessment and Management
Incompatible V_T, peak inspiratory flow rate, and respiratory rate controls	Check compatibility of V_T, peak inspiratory flow rate, and respiratory rate controls. Adjust as necessary.
	If V_T and RR are set correctly, adjust peak inspiratory flow rate to achieve desired I:E ratio.

Inoperative Ventilator/Machine Failure

A ventilator-inoperative alarm occurs when a fault is detected. A fault is a condition that jeopardizes the ventilator's ability to control the delivery of gas to the patient. When a ventilator is unable to provide ventilation to a patient reliably, the default response is usually either the opening of a safety valve to room air, enabling the patient to breathe unassisted by the ventilator, or the institution of a backup minimal ventilation mode. In addition, some microprocessor ventilators perform a power-on self-test (POST) in an effort to detect and correct the cause of the internal problem. During the POST, one of the two methods of ensuring a source of fresh gas to the patient is activated.

Cause	Assessment and Management
Loss of electrical power	Check electrical power cord for proper connection to working electrical outlet. The ventilator should always be plugged into an outlet that will be powered by a backup generator in the event of power outage.
	Provide manual ventilation until problem is corrected.
Loss of air or oxygen pressure	Check air and oxygen hose assemblies for proper connection and proper pressure.
	Provide manual ventilation until problem is corrected.
Internal hardware or micro-processor dysfunction	Provide manual ventilation and remove ventilator for servicing.

More Troubleshooting of Patient Problems

LOW PaO_2

A low PaO_2 is one that is less than 60 to 70 mm Hg with an oxygen saturation of 90% or less. The earliest warning signs of hypoxemia are changes in the clinical presentation of the patient. The patient may become restless, confused, and agitated; the heart rate, blood pressure, and respiratory rate may increase; dysrhythmias may develop; and the patient may complain of dyspnea. Ideally, this is the critical time to correct the hypoxemia, not when late signs and symptoms, such as cyanosis, bradycardia, and hypotension, or decreased S$\bar{v}O_2$, indicating inadequate tissue oxygenation, develop.

Objective early identification of oxygenation problems is most easily performed with a noninvasive monitor such as a pulse oximeter, especially in a patient with a tenuous oxygenation status. A change in the noninvasive value may be followed by rapid intervention to correct a readily identifiable cause of hypoxemia, or it may signal the need to obtain a blood gas. The PaO_2 and oxygen saturation are only part of an assessment of a patient's overall oxygenation status. To ensure adequate *tissue oxygenation*, one must achieve optimal oxygen delivery by ensuring an adequate hemoglobin and cardiac index by securing the physiologic state that promotes the release of oxygen at the tissue level and by reducing oxygen consumption.

Cause	Assessment and Management
Change in lung function, resulting in increased intrapulmonary shunt (e.g., atelectasis, secretions, bronchospasm, pneumonia, ARDS, pulmonary edema)	Assess patient rapidly for potential causes of hypoxemia that may be readily corrected, such as collected secretions, evident by coughing or increased rhonchi; or bronchospasm, evident by wheezing and elevated PIPs.
	Increase FIO_2 to prevent even transient hypoxemia until suctioning can be performed or a bronchodilator administered. To correct inadequate oxygenation, the primary two ventilator settings that are adjusted are the FIO_2 and the level of PEEP. The FIO_2 is generally increased in increments of 0.1 to 0.2. PEEP should be added in increments of 2.5 to 5 cm H_2O if the hypoxemia is refractory and the FIO_2 is reaching a toxic level (i.e., >0.5).
	Efforts to improve lung function, such as chest physiotherapy, high-frequency chest wall oscillation, positive expiratory pressure, suctioning, diuresis of edema, or administration of antibiotics, must be instituted simultaneously to making changes in the level of ventilatory support.
	Gather information to determine cause of increased shunting. For example, review the patient's history, perform a physical examination, obtain a chest x-ray film, and evaluate culture results.
	The hemoglobin should be checked for adequacy, and the patient should be prevented from fighting the ventilator.
Air leak, causing loss of PEEP	Low PEEP/CPAP alarm may sound. Use airway pressure manometer on ventilator to determine whether proper level of PEEP is being maintained. Troubleshoot source of air leak (around airway, ventilator circuitry, pleural space) and make correction.
Increase in intrapulmonary shunt as a result of a change in body position that places abnormal lung areas in the dependent position	Note body position in which decreased oxygenation became evident. Reposition patient.
	Correlate patient history with chest x-ray findings of area of abnormality (e.g., left chest wall bruising and rib fractures). Refrain from placing patient in bad lung-down position; use good lung down to achieve optimal ventilation/perfusion matching and thus oxygenation (see Chapter 2 regarding the effect of body position on $\dot{V}/\dot{Q}$ matching and Chapter 5 sections on positioning). Use pulse oximeter to determine trend in effect of body position on oxygenation.

Cause	Assessment and Management
ABG error; sample drawn incorrectly or too soon after patient-ventilator disconnection	Wait at least 15 to 20 minutes after ventilator setting changes or after secretions are suctioned before obtaining samples for ABG analysis. Eliminate excess heparin and air bubbles from specimen. Ensure that specimen container is capped tightly and kept on ice. Ensure that specimen is a pure arterial sample and contains no venous contamination.
Error in FIO_2, PEEP, inspiratory hold setting	Check vent systematically for correctness of settings and correct error.
Ventilator not delivering desired FIO_2	Low-oxygen or low-oxygen-pressure alarms may activate. Assess air and oxygen lines for proper connection. If oxygen source fails, provide oxygenation with portable oxygen source and manual resuscitation bag. Consider problems with oxygen blender, and use oxygen analyzer to confirm delivered FIO_2. Correct problem and reanalyze delivered oxygen.

HIGH Pao_2

In general, a Pao_2 of 100 mm Hg or greater is considered excessive and can be safely decreased.

Cause	Assessment and Management
Improvement in patient's lung function	Determination of whether to decrease the FIO_2 or the level of PEEP is based on the actual levels of these therapies being used. The FIO_2 should be decreased to nontoxic levels (i.e., 0.5 or less), followed by incremental decreases in the level of PEEP. If a prolonged inspiratory time is utilized, once the FIO_2 is 0.5 and the PEEP is 10 cm H_2O, the inspiratory time can be normalized. An inverse I:E ratio can be gradually reversed when the FIO_2 is 0.5, oxygenation is stabilized, and the underlying abnormality shows signs of resolution (e.g., improved chest x-ray findings, culture results, and measures of lung compliance).
Inaccurately high oxygen concentration setting on ventilator	High-oxygen alarm should sound. Correct setting.

RESPIRATORY ALKALOSIS

Respiratory alkalosis is confirmed by blood gas findings of pH more than 7.45 with $Paco_2$ less than 35 mm Hg. Because the $Paco_2$ is inversely proportional to the alveolar minute ventilation, $Paco_2$ is increased by manipulating factors that decrease alveolar $\dot{V}E$, as illustrated in the following formula:

$$\text{Alveolar } \dot{V}E = RR \times (VT - VD)$$

Where:
- Alveolar $\dot{V}E$ = alveolar minute ventilation
- RR = respiratory rate
- VT = tidal volume
- VD = dead-space volume

Therefore, alveolar $\dot{V}E$ is decreased by decreasing the respiratory rate or VT or increasing the dead space. Anatomic dead space remains relatively fixed in any given patient. Physiologic dead space is increased in pulmonary hypoperfusion, pulmonary embolus, and ARDS, and by overdistention of the alveolus with excessive PEEP or VTs. *Mechanical* dead space (the artificial airway and ventilator circuitry) is rarely manipulated during mechanical ventilation in an effort to alter the $Paco_2$.

Cause	Assessment and Management
Factors that increase the RR: anxiety, pain, hypoxemia, central nervous system abnormality	Confirm hyperventilation and respiratory alkalosis with ABG determinations. Reduce anxiety through calm, confident approach. Administer sedation and anxiolytic agent as needed to targeted sedation goals. Assess and control pain.
Inappropriate ventilator settings of VT, RR, or mode	Look at ventilator display panel for EVTs. Appropriate EVT varies based on lung compliance and whether lung protective strategy is employed. Range of appropriate values: 8 to 10 mL/kg for mandatory breaths (or lower for lung protection) and 5 mL/kg for spontaneous breaths. Decrease the EVT by decreasing the VT in a volume controlled mode (A/C or SIMV), or by decreasing the inspiratory pressure in a flow- or time-cycled mode (PS, PC). If SIMV and PS are in use, the EVT generated by each mode must be assessed and individually adjusted as necessary. If the ventilator's RR is too high, decrease the frequency of mandatory breaths in SIMV, V-A/C, or P-A/C mode. If the A/C mode is in use and the patient is hyperventilating by breathing over the set rate, the patient-related causes of increased RR must be ruled out and treated. If hyperventilation persists, then switch from A/C to SIMV or PS mode.
Ventilator self-cycling	Spontaneous breath indicator flashes when patient shows no evidence of respiratory effort. Ventilator initiates inspiration before pressure manometer gauge reaches trigger level (2 cm

Cause	Assessment and Management
	H_2O below baseline pressure). Sensitivity is set too high. Adjust sensitivity to 2 cm H_2O below baseline pressure.
	Vibration of excess condensation in ventilator tubing may be read by the ventilator as patient effort. Discard excess condensation, using universal precautions.

RESPIRATORY ACIDOSIS

Respiratory acidosis is confirmed by blood gas findings of a pH less than 7.35 with a $PaCO_2$ more than 45 mm Hg. A rising $PaCO_2$ may cause the physical signs and symptoms of somnolence, obtundation, warm skin, vascular dilation, and headache. The $PaCO_2$ is determined by, and inversely proportional to, the alveolar minute ventilation. Therefore, the $PaCO_2$ is decreased by manipulating factors that increase $\dot{V}E$: increasing the RR or V_T and decreasing the dead space. Anatomic dead space remains relatively fixed in any given patient. Physiologic dead space is increased in pulmonary hypoperfusion, pulmonary embolus, and ARDS, and by overdistention of the alveolus with excessive PEEP or V_T. *Mechanical* dead space (the artificial airway and ventilator circuitry) in the patient supported by mechanical ventilation may alter the $PaCO_2$.

Cause	Assessment and Management
Inadequate RR	Determine cause of decreased patient RR, such as acute neurologic event, oversedation, or metabolic alkalosis, and provide treatment. Increase RR setting on ventilator (assuming V_T is set appropriately).
Inadequate V_T	Monitor EV_T and compare with set V_T. If deviation of 50 mL or greater exists in an adult, evaluate cause of air loss, such as cuff leak, circuit leak, or pleural leak. Correct leak if possible. If leak is in pleural space, adjust V_T to compensate for loss. If increasing the V_T increases the air leak (by increasing bronchopleural pressure gradient), increase the RR to increase the $\dot{V}E$.
	If EV_T values are not 8 to 10 mL/kg for mandatory breaths (or lower for lung protection) and 5 to 8 mL/kg for spontaneous breaths, then (to increase V_T) increase the V_T setting in volume-cycled modes and increase inspiratory pressure in pressure- or flow-cycled modes.
Excess glucose loads in parenteral or enteral feeding solutions (As excess glucose is converted to fat, CO_2 production increases.)	Consider overfeeding as a potential cause of an unexplained, increased $\dot{V}E$ and/or failure of weaning. Patient who has limited ventilatory reserve will not be able to increase $\dot{V}E$

Cause	Assessment and Management
	sufficiently to blow off excess CO_2 being produced; the result will be respiratory acidosis.
	Calculate nutritional needs. With assistance of dietitian, evaluate amount and source of non-protein calories. Eliminate overfeeding. A high-fat, low-carbohydrate diet may be preferable for the patient with pulmonary disease because fat combustion yields less CO_2 than combustion of carbohydrates or protein.
Increased physiologic dead space	If caused by hyperinflation, chest x-ray film may show hyperinflation of nondiseased area of lung. Further evidence of increased physiologic dead space includes widened end-tidal to arterial CO_2 gradient and a decreased CO_2 after increasing the VT or level of PEEP. Correct the problem by decreasing the VT or level of PEEP, if possible.
	If lung disease is unilateral and good lung is being hyperinflated, consider independent lung ventilation.
	If cause is worsening pathologic condition, such as ARDS, the caregiver may have to consider tolerating elevated CO_2 through use of permissive hypercapnia (see Chapter 9).
	Confirm suspicions of pulmonary embolus through diagnostic testing and treat on the basis of severity of embolus.
Increased mechanical dead space	Remove dead space tubing if present. Cut off excess ETT at 1.5 inches from teeth or nares after confirmation of placement by chest x-ray film. If increased mechanical dead space is potential cause of inability to wean patient from ventilator, consider changing airway to a tracheostomy.

Patient Fighting Ventilator or Breathing Out of Synchrony with Ventilator

Ventilator synchrony is defined as the matching of the ventilator-delivered breath to the patient-demanded breath during assisted or supported ventilation. If the level of ventilator support is below that demanded by the patient, the result is significant imposed WOB and may result in acidosis and hypoxemia, increased oxygen consumption, and carbon dioxide production. Patient-ventilator interaction exists during all phases of the breath: trigger, cycle, and limit. Synchrony is improved by recognizing ventilator parameter deficiencies in relation to the patient's spontaneous need and adjusting the flow pattern, trigger, cycle, or limit to improve the interaction. Use of the pulmonary graphics described in Chapter 8 assists tremendously in recognition of problems and titration of parameters to patient-ventilator synchrony. Use of sedation should be considered only after ventilator adjustments are optimized.

"Fighting the ventilator" is a phrase often used to indicate that the patient is having acute respiratory distress and the patient and ventilator are breathing out of synchrony with each other. Another common term used when the patient and ventilator are breathing out of synchrony with each other is that the patient is "bucking" the ventilator. Signs and symptoms of acute respiratory distress include dyspnea, agitation, use of accessory ventilatory muscles, nasal flaring or wide-open-mouth inspiratory efforts, tachypnea, abdominal paradox, tachycardia, hypertension, agitation, expression of fear, and diaphoresis. Multiple ventilator alarms, including high-pressure limit and low V_T, may sound. A pulse oximeter may also warn of hypoxemia if the distress continues and cardiac monitors warn of hemodynamic instability and cardiac rhythm changes.

The primary goal of management of the patient in distress is to ensure adequate ventilation and oxygenation. The initial step is to disconnect the patient from the ventilator and provide manual ventilation with 100% oxygen. Rapid, systematic physical assessment and ventilator assessment should be performed to identify a cause of the distress. Acute distress in the patient usually involves the sensation of dyspnea, which needs to be explored by the clinician, using direct questions that the patient can answer with head nodding or pointing. Be cautious about releasing the restrained

TABLE 9-5	Potential Reasons for Patient to Have Acute Respiratory Distress and to "Fight the Ventilator"
Patient-Based Causes	**Ventilator-Based Causes**
Artificial airway problems	Sensitivity set too high or too low (trigger dyssynchrony)
Cuff herniation	
■ Upward migration	Inadequate peak inspiratory flow rate setting (flow dyssynchrony)
Sudden increase in airway resistance:	
■ Bronchospasm	Inadequate ventilatory support or inadequate delivery of oxygen
■ Secretions	
Acute change in lung compliance:	Large air leak in circuitry or patient-ventilator disconnection
■ Tension pneumothorax	
■ Pulmonary edema	
Acute agitation and anxiety, possibly because of inadequate sedation, emergence from street drugs, alcohol withdrawal, or pain	
Change in respiratory drive:	
■ Central neurogenic hyperventilation	
■ Fatigue	
Unknown development of auto-PEEP, which creates need for increased inspiratory effort, and thus work of breathing, to trigger ventilator	
Acute change in ventilation/perfusion matching:	
■ Pulmonary embolus	
■ Change in body position that leads to hypoxemia (e.g., lung with greatest abnormality placed in dependent position)	

hand of a patient who is fighting the ventilator because self-extubation may occur if the patient believes the airway is the cause of the sensation of dyspnea. Call for assistance as needed in maintaining patient stability, assessing the cause of distress, and implementing appropriate measures to alleviate distress.

If the initial step of disconnecting the patient from the ventilator and providing manual ventilation relieves the respiratory distress, the cause of the problem was likely within the ventilator. If the distress continues, the problem is probably patient based. Table 9-5 delineates some of the most common ventilator- and patient-related causes of patient-ventilator asynchrony.

RECOMMENDED READINGS

Amato MBP, Barbas CSV, Medeiros DM, et al. Effect of a protective-ventilation strategy on mortality in the acute respiratory distress syndrome. *N Engl J Med* 1998; 338:347–354.

American Association of Respiratory Care Mechanical Ventilation Guidelines Committee. AARC clinical practice guideline: Patient-ventilator system checks. *Respir Care* 1992; 37(8):882–886.

Brook AD, Ahrens TS, Schaiff R, et al. Effect of a nursing-implemented sedation protocol on the duration of mechanical ventilation. *Crit Care Med* 1999; 27:2609–2615.

Brower RG, Matthay MA, Morris A, et al. Ventilation with lower tidal volumes as compared with traditional tidal volumes for acute lung injury and the acute respiratory distress syndrome. *N Engl J Med* 2000; 342(18):1301–1308.

Centers for Disease Control and Prevention. Guidelines for preventing health-care-associated pneumonia. *MMWR* 2004(53):No. RR-3.

Drakulovic M, Torres A, Bauer T, et al. Supine body position as a risk factor for nosocomial pneumonia in mechanically ventilated patients: A randomized trial. *Lancet* 1999; 354:1851–1854.

Eisner MD, Thompson T, Hudson LD, et al. Efficacy of low tidal volume ventilation in patients with different clinical risk factors for acute lung injury and the acute respiratory distress syndrome. *Am J Respir Crit Care Med* 2001; 164:231–236.

Ferguson ND, Frutos-Vivar F, Esteban A, et al. Mechanical Ventilation International Study Group. Airway pressures, tidal volumes, and mortality in patients with acute respiratory distress syndrome. *Crit Care Med* 2005; 33:1141–1143.

Happ MB. Communicating with mechanically ventilated patients: State of the science. *AACN Clin Issues* 2001; 12(2):247–258.

Hess DR, Kacmarek RM. Ventilator induced lung injury. In DR Hess, RM Kacmarek (eds.), *Essentials of Mechanical Ventilation* (pp. 16–25). New York: McGraw-Hill, 2002.

Hess DR, Kallstrom TJ, Mottram CD, et al. Care of the ventilator circuit and its relation to ventilator-associated pneumonia. *Respir Care* 2003; 48(9):869–879.

Jacobi J, Fraser GL, Coursin DB, et al. Clinical practice guidelines for the sustained use of sedative and analgesics in the critically ill adult. *Crit Care Med* 2002; 30:119–141.

Kollef MH, Levy NT, Ahrens TS, et al. The use of continuous IV sedation is associated with prolongation of mechanical ventilation. *Chest* 1998; 114:541–548.

Kress JP, Pohlman AS, O'Connor MF, et al. Daily interruption of sedative infusions in critically ill patients undergoing mechanical ventilation. *N Engl J Med* 2000; 342:1471–1477.

Laffey JG, O'Croinin D, McLoughlin P, et al. Permissive hypercapnia—Role in protective lung ventilatory strategies. *Intensive Care Med* 2004; 30:347–356.

MacIntyre NR, Day S. Essentials for ventilator alarm systems. *Respir Care* 1992; 37(9):1108–1112.

Munroe CL, Grap MJ. Oral health care in the intensive care unit: State of the science. *Am J Crit Care* 2004; 13(1):25–34.

Mutlu GM, Mutlu EA, Factor P. Prevention and treatment of gastrointestinal complication in mechanical ventilation. *Am J Respir Med* 2003; 2(5):395–411.

Pilbeam SP. Introduction to ventilators: Part IV. Troubleshooting during mechanical ventilation. In JM Cairo, SP Pilbeam (eds.), *Mosby's Respiratory Care Equipment,* 7th ed. (pp. 372–390). St. Louis: Mosby, 2004.

Pingleton SK. Complications associated with mechanical ventilation. In MJ Tobin (ed.), *Principles and Practice of Mechanical Ventilation* (pp. 775–792). New York: McGraw-Hill, 1994.

Rello J, Ollendorf D, Oster G, et al. Epidemiology and outcomes of ventilator-associated pneumonia in a large US database. *Chest* 2002; 122:2115–2121.

Slutsky AS, Tremblay LN. Multiple system organ failure. Is mechanical ventilation a contributing factor? *Am J Respir Crit Care Med* 1998; 157:1721–1725.

Task Force on Guidelines, Society of Critical Care Medicine. Guidelines for standards of care for patients with acute respiratory failure on mechanical ventilatory support. *Crit Care Med* 1991; 19(2):275–278.

Villar J, Kacmarek RM, Perez-Mendez, et al. A high positive end-expiratory pressure, low tidal volume ventilatory strategy improves outcome in persistent acute respiratory distress syndrome: A randomized, controlled trial. *Crit Care Med*, 2006; 34:1311–1318.

Noninvasive Respiratory Monitoring and Invasive Monitoring of Direct and Derived Tissue Oxygenation Variables

Monitoring the patient's respiratory status is one of the primary functions of critical care practitioners. This chapter examines noninvasive and invasive methods for monitoring the patient's oxygenation and ventilation. The clinician must become thoroughly familiar with these commonly used techniques. When utilizing a pulse oximeter or end-tidal carbon dioxide monitor, one must know how to apply and troubleshoot the monitors correctly, interpret the data they provide, and respond appropriately to achieve optimal patient outcomes. Blood gas interpretation extends from analysis of the direct variables provided by the arterial and the mixed venous samples to the derived variables obtained with one or both of the samples. Invasive methods of monitoring tissue oxygenation with a variety of configurations of the pulmonary artery (PA) catheter are in widespread use. Understanding the direct and derived variables that these catheters provide is essential to reaching the ultimate goal: preservation of *tissue oxygenation.*

The best methods of monitoring, whatever techniques are employed, ideally provide the greatest accuracy with the least risk to the patient. When a knowledgeable practitioner manages the monitor, risk to the patient is minimized.

PULSE OXIMETRY: MEASURING OXYGEN SATURATION

Principles of Operation

Pulse oximetry is the continuous, noninvasive measurement of arterial oxygen saturation (Sao_2), which is the amount of oxygen carried by hemoglobin. When the Sao_2 is measured with a pulse oximeter, the abbreviation is Spo_2.

Spo_2 is measured by placing a probe on a finger, bridge of the nose, earlobe, or other translucent body part in which the pulsating arterial bed can be detected. The

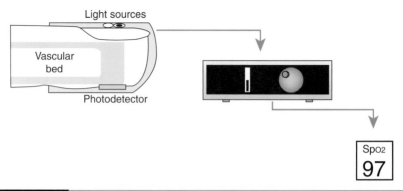

FIGURE 10-1

Light is transmitted through the translucent body part from light-emitting diodes (LEDs). A photodetector opposite the LEDs detects how much light passes through, unabsorbed by deoxygenated hemoglobin (Hb) or oxyhemoglobin (Hbo$_2$). See text for further explanation. *(Modified from Nellcor Inc., Pleasanton, Calif.)*

probe emits two wavelengths of light, red and infrared, from light-emitting diodes (LEDs). The light is transmitted through the body part and received by a photodetector (PD) on the other side. The PD uses the principles of spectrophotometry to determine the amount of light absorbed as it passes through the body part (Fig. 10-1). The red light is readily absorbed by deoxygenated (reduced) hemoglobin, and the infrared light is absorbed by the oxyhemoglobin (Hbo$_2$). This information is then carried to the pulse oximeter monitor, which performs a logarithmic computation and displays a digital readout of the ratio of saturated hemoglobin to total hemoglobin as illustrated in the following formula:

$$Spo_2 = \frac{Hbo_2}{Hb + Hbo_2}$$

The pulse oximeter measures the amount of deoxygenated hemoglobin (Hb) and oxygenated hemoglobin (Hbo$_2$). Total Hb is the sum of Hb and Hbo$_2$. The Spo$_2$ value is the percentage of total hemoglobin that is hemoglobin saturated with oxygen.

To differentiate arterial from venous blood, the pulse oximeter uses the principles of plethysmography to measure a change in volume. Identification of the arterial blood is accomplished by the recognition that arterial blood pulsates, whereas other optical components, such as venous blood and tissue, do not. The pulsating arterial bed dilates at systole, the blood volume increases, and so does the light absorption. Light absorbed by skin, bone, tissue, and venous blood is constant and therefore represents a baseline (Fig. 10-2). The pulse oximeter assumes that only pulsatile absorbance is arterial blood.

Most pulse oximeters have features that provide graphic information about the amplitude of the pulse signal being received and a real-time waveform that confirms reception of the arterial pulsation. Some oximeters provide auditory cues about pulse

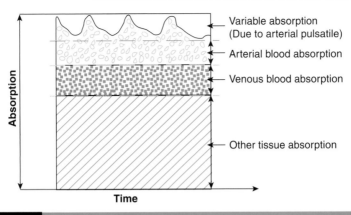

FIGURE 10-2

Absorption of light is translated into a plethysmographic waveform. Light absorption by venous blood and tissues is constant. Absorption of light by the arterial bed is variable because of the expanding vascular volume during systole. *(Modified from Petty TL. Clinical Pulse Oximetry. Monograph of the Webb-Waring Lung Institute, Denver, 1986.)*

amplitude. The intensity, or pitch, of a beep tone varies to correspond with pulse amplitude. Both methods, auditory and visual, may be present on some models. Verification of the adequacy of the pulse amplitude is essential for ensuring the accuracy of the SpO_2 value.

Accuracy

Investigators focusing on critically ill patients have concluded that pulse oximeters are accurate within 2% in the saturation range of 70% to 99.9%. Accurate oximeter readings can be obtained through dirty or burned skin.

Errors in SpO_2 measurement are introduced by several factors that either exceed the capabilities of, or interfere with, the instrument's two wavelengths of light or its spectrophotometric analysis. The presence of dysfunctional hemoglobins, notably carboxyhemoglobin (COHb) and methemoglobin, leads to falsely high and low SpO_2 values, respectively, as compared to cooximeter-assessed SaO_2. These hemoglobins are not detected by the two-wavelength system; therefore the total hemoglobin is incorrectly calculated. An instrument with four wavelengths of light is required to detect these abnormal hemoglobins. In cases of inhalation injury when the amount of COHb can be significant, the pulse oximeter, although accurately calculating SpO_2, may not be a reliable indicator of total oxygen saturation. When COHb is present, SpO_2 can be used to determine how well normal Hb is saturated and whether it is functioning optimally. A cooximeter SaO_2, however, must be intermittently assessed to determine the total Hb saturation.

Several other factors may affect light transmission, absorption, or analysis. Three vascular dyes—methylene blue, indigo carmine, and indocyanine green—all cause abrupt, transient decreases in SpO_2 measurements. In individuals with deeply pigmented skin, oximeter readings are slightly less accurate, and more technical problems may occur. Most nail polishes have no effect on oximeter readings, with the exception of black, brown, blue, green, and frosted, which cause erroneously low readings. Synthetic fingernails that are very thick may also adversely affect oximeter accuracy.

Error in SpO_2 measurement is also introduced by factors that dampen the plethysmographic signal. Any event that significantly reduces vascular pulsations reduces the instrument's ability to perform plethysmographic analysis. Such events include significant hypothermia, hemoglobin concentration, hypotension (mean blood pressure less than 50 mm Hg), infusion of vasoconstrictive drugs at high doses, and direct arterial compression, such as with application of a blood pressure cuff.

MOTION ARTIFACT

Outside the operating room, where pulse oximetry first became the standard of care, the patient's body motions create a technical challenge. Motions interfere with the accuracy of conventional pulse oximeters by being incorrectly interpreted as a pulse signal or by preventing accurate detection of the true pulse signal. False alarms and inaccurate measurement can desensitize clinicians to true alarm conditions. Newer generation pulse oximeters are designed to reduce motion sensitivity and thus fewer false alarms. This is achieved through improvements in the pulse signal algorithms. The exact approach to reducing motion artifact varies by manufacturer. Multiple algorithms are typically functioning simultaneously to track the pulse rate and saturation. Locking on to the pulse signal helps the oximeter provide accurate saturation values during motion and environmental noise.

The signal-average time represents the amount of time (in seconds) that the oximeter collects signals used to calculate and display the SpO_2. The shorter the signal-average time, the more sensitive the device is to changes in SpO_2, but the more prone it is to false alarms caused by artifact. Conversely, as the signal-average time is increased, the number of alarms caused by error or artifact is decreased. The instrument's reduced false-alarm rate may be achieved at the expense of an unreliable or delayed identification of hypoxemia and bradycardia. Because the SpO_2 values are averaged over a longer period, the amount of time needed to detect a true hypoxemia is also increased. In most of the new-generation pulse oximeters, signal-averaging times are short. This enhances detection of hypoxemia while simultaneously the enhanced algorithms filter out motion artifact caused by movement, thus helping to control for the increase in false alarms that accompany decreased signal-average times. In laboratory studies and clinical studies, all of the new-generation pulse oximeters performed better than any of the conventional devices to which they were compared.

Advantages and Limitations of Pulse Oximetry

Pulse oximetry has several advantages. It is noninvasive and therefore painless. It requires no calibration and minimal site preparation, making it quick and easy to apply. The measurement of SpO_2 is in real time and continuous, and therefore the time delay and sporadic monitoring associated with arterial blood gas (ABG) determination are eliminated. It is a valuable tool for routine monitoring of the

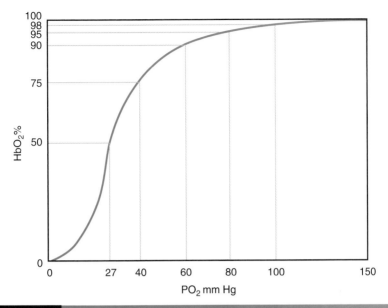

FIGURE 10-3

Oxygen-hemoglobin dissociation curve expresses the relationship between Sao$_2$ and Pao$_2$. *(Modified from Kacmarek RM, Stoller JK. Current Respiratory Care. Toronto: Decker, 1988.)*

patient at risk of hypoxemia. Its greatest advantage is as an early warning of hypoxemia because desaturation is detected earlier by pulse oximetry than by clinical observation.

The biggest dangers in applying pulse oximetry are in misinterpreting the value and in using it as a monitor of ventilation status. The relationship of SpO$_2$ to Pao$_2$ is expressed in the oxygen hemoglobin dissociation curve (Fig. 10-3). This is a sigmoid-shaped curve, and therefore SpO$_2$ and Pao$_2$ are not linearly related (see Chapter 2). When the SpO$_2$ is 90%, the Pao$_2$ is approximately 60 mm Hg under conditions of normal body temperature, pH, Paco$_2$, and blood levels of 2,3-diphosphoglycerate (2,3-DPG). Changes in these factors cause the curve to shift to the right or left. This increases or decreases, respectively, the affinity of oxygen to hemoglobin and therefore the relationship of Sao$_2$ to Pao$_2$. Correct interpretation of SpO$_2$ requires taking into consideration all factors present in the patient that may cause a shift in the oxyhemoglobin dissociation curve.

The pulse oximeter can be used for patients of any age. SpO$_2$ monitoring is the standard of care during anesthesia, during transport of patients from the operating room to the recovery room or from the intensive care unit (ICU) to a procedure site, postanesthesia, and for almost all patients in the ICU. In the critical care unit, pulse oximetry is useful in determining a patient's oxygenation status during procedures such as bronchoscopy, suctioning, and turning or while patients are undergoing oxygen therapy with low- or high-flow systems or mechanical ventilation; in any patient with a marginal or fluctuating oxygenation status; and for patients receiving sedation. It must be recognized that pulse oximetry alone may not be useful during the process of weaning from mechanical ventilation because it does not reflect changes in ventilation (Pa_{CO_2}). It is also useful for evaluation of patients with sleep-disordered breathing, in emergency medicine, and in dental and outpatient surgical settings. Pulse oximeters may also be used as an adjunct to monitor the adequacy of perfusion distal to a surgical or traumatic injury such as after digit or extremity reimplantation surgery.

Technical Limitations and Suggestions for Their Alleviation

There are technologic limitations to pulse oximeters, just as with any technology used in the ICU. Therefore it is important for the clinician to be able to troubleshoot problems that may occur and thus to maintain accuracy of the values obtained.

Optical interference occurs when ambient light is allowed to reach the PD. Ambient light detection by the PD creates inaccuracies or, sometimes, complete loss of measurement. Most oximeters are designed to reject ambient light; however, when the intensity of ambient light is high (as from a surgical light, infrared heating lamp, or from sunlight), the photodetector cannot sense the light transmitted through tissue or calculate Sp_{O_2}. The digital display may remain blank, the unit may show a falsely low pulse rate or Sp_{O_2}, or the unit may show by activation of an alarm that there was a loss of signal. Protecting the PD from bright light sources by covering it with an opaque material obviates the problem. Optical interference can also occur when the sensor's optical components are misplaced, such as when the sensor was applied too loosely.

Another technical problem that may occur during use of an oximeter is *optical shunting*. This occurs when part of the light from the LEDs reaches the photodetector without passing through the finger (i.e., it travels around the finger to the PD). The displayed saturation is a combination of the patient's actual saturation and the value the oximeter calculates when light directly travels from the LED to the PD. Correct alignment of the LED and the PD, so they are opposite each other and flush to the skin, eliminates optical shunting.

Incorrect choice or application of the oximeter probe may also lead to technical problems. Choosing the proper size and type of sensor for the patient helps eliminate optical interference, optical shunting, and loss of signal. Sensors may be reusable (durable) or single use (disposable) (Fig. 10-4). Cost, setting, and patient size are factors to consider when choosing a sensor. When applying the sensor, the clinician must be sure it is free of body oils or dirt that will affect its sensing capability. The sensor may be cleaned with alcohol as necessary.

Factors that lead to venous congestion or venous pulsation cause erroneously low Sp_{O_2} values to be reported because the venous bed is misinterpreted as arterial. The sensor should be applied snugly, but not too tightly, around the monitoring site. Ensure that the sensor is not constrictive, prevent dependent positioning of the monitored site, and avoid tight-fitting garments on a monitored extremity. Intraaortic balloon pumping represents a situation in which the action of the pump creates a rhythmic disturbance in the arterial waveform that is in synch with the cardiac cycle, making it difficult for the oximeter to distinguish the true arterial pulsation. Sp_{O_2} measurements should be used cautiously when pumping.

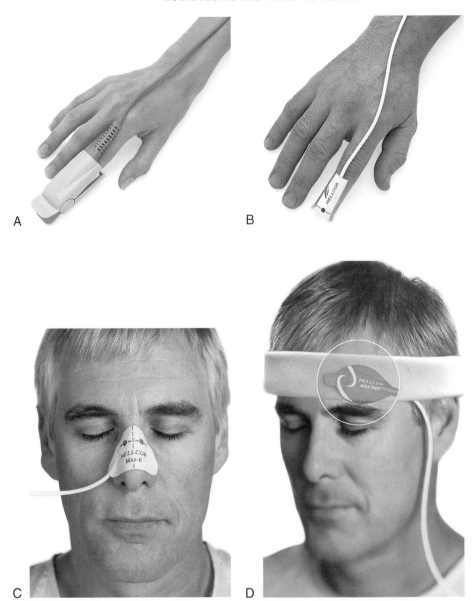

FIGURE 10-4

Reusable and disposable pulse oximeter sensors. **A,** Reusable clip-style finger sensor. **B,** Disposable, adult sterile adhesive sensor. **C,** Disposable, adult nasal sensor. **D,** Limited-reuse adult reflectance sensor. Application of sensor is to forehead. Sensor is effective in poor perfusion or low cardiac output states when obtaining SpO_2 from a digit is sometimes impossible. The manufacturer's directions for use of each sensor should be carefully followed for optimal performance. *(Photos courtesy Nellcor, Pleasanton, Calif.)*

Instituting Pulse Oximetry

After correctly choosing and applying the sensor probe, perform auditory and/or visual verification of the arterial signal to confirm that the pulse signal is adequate to provide accurate optical measurements. Obtain an ABG and compare the SpO_2 reading taken concurrently with the laboratory-determined SaO_2 to determine an acceptable correlation. To be considered accurate, the SpO_2 and SaO_2 values should be within 2% of each other. Troubleshoot larger than 2% disparities by checking the monitor for proper function and searching for the presence of factors that cause erroneous SpO_2 values. Set HIGH and LOW pulse and SpO_2 alarm parameters and alarm volume. Pulse alarms, if present, should be set at 10 beats/min above and below the patient's heart rate. The SpO_2 high alarm should be set at 100%, and the low alarm set at the minimum acceptable SpO_2 as determined by the physician's order or by institution standard of practice.

END-TIDAL CARBON DIOXIDE MONITORING

End-tidal carbon dioxide ($ETCO_2$) monitoring is the noninvasive trend measurement of alveolar carbon dioxide at the end of exhalation when carbon dioxide concentration is at its peak. It can be measured at the bedside with a monitor that both numerically and graphically displays values of exhaled carbon dioxide. The measurement and numeric display of the amount of carbon dioxide in respired gases is known as capnometry, whereas capnography is the measurement and graphic display of respired gases in a waveform known as a capnogram. Primary application of $ETCO_2$ monitoring is in the monitoring of the patient's ventilatory ($PaCO_2$) status.

Principles of Operation

Monitors that measure $ETCO_2$ use either of two methods of analyzing exhaled gases for carbon dioxide concentration: mass spectrometry or infrared absorption spectrophotometry. A mass spectrometer is an instrument capable of analyzing a gas sample for its concentrations of oxygen, carbon dioxide, nitrogen, and even anesthetic gases. Because mass spectrometers are highly sophisticated and expensive systems, they are usually used to monitor more than one patient. Gases are therefore sampled at the patient's airway and travel through special plumbing to the mass spectrometer for analysis. Because many patients may be monitored with one system, gas samples are typically taken from patients sequentially. Therefore, no patient is continuously monitored.

Infrared absorption spectrophotometry, the alternative to mass spectrometry, uses infrared light absorption to determine the concentration of carbon dioxide in the respired gases. The carbon dioxide concentration is determined by comparing the amount of light absorbed by the carbon dioxide in the exhaled sample with that absorbed by a reference sample free of carbon dioxide. Infrared analyzers are portable and less expensive to purchase and maintain, and they may provide continuous monitoring. For these reasons they are more commonly used in the intensive care setting (Fig. 10-5).

$ETCO_2$ monitors are further categorized by gas sampling techniques such as mainstream, proximal diverting, or sidestream (Fig. 10-6). *Mainstream* analyzers

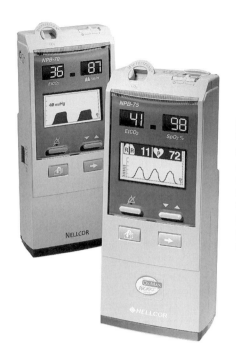

FIGURE 10-5

Portable, infrared mainstream end-tidal carbon dioxide ($ETCO_2$) monitor. Portable monitors expand use of $ETCO_2$ monitoring beyond the operating room or intensive care setting into the emergency department and recovery room and during transport. The monitor shown also performs the dual function of pulse oximetry.

(Photo courtesy Nellcor, Pleasanton, Calif.)

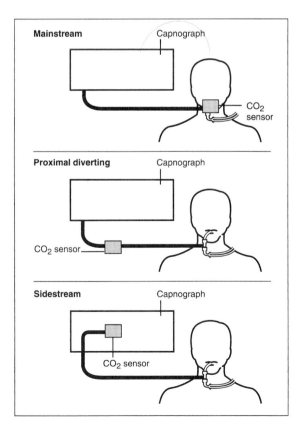

FIGURE 10-6

End-tidal carbon dioxide monitors may be categorized by gas sampling technique as mainstream, proximal diverting, or sidestream. See text for complete discussion.

(Reprinted with permission. Copyright Nellcor, Pleasanton, Calif.)

measure carbon dioxide directly at the airway. Analyzing carbon dioxide in this fashion requires heating the infrared device attached to the airway to avoid condensation on the sensor cells. The presence of condensation on the sensor cell can lead to erroneously high readings. Two of the advantages of mainstream analyzers are that they provide continuous monitoring of one patient and that testing of exhaled carbon dioxide is more rapid because transport of the gas sample to another site for analysis is avoided. Disadvantages are that placing the analyzer inline creates mechanical dead space and extra weight, and thus traction, on the patient's airway.

A *proximal diverting* system transports the gas sample a short distance from the airway to a site where the carbon dioxide sensor is housed. This method reduces bulk at the airway.

A *sidestream* analyzer aspirates a gas sample through small-bore tubing and transports it to the carbon dioxide sensor for analysis. An advantage is that no additional dead space or weight is added by the carbon dioxide sensor at the airway. Disadvantages include a time delay that occurs as the gas travels from the sample site to the analyzer; volume loss because the sample is aspirated from the airway, which affects measurement of total exhaled minute volume; and falsely low measurements because of potential moisture collection in the sample tubing. The sensor should be placed upright to keep moisture from interfering with accuracy. Some systems contain water traps or a purging mechanism to alleviate the latter problem. Regardless of the type of sampling technique, the sampling port should be placed as close as possible to the patient's airway. Technical problems that obviate accurate gas sampling must be eliminated by the clinician. These problems include gas leaks caused by poor connections, partial to complete obstruction of the gas sampling lines or sensors, and incorrect circuit assembly.

Carbon Dioxide Physiology

Essential to grasping the indications and uses of $ETCO_2$ monitoring and interpretation of the $ETCO_2$ variable is an understanding of the physiology of carbon dioxide elimination. Carbon dioxide, which is produced by the cells as a byproduct of metabolism, diffuses from the cells into the blood and is then carried to the lungs for elimination (Fig. 10-7). At the level of the lung, the carbon dioxide readily diffuses from the pulmonary capillaries into the alveoli, and therefore the amount of carbon dioxide in these two compartments reaches near equilibrium. Carbon dioxide is then eliminated from the body during the exhalation phase of the respiratory cycle (Fig. 10-8). At the beginning of exhalation, gases from the anatomic dead space that are free of carbon dioxide are exhaled. Carbon dioxide elimination rapidly rises, reaching a plateau as alveolar gases are exhaled. At the end of a tidal breath, the concentration of exhaled carbon dioxide is at its highest. Therefore, the measurement of the concentration of carbon dioxide at the end of a tidal breath provides a reflection of the alveolar carbon dioxide (P_{ACO_2}), which in turn reflects the arterial carbon dioxide (Pa_{CO_2}). Accordingly, $ETCO_2 \approx P_{ACO_2} \approx Pa_{CO_2}$.

Normally, Pa_{CO_2} is 35 to 45 mm Hg. Typically $ETCO_2$ values average 2 to 5 mm Hg less than the Pa_{CO_2} in individuals with normal ventilation and perfusion to the lung. Therefore, if the $ETCO_2$ is measured at the same time that a blood gas value is obtained, the $ETCO_2$ can be subtracted from the Pa_{CO_2}, providing an index known

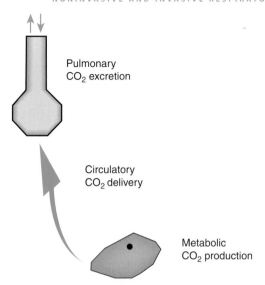

FIGURE 10-7

The amount of carbon dioxide in the exhaled gases is determined by metabolic rate, perfusion status, and alveolar ventilation. *(Modified from Hess D. Noninvasive respiratory monitoring during ventilatory support. Crit Care Nurs Clin North Am 1991; 3[4]:565–574.)*

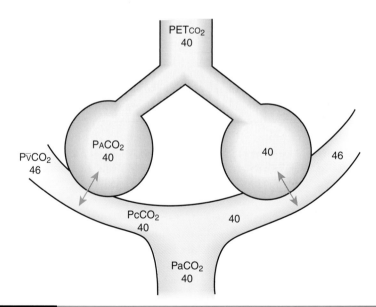

FIGURE 10-8

Normal partial pressure of carbon dioxide in the mixed venous ($P\bar{v}CO_2$) and arterial ($PaCO_2$) blood, the alveolus ($PACO_2$), and the exhaled gases ($PETCO_2$). *PcCO_2*, Partial pressure of carbon dioxide in capillary blood. *(Modified from Szaflarski NL, Cohen NH. Use of capnography in critically ill adults. Heart Lung 1991; 20[4]:363–372.)*

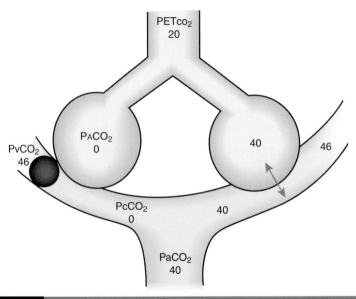

FIGURE 10-9

Model of lung unit with dead-space ventilation (*left*) demonstrates how the arterial-to-alveolar gradient for carbon dioxide widens under these conditions. PETco_2 is significantly lowered. *P*c*CO$_2$*, Partial pressure of carbon dioxide in capillary blood. *(Modified from Szaflarski NL, Cohen NH. Use of capnography in critically ill adults. Heart Lung 1991; 20[4]:363–372.)*

as the $Paco_2$-ETCO$_2$ gradient, or a-ADco_2. For example, if a blood gas is obtained and the $Paco_2$ is 39 and simultaneously the ETCO$_2$ is noted to be 35, the $Paco_2$-ETCO$_2$ gradient is +4. Knowing this gradient allows for noninvasive monitoring of the patient's ventilation by monitoring the ETCO$_2$ trend and by inferring the $Paco_2$ with the use of the gradient.

Circumstances that widen the a-ADco_2 gradient ($Paco_2$ rises, whereas ETCO$_2$ stays the same or decreases) are clinically significant. Knowing the factors that can alter the a-ADco_2 alerts the clinician to recheck the gradient when one of these conditions arises so accurate trend monitoring can be maintained. Conversely, understanding what causes a widened a-ADco_2 assists in interpreting what is occurring physiologically in a patient when a widened gradient is identified. The a-ADco_2 may be widened with increasing physiologic dead space because perfusion of the mixed venous carbon dioxide–rich blood to some of the ventilated alveoli is decreased or absent (Fig. 10-9). Exhaled gases from dead-space units "free" of carbon dioxide mix with those from lung units with a normal ventilation/perfusion ratio, "diluting" the ETCO$_2$ value. Box 10-1 further delineates causes of a widened a-ADco_2.

The most common pitfall of ETCO$_2$ monitoring is believing that ETCO$_2$ reflects the patient's ventilatory status alone. As Table 10-1 shows, changes in exhaled carbon dioxide levels may occur because of changes not only in ventilation but also in carbon dioxide production (metabolism), transport of carbon dioxide to the lung

BOX 10-1 — Causes of a Widened Arterial (Pa_{CO_2}) to Alveolar ($P_{A_{CO_2}}$) Gradient (a-aD_{CO_2})

INCREASED PHYSIOLOGIC DEAD SPACE

Pulmonary embolus (thromboembolic, fat, or air)
Pulmonary hypoperfusion (hypotension → cardiac arrest)
Excessive V_T or PEEP ventilation
Acute respiratory distress syndrome (ARDS)

INCOMPLETE ALVEOLAR EMPTYING

Severe hypoventilation
High rate/low V_T ventilation

POOR SAMPLING TECHNIQUE

Dilution of gas sample with carbon dioxide free gas (poorly fitting mask or mouth breathing when sampling is performed via nasal cannula setup, or sample site too far from airway and too close to fresh gas inlet)
Leakage of exhaled gas into the atmosphere (ETT cuff leak)

....

ETT, Endotracheal tube; *PEEP*, positive end-expiration pressure.

TABLE 10-1 — Causes of Alterations in End-Tidal Carbon Dioxide (ETCO₂)

Increased ETCO₂	Decreased ETCO₂
VENTILATION	
Mild hypoventilation	Moderate to extreme hypoventilation
Rebreathing, as when mechanical dead space is added to circuitry	Hyperventilation
	Airway obstruction
	Increased physiologic dead space (increase in amount of exhaled gas that has not interfaced with CO₂-laden blood)
PERFUSION	
Increased transport of CO₂ to lungs after perfusion has been impaired (e.g., after cardiopulmonary bypass, after arrest, or postshock state)	Impaired pulmonary perfusion (e.g., pulmonary embolus, state of decreased cardiac output up to and including cardiac arrest)
METABOLISM	
Increased CO₂ production, as in fever, pain, a hypermetabolic state such as after trauma, or increased muscle activity caused, for example, by seizures or shivering	Decreased CO₂ production, as in hypothermia, or decreased muscle activity caused, for example, by heavy sedation and/or paralytic agents
Injection of sodium bicarbonate (transient rise)	
Malignant hyperthermia	
EQUIPMENT	
Leak in ventilator circuit, resulting in reduced tidal volume delivery to patient	Poor sampling, such as when water is in sample line of sidestream system
Exhausted CO₂ absorber (anesthesia system)	Leak around endotracheal tube cuff, resulting in loss of exhaled gas to atmosphere
Reduced ventilation caused by partially obstructed airway	Ventilator disconnect
	Esophageal intubation or dislodged artificial airway
	Obstructed or kinked endotracheal tube

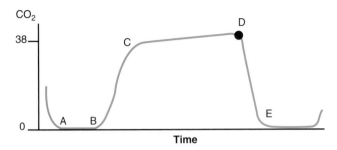

- Zero baseline (A-B)
- Rapid, sharp rise (B-C)
- Alveolar plateau (C-D)

- End-tidal value (D)
- Rapid, sharp downstroke (D-E)

FIGURE 10-10

Normal capnogram. See text for explanation. *(Modified from Nellcor, Inc., Pleasanton, Calif.)*

(pulmonary perfusion), and accuracy of equipment. If any three of these variables are held constant, a change in the carbon dioxide value reflects an alteration in the remaining variable. For example, if metabolism, cardiac output, and accuracy of monitoring are all held constant, the $ETCO_2$ concentration is inversely related to alveolar ventilation. An increase in the $ETCO_2$ value indicates hypoventilation, and a decrease in the value indicates hyperventilation.

Graphing the Exhaled Carbon Dioxide Waveform: Capnography

The capnogram is a tracing of the inhaled and exhaled concentrations of carbon dioxide with time (Fig. 10-10). In the normal capnogram, at the beginning of exhalation, the carbon dioxide value is zero as gas from the anatomic dead space leaves the airway (A-B). A sharp rise in the waveform, and thus in carbon dioxide elimination, occurs as alveolar air mixes with dead-space gas (B-C). Most of exhalation is represented by a leveling of the curve known as the alveolar plateau, which represents gas flow from the alveoli (C-D). The PCO_2 at the end of the plateau (D) is the $ETCO_2$, which is the highest concentration of exhaled alveolar carbon dioxide. The curve then takes a rapid, sharp downstroke as inspiration of carbon dioxide–free gas occurs (D-E). It is notable that on a capnogram, positive deflections represent expiration, whereas negative deflections represent inspiration (which is the opposite of most respiratory waveforms). The shape of the capnogram can be diagnostic of abnormal lung function or may indicate technical problems (Fig. 10-11, *A-J*). The capnogram provides critical information regarding the accuracy of the $ETCO_2$ value. Anytime the numerical value of $ETCO_2$ is questioned, the quality of the waveform should be inspected.

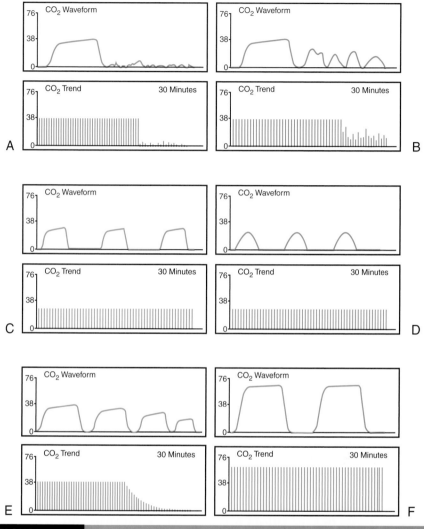

FIGURE 10-11

Abnormal capnographic waveforms: **A,** Sudden decrease in $ETCO_2$ to zero or near-zero value. Possible causes include airway disconnection; esophageal intubation; and dislodged, totally obstructed, or kinked ETT. **B,** Sudden decrease in $ETCO_2$ to low, nonzero value. Decrease may be caused by incomplete sampling, air leak in the system, such as around the mask or endotracheal tube or in the ventilator circuitry, or to partial airway obstruction. **C,** Persistent low $ETCO_2$ with good alveolar plateau. Possible causes include hyperventilation, hypothermia, sedation, anesthesia, and increased dead-space ventilation. **D,** Persistent low $ETCO_2$ without alveolar plateau. Possible causes include incomplete exhalation caused by kinking of the airway, bronchospasm, or mucous plugging, and poor sampling technique. **E,** Exponential decrease in $ETCO_2$. Possible causes include factors that decrease pulmonary blood flow, such as decreased cardiac output. **F,** Elevated $ETCO_2$ with good alveolar plateau. Possible causes include inadequate minute ventilation, combined with tidal volume sufficient to empty alveolar gas, and factors that increase the metabolic rate such as fever, pain, and shivering. *(Modified from Nellcor, Inc., Pleasanton, Calif.)*

Continued

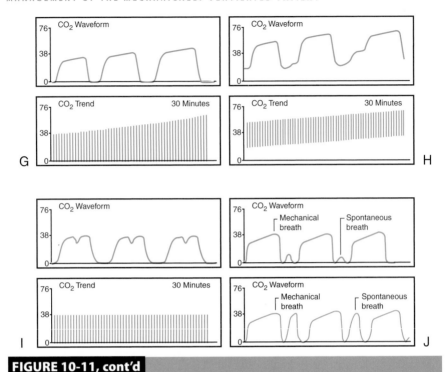

FIGURE 10-11, cont'd

Abnormal capnographic waveforms: **G,** Gradually increasing $ETCO_2$. Possible causes include hypoventilation, factors that increase the metabolic rate such as a rising body temperature, or malignant hyperthermia. **H,** Rise in baseline and $ETCO_2$. Possible causes include rebreathing of exhaled carbon dioxide, as in increased mechanical dead space; exhausted carbon dioxide absorber; sample cell needs cleaning; and need to recalibrate. **I,** Capnographic waveform, showing alveolar cleft, indicates inadequate neuromuscular blockade or emergence from blockade. **J,** Spontaneous breathing during mechanical ventilation. Spontaneous breaths of patient shown on *top* are shallower than those of patient shown on *bottom*. *(Modified from Nellcor, Inc., Pleasanton, Calif.)*

Applications of End Tidal Carbon Dioxide Monitoring

In addition to providing a reflection of the $Paco_2$ in patients with a stable respiratory pattern and perfusion status, other uses for $ETCO_2$ monitoring are identified. Detection of esophageal intubation may be achieved with the use of a disposable carbon dioxide detector. The $ETCO_2$ detector is a device that attaches between the manual resuscitation bag and the endotracheal tube (ETT). The instrument detects and, in some cases, provides an estimated measure of exhaled carbon dioxide (see Chapter 3). These disposable devices assist in determining correct placement of the ETT in patients in whom perfusion is present. They are useful, but not specific, for determining correct ETT placement in patients with cardiopulmonary arrest because, if circulation is not established, lack of carbon dioxide detection does not necessarily mean esophageal intubation.

The main use of $ETCO_2$ monitoring in the critical care unit is to determine the adequacy of ventilation in the patient supported by mechanical ventilation, especially during manipulation of the ventilator settings. It should be used with great caution because of the large number of factors that affect the variable. Acute increases in $Paco_2$, requiring adjustments in the ventilator settings, may occur in patients who are unable to increase their minute ventilation (e.g., in patients who are deeply sedated). Monitoring of $ETCO_2$ also provides continuous, noninvasive assessment of the patient when controlled hypocapnia is being used as a measure to decrease intracranial pressure.

In the operating room, the $ETCO_2$ monitor is very useful as an indicator of accidental ventilator disconnection. In the ICU, however, ventilators have sophisticated alarm systems that warn of disconnections, making the $ETCO_2$ an expensive additional alarm if it is being used only for this purpose. There are many uses for $ETCO_2$ monitoring in the postanesthesia recovery unit, including its use as an indicator of hypoventilation and apnea.

It is very important to understand that $ETCO_2$ monitoring is not useful as a monitor for weaning a patient from a ventilator. Many factors that can alter the $ETCO_2$ variable, such as changes in metabolic rate, may be present during a weaning trial. Therefore, $ETCO_2$ does not always reflect the patient's $Paco_2$ accurately during ventilator weaning.

Monitoring of exhaled carbon dioxide to assess the patient for the presence of perfusion is valuable during cardiopulmonary resuscitation (CPR). At the time of cardiac arrest, the $ETCO_2$ value falls to zero because there is a lack of pulmonary perfusion. The detection of exhaled carbon dioxide provides an indication of the adequacy of cardiac compressions and the return of spontaneous circulation.

To ensure accurate monitoring of $ETCO_2$ when it is first instituted, the practitioner must perform the required calibration routines as described in the operator's manual. Correct assembly of the airway adapter, exhaled carbon dioxide sensor, and display monitor is essential to prevent sampling errors. Proper connection to the patient's airway minimizes error caused by gas leaks. To decrease fluid accumulation in the sample line in a sidestream sampling device, ensure that the sampling port is placed at a right angle to the patient's airway. After setting up and connecting the $ETCO_2$ monitor correctly, obtain an ABG to compare the initial $ETCO_2$ reading with the laboratory-determined $Paco_2$. Troubleshoot greater than 5 mm Hg disparities by checking the monitor for proper function and searching for the presence of factors that can cause erroneous $ETCO_2$ values. Determine and document the a-$ADco_2$. Set HIGH and LOW $ETCO_2$ alarm parameters and alarm volume.

BLOOD GASES

Arterial Blood Gas

TECHNIQUE

Chapter 2 discussed normal values and the method of interpreting ABG values. This section presents the proper technique of obtaining the ABG sample so the patient has no complications and errors are not entered into the results.

The most common site for obtaining an ABG sample is the radial artery. In the adult, other sites are the brachial and femoral arteries. The latter is the most commonly

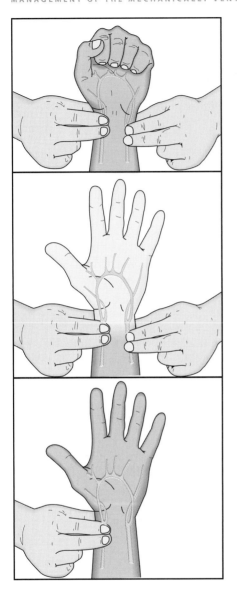

FIGURE 10-12

Modified Allen test used to assess adequacy of collateral circulation in the hand, via the ulnar artery, before performance of a radial arteriotomy. **A,** Elevate the hand and compress radial and ulnar arteries while the patient opens and closes fist until (**B**) the hand blanches. **C,** Release pressure from ulnar artery and evaluate for return of normal hand color. An erythematous blush is a positive Allen test result, whereas pallor is a negative result and indicates poor collateral circulation. Therefore arterial puncture should not be performed. *(Modified from Weilitz PB. Pocket Guide to Respiratory Care. St. Louis: Mosby, 1991.)*

used site in emergency settings because of its accessibility and the relative ease of palpating a weak pulse. Before an arterial puncture (arteriotomy) is performed, an assessment should be made of the adequacy of collateral circulation because if vessel disruption or hematoma formation leads to circulatory compromise, the result could be loss of the limb. Collateral hand circulation is assessed with a modified Allen test (Fig. 10-12).

Coagulopathy or medium- to high-dose anticoagulation therapy is a relative contraindication to arterial puncture. If necessary, then, adequate time should be allotted for the application of pressure to achieve hemostasis. Arterial puncture

BOX 10-2	Procedure for Arterial Puncture

1. Wash hands. Prepare heparinized syringe with a 22-gauge (or smaller) needle. Put on clean gloves.

2. Place the patient's wrist (for arterial puncture) or arm (for brachial puncture) in a hyperextended position.

3. Clean the skin with alcohol or povidone-iodine or chlorhexidine.

4. Palpate the pulse and insert the needle, bevel up, at a 45-degree angle to the skin (90 degrees for femoral puncture).

5. Observe for flash of blood at hub of needle. Pressure within the arterial system should allow the syringe to fill passively without aspiration. Withdraw approximately 3 mL of blood. Amount of blood needed depends on method of analysis.

6. Remove the needle and apply direct pressure for at least 5 minutes, longer if the patient has a history of anticoagulant therapy or coagulopathy.

7. While applying pressure, remove any bubbles from the syringe by holding it upright, allowing the air to float to the top, where it can be easily expelled.

8. Cap the syringe and immediately place it on ice.

9. Properly dispose of equipment and wash hands.

should not be performed distal to a surgical shunt or through an infected lesion. Repeated puncture of a single site should also be avoided because it increases the likelihood of hematoma formation, scarring, or laceration of the artery (Box 10-2).

If frequent ABG analysis or continuous monitoring of blood pressure is required, arterial cannulation should be performed. Patency of the arterial catheter is achieved with a continuous-flush device. All connections of such a device must be carefully secured because a loose connection could result in rapid blood loss.

When the specimen is obtained, precautions must be taken to handle it correctly for prevention of inaccurate results (Box 10-3). For prevention of clotting, liquid or powdered (lyophilized) heparin must be added to the syringe. Only a small amount of heparin should be used (the barrel of the syringe should be wet slightly and any excess heparin removed), or it may produce acidification of the sample because the pH of heparin is 7.0. The sample should be placed immediately in an ice bath to slow metabolism; otherwise, oxygen levels will be lowered and carbon dioxide levels elevated. If the specimen is held at 4°C, analysis may be performed for up to 1 hour. If it is held at room temperature, analysis should be performed within 15 minutes. The sample must be obtained anaerobically and any air bubbles rapidly expelled. Air bubbles will cause oxygen levels to be elevated and carbon dioxide levels to be lowered. The patient's body temperature should be taken at the time the specimen is obtained and recorded on the laboratory requisition. When the ABG is analyzed, a normal body temperature of 37°C is assumed. Temperature correction of the results can be performed by the laboratory if personnel are alerted to an abnormal body temperature. Temperatures higher than 37°C result in higher oxygen and carbon dioxide values, whereas temperatures lower than 37°C have the opposite effect (recall the concepts of the oxyhemoglobin dissociation curve). After the sample is obtained, pressure should be applied to the vessel for at least 5 minutes to achieve hemostasis.

BOX 10-3	Procedure for Obtaining an Arterial Blood Gas Specimen from an Indwelling Arterial Catheter

1. Wash hands. Prepare heparinized syringe. Put on clean gloves.

2. Remove dead-end cap from stopcock. Prevent contamination of cap.

3. Place nonheparinized syringe on stopcock.

4. Turn stopcock off to the flush device and open to the artery. Withdraw a sufficient amount of blood to ensure that line is free of flush solution, usually 2 to 3 mL. Conserve as much of the patient's blood as possible. Some systems are closed systems, avoiding the need to discard any blood.

5. Turn stopcock partially off to artery.

6. Remove syringe and discard blood and flush properly.

7. Place heparinized syringe on stopcock, open stopcock to artery, and withdraw approximately 3 mL of arterial blood. Amount of blood needed depends on method of analysis.

8. Turn stopcock off to artery, remove syringe, debubble, cap syringe, and immediately place syringe in ice bath.

9. Flush arterial line until free of blood. Always flush stopcock of residual blood and replace protective dead-end cap. Blood in line or stopcock provides an excellent culture medium for the growth of pathogens.

Mixed Venous Blood Gas

TECHNIQUE

Mixed venous blood gas analysis is performed to determine the adequacy of tissue oxygenation. The partial pressure of oxygen in mixed venous blood ($P\bar{v}o_2$) and saturation of hemoglobin with oxygen in mixed venous blood ($S\bar{v}o_2$) are also used to calculate additional tissue oxygenation variables (discussed in the following sections). Mixed venous blood can be obtained *only* from the distal port of a PA catheter (Box 10-4). It is at this point in the vasculature that the blood returning from all the venous beds of the body is thoroughly "mixed" in the right ventricle and therefore represents total-body venous blood (Fig. 10-13). Blood from the proximal port of the PA catheter, the right atrial (RA) port, is not true mixed venous blood because blood from the superior vena cava and that from the inferior vena cava are not yet adequately blended. Furthermore, blood from the coronary sinuses (which has a $P\bar{v}o_2$ of 23 mm Hg) empties into the RA; therefore, if the proximal sampling port were lying close to the coronary sinus, the sampled blood would be tainted and would certainly not reflect total-body venous oxygen values.

The same handling precautions that apply to arterial samples apply to mixed venous samples: Ensure that the specimen is free of bubbles, obtained anaerobically and capped, placed immediately on ice to slow metabolism, and analyzed with the use of the patient's body temperature at the time of sampling. Several calculations discussed in the following section require both an arterial and a mixed venous sample; therefore, the samples should be obtained in as close a time frame to each other as possible so changes in the patient's condition do not confound the results. Table 10-2 delineates the normal values for each sample.

BOX 10-4	Procedure for Obtaining a Mixed Venous Blood Gas Specimen from a Pulmonary Artery Catheter

1. Wash hands. Prepare heparinized syringe. Put on clean gloves.

2. Remove dead-end cap from stopcock. Prevent contamination of cap.

3. Place nonheparinized syringe on stopcock. Turn stopcock off to the flush device and slowly withdraw 3 mL of flush solution and blood for discard.

4. Turn stopcock partially off to pulmonary artery.

5. Remove syringe, and discard blood and flush properly.

6. Attach heparinized syringe, turn stopcock off to flush device, and *slowly* withdraw (over 1 minute) 1 to 3 mL of mixed venous blood. Too rapid withdrawal of blood may cause arterialized pulmonary capillary blood to flow retrograde, contaminating the sample. This would lead to $P\bar{v}_{O_2}/S\bar{v}_{O_2}$ readings higher than that of the true mixed venous blood.

7. Turn stopcock off to the sampling port and remove syringe. Debubble specimen, cap syringe, and immediately place syringe in ice bath.

8. Flush pulmonary artery catheter until free of blood. Always flush stopcock of residual blood and replace protective dead-end cap. Blood in line or stopcock provides an excellent culture medium for the growth of pathogens.

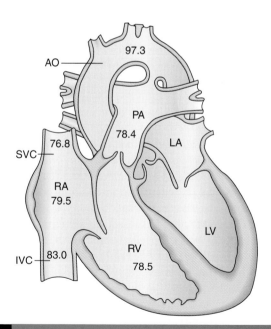

FIGURE 10-13

Normal values for oxygen saturation in the chambers of the heart and great vessels. *AO,* Aorta; *IVC,* inferior vena cava; *LA,* left atrium; *LV,* left ventricle; *PA,* pulmonary artery; *RA,* right atrium; *RV,* right ventricle; *SVC,* superior vena cava.

TABLE 10-2 Normal Values for Arterial and Mixed Venous Blood Gases

Component	Arterial	Mixed Venous
PH	7.35-7.45	7.30-7.37
P_{O_2} (mm Hg)	80-100	36-42
P_{CO_2} (mm Hg)	35-45	42-46
%Saturation	92-100	60-80
HCO_3^- (mEq/L)	22-26	24-28
Base excess (mEq/L)	−2 to +2	

INTERPRETATION OF MIXED VENOUS BLOOD GAS VALUES

Mixed venous blood samples are primarily used to determine the adequacy of tissue oxygenation in relation to tissue oxygen demand. The heart and lungs work together to deliver oxygenated blood to the tissues. At the tissue level, oxygen is normally consumed at a relatively constant rate. This relatively constant rate of consumption is maintained by a tissue extraction of approximately 25% of the oxygen delivered. If cardiac output falls, or if it fails to increase when arterial oxygen saturation decreases, then more than 25% of delivered oxygen has to be extracted to maintain a constant rate of tissue oxygen consumption ($\dot{V}_{O_2}$). Therefore, $P\bar{v}_{O_2}$ and $S\bar{v}_{O_2}$ values lower than normal, less than 35 mm Hg and less than 60%, respectively, are indicative of oxygen delivery that is inadequate in relation to oxygen demand. $P\bar{v}_{O_2}$ values less than 30 mm Hg are usually associated with lactate formation, an indication that tissue oxygenation is reaching critical levels and anaerobic metabolic pathways are being utilized. The clinician must then determine whether the oxygen delivery problem is cardiac or pulmonary in origin by systematically evaluating the adequacy of arterial oxygenation, hemoglobin, and cardiac output (heart rate, preload, afterload, and contractility).

$P\bar{v}_{O_2}$ and $S\bar{v}_{O_2}$ values that are higher than normal do not necessarily mean that tissue oxygenation is adequate. In fact, tissue hypoxia may be severe because of impaired *tissue utilization* of oxygen, as in severe sepsis. Therefore, the monitoring of $P\bar{v}_{O_2}$ and $S\bar{v}_{O_2}$ alone may be inadequate in complex critical illness, and more sophisticated indexes of tissue oxygenation may be necessary to complete the picture. These concepts are expanded further in subsequent sections.

Mixed venous blood gas values may also be utilized to evaluate whether an atrial or ventricular septal defect is present. When these clinical conditions are present, arterial blood from the higher-pressure left side of the heart combines with blood in the right side of the heart, resulting in higher than normal values for mixed venous oxygen saturation. As a standard PA catheter is passed, blood samples are obtained from the right atrium (RA), right ventricle (RV), and pulmonary arteries. As the fiberoptic $S\bar{v}_{O_2}$ PA catheter is passed, venous blood saturation in each chamber of the heart is recorded. An abnormal increase in mixed venous oxygen saturation as the catheter is passed into the RA or RV (abnormal "step-up") indicates a patent defect.

CONTINUOUS MONITORING OF MIXED VENOUS OXYGEN SATURATION

Mixed venous oxygen saturation ($S\bar{v}O_2$) is the flow-weighted average of the saturation of venous effluents from all of the body's perfused vascular beds. It does not reflect perfusion of any one organ, but rather reflects the balance of oxygen supply to oxygen demand within the entire organism. It is a cardiopulmonary variable, utilized to determine the adequacy of tissue oxygenation. $S\bar{v}O_2$ may be continuously monitored through the use of a fiberoptic PA catheter. The catheter does not provide any additional information about tissue oxygenation than the intermittent mixed venous blood sample does; however, continuous $S\bar{v}O_2$ monitoring provides real-time data reflecting the often ever-changing status of the critically ill adult.

Components of an $S\bar{v}O_2$ Monitoring System

The three components of an $S\bar{v}O_2$ monitoring system are the fiberoptic PA catheter, the optical module, and an accompanying monitor. The fiberoptic PA catheter uses the principles of reflectance spectrophotometry to determine $S\bar{v}O_2$ (Fig. 10-14).

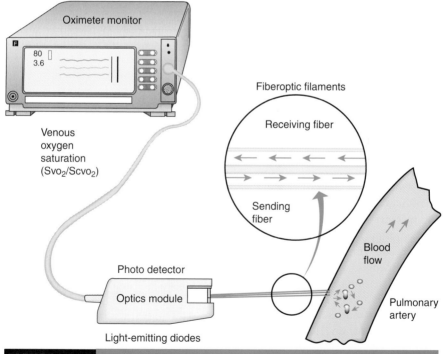

FIGURE 10-14

Principles of reflectance spectrophotometry. Fiberoptics transmit two or three wavelengths of light from light-emitting diodes. Another fiberoptic bundle sends information back to the photodetector about the amount of light reflected by the oxygenated and deoxygenated hemoglobin. The microprocessor then calculates the percentage of hemoglobin saturated with oxygen. *(Courtesy Edwards Lifesciences, Irvine, Calif.)*

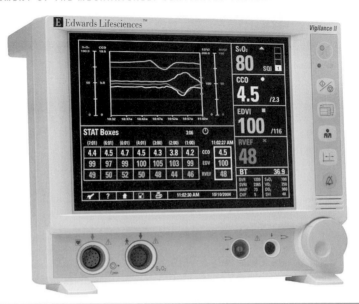

FIGURE 10-15

Microprocessor-based monitor that derives and reports continuous S$\bar{v}$O$_2$. Multiple hemodynamic parameters are also provided. *(Courtesy Edwards Lifesciences, Irvine, Calif.)*

Multiple wavelengths of light from LEDs in the optical module are transmitted into the PA blood through fiberoptic bundles. The amount of light reflected by oxygenated versus deoxygenated blood is carried back to a photodetector in the optical module via another fiberoptic filament. The microprocessor-based monitor then derives the oxyhemoglobin saturation by evaluating the ratio of transmitted to reflected light (Fig. 10-15). In addition to containing fiberoptics, the S$\bar{v}$O$_2$ PA catheter has PA and RA lumens for pressure readings, sampling, or infusion; a thermistor for measuring core body temperature and for thermodilution measurement of cardiac output; and a balloon lumen for measuring pulmonary capillary wedge pressure (PCWP). In addition, some catheters have the ability to perform continuous measurements of cardiac output and right ventricular volume measurements.

The microprocessor monitor continuously displays the S$\bar{v}$O$_2$ value and is capable of providing a trend graph of data during various time frames. Some monitors are capable of providing a printout of the trend data. Visual and audible alarms are available for low and high S$\bar{v}$O$_2$ values, with some systems providing additional alarm messages. The monitor also provides a display of intensity of the reflected light signal, which serves as a source of information about catheter position and system integrity and therefore about the accuracy of the reported S$\bar{v}$O$_2$ value. Light intensity problems should be corrected before the reported S$\bar{v}$O$_2$ value is accepted or calibration procedures are performed (Table 10-3). Accuracy is also determined by proper system calibration. There are two calibration methods: preinsertion and

| TABLE 10-3 | Troubleshooting Continuous $S\bar{v}O_2$ Monitoring Light Intensity Problems |

Problem	Potential Cause	Check and Adjust
High intensity	Catheter tip may be against vessel wall.	Check PA (pulmonary artery) pressure waveform for catheter position. Reposition catheter if it appears to be wedged. To move tip away from vessel wall, inflate balloon, flush catheter (with balloon down), or twist the catheter a quarter turn.
Low intensity	Loose connection at optical module, kink in catheter, clot at catheter tip, or break in fiberoptics may have occurred.	Secure connection between optical module and PA catheter. Straighten out any kinks. Ensure that distal lumen is patent by first aspirating blood to remove any clot and then flushing catheter. If fiberoptics are broken, catheter will have to be replaced.
Dampened or erratic intensity	Catheter has floated out too far or is in a wedged position, or clot is forming on the tip.	Check PA waveform for catheter position; reposition as necessary. Ensure that balloon is completely deflated. Ensure that distal lumen is patent by first aspirating blood to remove any clot and then gently flushing catheter. (Do not flush until catheter is pulled back from the wedge position.)

in vivo. Preinsertion calibration is performed to an optical reference and should always be performed. In vivo calibration should be performed if preinsertion calibration was inadvertently omitted, there is reason to suspect the oxygen saturation reading is incorrect, system integrity was disrupted, or at least every 24 hours.

Indications for Using Continuous $S\bar{v}O_2$ Monitoring

Monitoring of $S\bar{v}O_2$ is useful in that it provides an early warning of cardiopulmonary insufficiency, often before changes in the patient's hemodynamic status become evident. Interventions designed to achieve optimal tissue oxygen delivery or to decrease tissue oxygen demand can then be initiated before impairment in tissue oxygenation occurs. $S\bar{v}O_2$ monitoring is also useful as a patient management tool to monitor the effects of various interventions designed to increase tissue oxygen delivery or decrease tissue oxygen demand, such as volume loading, titration of vasoactive agents, or administration of sedation. Furthermore, cardiorespiratory tolerance of routine care such as positioning and various treatments (e.g., suctioning, turning, chest physiotherapy) can be assessed on a real-time basis so the plan of care can be altered immediately if necessary.

Despite the benefit of providing continuous insight into the patient's tissue oxygenation status, continuous $S\bar{v}O_2$ monitoring is not indicated in all critically ill patients. The risk/benefit ratio for invasive monitoring and the high cost associated with $S\bar{v}O_2$ monitoring must be factored into the decision to use this technology. In general, if it is anticipated that mixed venous blood gases will be drawn several times a day for evaluation of tissue oxygenation, the use of an $S\bar{v}O_2$ catheter may be cost effective. Each institution should develop indications for use of continuous $S\bar{v}O_2$ monitoring on the basis of its patient population. The following are examples of types of patients who may benefit from continuous $S\bar{v}O_2$ monitoring:

- Patients with severely compromised pulmonary function who require high levels of ventilatory support (e.g., more than 10 cm H_2O PEEP, FIO_2 >0.6) or who are undergoing modes of ventilation known to affect tissue oxygen delivery, such as pressure-control inverse inspiratory-to-expiratory (I:E) ratio ventilation
- Patients with severely compromised cardiac function, such as hemodynamically unstable patients receiving multiple vasopressor/inotropic agents or frequent titration or high doses of such agents, and patients undergoing massive volume resuscitation
- Patients with multiple organ dysfunction syndrome (MODS)
- Patients with systemic inflammatory response syndrome (SIRS), with sepsis, or in whom sepsis is suspected

Interpreting Changes in $S\bar{v}O_2$

NORMAL $S\bar{v}O_2$

The heart and lungs work together to deliver adequate, well-oxygenated blood to the tissues. Normal arterial oxygen saturation (SaO_2) is 95% to 100%, and normal $S\bar{v}O_2$ is 75%. These values indicate that 25% of all oxygen delivered is used by the tissues to maintain a constant state of $\dot{V}O_2$ via aerobic metabolic pathways (Fig. 10-16). Because 75% of the hemoglobin returning to the right side of the heart is still saturated with oxygen, some oxygen reserve is available for times of increased need, such as during

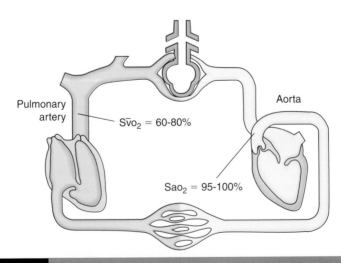

Pulmonary artery

Aorta

$S\bar{v}O_2 = 60\text{-}80\%$

$SaO_2 = 95\text{-}100\%$

FIGURE 10-16

Normal arterial and mixed venous blood oxygen saturations. Normally 25% of the available oxygen is used by the tissues, leaving an oxygen reserve for times of increased demand or physiologic stress. *(Courtesy Edwards Lifesciences, Irvine, Calif.)*

increased patient activity, episodes of fever, or administration of treatments such as suctioning or bathing.

The $S\overline{v}O_2$ value can be used as an indicator of available oxygen reserve. It is important to note that some tissue beds, such as the brain and heart, utilize more oxygen than others; the result is a much lower $S\overline{v}O_2$ value for these specific organs and therefore little oxygen reserve. Because present technology does not allow for monitoring the $S\overline{v}O_2$ of specific organs, we must rely on the $S\overline{v}O_2$ value, which reflects total body tissue utilization of oxygen, for clinical decision making about the adequacy of tissue oxygenation. An $S\overline{v}O_2$ greater than 65% indicates adequate reserve; 50% to 65%, limited reserve; 35% to 50%, inadequate reserve; and less than 35%, inadequate tissue oxygenation.

Prerequisite knowledge to an interpretation of a lower-than-normal $S\overline{v}O_2$ value (less than 60%) is an understanding of how the body responds when tissue oxygen needs exceed oxygen supply. Initially, tissue P_{O_2} will fall, resulting in a widened diffusion gradient between tissue and capillary, and promoting oxygen diffusion out of the capillary and into tissue. The falling Pa_{O_2} then prompts hemoglobin to begin unloading more oxygen. The increased use of oxygen by tissues is termed *increased extraction* or *increased utilization*. Its purpose is to maintain a level of $\dot{V}O_2$ that can maintain metabolic processes aerobically. An increase in the acidic chemical byproduct of aerobic metabolism, carbon dioxide (or lactate with anaerobic metabolism), stimulates chemoreceptors in the central nervous system to prompt a higher cardiac output (CO). This higher CO is mediated through the sympathetic nervous system. The goal is to deliver more oxygen to meet the increased demand. If the CO delivers enough oxygen each minute, an adequate capillary P_{O_2} is ensured and normal diffusion gradients are maintained. If the CO is not sufficient to deliver enough oxygen each minute, capillary P_{O_2} falls, prompting hemoglobin to unload more oxygen and leaving a lower-than-normal $S\overline{v}O_2$ (Fig. 10-17). Hence, a decreased $S\overline{v}O_2$ means that oxygen demand has exceeded the supply.

DECREASED $S\overline{v}O_2$

When a *decreased* $S\overline{v}O_2$ (<60%) is detected, the clinician must differentially determine, in a systematic fashion, whether the problem is cardiac or pulmonary in origin. If a pulse oximeter is in use, a quick look at the Sa_{O_2} will rule out a pulmonary cause for a decrease in tissue oxygen delivery. If the Sa_{O_2} is low, potential causes include a change in the underlying lung condition or a technical problem with the ventilator system, such as disconnection, loss of tidal volume or PEEP, or inaccurate setting of $F_{I_{O_2}}$. If the pulmonary system is ruled out as the cause of inadequate oxygen transport, the cardiac system is systematically evaluated. If the CO is low, analysis of the components of the CO—heart rate and stroke volume, specifically, preload, afterload, and contractility—will determine the cause of the low CO and necessary corrective action.

The low $S\overline{v}O_2$ state must be corrected or the body will convert to utilization of the much less efficient anaerobic metabolic pathways, resulting in lactic acid production. Metabolic acidosis will develop, and variable amounts of tissue ischemia will occur. What tissue beds in the body will experience hypoxia depends on the vulnerability of specific organs in regard to their need for oxygen.

Oxygen Balance

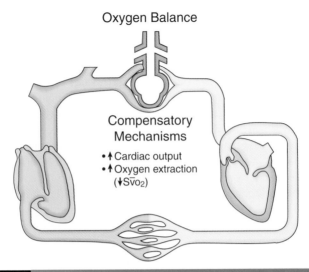

Compensatory
Mechanisms

- ↑ Cardiac output
- ↑ Oxygen extraction
  ($↓S\bar{v}o_2$)

FIGURE 10-17

The body utilizes two fundamental compensatory mechanisms in response to inadequate oxygen supply. The first one is to increase the cardiac output. The second is to increase the amount of oxygen extracted from the blood. *(Courtesy Edwards Lifesciences, Irvine, Calif.)*

Simultaneously to implementing interventions designed to achieve optimal tissue oxygen delivery, efforts should be made to decrease tissue oxygen demand, thereby balancing supply to demand. Factors that increase oxygen demand are those that increase the metabolic rate, such as fever, agitation, activity, pain, and seizures.

INCREASED $S\bar{v}o_2$

An *increased* $S\bar{v}o_2$, more than 80%, generally indicates an increased oxygen supply, a decreased demand for oxygen at the tissue level, or an inability of the tissues to utilize oxygen. Increased oxygen supply can occur with an increase in Sao_2, Pao_2, CO, or hemoglobin. Decreased tissue demand for oxygen occurs with conditions that decrease the metabolic rate, such as hypothermia, anesthesia, heavy sedation, barbiturate coma, and sleep. The more common, and potentially clinically ominous, cause of an increased $S\bar{v}o_2$ is tissue inability to utilize oxygen.

Decreased oxygen utilization occurs when there is an increased affinity of hemoglobin for oxygen (left shift of the oxyhemoglobin dissociation curve) because the tissues are not being offered the oxygen they need. Decreased oxygen utilization also occurs in vasodilated states (e.g., sepsis, distributive shock) that lead to a maldistribution of blood flow at the capillary level. Perfusion of oxygen-rich blood is adequate in areas not needing it and inadequate in areas of need. Toxic effects at the tissue level (e.g., thiocyanate toxicity, endotoxemia in septic syndrome) can also lead to decreased oxygen utilization and an increased $S\bar{v}o_2$. Calculation of $\dot{V}o_2$ and the oxygen utilization ratio (see Direct and Derived Variables of Tissue Oxygenation

Obtained with the Pulmonary Artery Catheter, later) assists in differentiating the cause of a tissue oxygenation defect when it is not apparent with the $S\overline{v}O_2$ alone and the patient has a complex critical illness.

Dual Oximetry

The simultaneous use of pulse oximetry and continuous $S\overline{v}O_2$ monitoring is termed *dual oximetry*. The main advantage of dual oximetry is that when a change in $S\overline{v}O_2$ occurs, the contribution of the pulmonary system to that change can be immediately, objectively evaluated and not speculated on or delayed while an ABG is obtained.

Dual oximetry can also be used to calculate the oxygen extraction index (O_2EI) and the intrapulmonary shunt. The O_2EI appears to be valid at an SpO_2 reading of 90% or greater. It is calculated as follows:

$$O_2EI = \frac{SpO_2 - S\overline{v}O_2}{SpO_2}$$

See the following section for interpretation of the oxygen extraction variable.

Calculation of the intrapulmonary shunt by dual oximetry may allow for continuous evaluation of pulmonary function during the titration of PEEP in a most cost-effective manner because multiple blood gas analyses may be eliminated. When the trend for intrapulmonary shunt is plotted by dual oximetry, the value is referred to as the ventilation perfusion index ($\dot{V}\dot{Q}I$). It is calculated as follows:

$$\dot{V}\dot{Q}I = \frac{1 - SpO_2}{1 - S\overline{v}O_2}$$

Even without performing calculations, dual oximetry provides immediately useful data regarding whether changes in $S\overline{v}O_2$ are caused by changes in cardiac performance or lung function. When the $S\overline{v}O_2$ decreases, a concurrent decrease in the SpO_2 indicates a defect in the pulmonary component of oxygen transport, whereas a stable SpO_2 indicates increased oxygen extraction, probably because of a decrease in cardiac performance.

CENTRAL VENOUS OXYGEN SATURATION

Central venous oxygen saturation ($ScvO_2$) is measured by a new technology using a modified central venous catheter with fiberoptic technology. $ScvO_2$ is a global indicator of balance between oxygen supply and demand that trends with $S\overline{v}O_2$. The normal value for $ScvO_2$ is more than 70%. $ScvO_2$ when compared to $S\overline{v}O_2$ is consistently higher by 5% to 18%, with an average of 7.5% in shock states. An $ScvO_2$ of 70% implies that the $S\overline{v}O_2$ is likely 60% to 65%. The central venous oximetric catheter is advocated as a surrogate for $S\overline{v}O_2$. Its use circumvents the need for flotation of a PA catheter, thereby increasing the in-hospital locations where a global tissue oxygenation parameter can be attained. For example, insertion of a PA catheter to attain $S\overline{v}O_2$ is not standard practice in the emergency department or on a nursing unit outside of the ICU, whereas insertion of a central venous catheter to obtain $ScvO_2$ is more easily performed in these areas. More studies are needed to determine the clinical implications and limitations of $ScvO_2$ and whether the value parallels other markers of tissue oxygenation such as serum lactate or base deficit.

DIRECT AND DERIVED VARIABLES OF TISSUE OXYGENATION OBTAINED WITH THE PULMONARY ARTERY CATHETER

Respiration has both external and internal components. External respiration is the movement of gases into and out of the lung and includes the exchange of gases at the alveolar-capillary membrane. Internal respiration is the exchange of gases between the capillaries and the cells of the body, the ultimate respiratory units. Internal respiration, also known as tissue oxygenation, is the focus of this section.

The primary goal of internal respiration is to maintain aerobic metabolism because the oxidative metabolic pathways are the most efficient method of energy production. At the cellular level within the mitochondria (the energy factories of the cell), oxygen is consumed to produce energy in the form of adenosine triphosphate (ATP). The production of ATP occurs in the citric acid (Krebs) cycle. Aerobic oxidation ceases, however, if the amount of oxygen transported to the cells falls to a critical level.

Hypoxia is a state of inadequate oxygen at the tissue level. When hypoxia is present, energy production continues because anaerobic glycolysis takes over; however, energy production then becomes much less efficient (Fig. 10-18). The byproduct of anaerobic metabolism, lactic acid, begins to rise, creating a base deficit or metabolic acidosis. Therefore, the patient's serum lactate level and pH are among the assessment parameters that may be used as indicators of the adequacy of tissue oxygenation (see section on serum lactate, later).

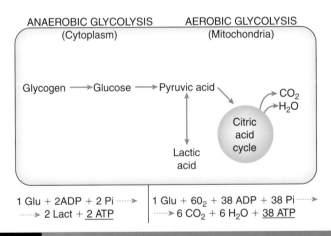

ANAEROBIC GLYCOLYSIS
(Cytoplasm)

AEROBIC GLYCOLYSIS
(Mitochondria)

Glycogen → Glucose → Pyruvic acid → Citric acid cycle → CO_2 → H_2O

Lactic acid

1 Glu + 2ADP + 2 Pi → 2 Lact + 2 ATP

$1 \text{ Glu} + 6O_2 + 38 \text{ ADP} + 38 \text{ Pi} \rightarrow 6 CO_2 + 6 H_2O + \underline{38 \text{ ATP}}$

FIGURE 10-18

Glucose metabolism in the presence, or relative absence, of oxygen. Anaerobic glycolysis is much less efficient than aerobic glycolysis, creating significantly fewer high-energy phosphate bonds and lactic acid as a metabolic byproduct. *(Modified from Mizock BA, Falk JL. Lactic acidosis in critical illness. Crit Care Med 1992; 20[2]:80–93.)*

Hypermetabolic and Hyperdynamic Response to Critical Illness

Recovery from critical illness requires a complex series of hemodynamic, metabolic, and immunologic adjustments. These adjustments provide the substrates needed to meet the body's high energy requirements for general maintenance of bodily functions, healing, immune system function, and so forth. During times of increased demand, large supplies of oxygen and substrates must be delivered to the cells for production of ATP via the oxidative pathways.

The body's response to the provoking stimuli of critical illness—such as surgery, trauma, fear, pain, inflammatory responses, wound healing, and infection—are mediated through the autonomic nervous system. Sympathetic nervous system stimulation results in an outpouring of catecholamines that increase ventilation, the amount of oxygen available in the blood, and the CO. These actions increase the delivery of available oxygen and thus the transport of oxygen to the tissues. Many hormonal processes are also called into play both to increase blood volume through the conservation of water and sodium and to stimulate the release of substrates, such as glucose, needed for growth and energy production. The goal of the body in activating all of its compensatory mechanisms is to maintain adequate tissue oxygenation. Soon after injury, the tissues have large oxygen demands because of the stress imposed by critical illness, a hypermetabolic state ensues, and the body develops a hyperdynamic response to meet the high oxygen demands.

The clinical goal for the practitioner is to support the process going on in the body and to augment it as needed when the patient's cardiopulmonary function limits the ability to mount a response sufficient to support the tissues. A prerequisite to appropriate patient intervention is an understanding of oxygen transport in the body and the ability to interpret tissue oxygenation variables.

Principle of Oxygen Supply and Demand

Formulating an understanding of oxygenation in terms of the principle of supply and demand provides a framework for the practitioner approaching the critically ill patient to determine the adequacy of tissue oxygenation. This framework also serves as a systematic way to determine which therapeutic measures should be taken to correct a state of inadequate tissue oxygenation.

COMPENSATORY RESPONSES TO INCREASED TISSUE OXYGEN DEMAND

A balance is ideally maintained between oxygen supply and oxygen demand in the body (Fig. 10-19). Both supply and demand can be monitored by objective measures of oxygen delivery (Do_2) and oxygen consumption ($\dot{V}o_2$), respectively. In response to increased oxygen demand by the tissues, the body activates compensatory responses mediated through the sympathetic nervous system. First, attempts to increase the oxygen supply, which include increasing the CO and increasing ventilation, are put into play. If attempts to increase the oxygen supply are unsatisfactory, the body then extracts a greater percentage of the available oxygen from the blood (see Fig. 10-17).

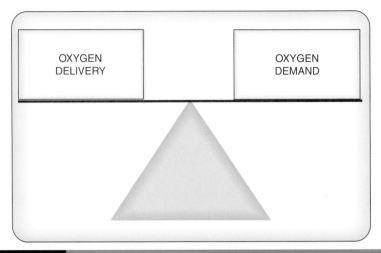

FIGURE 10-19

The primary function of the cardiopulmonary system is to provide an adequate supply of well-oxygenated blood to the tissues to meet tissue oxygen demand. The balance between oxygen delivery and oxygen demand can be monitored in the clinical setting with physiologic variables of oxygen transport and tissue oxygen utilization. *(Courtesy Edwards Lifesciences, Irvine, Calif.)*

This results in less oxygen return to the heart in the venous blood, as evidenced by a decrease in $P\bar{v}O_2$ and $S\bar{v}O_2$ mixed venous blood gas values. These decreased values indicate diminished oxygen reserves.

When DO_2 is inadequate, variable amounts of tissue injury occur, depending on the vulnerability of the tissues to hypoxia. Tissue hypoxia translates into cellular dysfunction when aerobic sources of energy fall below the level required by the metabolic processes of those tissues. Tissues at greatest risk are the central nervous system and the myocardium because these tissues use more oxygen than others in their resting state. When these vulnerable tissues must draw on reserve oxygen, little is available. Conversely, some tissues tolerate hypoxia better than others. In general, it depends on the metabolic activity level of the cells. Each organ that suffers cell death from hypoxia manifests its pathologic changes on the basis of the loss of the normal physiologic functions of that organ. Progressive damage, manifested by MODS, is extremely significant to patient outcome.

OXYGEN DEBT

The fact that the body is utilizing its oxygen reserves in an effort to meet tissue oxygen demand is an excellent compensatory response. However, because oxygen cannot be stored by the body for times of increased need, when demand continues to exceed supply, anaerobic metabolism ensues, lactic acid accumulates, and an actual oxygen debt accrues. The oxygen debt is the difference, with time, between the oxygen demand and the actual $\dot{V}O_2$ (Fig. 10-20). The debt will continue to grow if $\dot{V}O_2$ is

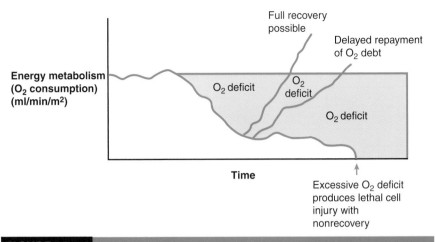

FIGURE 10-20

Oxygen debt (see text for discussion). *(Modified from Omert L.: Hemodynamic management. Crit Care Rep 1990; 1[3]:376.)*

limited by Do_2. If the oxygen supply is restored and the oxygen debt repaid before there is critical injury to tissue, then it is possible to preserve organ function. However, if the period of ischemia is prolonged, irreversible damage will result.

OXYGEN DELIVERY (Do_2): SUPPLY

The assessment of the patient begins with this question: Is adequate oxygen being delivered to the tissues? The amount of oxygen delivered to the tissues per minute depends on blood flow, CO or cardiac index (CI), and the oxygen content of the arterial blood (Cao_2) (Fig. 10-21). Therefore:

$$O_2 \text{ Delivery } Do_2 = CO \times Cao_2 \times 10$$
$$\text{Normal } Do_2 = 1000 \text{ mL } O_2/\text{min}$$

CO is the major determinant of Do_2. The CO occurs in response to metabolic demands, and individuals with an intact cardiovascular compensatory response to arterial desaturation or anemia will maintain Do_2. If the patient cannot mount a sufficient response because of new or preexisting myocardial dysfunction, then Do_2 falls. The clinician must then intervene to assist in augmenting the CO to maintain Do_2.

A systematic examination of oxygen supply requires a Cao_2 assessment, which requires an understanding of the components of Cao_2. The oxygen content is the actual amount of oxygen in the blood. Oxygen is carried in the arterial blood in two ways (Fig. 10-22): dissolved in the serum, which is assessed with the Pao_2, and in combination with hemoglobin (Hb), which is assessed with the Sao_2 (or the Spo_2 when measured with a pulse oximeter).

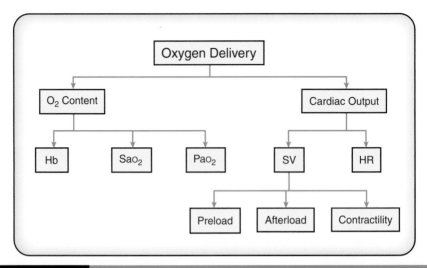

FIGURE 10-21

Oxygen delivery (Do_2) is determined by the adequacy of blood flow and the oxygen content of the blood. When optimizing Do_2 in the clinical setting, a systematic assessment of the pulmonary (Hb, Sao_2, Pao_2) and cardiac (SV, HR) aspects of delivery differentiates where therapeutic interventions will best be targeted. *Hb*, Hemoglobin; *HR*, heart rate; *SV*, stroke volume. *(Courtesy Edwards Lifesciences, Irvine, Calif.)*

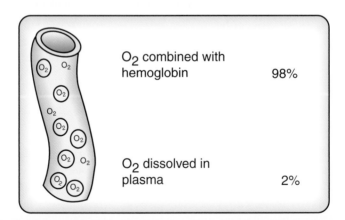

FIGURE 10-22

The majority of oxygen in the blood (98%) is carried in combination with hemoglobin and is assessed with the Sao_2. Only 2% to 3% is carried dissolved in the plasma. Dissolved oxygen is assessed with the Pao_2. *(Courtesy Edwards Lifesciences, Irvine, Calif.)*

The oxygen dissolved in the serum accounts for only 2% to 3% of the total oxygen transported in the blood: 0.0031 mL of oxygen per 1 mm Hg per 100 mL blood. Clearly, the PaO_2 provides information regarding only a very small part of the total CaO_2. If oxygen was carried in the blood only in this way, then the CO would have to be almost 160 L/min to deliver enough oxygen to the tissues to meet resting metabolic needs! The oxygen carried in combination with Hb accounts for 97% to 98% of transported oxygen. A total of 1.34 mL of oxygen is carried in combination with Hb per 100 mL of blood. Hb is therefore an important assessment factor because it plays a major role in the oxygen-carrying capacity of the blood. The relationship between Hb and oxygen is illustrated in the oxyhemoglobin dissociation curve (see Chapter 2).

Knowing how the blood carries oxygen and how to calculate the amount of oxygen carried by each method, the CaO_2 can be calculated as follows:

$$CaO_2 = (Hb \times 1.34 \times SaO_2) + (PaO_2 \times 0.0031)$$
$$\text{Normal } CaO_2 = 19 - 20 \text{ mL of } O_2 \text{ per dL of blood}$$

It should be evident from the previous discussion that Hb and SaO_2 are the primary determinants of CaO_2. If either of these components decreases, a compensatory increase in CO would be required if DO_2 was to remain adequate.

The oxygen content of the mixed venous blood, the $C\bar{v}O_2$, can also be calculated and then used in the computation of additional tissue oxygenation variables. For example, the difference between the oxygen contents of arterial and venous blood is used to determine *tissue utilization* of oxygen. The $C\bar{v}O_2$ value is calculated as follows:

$$C\bar{v}O_2 = (Hb \times 1.34 \times S\bar{v}O_2) + (P\bar{v}O_2 \times 0.0031)$$
$$\text{Normal } C\bar{v}O_2 = 14 - 15 \text{ mL of } O_2 \text{ per deciliter of blood}$$

OXYGEN CONSUMPTION ($\dot{V}O_2$): DEMAND

The most meaningful overall measurement of cellular metabolism is $\dot{V}O_2$. The $\dot{V}O_2$, the amount of oxygen consumed by the body per minute, represents the total of all oxidative metabolism. The amount of oxygen needed is determined by the metabolic rate. $\dot{V}O_2$ is calculated as follows:

$$\dot{V}O_2 = CO \times (CaO_2 - C\bar{v}O_2) \times 10$$
$$\text{Normal } \dot{V}O_2 = 200 - 250 \text{ mL of } O_2 \text{ per minute}$$

Flow-Dependent Oxygen Consumption

Under normal physiologic conditions, $\dot{V}O_2$ is independent of DO_2 (flow) and is maintained over wide variations in DO_2 because of the oxygen reserve in the blood. As delivery declines, $\dot{V}O_2$ is preserved through the activation of compensatory mechanisms, such as an increase in oxygen extraction. If delivery continues to fall, however, a point is reached where the ability to increase extraction further is exhausted. This point is termed the *critical delivery threshold* (Fig. 10-23). Below this threshold the ability of the tissues to consume oxygen depends on the flow of well-oxygenated

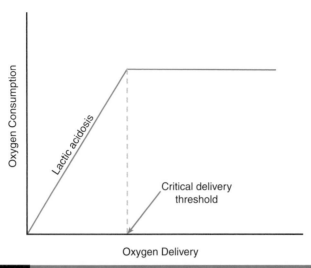

FIGURE 10-23

The relationship between oxygen delivery (Do_2) and oxygen consumption ($\dot{V}o_2$). The nonlinear response to decreases in oxygen supply is called oxygen regulation and is a normal physiologic phenomenon in humans. The plateau portion of the curve represents the supply independent region where ($\dot{V}o_2$) is maintained over a wide range of Do_2 as a result of vascular adaptations. Below the critical delivery threshold, ($\dot{V}o_2$) becomes dependent on Do_2 (flow-dependent oxygen consumption), the tissues must resort to anaerobic sources of energy production, and lactic acid ensues. See text for discussion. *(Modified from Mizock BA, Falk JL. Lactic acidosis in critical illness. Crit Care Med 1992; 20[2]:80–93.)*

blood. $\dot{V}o_2$ limited by Do_2 is known as flow-dependent, or supply-dependent, $\dot{V}o_2$; that is, the rate of oxygen consumed is limited by the rate of oxygen delivered to the tissues. In the supply-dependent region, as $\dot{V}o_2$ declines, anaerobic metabolism increases because $\dot{V}o_2$ no longer meets cellular energy requirements.

In the clinical setting, simultaneous increases in Do_2 and $\dot{V}o_2$ may indicate that a state of flow dependency is present and also provides useful information about the body's ability to further increase its $\dot{V}o_2$. Increases in Do_2 and $\dot{V}o_2$, but not in $S\bar{v}o_2$, indicate that tissue oxygen debt repayment is occurring. The $S\bar{v}o_2$ will not increase to normal values until the oxygen debt is repaid.

Causes of Abnormal $\dot{V}o_2$

LOW $\dot{V}o_2$

Potential causes of low $\dot{V}o_2$ include the following:

1. Inadequate delivery of oxygen. A state of flow- or supply-dependent $\dot{V}o_2$ (see previous section) may be present, commonly caused by a low CO state. Another example would be the early stage of hypovolemic or cardiogenic shock, in which sympathetic nervous system stimulation causes intense vasoconstriction in an effort to maintain blood pressure and venous return of blood to the heart.

Capillary perfusion is restricted, limiting the delivery of oxygen to some tissue beds in need of oxygen.

2. Tissue inability to utilize oxygen because of a defect in normal cellular metabolism. This may occur with thiocyanate toxicity (which may develop when high doses of sodium nitroprusside are used for a prolonged period) and sepsis-induced cytotoxic effects.

3. Maldistribution of capillary blood flow, primarily peripheral shunting of blood. In peripheral shunting of blood, the blood flows through capillary beds but no oxygen extraction occurs. For example, in sepsis, blood flow may be maldistributed to vasodilated areas and arterial-venous shunting occurs at the capillary level. In sepsis, oxygen extraction and consumption are reduced as a result of microcirculatory abnormalities caused by the presence of endotoxins or microemboli. Peripheral shunting also occurs with significant peripheral edema, which not only increases the diffusion distance for oxygen but may also impede capillary flow.

4. States that decrease $\dot{V}O_2$ because they decrease the metabolic rate. Examples include hypothermia, anesthesia, and use of paralytics.

HIGH $\dot{V}O_2$

Potential causes of high $\dot{V}O_2$ include the following:

1. States that increase $\dot{V}O_2$ because they increase the metabolic rate. Examples include the presence of fever, shivering, seizures, hyperthyroidism, healing, increased work of breathing (WOB), and patient care activities such as turning, chest physiotherapy (CPT), bathing, and suctioning.

2. Repayment of oxygen debt.

Relationship of $\dot{V}O_2$ to Survival

When $\dot{V}O_2$ is inadequate, an oxygen debt develops and various cells suffer ischemic damage depending on their vulnerability to hypoxia. Once the DO_2 improves, or the defect at the cellular level that is preventing oxygen extraction is corrected, $\dot{V}O_2$ exceeds the baseline demands for oxygen for a time. This excessive $\dot{V}O_2$ occurs to repay the oxygen debt and is a compensatory response with survival value. The increase in $\dot{V}O_2$ is a positive sign that the tissues are still able to use oxygen. Failure of the tissues to consume oxygen is an ominous sign that implies cellular defect and predicts a poor patient outcome. Inadequate cellular oxygenation results in MODS. Patients who present with MODS or who die have been shown to have had greater, and more prolonged, reduced or inadequate $\dot{V}O_2$ and a greater calculated oxygen debt than those who survive with or without organ failure. Therefore, the maintenance of optimal $\dot{V}O_2$ should be a high-priority therapeutic goal in the clinical setting.

TISSUE OXYGENATION VARIABLES

A firm understanding of oxygen supply-and-demand dynamics prepares the clinician to analyze tissue oxygenation variables further. After an answer is found to the question of whether oxygen delivery is adequate to meet tissue oxygen demand, the next assessment question becomes this: Is internal respiration adequate to maintain aerobic metabolism and prevent tissue hypoxia? Two variables, in addition to $\dot{V}O_2$ as previously described, are analyzed here in an attempt to answer this question: the arterial–mixed venous oxygen content difference (a-vDO$_2$) and the oxygen extraction ratio (O$_2$ER).

Arterial–Mixed Venous Oxygen Content Difference

The a-vDO$_2$ measures the degree of oxygen extraction by the tissues. It identifies the extent to which oxygen transport matches tissue oxygen demands. The a-vDO$_2$ is calculated as follows:

$$\text{a-vDO}_2 = \text{Cao}_2 - \text{C}\bar{\text{v}}\text{O}_2$$
$$\text{Normal a-vDO}_2 = 4\text{-}6 \text{ mL/dL}$$

Because the CO is the primary determinant of oxygen delivery, the a-vDO$_2$ has implications for flow and is often inversely proportional to the CO or CI. The following values, although not exact, are used for illustrative purposes:

a-vDO$_2$	Cardiac Index (CI)
>6	<2
<3	>5

HIGH a-vDO$_2$: MORE THAN 6 mL/dL

When the a-vDO$_2$ is high, the venous oxygen content is *decreased* because tissue oxygen extraction is increased. There is thus an inadequate supply of oxygen in relation to demand. Causes include the following:

1. Low flow states: decreased CO caused by problems with heart rate, preload, afterload, or contractility
2. Decreased arterial oxygen content caused by insufficient Hb or a defect in the pulmonary system resulting in a low Pao$_2$ or Sao$_2$
3. Increased oxygen demand because of fever, agitation, anxiety, pain, inflammatory processes, or healing; treatments such as weighing, bathing, or performing range-of-motion maneuvers; or interventions such as intubation, radiography, suctioning, or turning

LOW a-vDO$_2$: LESS THAN 4 mL/dL

When the a-vDO$_2$ is low, the venous oxygen content is *increased* because tissue oxygen extraction is decreased. There is poor utilization of oxygen. Potential causes include the following:

1. Tissues unable to utilize oxygen because of blockage of normal cellular metabolism, as may occur with thiocyanate toxicity or sepsis-induced cytotoxic effects.
2. Maldistribution of microcirculatory flow because of peripheral shunting of blood. In peripheral shunting of blood, the blood flows through capillary beds, but oxygen extraction does not occur. An example is in the stage of sepsis in which blood flow is redistributed to vasodilated areas, causing arterial-venous shunting to occur at the capillary level. In sepsis, oxygen extraction and consumption are reduced as a result of microcirculatory abnormalities caused by the presence of endotoxins or microemboli. Peripheral shunting also occurs with significant peripheral edema, which increases the diffusion distance for oxygen and impedes capillary flow.

3. Increased affinity of Hb for oxygen, that is, left shift of the oxyhemoglobin dissociation curve. This may occur with alkalosis, hypothermia, or administration of banked blood low in 2,3-DPG.
4. Error in mixed venous blood sampling. Aspirated blood is "arterialized" because the PA catheter is out too far or the sample was withdrawn too rapidly.
5. Oxygen delivery in excess of demand, such as when excessive supplemental oxygen is administered, hyperbaric oxygen therapy is given, or an induced high CO state is combined with a constant cellular demand.

Oxygen Extraction Ratio

The O_2ER is the percentage of oxygen delivered that is used by the tissues. This computation allows for the evaluation of the rate of $\dot{V}O_2$ normalized for the amount of oxygen transported. It is calculated as follows:

$$O_2ER = \frac{CaO_2 - C\bar{v}O_2}{CaO_2}$$

Normal range of O_2ER = 24%-28%

LOW OXYGEN EXTRACTION, OR UTILIZATION

Low oxygen extraction, or utilization, is an ominous sign, like low $\dot{V}O_2$, that may affect patient survival. The underlying defect needs to be identified and corrective action taken before cell death occurs. Causes of low oxygen extraction include the following:

1. Impaired ability of the tissues to utilize oxygen; blockage of normal cellular metabolism, as may occur with thiocyanate toxicity or microcirculatory abnormalities caused by sepsis.
2. Maldistribution of capillary blood flow, which may occur, for example, when doses of a vasopressor are used that result in intense vasoconstriction of some vascular beds. Because little or no blood flow is delivered to some areas, oxygen extraction cannot take place.
3. Increased affinity of Hb for oxygen, indicated by a left shift of the oxyhemoglobin dissociation curve. This may occur with alkalosis, hypothermia, or administration of banked blood low in 2,3-DPG.

HIGH OXYGEN EXTRACTION, OR UTILIZATION

High oxygen extraction indicates there is inadequate delivery in response to demand, and therefore the tissues are compensating by extracting more of the available oxygen in an attempt to maintain adequate consumption. Delivery needs to be improved so that tissues do not continue to utilize oxygen reserves.

Causes of high O_2ER may include the following:

1. Low hemoglobin concentration
2. Low PaO_2 or SaO_2 because of a pulmonary condition, such as acute respiratory distress syndrome (ARDS), pulmonary edema, an infiltrative-consolidative process, or pulmonary contusion; inappropriate ventilator settings; or technical problem with the patient-ventilator interface
3. Low CO because of a heart rate, preload, afterload, or contractility problem

Serum Lactate Concentration

A unifying factor in critically ill patients with inadequate tissue perfusion, whether it is caused by hypovolemic, cardiogenic, or distributive shock, is lactic acidosis. Serum lactate levels increase with anaerobic metabolism and are considered the clinical gold standard as a marker of inadequate cellular oxygenation. Lactate levels may also increase in a variety of other conditions. Lactic acidosis is therefore classified as either type A (clinical evidence of tissue hypoxia) or type B (no clinical evidence of tissue hypoxia). Examples of causes of type B lactic acidosis include liver disease, malignancy, diabetes mellitus, drugs or toxins such as ethanol or salicylates, and inborn errors of metabolism. This section focuses on type A lactic acidosis, resulting from an imbalance of oxygen supply and demand.

Lactate is primarily metabolized by the liver. The normal amount of lactate produced under aerobic conditions is generally sufficiently managed by the liver. Therefore, under the conditions of aerobic metabolism and good liver function, there is no significant accumulation of lactate in the blood. Under anaerobic conditions, however, the amount of lactate produced exceeds the liver's ability to metabolize it, resulting in a metabolic acidosis. The patient's baseline liver function also affects the efficiency of lactate clearance and should be taken into consideration when lactate levels are interpreted.

Confirmation of a state of inadequate tissue perfusion is assisted by obtaining a baseline lactate level drawn at the same time, or even before, the initial cardio-pulmonary profile is obtained. The amount of lactate gives an indication of the severity of oxygen debt. Serial lactate levels monitored with time are then useful to determine the effectiveness of resuscitative therapies. Ideally, a steady decrease in the lactate level should be seen. If not, then the therapeutic plan should be reevaluated systematically for ways to further increase Do_2 and decrease oxygen demand. Serial evaluation of the patient's pH and base deficit may also serve as indicators of the adequacy of tissue perfusion.

Base Deficit

The base deficit is a variable calculated from the ABG and is generally reported with the rest of the ABG results. Base deficit is defined as the amount of base, such as bicarbonate, required to titrate a liter of whole blood to a pH of 7.4 when the sample is fully saturated with oxygen at normal body temperature and a $Paco_2$ of 40 mm Hg. The normal value of base deficit is +2 to −2 mmol. The base deficit provides an estimate of acidosis and correlates fairly well with lactate. Severely abnormal base deficits at the time of ICU admission are correlated with ICU mortality. The base deficit, a sensitive measure of tissue resuscitation in trauma patients, is used as an endpoint in resuscitation in many trauma centers. It has the advantages of being easily measured and available to many ICUs with an ABG analyzer.

Several factors besides the adequacy of tissue oxygenation can affect the base deficit value. Conditions that result in an acidosis unrelated to perfusion defect also cause an increased base deficit. Examples are similar to causes of type B lactic

TABLE 10-4 Oxygen Transport and Oxygen Utilization Variables

Variable	Measurement or Calculation	Normal Value
Cardiac output (CO)	Direct measurement	4-8 L/min
Cardiac index (CI)	$\dfrac{CO}{\text{Body surface area}}$	2.5-4.0 L/min
Arterial O_2 content (Cao_2)	$Cao_2 = (Hb \times 1.34 \times Sao_2 + (Pao_2 \times 0.0031)$	19-20 mL O_2 per dL blood
Venous O_2 content ($C\bar{v}o_2$)	$C\bar{v}o_2 = (Hb \times 1.34 \times S\bar{v}o_2) + (P\bar{v}o_2 \times 0.0031)$	14-15 mL O_2 per dL blood
O_2 delivery (Do_2)	$Do_2 = Cao_2 \times CO \times 10$	1000 mL/min
O_2 delivery index	$Do_2 = Cao_2 \times CI \times 10$	520-720 mL/min/m^2
O_2 consumption ($\dot{V}o_2$)	$\dot{V}o_2 = CO \times (Cao_2 - C\bar{v}o_2) \times 10$	180-280 mL/min
O_2 consumption index	$\dot{V}o_2 = CI \times (Cao_2 - C\bar{v}o_2) \times 10$	130-160 mL/min/m^2
O_2 extraction ratio	$O_2ER = \dfrac{Cao_2 - C\bar{v}o_2}{Cao_2}$	24%-28%
Arterial-venous oxygen content difference	$a\text{-}vDo_2 = Cao_2 - C\bar{v}o_2$	4-6 mL/dL
Serum lactate		0.5-2.0 mEq/L

acidosis and include infusions of large volumes of normal saline resulting in a hyperchloremic acidosis, renal failure, acute ingestion of acids such as aspirin, and diabetic ketoacidosis.

TREATMENT OF TISSUE OXYGENATION IMBALANCES

Regardless of the type of shock a patient is experiencing, or the precipitating event, the common denominator is a disparity between the supply and demand of oxygen. This imbalance leads to inadequate oxygen consumption by the tissues. $\dot{V}o_2$ inadequate to meet tissue demand is related to decreased survival rates among patients with critical illness. Furthermore, persons who are critically ill often have increased oxygen needs because of a hypermetabolic state brought on by injury, inflammatory mediators, and the demands placed on the body for healing. Table 10-4 provides a quick reference of normal hemodynamic oxygen transport and oxygen utilization variables.

Optimize Do_2 and $\dot{V}o_2$

The goals of tissue resuscitation are to restore microcirculatory perfusion, stop the progression of oxygen debt, and repay any existing debt. The approach is to oxygenate, infuse, and perfuse. Sufficient Fio_2 should be used, possibly with mechanical ventilation, to ensure adequate oxygenation and ventilation and to maintain an Sao_2 of 92% or greater. The hemoglobin should be evaluated and packed red blood cells (PRBCs) administered as necessary to enhance oxygen transport.

The CI, and thus the Do_2, should be enhanced by first obtaining optimal preload. Fluid therapy titration should be based on improvements in oxygen transport (CI) and $\dot{V}o_2$, as well as physical assessment findings. Closely monitor the patient for signs of fluid overload, and if it seems that the optimal goals for volume resuscitation have been reached and Do_2 and $\dot{V}o_2$ are still inadequate, evaluate the need for pharmacologic support of the CI. Assess the hemodynamic profile to determine whether CI should be improved through agents that enhance preload, afterload, or contractility.

Contractility is enhanced with inotropic agents. An inotropic agent that increases CI without increasing systemic vascular resistance (SVR), such as dobutamine, is optimal because it increases $\dot{V}o_2$ not only by increasing Do_2 but also by promoting more even distribution of peripheral blood flow. If the mean arterial pressure (MAP) and SVR are high, indicating that a high afterload may be impairing the ability to reach optimal CI, then a vasodilator may be needed. First ensure that other common causes of elevated SVR, such as pain, hypovolemia, hypothermia, anxiety, agitation, and excessive catecholamine administration, are treated. If treatment of other causes of elevated SVR is unsuccessful and shock is still refractory, use of a vasodilator is indicated. Vasodilators allow for an improvement in stroke volume by reducing afterload. The appropriate dose improves CI, Do_2, and $\dot{V}o_2$ without precipitating hypotension. Finally, if perfusion deficit continues, the use of a vasopressor may be indicated. A vasopressor is used to increase the MAP and is most often needed in neurogenic, anaphylactic, or septic shock or in support of a patient in arrest. Its use is contraindicated if volume status is inadequate, and caution must be used to prevent renal or splanchnic ischemia and dysrhythmias.

Identify and Manage Underlying Pathologic Conditions

Patient management would be incomplete if the cardiopulmonary profile were the only focus. The underlying pathologic changes must be identified and the appropriate therapies initiated. The latter may include surgical drainage or debridement, antibiotic therapy, pulmonary hygiene, and a myriad of other interventions. Adequate nutrition must also be ensured. Substrates are needed to produce ATP, for healing, to maintain immunologic function, and to ensure that visceral stores are not utilized for these processes. The goal of nutritional assessment and intervention is an anabolic state of healing. The critically ill patient must be fed early in the course of the illness, before a significant negative nitrogen balance develops.

Reduce Oxygen Demand

Reduction of oxygen demands should be made, when possible, concurrently with the achievement of optimal Do_2 and $\bar{v}o_2$ and is done by administering sedation if the patient is agitated or active. Febrile states should be treated because for every 1°C rise in temperature, there is a 13% increase in metabolic rate, and for every 1°F rise, a 7% increase. Patient care activities should be organized to avoid excessive demands. The use of continuous $S\bar{v}o_2$ monitoring is particularly helpful in determining when activity, and thus oxygen demand, should be reduced.

Achieving maximal DO_2 in critically ill patients results in improved survival. Underlying oxygen deficits must be treated with the use of physiologic principles to ensure that adequate resuscitation has occurred at the cellular level, which is where the ultimate respiratory units lie.

APPLICATION OF TISSUE OXYGENATION VARIABLES: A CASE STUDY

A 52-year-old male pedestrian hit by a car was admitted to the trauma center. His injuries included a closed head injury; liver, renal vein, and superior mesenteric vein lacerations; an open fracture of the right femur; and multiple abrasions and lacerations. He was taken to the operating room, where an exploratory laparotomy was performed. Control of bleeding and repair of the liver, renal, and mesenteric lacerations was achieved. The right leg wound was irrigated and debrided, and a right tibial Steinmann pin was placed for application of traction and fracture reduction.

When the patient was admitted to the ICU, his Hb and hematocrit values were 9.7 and 27.8, with a platelet count of 54,000. The patient was putting out moderate to large amounts of bloody drainage via an abdominal drain. Oozing from the femur wound and multiple abrasions was also evident. Hemodynamics after administration of dobutamine, 14.0 mcg/kg/min, and epinephrine, 10 mcg/min, were as follows:

- Sinus tachycardia rate = 110 beats/min
- MAP = 65 mm Hg
- Central venous pressure (CVP) = 9
- PCWP = 11
- CI = 5.4 L/min/m^2

An ABG sample was drawn on the following ventilator settings: assist/control (A/C) of 14, FIO_2 0.6, 5 cm H_2O PEEP, and VT 900. The following values were revealed:

pH	7.19	$PaCO_2$	46			
PaO_2	144	HCO_3^-	18			
SaO_2	97.8%	Base excess (BE)	−9.9	Temperature	33.4°C	

Therefore, the pulmonary aspects of oxygen transport (PaO_2, SaO_2) were sufficient. The patient's ventilation ($PaCO_2$) needed to be improved to correct that portion of the acidosis attributable to the respiratory system. The therapeutic goal was to increase preload and to assist in the weaning of the vasopressor (epinephrine), which because of its intense vasoconstrictive effect would impair microcirculatory perfusion and $\dot{V}O_2$. The patient was given 1000 mL of 5% albumin and 2 units of PRBCs because of ongoing blood loss. Hypothermia was also noted to be a problem, and warming measures were instituted. It was recognized that returning the body temperature to normal would result in dilation of vasoconstricted vascular beds and possibly in a drop in blood pressure (BP) or CO.

After rewarming measures and volume administration, the epinephrine was reduced to 8.0 mcg/min and the MAP increased to 72 mm Hg. A cardiopulmonary profile was then obtained (normal values in parentheses):

a-vDO$_2$	2.4	(4-6)	CI	3.0
O$_2$ER	21	(24-28%)	BP	104/50 (72)
V̇O$_2$ (index)	124	(130-160)	PCWP	15
S̄vO$_2$	79	(60-80)	Hb	8.0
Lactate	8.2	(<2.0)	Temperature	36.9°C

ABG: 7.32/168/31/HCO$_3^-$ 16/BE – 8.2/SaO$_2$ 98% on A/C 14, FIO$_2$ 0.6, 5 cm H$_2$O PEEP, and VT 900

The following is the interpretation of the tabular material just shown: The a-vDO$_2$ is low, indicating that C̄vO$_2$ is increased, which is confirmed with an S̄vO$_2$ of 79%. The cause of the high C̄vO$_2$ is revealed by the low O$_2$ER. The V̇O$_2$ is low because the tissues are not extracting quite enough oxygen, probably because the oxygen supply is inadequate to meet the needs of this patient with huge oxygen demands. Regional oxygen supply is also being compromised peripherally because of the intense vasoconstriction caused by the epinephrine. Anaerobic metabolism is evident with the high lactate level.

Volume resuscitation continued, so that DO$_2$ could be increased further, with 250 mL additional 5% albumin, 2 units additional PRBCs, 4 units fresh-frozen plasma, and 6 platelet packs, until the CI continued to show no further improvement at 4.2 L/min/m^2. The epinephrine dosage was able to be reduced downward to 4 mcg/min. This hemodynamic state was maintained, and the trend of the progression was monitored with lactate levels. Within 7 hours, the lactate concentration was 4.0. Four hours later it was down to a normal level of 2.2. Throughout this resuscitation, oxygen demand was minimized through the use of deep sedation because the patient was very agitated. For a brief period of time, the use of a neuro-muscular blocking agent was also necessary.

SUMMARY

In the critical care setting, a plethora of variables may be monitored by the critical care clinician for the purposes of completing an advanced pulmonary assessment, determining where deficiencies lie, and intervening appropriately. The use of sophisticated physiologic variables of oxygen transport and consumption provides the clinician with the insight necessary to manage the resuscitation, not of the vital signs, but of the tissues. Timely resuscitation of states of oxygen deficiency reduces morbidity and mortality among critically ill persons.

It is imperative that the bedside practitioner understand how to interpret the data collected and what aspect of the cardiopulmonary system each variable assesses (Fig. 10-24). These variables, however, are useful only if collected with reliable equipment and interpreted in light of physical assessment of the patient.

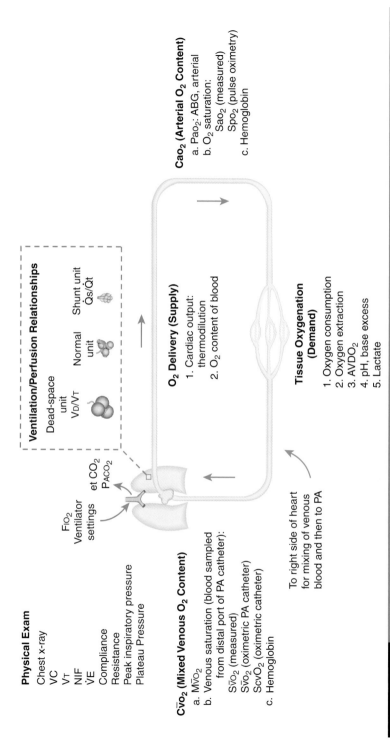

FIGURE 10-24

Pierce model of advanced cardiopulmonary assessment. Data guide evaluation of external and internal respiration. Understanding which aspect of respiration each variable assesses is essential.

RECOMMENDED READINGS

Adams KL. Hemodynamic assessment: The physiologic basis for turning data into clinical information. *AACN Clin Issues* 2004; 15(4):534–546.

Aoyagi T, Miyasaka K. Pulse oximetry: Its invention, contribution to medicine and future tasks. *Anesth Analg* 2002; 94(1 Suppl.):S1–S3.

Branson RD, Mannheimer PD. Forehead oximetry in critically ill patients: The case for a new monitoring site. *Respir Care Clin N Am* 2004; 10:359–367.

Bridges EJ. Monitoring pulmonary artery pressures: Just the facts. *Crit Care Nurse* 2000; 20(6):59–78.

Cairo JM. Assessment of pulmonary function. In JM Cairo, SP Pilbeam (eds.), *Mosby's Respiratory Care Equipment*, 7th ed. (pp. 215–253). St. Louis: Mosby, 2004.

Cardiopulmonary Diagnostics Guidelines Committee. AARC clinical practice guideline: Sampling for arterial blood gas analysis. *Respir Care* 1992; 37(8):913–917.

Darovic GO. *Hemodynamic Monitoring: Invasive and Noninvasive Clinical Application*, 3rd ed. Philadelphia: Saunders, 2002.

Dellinger RP, Carlet JM, Masur H, et al. Surviving sepsis campaign guidelines for management of severe sepsis and septic shock. *Crit Care Med* 2004; 32(3):858–873.

Dracup K, Bryan-Brown CW (eds.), $S\bar{v}o_2$ monitoring: Research and clinical applications [Symposium proceedings]. *Heart Lung* 1990; 19(5):Pt 2 [Suppl.].

Giuliano KK, Higgins TL. New-generation pulse oximetry in the care of critically ill patients. *Am J Crit Care* 2005; 14(1):26–39.

Grap MJ. Pulse oximetry. *Crit Care Nurse* 2002; 22(3):69–76.

Gutierrez G, Ronco JJ. Tissue gas exchange. In R Bone (ed.), *Pulmonary and Critical Care Medicine* (pp. 1–18). St. Louis: Mosby, 1995.

Hess D. Noninvasive respiratory monitoring during ventilatory support. *Crit Care Clin North Am* 1991; 3(4):565–574.

Johnson KL. Diagnostic measures to evaluate oxygenation in critically ill adults. *AACN Clin Issues* 2004; 15(4):5-6-524.

Levine RL. End-tidal CO_2: Physiology in pursuit of clinical applications. *Intensive Care Med* 2000; 26(11):1595–1597.

Mackersie RC, Karagianes TG. Use of end-tidal carbon dioxide tension for monitoring induced hypocapnia in head-injured patients. *Crit Care Med* 1990; 18(7):764–765.

McArthur CD. AARC Clinical Practice Guideline: Capnography/capnometry during mechanical ventilation. *Respir Care* 2003; 48(5):534–539.

Nellcor Inc. *Advanced Concepts in Capnography*. Pleasanton, Calif: Nellcor Inc., 2003.

Preuss T, Lynn-Hale Wiegand DJ. Blood sampling from a pulmonary artery catheter. In McHale DL, Carlson K (eds.), *AACN Procedure Manual for Critical Care*, 5th ed. (pp. 226–230). St. Louis: Saunders, 2005.

PACEP Collaborative. Pulmonary Artery Catheter Education Project. 2001-2006. http://www.pacep.org, accessed April 23, 2006.

Rivers EP, Ander DS, Powell D. Central venous oxygen saturation monitoring in the critically ill patient. *Curr Opin Crit Care* 2001; 7:204–211.

Scanlan CL, Wilkins RL. Analysis and monitoring of gas exchange. In RL Wilkins, JK Stoller, CL Scanlan (eds.), *Egan's Fundamentals of Respiratory Care*, 8th ed. (pp. 355–389). St. Louis: Mosby, 2003.

Shaffer RB. Blood sampling from an arterial catheter. In DJ Lynn-Hale Wiegand, KK Carlson (eds.), *AACN Procedure Manual for Critical Care* (pp. 465–471). St. Louis: Saunders, 2005.

Shoemaker WC. Monitoring and management of acute circulatory problems: The expanded role of the physiologically oriented critical care nurse. *Am J Crit Care* 1992; 1(1):38–53.

Smith I, Kumar P, Molloy S, et al. Base excess and lactate as prognostic indicators for patients admitted to intensive care. *Intensive Care Med* 2001; 27:74–83.

St. John RE. End-tidal carbon dioxide monitoring. *Crit Care Nurse* 2003; 23(4):83–88.

Swedlow DB. Capnometry and capnography: The anesthesia disaster early warning system. *Semin Anesth* 1986; 5(3):194–205.

Szaflarski NL, Cohen NH. Use of capnography in critically ill adults. *Heart Lung* 1991; 20(4):363–372.

Tobin MJ. Respiratory monitoring in the intensive care unit. *Am Rev Respir Dis* 1988; 138:1625–1642.

Van de Louw A, Cracco C, Cerf C, et al. Accuracy of pulse oximetry in the intensive care unit. *Intensive Care Med* 2001; 27:1606–1613.

Varon AJ, Morrina J, Civetta JM. Clinical utility of a calorimetric end-tidal CO_2 detector in cardiopulmonary resuscitation and emergency intubation. *J Clin Monit* 1991; 7(4):289–293.

Weaning from Mechanical Ventilation

Suzanne M. Burns

The process of liberating patients from mechanical ventilatory support is referred to as *weaning*. Most patients are rapidly weaned once they recover from the condition that initially necessitates mechanical ventilation. In some cases, however, mechanical ventilation is required for prolonged periods of time and withdrawal of the support is more difficult. The process is often referred to as weaning from long-term mechanical ventilation (LTMV), and to be successful, it requires a thoughtful and orderly approach.

Although most patients who require mechanical ventilatory support suffer no ill effects from the therapy, those who require mechanical ventilation for longer than 3 consecutive days are at risk for iatrogenic illnesses and complications including pneumothorax, ventilator-associated pneumonia (VAP), deep vein thrombosis, urinary tract infection, and immobility. All these complications can result in prolonged ventilator duration and intensive care unit (ICU) and hospital length of stay (LOS), increased mortality (40% or higher), and increased costs. Hospitals charged with the care of the patients experience financial losses because reimbursement is commonly less than the incurred costs. Although units and centers specifically designed to wean patients who require LTMV offer a reasonable and cost-effective alternative to long stays in critical care, the units are relatively rare, and most weaning still occurs in critical care units and step-down units.

For all these reasons, clinicians, researchers, and institutions are extremely interested in finding the best method to liberate patients from the ventilator. To that end, this chapter focuses on evidence-based information related to the weaning process. Key concepts such as respiratory muscle work, rest, conditioning, and fatigue are covered in addition to weaning assessment, prevention of selected complications, weaning modes and techniques, and systematic approaches. Where applicable, unique strategies for weaning the patient who requires short-term mechanical ventilation (STMV) versus LTMV are differentiated.

Short-Term and Long-Term Mechanical Ventilation

As just described, mechanical ventilation provided for less than 3 consecutive days is commonly referred to as short-term mechanical ventilation (STMV), whereas ventilation beyond 3 days is referred to as long-term mechanical ventilation (LTMV).

Weaning, or the process of gradual ventilator liberation, is rarely required for those patients who are ventilated short term. For example, many patients are intubated for general anesthesia, and once fully awake, they are quickly extubated. Regardless, in all ventilated patients, appropriate and timely evaluations and interventions are necessary to prevent unnecessary ventilator duration. The longer the patient requires mechanical ventilation, the higher the risk of excessively long and costly stays. Early identification of patients at risk for prolonged ventilation is especially important so that strategies to prevent the associated complications such as VAP can be implemented immediately. Patients requiring LTMV transition through multiple stages of illness or acuity, and associated interventions vary dependent on the stages of the weaning process, described next.

Stages of the Weaning Process

The AACN Weaning Continuum Model was introduced in 1994 and refined in 1998. The model described three stages of weaning categorized as the prewean, wean, and outcome stages. Subsequently, Burns and colleagues identified an additional stage called the acute stage, which precedes the prewean stage. Although many clinicians think the stages of weaning are theoretical, a number of studies suggest they are real and identifiable. The identification of the stages is helpful to consider the timing of interventions. Thus, to help categorize such interventions, the stages of weaning include the acute, prewean, weaning, and outcome stages and are described here. Unlike STMV patients, LTMV patients often do not often progress in a linear manner through the stages; instead, they may revisit stages during their time on the ventilator. Their weaning trajectory is one of peaks and valleys until an outcome is reached.

The *acute stage* is that time, generally the first 24 to 72 hours, when the patient is initially placed on a ventilator and is unstable. Some patients improve rapidly and are extubated; others progress slowly and/or irregularly and may die. The acute stage is marked by the use of a high level of ventilatory support and often hemodynamic support as well. Weaning is not a reasonable expectation, and the ventilator parameters are adjusted to protect the lung and/or to ensure adequate yet noninjurious oxygenation, ventilation, and acid-base status. Other interventions are focused on correction of the condition necessitating mechanical ventilation.

In the *prewean stage*, the patient is stable yet may still require a high level of care. During this stage, high-level cardiopulmonary support is not necessary; ventilatory settings are selected to enhance patient interaction on modes such as pressure support ventilation (PSV) and lower levels of oxygen and positive end-expiratory pressure (PEEP). Regular assessing and testing of "weaning ability" may occur during this stage, and clinical interventions are aimed at restoring or improving baseline status. In fact, the weaning trials may be used to restore ventilatory muscle strength and endurance; therefore, modes and methods are selected accordingly.

The *weaning stage* is generally short with rapid progress over consecutive days. It is marked by physiologic stability and attempts to withdraw ventilatory support with aggressive weaning trials. Modes such as continuous positive airway pressure (CPAP) and PSV are commonly used for trials with the goal being a predetermined duration of spontaneous breathing without evidence of intolerance. Once the goal is reached, a decision is made to extubate, or in the case of a tracheostomy patient, to attempt prolonged trials of spontaneous breathing (24 hours). When a tracheostomy tube is in place, specific techniques may be employed to enhance weaning and include short periods of capping the tracheostomy tube, use of speaking valves, and tube downsizing (discussed later in this chapter). Complete weaning, generally defined as breathing spontaneously for 24 consecutive hours, is one outcome of the weaning process, but other outcomes are possible, and are described later.

The *outcome stage,* the final stage of the weaning process, consists of complete weaning with removal of the artificial airway, complete weaning with an artificial airway still necessary, incomplete weaning with partial ventilatory support required, full ventilatory support required, or death. Although the definition and goal of weaning generally is complete withdrawal of ventilatory support with the removal of the artificial airway, for some patients this is not achievable. They may require the airway indefinitely or may require some degree of ongoing ventilatory support. Patients with high levels of spinal cord injury, advanced chronic obstructive lung disease, and neuromuscular diseases such as acute amyotrophic lateral sclerosis are examples.

Deciding When to Wean: Weaning Readiness

Deciding when to begin the weaning process is more complex for those requiring LTMV than those requiring STMV. All weaning generally begins with an assessment of whether or not the condition that necessitated mechanical ventilation has resolved. The primary condition may be a rapidly reversible nonpulmonary condition such as diabetic ketoacidosis or a pulmonary one such as pulmonary edema. If the condition is fully corrected and the patient is alert and able to breathe spontaneously, extubation may be the next step. In the LTMV patient, however, resolution of the primary condition may not be sufficient to ensure successful weaning and the weaning process may be very long. When mechanical ventilation is prolonged, patients often become physically debilitated and malnourished, and may sustain iatrogenic complications such as those noted previously. In addition, patients may become discouraged and demoralized. Although to date no one single factor appears to be solely responsible for the inability to wean, evidence suggests that a comprehensive approach to correcting these physiologic factors improves the potential for successful weaning. One important aspect of weaning is to prevent complications associated with prolonged ventilator duration and critical illness.

Preventing Complications

All complications associated with critical illness contribute directly or indirectly to prolonged ventilator time, increased ICU and hospital LOS, and death. Many are covered elsewhere in this book, and some are very briefly discussed later in this chapter. However, one complication in particular, respiratory muscle fatigue, is important to successful weaning trial outcomes and is described along with the related concepts of respiratory muscle work and rest. Successful weaning protocols integrate these concepts.

Respiratory Muscle Fatigue, Rest, and Work

FATIGUE

All muscles can be made to fatigue. If work is excessive (muscle loading), mitochondrial stores are depleted and effective muscle contraction cannot occur. The muscles of respiration are no exception. When they fatigue, respiratory failure ensues with resultant hypercarbia and acidosis. Mechanical ventilation can be lifesaving, and, applied correctly, it can offset the work and allow the muscles to rest, thus restoring them to their prefatigued state. Patients who are especially at risk for fatigue are those who suffer from respiratory conditions such as pneumonia, chronic obstructive pulmonary disease (COPD), and asthma, in addition to those who are debilitated and malnourished.

Signs and symptoms associated with fatigue include dyspnea, tachypnea, chest-abdominal asynchrony, and hypercarbia (a late sign). Both rapid, shallow breathing and chest-abdominal asynchrony emerge as compensatory mechanisms; fatigue and hypercarbic respiratory failure ensue if the workload continues.

Although studies suggest that various pharmacologic agents such as β-agonists, aminophylline, and low-dose dopamine and dobutamine may offset fatigue and/or reduce it, the dominant approach to restoring the respiratory muscles to a prefatigue state is to rest the patient on the ventilator.

REST

The first study demonstrating that the respiratory muscles could be rested with mechanical ventilation was accomplished with an iron lung. It was determined that if the patient was mechanically rested for 12 to 24 hours, fatigue would dissipate and the muscles could once again optimally contract. Since then, the question of how best to rest patients on mechanical ventilation so that fatigue is prevented or reversed has been a focus of debate.

Marini and colleagues studied patients on assist/control (A/C) ventilation and demonstrated that with initiation of a spontaneous breath, respiratory muscle work continues even if a machine breath is delivered simultaneously. In fact, with volume modes such as A/C and intermittent mandatory ventilation (IMV), true respiratory muscle rest is not attained without cessation of patient effort. Thus, if the clinical goal is to rest the respiratory muscles with a volume mode of ventilation, the patient will require either sedation and/or an increase in the mandatory breaths so that the drive to breathe is obliterated.

PSV, in contrast to volume ventilator modes, requires the patient to initiate respiration. Because PSV augments inspiratory effort, increasing the PSV level can reduce the workload substantially. Brochard and colleagues suggest that respiratory muscle unloading occurs when the PSV level is increased to that level required to eliminate accessory muscle use and to decrease the spontaneous respiratory rate (RR) (i.e., between 15 and 20 breaths per minute). Thus, to offset or prevent potential fatigue, an understanding of respiratory muscle rest is necessary.

WORK (AND CONDITIONING)

With prolonged mechanical ventilation, respiratory muscles can become deconditioned and in some cases may atrophy. This is especially true if paralytic agents, steroids, and/or high levels of sedation are used. Although possible under these conditions, it is indeed rare that a patient does not work at all while on the ventilator. Further, it is unclear exactly how much work is too much work. At what point does reconditioning work become fatiguing? Answers are as yet not definitive, but studies suggest that the type of muscle work (endurance or strengthening) may dictate the application of conditioning regimens.

Strengthening conditioning is generally described as moving a large force a short distance. As in weight lifting, such conditioning activity works muscles to extreme, indeed to fatigue. The muscle fibers sustain small muscle tears, and lactic acid production is expected. The fatigued muscles are then rested for greater than 24 hours to optimize the training effect (in weight lifting, the muscles are worked on an every-other-day schedule, never on 2 consecutive days). If done correctly, the conditioning technique builds sarcomeres and strength. If the concept of strengthening conditioning is applied to the respiratory muscles of a ventilated patient, modes and methods that require high-pressure, low-volume work most closely simulate such conditioning. Further, to ensure that optimal training effect occurs, the conditioning episodes need to work the muscles just to fatigue, but not beyond. Rest episodes are also provided. The strengthening episodes are of short duration and high intensity. CPAP, T-piece, and blow-by are examples of modes and methods that provide this type of work.

Endurance conditioning requires that the workload be gradually increased over time. Similar to endurance conditioning of other large muscles, this kind of conditioning may be done every day. The muscles are not worked to fatigue; instead, the work is increased slowly and steadily as endurance increases. A form of ventilatory endurance conditioning is PSV, which can be gradually decreased as the patient assumes more and more of the workload.

Although the concepts do make sense and are borrowed from the discipline of exercise physiology, the specifics of how long and how fast to progress conditioning intervals and how best to rest the respiratory muscles are as yet undetermined. However, studies exploring the superiority of weaning modes and methods suggest that short-duration CPAP or T-piece trials (1 hour, once per day) followed by rest are superior to other methods. The authors and critics of the studies concluded that the work-to-rest ratio in the studies may have lent to superior training effect and better outcomes (i.e., shorter weaning time) in the patients. Since the publication of the studies, protocols using short-duration trials of T-piece or CPAP have become popular and are common in critical care. How these concepts are applied into an integrated weaning plan is described later in this chapter in conjunction with protocols.

ASSESSING WEANING READINESS

Determining when a patient is ready to wean continues to be a concern of clinicians and investigators. Premature attempts at weaning and extubation can be deleterious to a patient's physiologic and psychological well-being. For example, unsuccessful extubation is linked to longer ventilator duration and ICU and hospital LOS. In addition, the risk of aspiration and subsequent pneumonia increases, placing the patient at greater risk of death. Cost of care is also adversely affected. As a result, many have attempted to design weaning predictors to help determine the timing of weaning trails and extubation. Despite the popularity of many of the predictors, little evidence indicates that they are in fact predictive. Cook and colleagues, in a large-scale review of weaning predictors, noted that they are not predictive. In general, they are good negative predictors (they tell us that the patient will not be successful) but poor positive predictors (if the score is good, they do not predict that the patient will wean).

Criticism of weaning predictors centers around three important concerns. The first is that the vast majority of weaning predictors are composed of pulmonary factors to the exclusion of nonpulmonary factors. This is despite the fact that non-pulmonary factors such as total body water, which is linked to unsuccessful weaning and death, are rarely included.

The second concern is that most predictors are designed to be tested at a "point in time," generally at the end of the process of recovery when the patient is deemed stable and ready to wean. Unfortunately, when used in this way, the predictor results are somewhat of a self-fulfilling prophesy. In a study by Burns and colleagues, four pulmonary point-in-time predictors were measured every other day until weaning occurred in patients ventilated for greater than 2 weeks. The predictors were compared to a multidimensional weaning tool, the Burns Wean Assessment Program (BWAP) (Fig. 11-1). Interestingly, none of the pulmonary-specific predictors changed over time, suggesting that their final predictor score is not predictive. The BWAP did change, however, and reflected the improvement of many factors over the course of time.

The last concern related to the usefulness of predictors is that studies using predictors are not stratified by condition, diagnosis, or the reason for mechanical ventilation. Although some studies on STMV patients stratified them by disease or condition (i.e., coronary artery bypass graft), studies in LTMV patients are rare. True stratification in LTMV patients will be difficult to do because patients who require LTMV have often recovered from the condition or disease that initially resulted in mechanical ventilation. Reasons for LTMV may have less to do with the primary problem or diagnosis than the resultant debilitated state. Thus, stratification of LTMV patients by disease, diagnosis, or reasons for long-term mechanical venti-lation may not be helpful.

Both Cook and colleagues and MacIntyre and colleagues, in large-scale reviews on predictors and weaning techniques, concluded that although predictors are not predictive, they may be helpful in assessing the components important to weaning success (e.g., muscle strength, endurance). To that end, they stressed that systematic attention to factors important to weaning and approaches that decrease variation in the weaning process, such as protocols for weaning and other multidisciplinary approaches, are essential to positive weaning outcomes. Given the state of the science to date on predictors, a discussion of some of the most popular predictors is described here so that they may be used as data points in an integrated compre-hensive weaning assessment.

BURNS' WEAN ASSESSMENT PROGRAM (BWAP)

Patient Name _____   **Patient History Number**_____

Patient Weight _____**kg**

I. GENERAL ASSESSMENT

YES	NO	NOT ASSESSED		
—	—	—	1.	Hemodynamically stable? (pulse rate, cardiac output)
—	—	—	2.	Free from factors that increase or decrease metabolic rate (seizures, temperature, sepsis, bacteremia, hypo/hyperthyroid)?
—	—	—	3.	Hematocrit >25% (or baseline)?
—	—	—	4.	Systemically hydrated? (weight at or near baseline, balanced intake and output)?
—	—	—	5.	Nourished? (albumin >2.5, parenteral/enteral feeding maximized) If albumin is low and anasarca or third spacing is present, score for hydration should be "no."
—	—	—	6.	Electrolytes within normal limits? (including Ca^{++}, Mg^+, PO_4). * Correct Ca^{++} for albumin level.
—	—	—	7.	Pain controlled? (subjective determination)
—	—	—	8.	Adequate sleep/rest? (subjective determination)
—	—	—	9.	Appropriate level of anxiety and nervousness? (subjective determination)
—	—	—	10.	Absence of bowel problems (diarrhea, constipation, ileus)?
—	—	—	11.	Improved general body strength/endurance? (i.e., out of bed in chair, *progressive* activity program)?
—	—	—	12.	Chest x-ray improving or returned to baseline?

FIGURE 11-1

Burns Wean Assessment Program (BWAP). *(Copyright Burns ©1990.)*

II.   RESPIRATORY ASSESSMENT

Gas Flow and Work of Breathing

YES	NO	NOT ASSESSED		
—	—	—	13.	Eupneic repiratory rate and pattern (spontaneous RR <25, without dyspnea, absence of accessory muscle use). * This is assessed off the ventilator while measuring #20-23. RR = ___
—	—	—	14.	Absence of adventitious breath sounds (rhonchi, rales, wheezing)?
—	—	—	15.	Secretions thin and minimal?
—	—	—	16.	Absence of neuromuscular disease/deformity?
—	—	—	17.	Absence of abdominal distention/obesity/ascites?
—	—	—	18.	Oral ETT >#7.5 or trach >#6.0 (ID)

Airway Clearance

—	—	—	19.	Cough and swallow reflexes adequate?

Strength

—	—	—	20.	NIP <−20 (negative inspiratory pressure) NIP = ___
—	—	—	21.	PEP >+30 (positive expiratory pressure) PEP = ___

Endurance

—	—	—	22.	STV >5 mL/kg (spontaneous tidal volume)? Spont VT = _____ STV/BW in kg = _____
—	—	—	23.	VC >10-15 mL/kg (vital capacity)? VC = _____

ABGs

—	—	—	24.	pH 7.30-7.45
—	—	—	25.	$PaCO_2 \sim 40$ mm Hg (or baseline) with M.V. <10 L/min * This is evaluated while on ventilator. $PaCO_2$ = _____ MV = ___
—	—	—	26.	PaO_2 >60 on FiO_2 <40%

FIGURE 11-1, cont'd

Burns Wean Assessment Program (BWAP). *(Copyright Burns ©1990.)*

Traditional (Standard) Weaning Predictors

The oldest and most commonly measured bedside predictors are discussed next. An inflated endotracheal tube (ETT) or tracheostomy tube cuff and a minimum level of sedation are required for the measurements to be accurate. Some also require that the patient be able to follow commands. In addition, studies demonstrate a considerable variation in interrater reliability between testers. To that end, those performing the measurements must be trained to be consistent in their technique.

NEGATIVE INSPIRATORY PRESSURE

Negative inspiratory pressure (NIP), also known as negative inspiratory force (Fig. 11-2), is considered the least effort dependent (the patient does not have to cooperate to do the study) of the traditional weaning predictors. As a result, it is the most frequently used. It is measured by connecting a series of one-way valves to a manometer and adjusting the device so the patient inspires against a closed system. The patient generally is taken off the ventilator for this test, although some of the newer ventilators allow for the measurement to be done while still connected. The patient is coached to inspire forcefully and may do so repeatedly up to a maximum of 20 seconds, if tolerated. The patient's best effort is recorded. The commonly cited threshold for NIP is −20 cm H_2O or less. The goal is a number more negative than −20 cm H_2O. Because the patient is breathing against a closed system, the best effort often occurs toward the end of the 20 seconds as the patient becomes progressively more stressed. Because the test can make the patient very anxious, an explanation must be given before testing, and coaching and encouragement should be given throughout the testing. The NIP can be done on unconscious patients unless they have central drive defects or are sedated; their response should be similar to a conscious patient. The NIP tests the strength of the inspiratory muscles. Although the threshold level of −20 cm H_2O or less is widely cited, studies demonstrated that many patients who cannot wean may generate NIPs that meet or exceed this threshold (i.e., of −45 cm H_2O or less). Thus, an NIP of −20 cm H_2O or less is not a reliable predictor of weaning.

POSITIVE EXPIRATORY PRESSURE

The positive expiratory pressure (PEP) measurement, also known as positive expiratory force, requires that the patient inhale maximally and breathe out forcefully against a closed system. The technique is similar to that used for the measurement of NIP. The difference is in the configuration of the one-way valves and the directions given to the patient. The traditional threshold for this measurement is +30 cm H_2O or more. The PEP measures expiratory muscle strength. It is also a good correlate of cough effectiveness because it employs activation of the abdominal muscles in addition to other muscles of expiration. Because this test is effort dependent, results are not always reliable.

SPONTANEOUS TIDAL VOLUME

For the spontaneous tidal volume (SVT) test, a spirometer is used and the patient is taken off the ventilator to accomplish the measurement. Or, alternately, the patient may be assessed while breathing on zero CPAP while still connected to the ventilator.

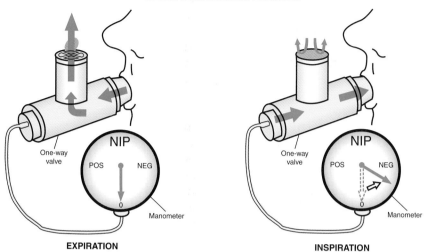

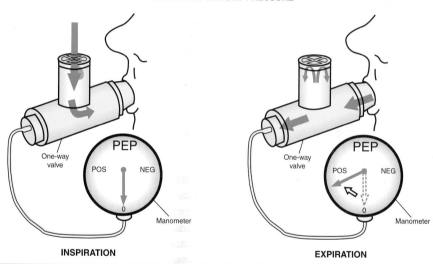

FIGURE 11-2

Negative inspiratory pressure and positive expiratory pressure. *(From Burns SM. Weaning Criteria: Negative Inspiratory Pressure, Positive Expiratory Pressure, Spontaneous Tidal Volume, and Vital Capacity Measurement. In McHale DL, Carlson K [eds]. AACN Procedure Manual for Critical Care, 5th ed. [pp. 226–230]. St. Louis: Saunders, 2005.)*

The patient is asked to breathe normally for 1 minute, and an average VT is calculated (minute ventilation divided by rate). A threshold of 5 mL/kg or more is expected. Smaller numbers may indicate respiratory muscle weakness, restrictive lung disease, oversedation, or noncompliance of the patient with the procedure.

The ability to maintain an adequate SVT over time is a good measure of respiratory muscle endurance. It is important to observe the patient carefully during the measurement of this test. For example, initially the patient may breathe slowly and shallowly but gradually increase the volume of each breath and be comfortable throughout. Conversely, the patient may increase the RR and decrease VT with each breath, indicating intolerance of the test and a fatiguing respiratory pattern.

VITAL CAPACITY

Although often regarded as one of the standard weaning criteria, the vital capacity (VC) measurement is difficult to do on an intubated patient. It requires that the patient take a maximum inspiration followed by a maximum exhalation. The VC can be measured with a spirometer with the patient off the ventilator or on the ventilator with the CPAP at zero. The minimum value for weaning is cited as 10 to 15 mL/kg.

If it can be measured, VC is a good indication of pulmonary reserve. The VC is normally at least three times that of the SVT. In those with limited reserve (i.e., myasthenia gravis, Guillain-Barré syndrome), a relatively normal SVT may be maintained for a long time at rest. However, if stressed, or even under conditions in which a bigger breath is necessary, such as in rising from a chair or in walking, the patient with little reserve will be unable to generate the volume necessary to match cardiac output and will experience dyspnea.

RAPID SHALLOW BREATHING INDEX

The rapid shallow breathing index (f:VT) predictor, first described by Yang and Tobin in 1991, combines RR and VT in a pulmonary-specific weaning index. Although early reports of the index's ability to predict were favorable, subsequent use was less convincing. Regardless, the value of the index is its ease of use and the fact that it describes a pattern of breathing consistent with an increase in workload and the potential for fatigue. The index can be measured either off or on the ventilator at zero CPAP, as just described for SVT. The index is derived by dividing the spontaneous RR by the spontaneous VT volume in liters. The thresholds for the f:VT are wean success, 105 or less; wean failure, 105 or more. A study testing the efficacy of the index in patients older than 65 years suggests that 130 or less is a more realistic threshold for this age patient.

MULTIDIMENSIONAL ASSESSMENT PREDICTORS

Two multidimensional predictors are reported in the literature. The first is a tool designed by Morganroth and colleagues that retrospectively measured multiple pulmonary and nonpulmonary factors in 11 LTMV patients. The factors in the tool were all weighted, and a final score was derived from the sum of the scores. The investigators demonstrated that the combination of the pulmonary and non-pulmonary scores was more predictive than either separately, and both were better than standard weaning predictors. Additionally, they noted the very uneven trajectory of weaning in the LTMV patients. The investigators suggested that by using a multidimensional predictive model, weaning prediction might be improved, and concurrently, the weaning plan might be adjusted appropriately based on the patient's status. A description of a similar but prospectively tested multidimensional model, the BWAP, follows.

The BWAP is composed of two parts: a personal digital assistant (PDA) application and a bedside worksheet (see Fig. 11-1). The PDA application contains an electronic copy of the worksheet in addition to extensive descriptions of the BWAP factors and their importance to the weaning process. In addition to the educational focus of the BWAP, the BWAP score, derived by dividing the total number of factors scored as "yes" by 26 (the total number of factors), may be used to track the progress of the patient and as a reference for the health care team to address collaboratively the impediments to weaning and to adjust weaning plans.

The BWAP score was tested in a prospective study of 37 patients to determine its predictive potential. As noted earlier, in contrast to four popular pulmonary-specific indices to which the BWAP was compared, the BWAP changed over the course of the weaning continuum and was more predicative than any of the other predictors. More recently, this was confirmed by Burns and colleagues in a larger study of 1500 LTMV patients. Despite the potential value of the BWAP as a weaning predictor, the more important use of such a tool is that it provides a method for assessing the LTMV patient comprehensively. This systematic approach to assessment decreases variation and prevents gaps in care delivery.

The Importance of Pulmonary and Nonpulmonary Factors

Although a comprehensive discussion of the multiple factors that affect weaning outcomes is beyond the scope of this chapter, developing a systematic approach to the evaluation of these factors and addressing those that are impediments to weaning are important goals. The clinician must ensure that systematic assessment of factors important to weaning occurs so that timely interventions can be implemented. A brief discussion of some selected BWAP nonpulmonary and pulmonary factors that are not addressed elsewhere in this chapter follow.

- *Hemodynamic and metabolic stability.* Both these factors are serious impediments to weaning and should be corrected before weaning trials ensue. Hemodynamic instability results in compromised oxygen transport. Patients experiencing sepsis, bacteremia, fever, or seizures have a greatly increased metabolic rate. By controlling or normalizing these factors, oxygen consumption and carbon dioxide production decrease.

- *Hematocrit.* A very low hematocrit, especially as a result of an acute hemorrhage, affects oxygen-carrying capacity, and an imbalance between supply and demand is created. In the weaning patient, oxygen consumption secondary to the work of breathing (WOB) can further magnify this imbalance. Decreased oxygen delivery to vital organs such as the heart increases the risk of ischemic injury and complications that will further impede weaning.

- *Fluids, electrolytes, and nutrition.* Fluctuations in intravascular volume may result in compromised pulmonary, cardiac, renal, and cerebral function, making weaning difficult. Electrolyte alterations affect cardiac and respiratory muscle function and can lead to muscle fatigue, decreased muscular contractility, and dysrhythmias. Especially important are potassium, magnesium, phosphate, and calcium because they are required for adequate respiratory muscle function and overall muscular strength and endurance.

- Malnutrition may result in a diminished immune response, respiratory muscle fatigue, electrolyte disturbances, inefficient gas transport, and weakness. In critically ill patients, metabolic requirements often exceed available energy stores. Low albumin stores also result in low intravascular oncotic pressures and third spacing of fluid.

- In general, enteral nutrition is preferable to hyperalimentation. It is hypothesized that even so-called trophic feedings (very small amounts) may prevent translocation of bacteria and subsequent sepsis. Use the gut whenever possible!

- *Anxiety, pain, and rest.* These three subjective symptoms are important to consider in any weaning patient. The invasive nature of procedures and treatments, noise, and lack of familiar surroundings and loved ones in the ICU all contribute and should be routinely addressed.

- *Bowel function.* Bowel elimination problems (e.g., diarrhea, constipation, ileus) result in inadequate enteral alimentation, discomfort, and inefficient respiratory muscle function, which make weaning difficult.

- *Physical conditioning and mobility.* Although little data exist that tell us that patients who are mobilized wean more quickly or have better clinical outcomes than those who do not, there are related data that suggest deconditioning occurs rapidly with negative results. For example, it is well known that within 2 to 3 days of recumbency, skeletal muscle atrophies and balance difficulties emerge. Rehabilitation takes longer and weaning is more difficult when the patient is weak. Thus, general body conditioning starts with sitting and balancing on the side of the bed and progresses to weight-bearing activities.

- It is also important to remember that while actively conditioning, ventilatory support may prevent excessive shortness of breath and promote better gains in conditioning. It is likely that while actively exercising the large muscles of the body, conditioning of the respiratory muscles will happen concurrently.

Pulmonary-Specific Factors

- *RR and pattern.* As described in the section on fatigue, chest-abdominal asynchrony and rapid, shallow breathing patterns herald an increased WOB and potential fatigue.

- *Secretions.* Secretions increase the resistive workload of the patient.

- *Neuromuscular disease and deformities.* The WOB may be greatly increased in patients with neuromuscular diseases and/or deformities. Weaning modes and methods that gently and gradually build endurance and strength are helpful interventions.

- *Airway size.* Tube diameter dramatically affects gas flow. As diameter decreases, resistance increases. Nasal passages may impinge on the diameter of the nasal tube and cause an increased resistance to flow. Nasotracheal tubes also increase the risk of sinusitis and VAP.

▓ *Airway clearance.* Absence of a strong cough, swallow, or gag may not prevent weaning; however, these findings herald potential problems with airway clearance. Gag is the least predictive of the three in evaluating a patient's ability to protect the airway. Patients with these deficits may wean, but once extubated they will be unable to clear secretions adequately.

▓ *ABGs.* Although ABGs are the gold standard for evaluating acid-base status, it is also important to consider the concomitant physical signs and symptoms. For example, minute ventilation (MV) should be considered when evaluating $PaCO_2$. As noted earlier, MV is the product of RR × tidal volume. A minute ventilation of greater than 10 L/min may indicate inefficient gas exchange. Occasionally, however, the MV is high secondary to a neurologic cause. In these cases, the $PaCO_2$ is low (reflective of the high MV). This is in contrast to a normal or high $PaCO_2$ and a high MV, which indicates a dead-space abnormality or increased carbon dioxide production.

Attention to multiple factors that affect weaning outcomes, such as those just described, go a long way to preventing gaps in care. These factors should be addressed before beginning weaning trials. As discussed later in the chapter, such a systematic approach is also likely to improve clinical outcomes.

WEANING TRIALS: MODES AND METHODS

To date, no one mode or method of weaning appears to be superior. Although two similarly designed randomized controlled trials were done seeking to determine the so-called best mode or method for weaning, the results were not conclusive. In the studies by both Brochard and colleagues and Esteban and colleagues, patients who met similar criteria for entry (parameters that suggested stability) were assigned to a trial of spontaneous breathing for up to 2 hours. If no signs of intolerance emerged, the patient was extubated. Patients who did not tolerate the trial were considered "wean failures" and randomly assigned to weaning based on protocols with PSV, IMV, and spontaneous breathing methods. Brochard's study suggested that PSV results in shorter weaning duration; Esteban's study suggested that once-a-day trials of spontaneous breathing (for up to 2 hours) results in the better outcome. Critiques of the studies point to differences in how the weaning trial progression was designed for the different modes in addition to how the patients were worked and rested following the trials. Although definitive answers about which mode or weaning method is best continues to be elusive, these studies demonstrated the efficacy of weaning protocols as part of the process.

Ely and colleagues were intrigued with the work just described. In particular, the investigators had noted that a 20% reintubation rate was present in those patients who met the initial entry "weaning screen" criteria and subsequently were extubated after successfully concluding the 2-hour spontaneous breathing trial. The investigators designed a randomized controlled trial to test the efficacy and safety of weaning based on protocols in coronary care and medical intensive care unit (MICU) patients. Managed by a nurse and a respiratory therapist, the protocol included similar components to those described by Esteban. Criteria for entry (weaning screen), a 2-hour spontaneous breathing trial, and definitions of intolerance (when to stop the trial) were all defined. Ventilator duration and other clinical variables of interest such as the reintubation rate and avoidance of tracheostomy were positively affected (statistically significant) in the patients assigned to the protocol. The authors concluded that weaning by protocol was both safe and effective.

In another randomized controlled trial, Kollef and colleagues tested the efficacy of a weaning protocol managed by nurses and therapists as compared to traditional weaning as planned by ICU physicians. Statistically significant improvements in ventilator duration and ICU and hospital LOS were demonstrated in the patients managed by the nurse-and-therapist weaning protocol.

Since the publication of these key articles, protocols for weaning both short- and long-term ventilated patients have been widely applied in critical care and step-down units. The protocols decrease variation in the weaning process by ensuring aggressive (and often early) testing of readiness, provide for scheduled work and rest intervals, and define intolerance so the trial is truncated as appropriate to prevent fatigue.

WEANING PROTOCOLS: THE COMPONENTS

As described, weaning protocols, or guidelines, give direction to caregivers in the gradual withdrawal of mechanical ventilation. But to be useful, they need to be clear, directive, and easy to apply. Box 11-1 provides an example of a protocol incorporating all the described components, and Box 11-2 summarizes the steps to consider when planning weaning. Both may be used with both STMV and LTMV patients.

BOX 11-1 — "When to Go" and "When to Stop": Example of Weaning Trial Protocol Components

WEANING TRIAL SCREEN: ASSESSED DAILY

1. Hemodynamic stability (no dysrhythmias, HR ≤120, absence of vasopressors: low-dose dopamine and dobutamine are exceptions).

2. FiO_2 ≤.5.

3. PEEP ≤8 cm H_2O.

4. BWAP >45% (in patients ventilated less than 3 days, a BWAP assessment is not necessary).

5. If the patient meets all these criteria, a *wean trial protocol* is initiated following a discussion with the multidisciplinary team.

WEAN TRIAL PROTOCOL: CPAP (1 TRIAL: 1-HOUR DURATION)

1. One trial of CPAP is attempted daily. The trial may last *no more than* 1 hour total unless previously negotiated with health care team.

2. With any signs of intolerance (see definition below), the trial is discontinued and the patient is returned to a resting mode until the next trial.

BOX 11-1 "When to Go" and "When to Stop": Example of Weaning Trial Protocol Components—cont'd

3. When the complete trial is sustained without signs of intolerance, the team is approached and extubation is discussed.

4. Full respiratory muscle rest is provided between trials and at night.

or

WEAN TRIAL PROTOCOL: PSV (2 TRIALS: 4-HOUR DURATION)

1. Start at PSV max level (level to attain RR ≤20 with V_T of 8-10 mL/kg).

2. Decrease PSV by 5 cm H_2O.

3. If no signs of intolerance are evident during the first 4-hour trial, the PSV is decreased by another 5 cm H_2O for the second trial.

4. With any signs of intolerance during trials, the patient is returned to previous level for the next 4-hour trial.

5. If unable to tolerate, the patient is fully rested until the next day when the process begins again.

6. Once the patient is able to sustain 5 to 6 cm PSV without signs of intolerance (for 4 hours), the team is approached and extubation is discussed.

Intolerance for either protocol is defined as *any* of the following (3-5 minutes sustained):

1. RR ≥35 for 5 min

2. O_2 saturation ≤90% or a decrease of 4%

3. HR ≥140 and/or a 20% sustained change of HR in either direction

4. Systolic BP ≥180, ≤90 mm Hg

5. Excessive anxiety or agitation

6. Diaphoresis

REST FOR EITHER PROTOCOL

1. PSV max: PSV max is that pressure level required to attain a RR of 20 or less and a V_T of 8-10 mL/kg. Respiratory pattern should be synchronous and there should be no accessory muscle use.

2. Other modes: With volume modes such as assist/control (A/C) or intermittent mandatory ventilation (IMV), respiratory muscle rest is not ensured unless there is cessation of respiratory muscle activity. Therefore, rest is considered that level of support required to prevent patient-initiated breaths. When IMV is used, PSV may be added for protection (i.e., as a "safety"). Regardless, the goal is cessation of spontaneous effort.

....

BWAP, Burns Wean Assessment Program; *CPAP,* continuous positive airway pressure; F_{IO_2}, fraction of oxygen in inspired gas; *HR,* heart rate; *PEEP,* positive end-expiratory pressure; *PSV,* pressure support ventilation; *RR,* respiratory rate; V_T, tidal volume.
Adapted from University of Virginia Health System MICU weaning protocol (©2002 by the Rector and Board of Visitors of the University of Virginia).

BOX 11-2 Summary of Steps to Consider for Weaning Patients

VENTILATED SHORT TERM OR LONG TERM

Is the patient stable, and is the underlying disease or condition that resulted in mechanical ventilation resolved?

- If "no": Focus of care is on improvement of the condition.
  - Adjust ventilator parameters to ensure lung protection and adequate acid-base status.
  - Care planning should include a focus on the prevention of complications such as infections (tight glucose control), deep vein thrombosis, sinusitis, ventilator-associated pneumonia, and malnutrition.

- If "yes": Short-term ventilation (<3 days)
  - Weaning parameters may be helpful to assess respiratory muscle strength and endurance.
  - Is the patient awake and able to protect his or her airway?
  - *Yes:* Consider short-duration spontaneous breathing trial or aggressive staged reduction of ventilatory support. Once the patient is able to sustain between a half hour and 2 hours of spontaneous breathing, consider extubation.
  - *No:* Address the need for additional interventions (withdrawal of sedation, etc.) and/or the potential need for tracheostomy.

- If "yes": Long-term ventilation (>3 days)
  - Assess overall weaning readiness with selected weaning predictors and a comprehensive assessment tool such as the BWAP: Work on interventions systematically to correct impediments to weaning.
  - Perform a weaning screen daily until criteria are met.
  - Once wean screen criteria are met, assign to weaning protocol.
  - If the patient successfully completes the weaning trial criteria, consider extubation *if the patient can protect his or her airway.*
  - *If unable to protect airway:* Address need for additional interventions and/or the need for a tracheostomy.

- If tracheostomy is required:
  - Assess overall weaning readiness on a regular basis (predetermined frequency) to ensure that impediments are addressed.
  - Design a plan for tracheostomy trials with progressively longer spontaneous breathing episodes. Use intolerance criteria to stop the trials and modes and method of ensuring rest.
  - Extend trials until successfully breathing for 24 hours.
  - Consider decannulation, downsizing, or tracheostomy tube capping.
  - If not successful: Consider need for permanent tracheostomy and/or ventilation.

Criteria for Entry (The "Wean Screen" or "When to Go")

The first component of a successful protocol, the "wean screen," consists of physiologic criteria that suggest patient stability and readiness to begin a weaning trial. Examples include thresholds for a minimum number of variables such as FIO_2, PEEP, minute ventilation, hemodynamic status (the absence of aggressive titration of vasoactive infusions, stable heart rate, and rhythm, etc.), and secretion clearance, to name just a few. Others, such as those for patients who require prolonged ventilation, may be more comprehensive and require a full BWAP assessment and a threshold score for the BWAP. The decision about what wean screen variables are required depends on whether the patient has been on STMV or LTMV. Patients ventilated for less than 3 days generally have fewer physiologic factors that affect weaning such as inadequate nutrition and profound deconditioning. Once the patient meets the wean screen criteria, the protocol moves the patient to the next step. In most cases this is assignment to a weaning trial by a specific mode or method. The key is that the patient's ability to wean is tested as early as possible.

Protocol Weaning Trials

Depending on a number of factors, weaning trials vary in length and duration. For example, tracheostomy patients may have longer trials and use different techniques than those without a tracheostomy. Regardless, protocols for weaning trials for STMV or LTMV (with or without a tracheostomy), if they are to be useful, should have "when to go" and "when to stop" trial criteria clearly defined (see Box 11-1).

Esteban and colleagues, in a follow-up to their earlier study using 2-hour spontaneous breathing trials for weaning, demonstrated that a half-hour spontaneous breathing trial was as effective in determining weaning trial outcome as a 2-hour trial. The authors noted that signs of fatigue (i.e., intolerance) generally appear within the first half hour and that additional time at that workload may be counterproductive. Thus, the duration of a trial using CPAP or T-piece is best kept relatively short in duration (e.g., between a half hour to 2 hours).

If PSV is selected as a weaning mode, the workload is gradually increased over time by decreasing the support level. Protocols using PSV may have longer duration trials than when CPAP is used. Once an endpoint or the lowest PSV level is reached successfully, extubation is attempted. PSV is an especially good mode option for those who are profoundly weak or those with poor cardiac reserves in whom the stress of a CPAP trial is poorly tolerated.

Application of concepts described earlier related to respiratory muscle conditioning is helpful in determining weaning trial duration and the mode of ventilation selected. For example, if CPAP or T-piece is selected, a form of "strengthening" workload is provided. The high-pressure, low-volume workload may induce fatigue after a relatively short time interval. Studies on the use of CPAP suggest the work is indeed more fatiguing than other modes. Optimal training affect is enhanced if "rest" follows such a training interval.

Patients with congestive heart failure pose a special challenge. When positive pressure is removed, as during extubation, venous return increases and the increased volume may exceed the heart's ability to compensate; pulmonary edema may result. An unsuccessful weaning trial in these cases is actually a cardiac failure. Appropriate pharmacologic preload and afterload reduction interventions must be provided prior to trial initiation. Also, once the lowest level of a weaning mode such as PSV is reached, it is helpful to test the patient's ability to tolerate complete removal of positive pressure before extubation is attempted with a trial of zero CPAP or T-piece.

Many clinicians use a combination of modes for weaning trials. IMV in conjunction with pressure support is one such combined mode. Although for some this mode may be useful, at least one study suggests that the combined mode, when used for weaning, may prolong weaning duration. The study was a survey of weaning methods in Spanish hospitals in 1994. To date, no studies have been done to test the validity of this finding. Since then, ventilators have become more responsive to patient triggering and inspiratory effort, and clinicians are more seasoned in the use of PSV and other mode options such as flow-by. It is difficult to know if the results would be the same if tested using a protocol or with other mode options. Regardless, this author believes that the combination mode, although not inherently bad, may indeed add potential and unintended variability to the weaning process. This so-called fiddle factor is defined as the amount of adjusting, that is, the fiddling that ensues when mixed modes are used. The decision to decrease or increase support is more complex because decisions about both IMV rate and PSV level must be made. Also, the choices are rarely as aggressive as when CPAP is used, for example. Further, it is difficult to determine clear intolerance thresholds for the combination modes. If the combined modes are used, the protocol must be constructed carefully so the patient is advanced as aggressively as possible and clear definitions for all protocol components are present.

Protocol Weaning Trials: Patients with a Tracheostomy

Patients with a tracheostomy also benefit from protocol weaning trials, but they differ substantively from those designed for use in patients with ETTs. These special considerations warrant discussion.

Patients receive a tracheostomy for many reasons. Conditions that preclude extubation such as high-level spinal cord injuries and some neuromuscular diseases are anticipated reasons. Other conditions render the patient unable to protect the airway, and in some, very lengthy stays on the ventilator or numerous unsuccessful attempts at extubation require that a tracheostomy be placed. A tracheostomy is often more comfortable for the patient who requires LTMV because the patient is able to eat, mobilization can be accomplished more safely, and communication is enhanced with the addition of speaking valves. Unfortunately, these patients require some of the longest ICU and hospital LOS. Weaning trials are approached somewhat differently, in part because the tracheostomy affords a degree of safety that is unavailable with an ETT. As with an ETT, removal of the airway is not necessary for testing whether the patient can sustain a 24- to 48-hour trial of spontaneous breathing. Furthermore, progression toward removal of the tracheostomy can occur in steps, allowing a fail-safe airway should one be required.

Weaning trials may progress from a supportive ventilatory mode (assist control, IMV plus PSV, etc.) to PSV, but most eventually transition to weaning trials of spontaneous breathing trials on CPAP, T-piece, or trach collar. Weaning protocols written for the patient with a tracheostomy are less prescriptive than for those who are being weaned with an ETT in place. Instead, plans for weaning trials tend to be more individualized. Regardless, the components of weaning based on protocols are helpful to include so the process of weaning is not subject to excessive variation and resultant delays. The patients are often very debilitated, weak, and discouraged, making consistency in care planning especially important.

Definitions for when to stop a trial and how to rest the respiratory muscles are important and should be clear to the caregivers. Tracheostomy tube trials generally consist of spontaneous breathing trials (CPAP, T-piece, or trach collar) that are gradually lengthened in duration until they reach a predetermined time interval of uninterrupted spontaneous breathing. At that point a decision is made to allow for nighttime sleep without ventilatory support. Until this point is reached, rest on mechanical ventilation is provided between trials of spontaneous breathing.

The exact pattern of spontaneous breathing trials varies. One example is to begin with two daily trials of 2 hours each (if no signs of intolerance emerge), and if both intervals are successfully reached, the trial intervals are lengthened until they merge and constitute a continuous 10-to 12-hour daytime trial. At that point a decision is made to extend the trial throughout the night with the disclaimer that if the patient evidences intolerance, ventilatory support will be provided. Once the patient successfully completes a 24- to 48-hour interval of spontaneous breathing without showing signs of intolerance, decisions are made related to downsizing, decannulation, tracheostomy tube capping, and, in some cases, the need to maintain the tracheostomy permanently.

Speaking valves, in addition to assisting with ease of communication and a feeling of normalcy, may also serve another important function in the patient with a tracheostomy. Generally, speaking valves use a one-way valve to allow air to flow into the trachea on inspiration. With expiration the valve closes so air is forced past the vocal cords for speaking. Some speaking valves also allow for oxygen to be bled into the trachea. Anecdotal reports suggest that in addition to supporting oxygenation, these devices may also create "back pressure" and restore functional residual capacity, thus making spontaneous breathing trials more successful. However, caution must be exercised because the speaking valves using oxygen may contribute to dry secretions and occlusion of the airway.

Definition of "Intolerance" or "When to Stop"

Applying the concepts described in the section on fatigue, selected signs and symptoms of intolerance are used to determine when to abort a weaning trial (see Box 11-1). For example, RR and pattern, dyspnea, diaphoresis, blood pressure levels, and heart rate changes may all be used. Thresholds for the criteria are essential if the caregivers are to interpret the criteria correctly and take the appropriate action. Note that the trial of weaning is considered a training (or work) episode, and some work is expected. Unlike the "rest" criteria, the criteria for intolerance are a bit more aggressive. For example, a RR of 30 may be acceptable for a training episode, but during a "rest" period, the threshold would be considerably lower (e.g., 15 to 20). All caregivers who work with the patients need to understand the thresholds and when to intervene (i.e., "when to stop"), regardless of the duration of the trial (5 minutes or 1 hour). Stopping the trials in a timely fashion is important to prevent fatigue and failure and to promote the patient's trust in the caregiver.

Definition of Rest

Although different definitions of rest exist, and many are anecdotal, only those discussed earlier in this chapter based on studies of volume and pressure ventilation are applied here. These are described in combination with the evidence related to respiratory muscle rest.

As noted earlier, fatigue may occur with excessive muscle activity. Because weaning trial episodes can result in fatigue, providing rest periods lasting 12 to 24 hours is a reasonable approach to offset or to prevent fatigue in the ventilated weaning patient. Not all patients who demonstrate signs and symptoms of dyspnea, tachypnea, and chest-abdominal asynchrony have fatigued muscles. But the emergence of such criteria indicates that the workload is high and the muscles are compensating. Continued work at the same level may progress to fatigue. Thus, erring on the conservative side and ensuring that patients are adequately rested between weaning trials is a prudent approach.

When volume modes of ventilation are selected to rest the patient, the mandatory (or set rate) is adjusted to ensure total cessation of respiratory muscle activity. In contrast, when using PSV, the level of PSV is increased to attain a spontaneous RR of between 15 and 20 and no evidence of accessory muscle use.

No data exist to help define how the combined IMV plus PSV mode might be used to ensure muscle rest. Regardless, if used, one approach would be to set the IMV rate so the patient rarely if ever initiates a breath and the PSV level to that level high enough that if a breath is initiated, the effort is minimal. In this case, the PSV is set as a "safety." This technique might be especially helpful in hospitals where a more flexible protocol (that allows nurses and therapists to adjust the levels as necessary) is not available.

The duration of rest can easily be timed so it corresponds with the patient's nighttime rest period. The coordination of both enhances a more restful and comfortable night's sleep. The same definition of rest is also used between daytime trials. Box 11-1 provides an example of how this information may be integrated into a weaning protocol.

The Case for Protocols Continues: It's Not Just What You Do with the Ventilator!

Of interest, protocols for use with ventilated patients are not limited to weaning. As described earlier, weaning from mechanical ventilation, especially LTMV, is expedited with a comprehensive approach to the assessment of impediments to weaning and a systematic approach to addressing the impediments. Furthermore, different elements by stage of the weaning continuum are important to address; what is done in the acute stage, for example, affects outcomes such as ventilator duration, LOS, and mortality.

Although the multiple factors listed in the BWAP are important to address before beginning weaning trials (i.e., the prewean stage), there are some factors present in the acute stage of the patient's ventilatory course that impact greatly on outcomes. Two acute conditions, acute respiratory distress syndrome (ARDS) and acute asthma, require that airway protective strategies, management of sedation infusions and paralytic agents (especially used in conjunction with steroids as in the case of the asthmatic patient), and the maintenance of tight glucose control be considered.

LUNG-PROTECTIVE STRATEGIES

In 1999, the ARDS Network of the National Institutes of Health (NIH) reported on study outcomes associated with low volume (6 mL/kg) ventilation compared to traditional volume (12 mL/kg) ventilation in patients with ARDS. Following an analysis of the first 800 patients, the study was stopped prematurely because mortality was 25% less in those randomized to the low lung volume ventilation intervention. Although some controversy exists related to the study results, to date no other study demonstrates as dramatic a difference in this category of patient. If weaning outcomes are to be optimized, attention to how patients are ventilated in the acute stage is essential for the lung to be protected. Use of the ARDS Network algorithm as a guideline for ventilatory management in patients with ARDS will promote lung protection and optimize weaning outcomes. Additional lung-protective strategies are described in detail in other chapters and include the use of PEEP and prone positioning.

Although asthma is an obstructive disease and ARDS is a restrictive disease, many elements of ventilatory management are similar in the acute stage. For example, although the reason for using low lung ventilation is to prevent volutrauma (see Chapter 9) in the patient with ARDS, low lung ventilation may also be necessary in the acute asthma patient to prevent dynamic hyperinflation and resultant circulatory compromise.

PARALYTIC AGENTS AND STEROIDS

The effect of paralytic agents on weaning outcomes is well described. Although paralytic agents are often necessary, indeed lifesaving in some acutely ill ventilated patients, the long-term effect of paralytics, especially used in conjunction with steroids as in acute asthma, may result in profound and debilitating myopathies and neuropathies; prolonged ventilation and long rehabilitation duration often result. A thoughtful and conservative approach to the use of paralytic agents and protocols for stopping the drug daily and or minimizing use are important interventions. In addition, for those who required the drugs at some time during their hospitalization, a high index of suspicion for neuropathies is warranted. Then an aggressive physical therapy program may be initiated and weaning trial mode selection appropriately made.

SEDATION INFUSIONS

Much attention now focuses on the role of sedation (specifically intravenous sedation infusions) on mechanical ventilation outcomes. In randomized controlled studies of sedation management by Brook and colleagues and by Kress and colleagues, a nurse-managed algorithm for sedation management and a protocol for daily interruption of sedative infusions, respectively, resulted in shorter ventilator duration and LOS. Although the results of the studies provide convincing evidence on how sedation infusions adversely affect weaning and other related clinical outcomes, some have suggested the infusions may be necessary to prevent psychological harm. Especially questioned was the method of sedation withdrawal employed by Kress and

TABLE 11-1 Effect of Protocols for Weaning and Sedation Management on Selected Outcomes by Author				
Author (Type of Protocol)	**Vent Duration**	**ICU LOS**	**Hospital LOS**	**Mortality**
Kollef et al. (wean trial protocol)	Yes*	NA	No	No
Ely et al. (wean trial protocol)	Yes*	No	No	No
Kress et al. (sedation management protocol)	Yes*	Yes*	No	No
Brook et al. (sedation management protocol)	Yes*	Yes*	Yes*	No

From Burns SM. The Science of Weaning: when and how? *Crit Care Nurs Clin North Am* 2004; 16; 379–386.
*Statistically significant.
ICU, Intensive care unit; *LOS,* length of stay.

colleagues. In their study, sedative infusions (defined as sedatives and narcotics) were stopped daily. Some wondered if this abrupt withdrawal might be especially harmful and result in a stress reaction similar to posttraumatic stress disorder (PTSD).

To determine the effect of the intervention, the investigators performed a follow-up study of the control and intervention groups. Intriguingly, the results demonstrated that sedative interruption did not result in adverse psychological outcomes; instead, those assigned to the protocol were likely to have fewer symptoms of PTSD than the control group. The study suggests that the rapid removal of the sedatives is beneficial both psychologically and clinically. Table 11-1 presents the effect of sedation management and weaning trial protocols on ventilatory weaning outcomes.

TIGHT GLUCOSE CONTROL

For some time, the relationship of high glucose levels on wound healing has been well documented. Yet rarely has so-called tight glucose control been rigorously pursued in the critically ill. Van den Berghe and colleagues tested the hypothesis that outcomes would be better in critically ill cardiovascular patients randomly assigned to tight glucose control compared to those not assigned. The results of the study demonstrated that variables of interest (mortality, wound infections, time on the ventilator, and ICU and hospital LOS) were all statistically significantly better in the intervention group.

Clearly, then, weaning and weaning outcomes are not just a result of ventilator manipulations. Recognizing patients at risk for LTMV is an important first step in the weaning process. And for weaning to be successful, attention to the course of the weaning continuum, by stage, is essential. Weaning is affected by numerous factors, all of which have to be managed if good outcomes are to result. Weaning is not just what we do with the ventilator. Given the complexity of the patients and the diversity of the diseases and co-morbid conditions affecting them, it is not surprising that comprehensive approaches work well. Systematic approaches to weaning are often inclusive of multiple components, such as the ones just described, that affect weaning outcomes. The focus of the initiatives is to decrease variation and ensure that, when possible, evidence-based practice is provided. Examples of successful systematic multidisciplinary approaches are described next.

SYSTEMATIC APPROACHES TO CARING FOR THE LTMV PATIENT POPULATION

Given all that was discussed earlier in this chapter related to the importance of systematic assessment and care planning, it is no surprise that many have taken a very comprehensive approach to the care for the LTMV patient. Solutions to reduce variation and promote standardization such as weaning teams and other unique institutional initiatives are implemented to assure that best practices are adhered to and good outcomes result.

Cohen and colleagues compared patients weaned by the critical care house staff to those weaned by a wean team composed of a critical care physician, a nurse, and a respiratory therapist. They found that care provided by the team was more effective (shorter ventilator duration) and more cost effective than that provided by the house staff. They attributed the positive outcomes to improved communication, comprehensive plans for weaning, and the team's use of clinical assessment versus the reliance on ABGs as reasons for shorter ventilator duration and cost savings.

Henneman and colleagues used a grease board on which the multidisciplinary team wrote the daily plan of care for weaning patients in a MICU. The investigators compared results of the intervention to outcomes of interest for the preceding year and showed a difference in ventilator duration and ICU LOS between groups.

In a more comprehensive approach, Smyrnios showed that outcomes could be improved by using an algorithmic approach to weaning managed by nurses in three adult ICUs. Finally, Burns and colleagues demonstrated that care managed and monitored by advanced practice nurses (called outcomes managers) using a multidisciplinary clinical pathway and protocols for the weaning of sedation and weaning trials was both clinically and cost effective. The two studies demonstrated that statistically significant positive differences in most variables of interest were attainable with the approaches. Table 11-2 displays outcomes associated with these initiatives.

The health care environment is often chaotic. Short LOS and decreased staffing levels affect the continuity of care and lead to gaps in practice and care planning. Given the complexity of the ventilated patient, it is clear that approaches to care that decrease variation will improve patient outcomes. To that end, the reader is encouraged to implement systematic processes of care for this patient population.

SUMMARY

Weaning, whether from STMV or LTMV, is a process that is greatly enhanced with approaches that decrease variation. The longer the patient is on the ventilator, the greater the potential for iatrogenic complications and poor clinical outcomes. This

TABLE 11-2	Effect of Three Systematic Multidisciplinary Approaches to Weaning by Author, on Outcome Variables				
Author/Population/Design	Ventilator Time	ICU LOS	Hospital LOS	Mortality	Cost
Henneman et al. (MICU, pre-post design)	Yes*	Yes*	No	No	No
Smyrnios et al. (MICU/SICU/CCU, prospective)	Yes*	Yes*	Yes*	No	Yes
Burns et al. (MICU, STICU, TCV-ICU, CCU, NICU, prospective)	Yes*	Yes*	Yes*	Yes*	Yes

From Burns SM. The Science of Weaning: when and how? *Crit Care Nurs Clin North Am* 2004; 16; 379–386.
*Statistically significant.
CCU, Coronary care unit; *ICU,* intensive care unit; *LOS,* length of stay; *MICU:* medical intensive care unit;
NICU: neuroscience intensive care unit; *SICU:* surgical intensive care unit; *STICU:* surgical-trauma intensive care unit;
TCV-ICU: thoracic-cardiovascular intensive care unit.

chapter discussed the importance of systematic assessments and modes and methods such as the use of protocols to facilitate the weaning process. Given the complexity of the health care environment and the multiple reasons patients require mechanical ventilation, it is important that clinicians use an evidence-based approach to weaning. Weaning is not just what we do with the ventilator!

RECOMMENDED READINGS

Bellemare F, Grassiino A. Evaluation of human diaphragm fatigue. *J Appl Physiol* 1982; 53:1196–1206.

Brochard L, RaussA, Benito S, et al. Comparison of three methods of gradual ventilatory support during weaning from mechanical ventilation. *Am J Respir Crit Care Med* 1994; 150:896–903.

Brook AD, Ahrens TS, Schaff R, et al. Effect of a nursing-implemented sedation protocol on the duration of mechanical ventilation. *Crit Care Med* 1999; 27:2609–2615.

Burns SM, Burns JE, Truwit JD. Comparison of five clinical weaning indices. *Am J Crit Care* 1994; 3:342–352.

Burns SM, Clochesy JM, Goodnough-Hanneman SK, et al. Weaning from long-term mechanical ventilation. *Am J Crit Care* 1995; 4:4–22.

Burns SM, Earven D, Fisher C, et al. Implementation of an institutional program to improve clinical and financial outcomes of patients requiring mechanical ventilation: One year outcomes and lessons learned. *Crit Care Med* 2003; 31:2752–2763

Burns SM, Marshall M, Burns JE, et al. Design, testing, and results of an outcomes-managed approach to patients requiring prolonged mechanical ventilation. *Am J Crit Care* 1998; 7:45–57.

Burns SM, Ryan B, Burns JE. The weaning continuum: Use of APACHE III, BWAP, TISS, and WI scores to establish stages of weaning. *Crit Care Med* 2000; 28:2259–2267.

Cohen CA, Zagelbaum G, Gross D, et al. Clinical manifestations of inspiratory muscle fatigue. *Am J Med* 1982; 73:308–316.

Cohen IL, Bari N, Strosberg MA, et al. Reduction of duration and cost of mechanical ventilation in an intensive care unit by use of a ventilatory management team. *Crit Care Med* 1991; 19:1278–1284.

Cook D, Meade M, Guyatt G, et al. *Evidence Report on Criteria for Weaning from Mechanical Ventilation.* November 1999. Contract No. 290-97-0017. Agency for Health Care Policy and Research, 6010 Executive Blvd., Suite 300, Rockville, Md, 20852.

Curley, MAQ, Fackler JC. Weaning from mechanical ventilation: Patterns in young children recovering from acute hypoxemic respiratory failure. *Am J Crit Care* 1998; 7:335–345.

Douglas PS, Rosen RL, Butler PW, et al. DRG payment for long term ventilator dependent patients: Implications and recommendations. *Chest* 1987; 91:413–417.

Douglas SL, Daly BJ, Gordon N, et al. Survival and quality of life: Short-term versus long-term ventilator patients. *Crit Care Med* 2002; 30:2655–2662.

Elpern EH, Silver MR, Bone RL, et al. The non-invasive respiratory care unit: Patterns of use and financial implications. *Chest* 1991; 99:205–208.

Ely EW, Baker AM, Dunagan DP, et al. Effect on the duration of mechanical ventilation of identifying patients capable of breathing spontaneously. *N Engl J Med* 1996; 335:1864–1869.

Ely EW, Bennett PA, Bowton DL, et al. Large scale implementation of a respiratory therapist-driven protocol for ventilator weaning. *Am J Respir Crit Care Med* 1999; 159:439–446.

Esteban A, Alia I, Ibanez J, et al. Modes of mechanical ventilation and weaning: A national survey of Spanish hospitals. *Chest* 1994; 106:1188–1193.

Esteban A, Alia I, Tobin MJ, et al. Effect of spontaneous breathing trial duration on outcome of attempts to discontinue mechanical ventilation. *Am J Respir Crit Care Med* 1999; 159:512–518.

Esteban A, Frutos F, Tobin MJ, et al. A comparison of four methods of weaning patients from mechanical ventilation. *N Engl J Med* 1995; 332:345–350.

Goodnough-Hanneman SK. Multidimensional predictors of success or failure with early weaning from mechanical ventilation after cardiac surgery. *Nurs Res* 1994; 43:4–10.

Goodnough-Hanneman SK, Ingersoll GL, Knebel AR, et al. Weaning from short-term mechanical ventilation: A review. *Am J Crit Care* 1994; 3:421–443.

Henneman E, Dracup K, Ganz T, et al. Effect of a collaborative weaning plan on patient outcome in the critical care setting. *Crit Care Med* 2001; 29:297–303.

Henneman E, Dracup K, Ganz T, et al. Using a collaborative weaning plan to decrease duration of mechanical ventilation and length of stay in the intensive care unit for patients receiving long-term mechanical ventilation. *Am J Crit Care* 2002; 11:132–140.

Knebel AR, Shekelton ME, Burns S, et al. Weaning from mechanical ventilation: Concept development. *Am J Crit Care* 1994; 3:416–420.

Knebel A, Shekleton MD, Burns S, et al. Weaning from mechanical ventilatory support: Refinement of a model. *Am J Crit Care* 1998; 7:149–152.

Kollef MH, Shapiro SD, Silver P, et al. A randomized, controlled trial of protocol-directed versus physician-directed weaning from mechanical ventilation. *Crit Care Med* 1997; 25:567–574.

Krieger BP, Isber J, Breitenbucher A, et al. Serial measurements of the rapid-shallow-breathing index as a predictor of weaning outcome in elderly medical patients. *Chest* 1997; 112(4):1029–1034.

Kress JP, Gehlbach, Lacy M, et al. The long-term psychological effects of daily sedative interruption on critically ill patients. *Am J Respir Crit Care Med* 2003; 168:1457–1461.

Kress JP, Pohlman, O'Connor MF, et al. Daily interruption of sedative infusions in critically ill patients undergoing mechanical ventilation. *N Engl J Med* 2000; 342:1471–1477.

MacIntyre NR. Weaning from mechanical ventilatory support: Volume-assisting intermittent breaths versus pressure-assisting every breath. *Respir Care* 1988; 83:121–125.

MacIntyre NR, Cook DJ, Ely EW Jr, et al. Evidence-based guidelines for weaning and discontinuing ventilatory support: A collective task force facilitated by the American College of Chest Physicians; the American Association for Respiratory Care; and the American College of Critical Care Medicine. *Chest* 2001; 20(6 Suppl.):375S–395S.

Mensies R, Gibbons W, Goldberg P. Determinants of weaning and survival among patients with COPD who require mechanical ventilation for acute respiratory failure. *Chest* 1989; 95:398–405.

Morganroth ML, Morganroth JL, Nett LM, et al. Criteria for weaning from prolonged mechanical ventilation. *Arch Intern Med* 1984; 144:1012–1016.

Pepe PE, Marini JJ. Occult positive end-expiratory pressure in mechanically ventilated patients with airflow obstruction. *Am Rev Respir Dis* 1982; 126:166–170.

Sahn SA, Lakshminarayan S. Bedside criteria for discontinuation of mechanical ventilation. *Chest* 1983; 63: 1002–1005.

Sahn SA, Lakshminarayan S, Petty TL. Weaning form mechanical ventilation. *JAMA* 1976; 235:2208–2212.

Sassoon CSH, Mahutte CK. Airway occlusion and breathing pattern as predictors of weaning outcome. *Am Rev Respir Dis* 1993; 143:860–866.

Sassoon CSH, Te TT, Mahutte CK, et al. Airway occlusion pressure: An important indicator for successful weaning in patients with chronic obstructive pulmonary disease. *Am Rev Respir Dis* 1987; 135:107–113.

Scheinhorn DJ, Chao DC, Stearn-Hassenpflug M, et al. Post-ICU mechanical ventilation: Treatment of 1,123 patients at a regional weaning center. *Chest* 1997; 111:1654–1649.

Sereika SM, Clochesy JM. Left ventricular dysfunction and duration of mechanical ventilatory support in the chronically critically ill: A survival analysis. *Heart Lung* 1996; 25:45–51.

Smyrnios NA, Connolly A, Wilson MM, et al. Effects of a multifaceted, multidisciplinary, hospital-wide quality improvement program on weaning from mechanical ventilation. *Crit Care Med* 2002; 30:1224–1230.

The Acute Respiratory Distress Syndrome Network. Ventilation with lower tidal volumes as compared with traditional tidal volumes for acute lung injury and the acute respiratory distress syndrome. *N Engl J Med* 2000; 342:1301–1307.

Tobin MJ, Guenther S, Perez W, et al. Konno-Mead analysis of ribcage-abdominal motion during successful and unsuccessful trials of weaning from mechanical ventilation. *Am Rev Respir Dis* 1987; 135:1320–1328.

Tobin MJ, Perez W, Guenther SM, et al. The pattern of breathing during successful and unsuccessful trials of weaning from mechanical ventilation. *Am Rev Respir Dis* 1986; 134:1111–1118.

Truwit JD, Rochester DF. Monitoring the respiratory system of the mechanically ventilated patient. *New Horizons* 1994; 2(1):94–106.

Van den Berghe G, Wouters PJ, Bouillon R, et al. Outcome benefits of intensive insulin therapy in the critically ill: Insulin dose versus glycemic control. *Crit Care Med* 2003; 31:359–366.

Vitacca M, Vianello A, Colombo D, et al. Comparison of two methods for weaning COPD patients requiring mechanical ventilation for more than 15 days. *Am J Respir Crit Care Med* 2001; 164: 225–230.

Yang KL, Tobin MJ. A prospective study of indexes predicting the outcomes of trials of weaning from mechanical ventilation. *N Engl J Med* 1991; 324:1445–1450.

Specialized Techniques in Mechanical Ventilation

Sherry M. Nelles and Michael A. Gentile

The application of positive-pressure mechanical ventilation is one of the cornerstones of support for patients with acute respiratory failure. Unfortunately, the condition of some patients does not improve despite escalating ventilatory support. Indeed, the condition of some patients may actually deteriorate when high levels of positive end-expiratory pressure (PEEP) and large tidal volumes (VTs) are used in an attempt to improve oxygenation. Research demonstrates that high PEEP and VT lead to barotrauma and to what is commonly referred to as ventilator-induced lung injury (VILI). Alternative modes of mechanical ventilation are being explored that use lung-protective strategies that support oxygenation and ventilation without causing further damage to an already-injured lung. A growing body of evidence suggests that alternative modes of ventilation in the patient with acute respiratory failure (ARF) may influence outcomes, including morbidity and mortality. In particular, adults with acute lung injury (ALI) or acute respiratory distress syndrome (ARDS) are showing beneficial results when lung-protective strategies are employed. As specific techniques continue to evolve, the practitioner should have a clear understanding of the modes, terminology, and scientific basis when undertaking the challenge of caring for these critical patients. This chapter discusses nonconventional modes of mechanical ventilation that include high-frequency ventilation (HFV), with particular emphasis on high-frequency oscillatory ventilation (HFOV) and independent lung ventilation. Also reviewed in this chapter are adjunct therapies to mechanical ventilation. These include heliox, inhaled nitric oxide (iNO), and extracorporeal membrane oxygenation (ECMO).

HIGH-FREQUENCY VENTILATION

Despite advances in mechanical ventilation, achieving adequate gas exchange in the diseased lung may contribute to a cascade of lung and systemic inflammatory responses seen in ARF. Lung injury can result from air escaping the alveolar space and migrating into extrapulmonary compartments (barotrauma), diffuse alveolar damage by overinflation (volutrauma), and shear stress when atelectatic collapsed lung units repeatedly open and close (atelectrauma). Growing appreciation for VILI has placed an emphasis on avoiding both alveolar overdistension and cyclic alveolar collapse and reexpansion, as well as opening closed alveoli and maintaining alveolar recruitment. In 2000, the National Institutes of Health (NIH) ARDS Network completed a multicenter, randomized trial of 861 patients with ARDS/ALI, comparing "lung-protective strategies" of smaller VTs (6 mL/kg vs. 12 mL/kg) and lower plateau pressures (less than 30 cm H_2O). In summary, the trial reported a statistically significant 22% reduction in 28-day mortality rates with the low VT strategy group. The results placed an emphasis on the need to avoid lung overdistention.

HFV is a ventilator strategy that delivers small VTs (1 mL/kg) at very fast rates with frequencies ranging from 1 to 15 Hz (1 Hz = 60 breaths per minute). HFOV is a mode of mechanical ventilation in which lung volume is adjusted and maintained to a continuous distending pressure. Superimposed small oscillations of gas flow close to or less than physiologic dead space provide gas exchange. HFV provides maintenance of high mean airway pressure (mPaw) with small tidal excursion while avoiding lung overdistention or expiratory collapse. Invented and patented in 1959 by Emerson, HFV was historically described in pediatric and neonatal respiratory failure until its introduction into the adult care arena.

Classification of HFV falls into four general categories: high-frequency jet ventilation (HFJV), high-frequency positive-pressure ventilation (HFPPV), high-frequency flow interrupter ventilation (HFFIV), and HFOV. HFOV is the most widely used of the HFV modes in the treatment of ALI and ARDS.

HIGH-FREQUENCY OSCILLATORY VENTILATION

HFOV is differentiated from other HFV modes primarily by three mechanisms: (1) gas is actively pushed into the lung and actively withdrawn; (2) the airway pressure during active exhalation may generate large subatmospheric pressures versus approximate atmospheric pressure; and (3) the humidification system is incorporated into the bias flow circuit. Active expiration enables control of lung volumes, decreasing the risk of air trapping and overdistention of air spaces. The SensorMedics 3100B (Viasys Healthcare, Yorba Linda, Calif) HFOV uses piston pumps or vibrating diaphragms to produce frequencies ranging from 1 to 50 Hz (60 to 3000 bpm). Amplitude is achieved by the power setting, which in turn sends an electronic signal to move the piston during inspiration and expiration and facilitates removal of carbon dioxide. Continuous warm, humidified flow of fresh gas (bias flow) through the respiratory circuit facilitates carbon dioxide removal from the system and lessens desiccation of lung mucosa and secretions.

The theoretic advantages of HFOV are that the elevated mPaw maintains the lung in an open recruited state, decreasing atelectatic trauma from minimal repetitive opening and closing of alveolar units, and facilitates the maintenance of end-expiratory lung volume, which improves oxygenation. Stretch injury is reduced because the smaller VTs minimize volutrauma and atelectrauma.

History and Clinical Studies

In the early 1970s, Lunkenheimer and colleagues were studying cardiac impedance in apneic dogs when they discovered that significant carbon dioxide removal occurred when oscillating small volumes of air at frequencies of 23 to 40 Hz in the animals' airways. At the same time, Bryan and colleagues found that while using a form of oscillation to measure lung impedance during anesthesia, carbon dioxide was eliminated. Optimal gas exchange was identified at approximately 15 Hz by Bohn and colleagues in 1979 when they were ventilating apneic dogs using a piston-driven oscillator with V_{TS} of 2 to 3 mL/kg with frequencies ranging from 5 to 30 Hz. Over the following years, multiple investigators concentrated on optimal gas exchange and the relationship of V_T and frequencies on carbon dioxide clearance with animals.

In the late 1980s, randomized, controlled clinical trials were conducted in neonates and preterm infants. Initially, the investigators in the NIH HIFI study comparing HFOV with conventional ventilation in 673 neonates and preterm infants with respiratory distress syndrome (RDS) found no significant differences with regard to oxygenation, lung disease, or mortality between HFOV and conventional mechanical ventilation. They did, however, find an increase in intraventricular hemorrhage and periventricular leukomalacia in the HFOV group. Subsequent review of the clinical trial questioned the methodology used in weaning, recruitment, and duration of conventional mechanical ventilation strategies. Despite these concerns, further studies were conducted to explore the possibility of HFOV. Clark and colleagues in the 1990s continued trials in premature infants and found no significant differences in outcomes between the HFOV and conventional mechanical ventilation groups. Also, they reported no increased incidence of intraventricular hemorrhage. Gerstman and colleagues in the Provo trial, conducted in 125 premature infants with RDS, found that HFOV with a lung recruitment strategy improved partial pressure of oxygen in arterial blood (Pa_{O_2}) and lowered the incidence of chronic lung disease when compared with conventional mechanical ventilation. Further neonatal and pediatric studies addressed early intervention of HFOV in RDS, lung recruitment strategies, and combination therapy with iNO.

Currently, HFOV is a standard modality in most neonatal and pediatric intensive care units for the treatment of respiratory failure. With the development of devices that have the capability of supporting larger patients, investigational HFOV trials for adults with ARF began in the 1990s. In 1997, Fort and colleagues published a nonrandomized pilot study on adult patients with severe ARDS failing conventional mechanical ventilation that observed a reduction in oxygenation index ($F_{IO_2} \times mPaw/Pa_{O_2}$) after starting HFOV. Also, there was no significant decrease in cardiac output despite significant increases in mPaw. The overall survival rate was 47%, and the number of prior days on conventional mechanical ventilation before initiating HFOV was associated with mortality. Mehta and colleagues, in a prospective study, reported that early institution of HFOV was a significant factor for reducing mortality. Derdak and colleagues in the first randomized, controlled trial in adults with ARDS found that 30-day mortality was 37% in the HFOV group and 52% in the conventional mechanical ventilation group. Also, there were no significant differences in hemodynamics, oxygenation, ventilation failure, barotraumas, or airway obstruction between the two groups (Table 12-1). Further research is needed to define the role of HFOV in ALI and ARDS before extensive lung injury occurs.

TABLE 12-1 Published Adult HFOV Clinical Studies

Study	Design	Population	Major Results and Outcomes
Fort et al. *Crit Care Med* 1997; 25(6):937–947.	Prospective, observational	17 ARDS patients. Lung Injury Score of 3.81 ± 0.23; failing inverse ratio on CMV (Pao_2/Fio_2) ratio 68.2 ± 21.6 mm Hg, peak inspiratory pressure 54.3 ± 12.7 cm H_2O, end-expiratory pressure 18.2 ± 6.9 cm H_2O. OI, 48.6 Apache II score, 23.3	Reductions in the OI ($P < .01$) and Fio_2 ($P < .02$) 12, 24, and 48 hours after starting HFOV. Pao_2/Fio_2 with HFOV was comparable to CMV. Overall 30-day survival 47%. Prior days on CMV, 2.5 days in survivors vs. >7 days in nonsurvivors suggested that earlier intervention in the course of ARDS with HFOV might be more beneficial. No significant compromise in cardiac output was noted despite significant increases in mPaw.
Mehta et al. *Crit Care Med* 2001; 29(7):1360–1369.	Prospective, observational	24 ARDS patients. Pao_2/Fio_2 98.8 ± 39.0 mm Hg, OI 32.5 ± 19.6. APACHE II score, 21.5	HFOV survival at 30 days; 33% with survivors on CMV for fewer days before institution of HFOV compared with nonsurvivors (1.6 ± 1.2 vs. 7.8 ± 5.8 days; $P = .001$). Increase in PAOP (at 8 and 40 hr) and CVP (at 16 and 40 hr) after HFOV initiated. No significant changes in systemic and pulmonary pressures associated with initiation and maintenance of HFOV. Complications: One patient with intermittent desaturation because of mucus plugs; two patients with pneumothoraces. Beneficial effect on oxygenation and ventilation when instituted early. May be a safe and effective rescue therapy for patients with severe oxygenation issues.
Derdak et al. *Am J Respir Crit Care Med* 2002; 166, 801–808.	Randomized, controlled	148 ARDS patients. Pao_2/Fio_2 ratio 112.5 on 10 or more cm H_2O PEEP. OI, 25.2 APACHE II score, 22	HFOV showed early improvement (<16 hr) in Pao_2/Fio_2 compared with CMV group; difference did not persist beyond 24 hr. OI decreased similarly over the first 72 hr in both groups. Thirty-day mortality: 37% with HFOV, 52% with CMV ($P = 0.102$). No significant differences in hemodynamic variables, oxygenation, ventilation failure, barotraumas. HFOV is a safe and effective mode of ventilation for treatment of ARDS in adults.

APACHE, Acute Physiology and Chronic Health Evaluation; *ARDS,* acute respiratory distress syndrome; *CMV,* conventional mechanical ventilation; *CVP,* central venous pressure; *Fio₂,* fraction of oxygen in inspired gas; *HFOV,* high-frequency oscillatory ventilation; *OI,* oxygenation index; *Pao₂,* partial pressure of oxygen in arterial blood; *PAOP,* pulmonary artery occlusive pressure; *mPaw,* mean airway pressure; *PEEP,* positive end-expiratory pressure.

TABLE 12-2	Differences Between High-Frequency Oscillators and Conventional Mechanical Ventilation	
Characteristic	CMV	HFO
Frequencies available	2-60 bpm	300-3000 bpm
Target delivered volumes	50-2500 mL	1-2 mL/kg
Expiration	Passive	Active
Baseline pressure manipulated by	Extrinsic PEEP	Bias flow
f × VT product for effective VA	Necessary	Not necessary

Modified from Macintyre NR. *Mechanical Ventilation* (p. 416). Philadelphia: Saunders, 2001.
bpm, Breaths per minute; *CMV*, conventional mechanical ventilation; *HFO*, high-frequency oscillator; *f*, frequency; *VA*, alveolar ventilation; *VT*, tidal volume.

Mechanisms of Gas Exchange

VTS generated by HFOV are small as compared to CMV. Whereas patients being managed on CMV may have a VT volume of 6 to 10 mL/kg, those managed on HFOV experience volumes of 1 to 2 mL/kg. Essentially, VT is less than dead space during HFOV (Table 12-2). Mechanisms of gas exchange in HFV were described as early as 1915. Henderson asserted that VT less than dead space could support life. Several theories are proposed to explain the mechanism of gas exchange during HFOV (Fig. 12-1).

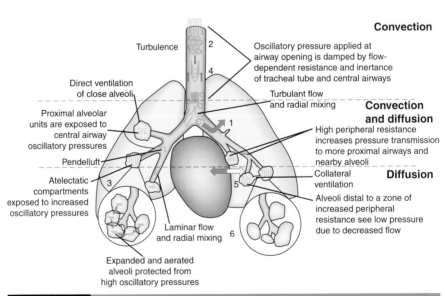

FIGURE 12-1

Mechanisms of gas exchange during HFOV. Proposed mechanisms of gas transport during HFV: **1,** bulk flow; **2,** Taylor dispersion; **3,** Pendelluft; **4,** asymmetric velocity profiles/coaxial flow; **5,** cardiogenic mixing; **6,** molecular diffusion. See text for further discussion.

BULK FLOW

Similar to CMV, bulk flow describes the direct flow of inspired gas delivered to alveoli close to the tracheobronchial tree. The process results in gas exchange by the mechanism of convective flow.

TAYLOR DISPERSION

Taylor dispersion is the mixing of residual with fresh gas as it passes through the airway lumen. This complex concept takes place on the front end of the gas flowing at high velocity and may augment bulk flow ventilation.

PENDELLUFT

Pendelluft refers to gas mixing between lung regions having different impedances. In diseased lungs with variable impedances, the Pendelluft effect can contribute to effective alveolar ventilation during HFOV.

ASYMMETRIC VELOCITY PROFILES/COAXIAL FLOW

The shape of gas delivered to the lung is altered during HFOV. In the airway, a cone-shaped profile occurs during inspiration with the center of the gas having the quickest velocity. Slower flow rates on the fringes of the gas profile return in the airways toward the mouth. This phenomenon creates a virtual two-way street, as it were, with the center of the breath participating in inspiration and the outside of the gas profile involved in expiration.

CARDIOGENIC MIXING

Lung units in close proximity to the heart may benefit from mechanical movement of the cardiac cycle.

MOLECULAR DIFFUSION

Molecular diffusion is the mechanism responsible for mixing of air in small bronchioles and alveoli close to the alveolar-capillary membrane. Molecular diffusion takes place during both CMV and HFOV.

The HFOV Therapeutic System

The SensorMedics 3100B (Viasys Healthcare, Yorba Linda, Calif) high-frequency oscillatory ventilator (Fig. 12-2) was approved in November 2001 by the Food and Drug Administration (FDA) for use in adults and children weighing more than 35 kg in ARF. The 3100B is an electronically powered, microprocessor-controlled, piston-driven mechanical ventilator. The piston rapidly moves in both a forward and backward motion, which displaces a flexible diaphragm and produces a square wave–shaped flow pattern. These oscillations are superimposed on a baseline mPaw. End-expiratory lung volume is determined by the mPaw and remains continuous throughout the respiratory cycle. The mPaw is controlled by adjusting flow in and out of the patient ventilator circuit. Exhalation is active because of the backward movement of the piston, which creates a biphasic pressure waveform. The clinician can adjust the mPaw (5 to 55 cm H_2O), pressure amplitude (6 to 130 cm H_2O), ventilator frequency (3 to 15), and percentage of inspiratory time (30% to 50%).

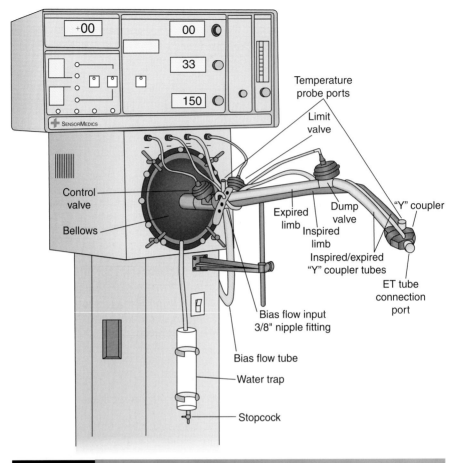

FIGURE 12-2

Details of SensorMedics 3100B patient circuit. *(From SensorMedics Critical Care Corporation: 3100B High Frequency Oscillatory Ventilator Operator's Manual [p. 28], 1999.)*

Amplitude is a monitored variable reflective of respiratory system resistance and compliance.

The 3100B ventilator is composed of six separate systems to make up the HFOV system: pneumatic, patient circuit, oscillator, pressure monitoring, electrical, and alarms. The pneumatic system controls four variables: bias flow, mPaw, mPaw limit, and circuit calibration. The bias flow is humidified, oxygen-enriched gas that provides continuous flow through the circuit. The mPaw adjustment controls the size of a mushroom-type valve in the expiratory side of the circuit and thus creates an expiratory restriction. The mPaw limit determines the maximum airway pressure allowed in the patient circuit. The patient circuit calibration is an adjustment used to set the mean pressure limit.

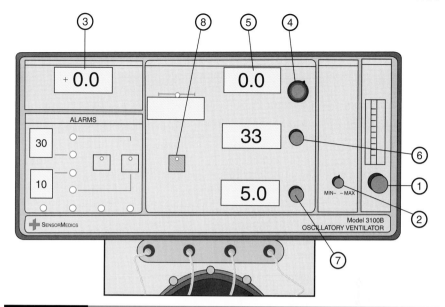

FIGURE 12-3

SensorMedics 3100B front control panel. *(From SensorMedics Critical Care Corporation: 3100B High Frequency Oscillatory Ventilator Operator's Manual [p. 42], 1999.)*

The patient circuit provides the path for the bias gas flow to travel from the ventilator to the patient. At the end of the expiratory limb is the pressure control valve, just discussed, which adjusts mPaw. Two other mushroom valves are located within the circuit to limit circuit pressure and provide a safety "dump" valve that allows a patient to breathe room air in the case of mPaw more than 60 cm H_2O or mPaw less than 20% of set maximum mPaw. Temperature and humidity of the inspired gas are controlled by a heated wire circuit.

The oscillator system includes the electronic controls (Fig. 12-3) that drive the motor and piston assembly to produce gas movement. The operator sets the power setting, which creates an electronic signal delivered to the piston and determines the amount of piston movement. When the piston moves forward, inspiration occurs. Expiration takes place as the piston moves backward. The percentage inspiratory time is the relative duration of the forward movement of the piston. As frequency is decreased, volume displacement of the piston increases, resulting in a larger delivered V_T.

The electrical and alarm systems monitor the system for abnormalities. In the event of an alarm condition, an audible signal sounds, alerting caregivers to investigate and correct the condition.

Management and Weaning During HFOV

Box 12-1 outlines the indications for HFOV. Once the decision is made to place a patient on HFOV, care must be taken to manage patients from the acute stage

| **BOX 12-1** | Indications for High-Frequency Oscillation Ventilation |

Patients may be candidates for high-frequency oscillation ventilation (HFOV) if their oxygenation status is inadequate and not amenable to conventional mandatory ventilation as evidenced by the presence of three or more of the following:

1. $FiO_2 \geq 50\%$

2. Plateau pressure ≥ 30 cm H_2O

3. Presence of bilateral infiltrates consistent with acute respiratory distress syndrome (ARDS)

4. Presence of gross air leak with inability to expand alveoli adequately

HFOV Protocol, Duke University Medical Center Respiratory Care Services, 2004.

| **TABLE 12-3** | Terminology and Definitions of HFOV Controls |

Terminology	Definition
Hertz (Hz)	Sets the oscillator frequency in Hertz (Hz). 1 Hz = 60 breaths per minute. Range: 3-15 Hz. A decrease in Hz = increased VT and MV.
mPaw	Mean airway pressure. Initial setting is slightly higher than conventional ventilation. Directly affects oxygenation and lung recruitment.
ΔP and amplitude	The amount of power (ΔP) that is driving the oscillator piston during inspiration and expiration. The power setting ranges from 1 to 10. The corresponding display of amplitude ranges from 0% to 100%.
I time	% respiratory cycle spent in inspiration. Longer I-time facilitates ventilation and carbon dioxide removal.
Bias flow	Controls and indicates the rate of continuous flow of humidified blended gas through the patient circuit. Range is 25-40 LPM. The control sets the flow of blended gas that continuously moves past the patient airways. Higher flows could indirectly affect mPaw and $PaCO_2$ clearance.

through weaning with a thorough knowledge of how to apply HFOV and adjust the settings based on assessment findings. First the HFOV equipment must be calibrated prior to initiation on a patient. Calibration is a relatively quick procedure and ensures proper machine function. The calibration procedure is described in the device operating manual.

The settings adjusted during HFOV are FiO_2, mPaw, Hz, percentage inspiratory time, power setting (amplitude), and bias flow (Table 12-3). Alarms to be set and adjusted accordingly to patient response are for high/low mPaw and FiO_2.

Because the most common reason to place a patient on HFOV is oxygenation impairment, the first considerations in HFOV management and implementation should always be FiO_2 and mPaw. FiO_2 is most usually started at 1.0 and weaned when the patient's gas exchange is deemed stable. mPaw is started at 5 cm H_2O above the monitored mPaw prior to switching to HFOV.

The frequency or Hz setting is usually started at 5 Hz and adjusted according to targeted $PaCO_2$ and pH values. Inspiratory time percentage (I time%) is typically

TABLE 12-4	Clinical Protocol for High-Frequency Oscillation Ventilation Initiation

GOALS

To maintain the patient's arterial pH between 7.20 and 7.50

To maintain the patient's Pao_2 between 55 and 80 mm Hg

To maintain the patient's Spo_2 between 88% and 95%

INITIAL SETTINGS/ACTIONS

Fio_2	1.0
Frequency	5 Hz (300 breaths per minute)
Bias flow	30 L/min
% Inspiratory time	33%
Power setting	Start at 6.0 and adjust to achieve an adequate wiggle (from clavicle to mid thigh). Initial amplitude: 70%-90%.
Mean airway pressure (mPaw)	5 cm H_2O above mean airway pressure on the conventional mechanical ventilation
Humidified temperature	38.5°-39°C.
Perform a recruitment maneuver (see Box 12-2).	

ASSESSMENT

Perform initial assessment of the patient immediately after initiating HFOV. Check BP, chest wiggle, oxygenation.

Obtain an ABG within 30 minutes and a chest radiograph within 2 hours after initiating HFOV.

ABG, Arterial blood gas; *BP,* blood pressure; *mPaw,* mean airway pressure.
HFOV Protocol, Duke University Medical Center Respiratory Care Services, 2004.

started and maintained at 33%, resulting in a 1:2 inspiratory-to-expiratory (I:E) ratio. The power setting creates an electric signal delivered to the piston to determine amount of piston movement. The corresponding display of amplitude is a function of resistance and compliance of the entire respiratory system from endotracheal tube (ETT) to alveolus. The power setting is started at the dial position 6. Table 12-4 summarizes the goals and initial settings of HFOV.

Once on HFOV, many centers perform a recruitment maneuver (RM) to open the lung and optimize gas exchange (Box 12-2). The RM should be done under close observation because of the possibility of transient hypotension. The increase in mPaw (up to 40 cm H_2O for 40 seconds) is the physiologic cause of hypotension because it creates increased intrathoracic pressure, which in turn reduces venous return to the right ventricle. Thus, the patient must have all cardiorespiratory parameters closely monitored during an RM to ensure the safety and effectiveness of such an intervention.

mPaw should be adjusted quickly in increments of 3 to 5 cm H_2O after a patient is placed on HFOV while observing pulse oximetry, heart rate, and arterial blood pressure. Power setting is adjusted to obtain a "chest wiggle factor" of movement

---

BOX 12-2 Recruitment Maneuver for Adult Patients Supported by High-Frequency Oscillatory Ventilation

PROCEDURAL STEPS

- FiO_2 1.0.
- Inflate cuff.
- Stop oscillations.
- Increase the mPaw to 40 cm H_2O; then maintain that pressure for 40 seconds.
- Return to previous oscillator settings.
  - Reestablish previous cuff leak.
  - Resume oscillations.
  - Decrease mPaw.

RECRUITMENT MANEUVER GUIDELINES

- Perform after any circuit disconnect.
- Perform twice daily as long as FiO_2 >0.4 and there is an increase in SpO_2 associated with the maneuver (even if transient).
  Caution: Do *not* perform a recruitment maneuver if:
- Pneumothorax is present with active air leak.
- Patient is hemodynamically unstable. For example,
  - MAP <60 mm Hg or MAP falls >20 mm Hg during the maneuver.
  - Heart rate >140 or <60.
  - New dysrhythmias are noted.
  - SpO_2 <85%.

....

MAP, Mean arterial pressure; *mPaw*, Mean airway pressure; *FiO_2*, fraction of oxygen in inspired air; *SpO_2*, saturation of hemoglobin with oxygen measured by pulse oximetry.
HFOV Protocol, Duke University Medical Center Respiratory Care Services, 2004.

---

from chest to midthigh level. Within 30 minutes of initiating HFOV, obtaining an arterial blood gas (ABG) determines the adjustments needed to maximize oxygenation and/or ventilation.

It is imperative to consider HFOV in two separate modalities: oxygenation and ventilation. Adjustments in ventilator settings are made separately for any desired result. Oxygenation is monitored by PaO_2 and SpO_2 and controlled by FiO_2 and mPaw, whereas ventilation is monitored by assessments of $PaCO_2$ and pH and can be altered by amplitude, Hz, and I time%. The active withdrawal of gas (carbon dioxide) is primarily controlled by adjustments to the power amplitude and the frequency. Carbon dioxide removal is facilitated by increasing the power setting, whereas lowering the frequency holds on to carbon dioxide. Failure to improve oxygenation in the first 24 to 48 hours of HFOV is indicative of a poor prognosis.

Once the patient stabilizes or improves, weaning of HFOV takes place in a systematic fashion. When patients respond to HFOV with improvements in oxygenation, FiO_2 is weaned from 1.0 to a level resulting in a SpO_2 of 90%. FiO_2 must be sufficiently weaned prior to any reduction in mPaw. To maximize alveolar recruitment, the mPaw is usually not weaned for the first 24 hours. Subsequent weaning of the mPaw is usually accomplished in steps of 1 to 2 cm H_2O every 4 to 12 hours as tolerated. Box 12-3 delineates the management strategies for oxygenation and acid-base problems.

BOX 12-3	High-Frequency Oscillation Ventilation (HFOV) Oxygenation and Acid-Base Management Strategy

OXYGENATION MANAGEMENT STRATEGY

During the first 24 hours after initiation of HFOV:
- Do not decrease mPaw.
- Wean F_{IO_2} if Pao_2 >80 mm Hg or Spo_2 >95.

After the initial 24 hours of HFOV:
- Consult with the medical team and titrate the mPaw and F_{IO_2} according to the following table:
  - Changes in mPaw and F_{IO_2} should fall within the established bands.
  - Any increase in mPaw should be preceded by a recruitment maneuver (see Box 12-2).
  - Note: Decreases in oxygenation may be caused by an airway obstruction because of increased secretions. Before increasing mPaw, assess for chest wiggle and the possible need for secretion clearance.

Mean Airway Pressure/F_{IO_2} Table

GOAL: Pao_2 55-80 mm Hg
GOAL: Spo_2 88%-95%
GOAL: $88 \leq Spo_2 \leq 95$

Mean Airway Pressure	F_{IO_2}
<25	0.4-0.5
25-30	0.5-0.8
31-39	0.8-1.0
40-45	1.0

ACID-BASE MANAGEMENT STRATEGY

For pH <7.20:
- Decrease frequency in increments of 0.5 Hz (to a minimum of 3 Hz).
- Increase power setting in increments of 0.5 to a maximum of 10.
- Increase % inspiratory time (IT) to 50%. Note: If an increase in % IT results in an increase in $Paco_2$, return to a % IT of 33%.
  - Increase cuff leak to allow more passive exhalation. Initiating a cuff leak may result in a decrease in mPaw. If this occurs, increase the bias flow to maintain the desired mPaw.

For pH >7.50:
- Decrease power setting in increments of 0.5.
- Increase frequency in increments of 0.5 Hz.
- Increase % IT to 33%.
- Decrease cuff leak.
  - Decreasing the cuff leak may increase mPaw. If this occurs, decrease the bias flow to maintain the desired mPaw.

From HFOV Protocol, Duke University Medical Center Respiratory Care Services, 2004.

The exact time to transition patients from HFOV to CMV remains unclear. Once the patient is stable on a F_{IO_2} of 0.40 and mPaw of 20 to 22 cm H_2O, a trial of CMV may be warranted. The CMV must be set up to support gas exchange adequately but not exceed the parameters believed to inflict VILI. Attention must be given to F_{IO_2}, plateau pressure, and V_T.

Potential Complications During HFOV

Potential problems may occur with HFOV; therefore, the practitioner must be vigilant in detecting possible complications. Classic auscultatory findings are absent because of diffuse breath sounds and the background noise of the oscillator. The following sections identify potential complications and the assessment necessary for diagnosis and clinical management.

HYPOTENSION

Hypotension may occur with some patients when transitioning from CMV to HFOV because of the increase in the mPaw and its relationship to the patient's intravascular volume status. When assessing hemodynamics, consider the possible effect of the elevated mPaw, especially when high (e.g., 30 to 35 cm H_2O), being transmitted to the vascular compartment, and reflected in the central venous pressure (CVP) or pulmonary artery occlusion pressure (PAOP). See Chapter 9 for management of hypotension and low cardiac output secondary to elevated mPaw.

PNEUMOTHORAX

When a tension pneumothorax occurs during HFOV, changes in mPaw and amplitude may not be evident initially. The first indication of pneumothorax, as with CMV, may be the clinical signs: hypotension, tachycardia, hypoxemia, tracheal deviation, subcutaneous emphysema, and asymmetry of the chest wall. An additional sign for the patient on HFOV is loss of chest wiggle on the affected side. When a pneumothorax is suspected, if patient stability permits, an immediate portable chest radiograph is obtained. When patient instability precludes getting a chest radiograph, a chest tube is placed on the suspected side. Once a chest tube is placed, adjustments in mPaw, amplitude, and Hz may be required.

MAIN-STEM INTUBATION

Acute unilateral reduction in chest wiggle and a sudden increase in amplitude with no change in mPaw may indicate right main-stem intubation. Auscultation of bilateral breath sounds will show a decrease in transmission of oscillatory sounds on the left side. If patient stability allows, obtain a chest radiograph to identify location of the ETT. If patient instability precludes this option, the ETT should be pulled out 1 to 2 cm until lateral chest wall wiggle returns, and then followed up with a chest radiograph.

ENDOTRACHEAL OBSTRUCTION

A sudden rise in $Paco_2$, an increase in amplitude, and/or an abrupt stop or diminishment bilaterally of chest wiggle are clinical signs of obstruction or narrowing of the ETT lumen with secretions. Endotracheal suctioning with a closed suction system should be performed immediately to ensure the tube is patent. A bronchoscopy to inspect the airways visually can be performed during HFOV.

OSCILLATOR MECHANICAL FAILURE

A sudden cessation of the HFOV can occur with decompression of the circuit secondary to a pressure-regulating valve or any external connection becoming loose or disconnected. The patient should be disconnected from the HFOV and immediately ventilated using a resuscitative bag with a PEEP valve. Appropriately trained personnel will be needed to troubleshoot and/or replace the HFOV. Once the patient is placed back on the oscillator, to minimize the effect of alveolar derecruitment, the clinician should consider performing an RM on the patient.

Patient Care Considerations for the Patient Undergoing HFOV

Collaboration between the bedside registered nurse and the respiratory therapist is critical in delivering safe, appropriate ventilator care to the HFOV patient. The patient's plan of care should be discussed intermittently throughout the day by the multiprofessional team, including medicine, nursing, and respiratory therapy, so oscillator management, concerns, and goals are clearly understood by those caring for the patient at the bedside. Team rounds should include a review of ABGs, chest radiographs, oxygenation response to care procedures, dyssynchrony events, F_{IO_2} and mPaw weaning parameters, outcome of RMs, and an assessment of bilateral oscillatory lung sounds and endotracheal secretions. A systematic discussion regarding all body systems should be undertaken to ensure the current plan addresses all problems and to prevent the development of complications.

PATIENT-VENTILATOR SYSTEM MONITORING

Because of the uniqueness of the method of providing ventilatory support with HFOV, patient management principles also differ in some aspects from those applied during conventional ventilation. Collaboration among physicians, nurses, and respiratory therapists is imperative in delivering care to these patients.

An extensive knowledge base of the patient-ventilator system is required for practitioners to be skilled at delivering appropriate safe care. A thorough understanding of oxygenation and ventilation principles and the corresponding therapeutic interventions (e.g., mPaw, pressure amplitude of oscillation [ΔP]) and treatment rationale of the HFOV is essential. The practitioner should be capable of monitoring the following oscillator settings: mPaw, ΔP, Hz, allotted time for inspiration (I time%), and bias flow. The clinician should also be capable of rapidly assessing and detecting the following subtle and or abrupt changes in patient conditions: hypoxemia, pneumothorax, and airway obstruction.

SEDATION AND PARALYTICS

Patients with severe respiratory failure require high inspiratory flow and mPaws that may lead to discomfort and possibly dyspnea with spontaneous inspirations. Patient-initiated efforts to breathe while on the ventilator may cause agitation and anxiety, resulting in the inability to facilitate adequate ventilation and ventilator dyssynchrony. An analgesic is the appropriate initial therapy when pain is suspected. Although analgesics do have some sedative effects, they do not diminish the patient's awareness of stressful events. Sedatives are needed in conjunction with analgesics to ensure comfort and relief from anxiety. A continuous infusion of analgesics and sedatives is essential to the therapeutic plan of care when patients are suffering from severe respiratory failure.

Before transitioning to HFOV, adequate titration of sedation and analgesia is assessed while still on conventional ventilation. The degree of sedation is determined by a defined goal of therapy and assessed by utilizing a sedation scale that is simple to use and has well-defined categories that accurately describe the degree of sedation. Several objective sedation assessment scales show reliability for use in the critical care patient (e.g., Ramsey scale, Riker Sedation-Agitation Scale [SAS], Motor Activity Assessment Scale [MAAS]). The Bispectral (BIS) device may be useful in assessing sedation and analgesia needs for the paralyzed patient. The BIS device converts electroencephalographic signals into a continuously displayed digital value from 100 (fully awake) to 0 (isoelectric electroencephalogram). The value reflects the level of sedation/cerebral arousal. Widespread use of the BIS in ICU patients has been limited secondary to the BIS index values varying widely, even in the paralyzed patient. However, recent improvements in the BIS device, particularly with artifact reduction have improved the correlation between BIS index values and various sedation measures.

Once adequate sedation and analgesia are determined, prior to initiating HFOV, the patient is started on a long-acting neuromuscular blocking agent (e.g., pancuronium, cisatracurium) to suppress spontaneous respiration and diaphragm movement. A bolus based on the patient's weight is given and a continuous infusion is started. Prior to starting the neuromuscular blockade, a peripheral nerve stimulator is used to determine the milliamperes necessary to stimulate a nerve to twitch. The stimulator provides a small electrical current to a preselected nerve (e.g., ulnar, facial, posterior tibial, peroneal) that produces four twitches of the nerve in the nonparalyzed patient. In the HFOV patient, usually the paralysis therapy goal is two twitches, which is indicative of an 85% to 90% blockade and absence of respiratory effort. In the absence of movement in the paralyzed patient, sinus tachycardia and hypertension may be the only clinical signs that the patient is not receiving adequate pain relief or sedation. Also, an increased mPaw on the oscillator may be indicative of the patients' need for additional sedation or paralytics. Prior to any position changes, the patient is assessed for the need of additional sedation and analgesic to ensure patient comfort as well as to decrease oxygen consumption and decrease ventilator dyssynchrony with movement.

Because of the complications (e.g., prolonged skeletal muscle weakness, persistent paralysis) associated with excessive and prolonged paralysis, patient management with deep sedation versus NMBs (intermittent and continuous) should be considered. Once the patient is stabilized on the HFOV, the practitioner should use the minimal doses of sedative, analgesic, and NMBs necessary to facilitate oxygenation and ventilation. Attempts to wean off the neuromuscular blockade should routinely be made. During daily patient rounds with the health care team, sedation and paralytic goals should be discussed and a plan of care initiated.

AIRWAY AND VENTILATION MANAGEMENT

The security of the ETT is assessed routinely and ETT position to lip/teeth recorded to ensure placement and no migration of the ETT into the right main-stem bronchus secondary to the continuous chest wall movement. The HFOV patient may require a full or partial endotracheal cuff leak to help facilitate carbon dioxide removal. The practitioner should be aware of its presence and note any cuff leak changes because carbon dioxide removal could be affected. Daily chest radiographs are obtained to assess ETT placement, fluid status of lung fields, atelectasis, presence of infiltrates, and alveolar overdistention/hyperinflation evident by flattening of the diaphragm below the ninth thoracic rib margin.

Endotracheal suctioning should be done prior to initiation of HFOV and then delayed when possible for 24 hours to minimize a reduction in mPaws leading to alveolar derecruitment. After 24 hours, endotracheal suctioning should be done only when clinically indicated as described later. Lung auscultation is challenging because of the continuous chest wall movement and noise of the oscillator. Routine auscultation of bilateral lung sounds to assess equal transmission of oscillatory sounds throughout all lobes detects subtle changes in narrowing or obstructing airways caused by secretions. Ongoing assessments for changes in the chest wiggle and variations in oscillator amplitude also assist the practitioner in determining if secretions are decreasing lung compliance. The respiratory care team should evaluate the need for endotracheal suctioning every 6 hours and as indicated (e.g., abrupt increase in amplitude with decreased chest wiggle, unexplained hypercapnia, or increasing oxygen requirements). Placing a closed inline suction catheter system may lessen alveolar derecruitment. If needed to visualize the airways, a bronchoscopy should be done through a circuit inline adapter while the patient is on the oscillator. A resuscitative bag with PEEP valve should be maintained at the bedside for emergent situations when the patient may need to be disconnected from the oscillator. An RM should be performed after any oscillator disconnect and twice daily as long as FIO_2 is more than 0.4 and there is an increase in SpO_2 associated with the maneuver unless a contraindication to performing an RM is present.

During the first 24 hours after initiation of HFOV, patient movement should be minimal to maximize alveolar recruitment, which can take 24 to 48 hours in a patient with ALI. The respiratory therapist is present during position changes to focus on airway security and to reassess oscillator parameters, chest wiggle, presence of a cuff leak, and oxygenation after position change. To promote an increase in lung compliance, the abdomen is kept off the lungs by elevating the head of bed (HOB) 30 degrees using the reverse Trendelenburg position. Continuous lateral rotation should be initiated when the patient's oxygenation levels tolerate position changes.

Continuous pulse oximetry is monitored with target goals of 88% to 92%. ABGs should be obtained at least every 4 hours for the first 24 hours after initiation of the oscillator. Thereafter, an ABG is indicated within 30 to 60 minutes of making any adjustments in oscillator parameters such as mPaw, amplitude, and FIO_2, with any acute changes in patient condition, chest wiggle, or SpO_2. Trending values of mPaw and amplitude should be documented every 2 hours to provide valuable information regarding lung compliance. In the neuromuscular blockade and/or sedated patient, safety alarms on the ventilator and continuous patient observation/ monitoring is imperative in case of ventilator disconnect or airway mishap.

INFECTION CONTROL

Unlike conventional mechanical ventilators, the HFOV constantly vents gas out of the mean airway pressure control diaphragm. The inability of the SensorMedics

3100B circuit to adequately filter exhaled respiratory secretions being aerosolized into the room places an occupational risk on the clinician. One institution uses various degrees of precautionary measures dependent on whether the patient has an undifferentiated febrile respiratory illness or a known noninfectious case of ARDS. Depending on patient diagnosis, precautions include (1) patient placed in a single room with negative-pressure ventilation with clinicians using protective equipment such as goggles, N95 mask, gown, and gloves; or (2) droplet precautions with clinicians using a surgical mask, goggles, and gloves.

The severe acute respiratory syndrome (SARS) outbreak brought to the forefront the need to develop scavenger devices on the HFOV circuit to protect clinicians. Currently SensorMedics 3100B has a scavenger cap (Viasys Healthcare, Yorba Linda, Calif.) that is attached over the mean airway pressure control diaphragm and then, in turn, connected to a high-efficiency filter and wall suction. At this time, only a few institutions are incorporating this system into their practice. Several scavenger devices and filters are being trialed; however, they are not currently available in the United States.

PREVENTIVE CARE

Preventive care management of the HFOV patient incorporates a number of interventions beyond the respiratory plan of care. Lack of patient mobility because of oxygenation requirements, sedation, and paralysis places the patients at risk for complications related to deep vein thrombosis (DVT), reduced gastric motility, and skin breakdown. Emphases on ophthalmic and auditory protection need consideration. As with all patients undergoing mechanical ventilation, the HFOV patient must have adequate DVT and stress ulcer disease prophylaxis.

Prior to implementing HFOV, a small-bore small bowel enteral feeding tube for nutrition to prevent possible aspiration should be considered. Pharmacologic gastroprokinetic agents should be started to establish a bowel regimen that uses a rectal tube if the patient has poor oxygenation and is unable to turn routinely. This also prevents sacral skin breakdown.

To increase mobility and thereby reduce skin breakdown and to improve pulmonary function, continuous lateral rotation therapy is indicated. It is initiated after the patient is on the oscillator for 24 hours with adequate oxygenation with a gradual increase to 50% to 70% degree turn and a frequency of 2 minutes on each side and 3 to 5 minutes in the center. The practitioner must be cognizant of the placement of oscillator circuit tubing to keep it from pulling on the ETT and keep tubing free of kinks during rotational therapy.

Ophthalmic lubrication ointment every 4 hours is necessary to decrease the risk of developing keratitis, conjunctivitis, and corneal abrasions while the patient is on neuromuscular blockade. In HFOV studies on noise measurement, the HFOV was cited as approximately twice as loud as a conventional ventilator. Although the oscillator noise was not enough to exceed occupational and safety standards, reducing auditory patient sensory overload needs to be considered whenever possible. Moving the oscillator to the HOB may lessen some of the direct noise impact on the patient.

Summary and Future Direction

HFOV is a viable alternative method of mechanical ventilation for patients with ARDS because it improves $\dot{V}/\dot{Q}$ matching and provides a lung-protective strategy of reduced Vts and distending pressure swings in conjunction with elevated mPaw to promote lung recruitment and oxygenation. It should be considered when escalating CMV support yields little improvement in gas exchange or settings are considered toxic and therefore may be inflicting VILI. Although HFOV is used routinely for neonate and pediatric patients with ARDS, its use in adults is relatively new. Randomized, controlled trails have yielded a trend toward improved outcomes, but the widespread use of HFOV in adults with ARDS remains limited. Fundamental education is required for caregivers to understand and use HFOV technology effectively. Care must be taken before, during, and after the use of HFOV to ensure safe and effective use of this complex technology. The future of HFOV will focus on large randomized, controlled trials investigating mortality. Evaluation of conjunctive and synergistic therapies such as iNO, prone positioning, instilled surfactant, and aerosolized prostacyclin will also be undertaken.

INDEPENDENT LUNG VENTILATION

The patient with pulmonary disease that is more predominant in one lung than the other illustrates a situation in which inadequate oxygenation may persist despite conventional methods of treatment. In fact, in patients with predominantly unilateral lung disease (ULD), traditional methods of conventional mechanical ventilation that apply the same flow and pressure to both lungs could result in deterioration of gas exchange and VILI to the noninvolved lung. One approach to the problem of ULD is the role of lateral decubitus positioning where the patient is positioned with the involved lung placed in the nondependent position. This maneuver presents a quick, simple method to possibly improve gas exchange that is inadequately managed on conventional ventilation. See Chapter 2 for further discussion on the effect of body positioning on best matching of ventilation and perfusion. Another approach uses a double-lumen endobronchial tube that allows independent ventilation with different support strategies (e.g., PEEP, Vt) to each lung. This method of ventilation is known as independent lung ventilation (ILV). *Simultaneous independent lung ventilation* (SILV) is the term used when the timing of inspiration is synchronized between the two lungs. With the possibility of hyperinflation and VILI to the noninvolved lung, practitioners are now using asynchronous independent lung ventilation (AILV) in which no concern is given to the timing of inspiration and expiration between the two lungs. Particular emphasis will be placed on asynchronous ILV in which different ventilator settings and possibly modes of ventilation will be adapted to each lung to optimize oxygenation and gas exchange.

History and Indications

In 1949, Eric Carlens described a double-lumen endobronchial tube that he had developed for use with differential bronchospirometry. The Carlens double-lumen tube (DLT) was adapted to prevent the spread of secretions from one lung to the other during pulmonary resection. By the 1960s, the Carlens DLT had proved useful in all types of thoracic surgery.

The Carlens tube was made of red rubber and had a small carinal hook, which, when properly placed, engaged the carina and promoted tube stabilization. The distal lumen opened to aerate the left lung, and the proximal lumen opened to aerate the right lung. The tube had two cuffs, the distal cuff lying in the left bronchus and the proximal in the trachea. Although the Carlens DLT was significant in the advancement of independent lung ventilation, many problems limited its use in the operating room and in intensive care settings. These problems included laryngeal/tracheal injury produced by the carinal hook; mucosal irritation caused by tube composition; increased resistance to airflow secondary to the small lumen; airway occlusion from lack of secretion mobilization; unreliable low-volume, high-pressure cuffs; tracheal dislodgement; and difficulty with right upper lobe ventilation because of the distal endobronchial cuff placement. The development of the White endobronchial tube in 1960 provided cuff placement in the bronchus just distal of the carina, which enabled tenuous ventilation to the right upper lobe through a side port in the lumen. The Robertshaw DLT design included a slotted endobronchial cuff that provided right upper lobe ventilation (Fig. 12-4). In the mid-1970s, ILV was extended to the postoperative and critical care settings in patients with ULD and unilateral pneumonia.

Advances in materials and tube design led to flexible, transparent polyvinyl chloride (PVC) tubes that allowed visualization of the bright blue endobronchial cuff position by fiberoptic bronchoscopy; removal of the carinal hook to decrease endobronchial trauma; increase in tube and lumen sizes resulting in decreased airway resistance and facilitation of secretion removal; transition to low-volume, high-compliance cuffs; radiopaque markers at the tracheal and bronchial orifices providing radiographic verification of tube position; and ventilator DLT Y-adapters that lessen the loss of ventilator airway pressures during bronchoscopy. Several DLTs exist today, including the Broncho-Cath I, II (Mallinckrodt Critical Care, Argyle, NY); Portex (Portex, Keene, NH); Robertshaw (Promedica, Preston, Lancashire, UK); Rusch endobronchial tube (Rusch, NY); and Sheridan Broncho-Trach (Sheridan, Argyle, NY).

The development of a better DLT led to the evolution of many applications. It is generally agreed that ILV is indicated when conventional ventilatory support fails in the presence of asymmetric or unilateral lung disease. Other possible indications include massive hemoptysis, massive unilateral pulmonary embolism, pulmonary alveolar proteinosis, single lung transplant, aspiration, pulmonary contusions, refractory unilateral atelectasis, bronchopleural fistulas or massive air leaks, and ARDS (Table 12-5).

Cited criteria for the possible use of ILV with radiographic-apparent ULD includes one or more of the following: inability to achieve adequate gas exchange when using high levels of PEEP and F_{IO_2}; a Pa_{O_2}/F_{IO_2} ratio less than 150; PEEP-induced hypoxemia or shunt fraction; and overinflation of the noninvolved lung with or without collapse of the involved lung (Box 12-4). In addition, the use of ILV depends on equipment resources and ultimately the availability, proficiency,

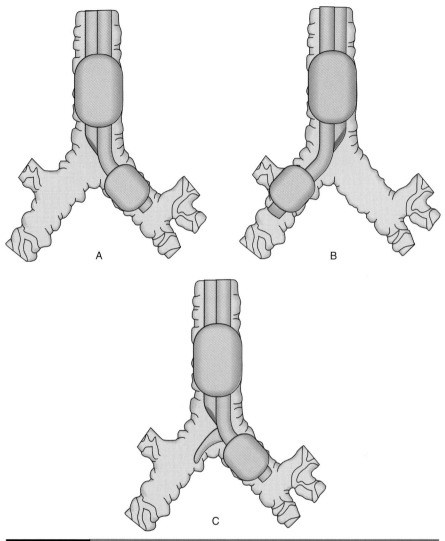

A

B

C

FIGURE 12-4

Design of the (**A**) left- and (**B**) right-sided Robertshaw and the (**C**) Carlens double-lumen endotracheal tubes showing relative placement of the two cuffs in the airways for each design as well as the carinal hook characteristic of the Carlens tube. The small hook engages the carina to promote tube stabilization. *(From Thomas AR. Ventilation in the patient with unilateral lung disease. Crit Care Clin 1998; 14[4]:743–773.)*

TABLE 12-5 Unilateral Lung Disease Associated with Respiratory Failure

Category of Unilateral Disease	Specific Disease Processes
Unilateral parenchymal disease with decreased compliance of the involved lung	Pulmonary contusion
	Unilateral pneumonia
	Reexpansion edema
	Reperfusion edema
	Aspiration
	Refractory atelectasis
	Massive hemorrhage
Unilateral lung problems associated with increased compliance of the involved lung	Bronchopleural fistula
	Single-lung transplant in obstructive lung disease
	Unilateral hyperinflation
Other reported unilateral problems	Massive unilateral pulmonary embolism
	Large pleural effusions

From Thomas A, Bryce T. Ventilation in the patient with unilateral lung disease. *Crit Care Clin* 1998; 14(4):743–773.

BOX 12-4 Criteria for Initiating Independent-Lung Ventilation in Unilateral Lung Disease

Radiographically apparent unilateral or asymmetrical lung disease with one of the following:

1. Hypoxemia refractory to high FiO_2 and generalized PEEP.

2. PEEP-induced deterioration in oxygenation or shunt fraction.

3. Overinflation of the noninvolved lung with or without collapse of the involved lung.

4. Significant deterioration in circulatory status in response to PEEP.

FiO_2, Fraction of oxygen in inspired gas; *PEEP,* positive end-expiratory pressure.
From Thomas A, Bryce T. Ventilation in the patient with unilateral lung disease. *Crit Care Clin* 1998; 14(4):743–773.

and experience of the health care team (nursing, respiratory, physician) to provide adequate monitoring, ongoing assessments, and capable response to emergencies.

Pathophysiology of Asymmetric Lung Disease

Full appreciation of the indications for ILV is achieved through an understanding of the regional maldistribution of ventilation and perfusion in the lung under the conditions of mechanical ventilation and ULD. When a patient is being mechanically ventilated, the volume of gas received by different regions of the lung depends on regional compliance and resistance differences. Areas of the lung with decreased compliance and increased resistance are relatively underventilated in comparison with normal lung regions. The patient with unilateral, or asymmetric, lung disease presents a classic example of the situation in which ventilation is maldistributed because the two lungs demonstrate significantly different time constants.

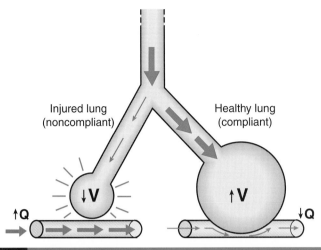

FIGURE 12-5

Maldistribution of ventilation and perfusion during conventional ventilation with asymmetric lung disease. Tidal volume is preferentially distributed to the more compliant lung, overdistending the alveoli (*right*). Compression of adjacent pulmonary capillaries increases pulmonary vascular resistance and shifts pulmonary blood flow to the poorly ventilated, less compliant lung (*left*). $\dot{V}/\dot{Q}$ mismatch is increased with overventilation of the compliant lung (increased dead space and therefore increased $Paco_2$) and overperfusion of the noncompliant lung (increased shunt and therefore hypoxemia). *(From Simon B, Borg U. Independent lung ventilation. Crit Care Report 1990; 1[3]:398–407.)*

In ULD, when parallel (conventional) ventilation is applied, the diseased lung receives a smaller portion of the V_T because of its decreased compliance and increased resistance. The less diseased lung, because it is more compliant and has a lower airway resistance, receives a greater portion of the V_T. The delivered V_T is therefore unevenly distributed to the more normal lung while the affected lung, because of its longer time constant, receives proportionately less volume. Maldistribution of the V_T leads to overdistention of the more compliant lung. Hyperinflation causes the airway pressures to rise and results in an increased potential for barotrauma in the more compliant lung. The high pressure within the overinflated alveoli is transmitted to the alveolar capillary bed, compressing the alveoli so that blood flow through them is minimal to absent. These areas of high $\dot{V}/\dot{Q}$ or dead space, predominant in the more compliant lung, are clinically manifested by a rising $Paco_2$.

The compression of the pulmonary capillary bed in the hyperinflated normal lung, together with the regional increase in the pulmonary vascular resistance, causes a diversion of blood to lower-resistance capillary beds in the pathologic lung. Blood flow, being shifted to the relatively underventilated diseased lung, creates low $\dot{V}/\dot{Q}$ or intrapulmonary shunt ($\dot{Q}s/\dot{Q}T$) areas, which are clinically manifested by failing oxygenation despite the delivered Fio_2 (Fig. 12-5). In an effort to improve oxygenation, the application of PEEP worsens the hyperinflation of the good lung and the diversion of blood to the bad lung. The therapeutic paradox in ULD, therefore, is that volume and pressure are necessary to ventilate the less compliant lung; yet these same required volumes and pressures increase pulmonary barotrauma and volutrauma by overdistending the more compliant lung and worsening overall $\dot{V}/\dot{Q}$ matching.

Criteria for Determining Asymmetric Lung Disease

The criteria for determining ULD and thus whether the patient may benefit from ILV can be divided into clinical findings and physiologic criteria. The chest radiograph film may provide anatomic evidence of the presence of asymmetric or unilateral pathologic changes. However, physiologic asymmetry may not always be apparent radiographically. An asymmetric pattern becomes apparent on occasion *after* PEEP is applied when the nondiseased lung demonstrates hyperinflation and there is a shifting of the cardiac silhouette to the opposite hemithorax.

An asymmetric pattern of thoracic injury may create a high index of suspicion that the pulmonary pathologic changes are predominantly unilateral. Examples of such patterns are prevalent in the thoracic trauma population and include an injury such as flail chest and pulmonary contusion in one hemithorax.

Physiologically, asymmetric abnormality may be confirmed by measuring the compliance of each lung. This requires the placement of an endobronchial tube to isolate each lung and therefore is not practical as a means of deciding whether ILV is indicated. A maneuver more realistically performed in the clinical setting is the determination of oxygenation in each lateral decubitus position. If a disparity exists, the lung disease is likely asymmetric. Patients with asymmetric lung disease demonstrate their best oxygenation in the position where the better lung is dependent because in this position there is the best matching of ventilation and perfusion. In the good-lung-down (GLD) position, ventilation is greatest in the dependent lung because it has the best compliance. Perfusion, being affected by gravity, is also best in this dependent lung. This optimal $\dot{V}/\dot{Q}$ matching in the GLD position results in the best oxygenation. See Chapter 2 for further discussion on the effect of body position on $\dot{V}/\dot{Q}$ matching.

Asynchronous Independent Lung Ventilation Therapeutic System

DOUBLE-LUMEN TUBE

After determining that the patient's lung disease is asymmetric and that conventional ventilatory support has failed to improve oxygenation, the practitioner can make the decision to use ILV to improve $\dot{V}/\dot{Q}$ matching. Necessary for the institution of ILV is independent access to each lung by placement of a DLT. Two tubes are bonded together with one tube shorter providing ventilation to the trachea and the longer tube going into the main-stem bronchus. DLTs are available in five sizes: Nos. 28, 35, 37, 39, and 41 French. Most adult men accommodate a No. 41 French, and women usually accept a No. 39 French. DLTs can be right - or left-side angled for cannulation of the right or left main-stem bronchus. The endobronchial tube has two cuffs. The proximal cuff is situated in the usual tracheal position. The proximal lumen opens into the airway below the tracheal cuff and just above the carina. The distal cuff is on the bronchial extension of the tube. The distal airway lumen opens at the end of the

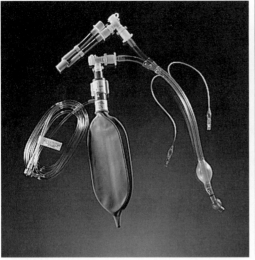
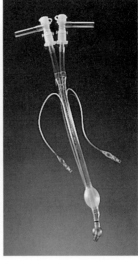

A   B

FIGURE 12-6

Broncho-Cath endobronchial tubes. The double-lumen design permits an airtight seal of the trachea and one bronchus. **A,** Left-angled double-lumen endobronchial tube. **B,** Right-angled endobronchial tube. The right-angled tube has a specifically designed bronchial cuff and fenestrated bronchial lumen to allow ventilation of the right upper lobe. Both tubes come in a variety of sizes measured in French units. Color-coded cuffs, pilot balloons, and proximal lumens help identify bronchial and tracheal lumens. *(Courtesy of Mallinckrodt Critical Care, Argyle, NY.)*

bronchial extension. Inflation of the bronchial cuff allows for differential ventilation. The cuffs, pilot balloons, and airway extensions are color coded for rapid differentiation between bronchial and tracheal lumens (Fig. 12-6).

TWO VENTILATORS
Each endobronchial tube lumen is usually attached to a separate ventilator circuitry attached to its own ventilator. The two ventilators provide asynchronous ILV with no attempt to synchronize the inspiratory cycles. Each system is independent, enabling different types of ventilators (e.g., continuous positive airway pressure [CPAP], HFOV) to be used to maximize response in each lung. Pulmonary artery and occlusion pressures are difficult to interpret during asynchronous ventilation. Systemic pressures and cardiac outputs are comparable to values obtained prior to instituting AILV. Individual ventilator settings are dictated by the particular lung mechanics demonstrated by each lung. It is feasible to have a variance between the two lungs in the delivery of frequencies, VT, level of PEEP, I:E ratio, and ventilatory mode.

Institution of Independent Lung Ventilation
The purpose of ILV is to provide therapy that will optimize $\dot{V}/\dot{Q}$ matching in each lung. Isolating each lung allows for the delivery of sufficient PEEP and VT to the affected lung to promote its reexpansion. Hyperinflation of the good lung and the resulting diversion of perfusion to the affected lung are also avoided.

BOX 12-5 Criteria for Terminating Independent-Lung Ventilation

1. Difference in PEEP in two circuits <5 cm H_2O with stable PaO_2

2. PIP difference <5 cm H_2O on identical settings in both circuits

3. Compliance difference between the two lungs <10 mL/cm H_2O

4. Ratio of end-tidal CO_2 ($ETCO_2$) or CO_2 production ($\dot{V}CO_2$) ≥ 0.88

5. Total minute ventilation <12 L/min (sum of the two systems)

6. Radiographic improvement with decreased asymmetry

....

From Thomas A, Bryce T: Ventilation in the patient with unilateral lung disease. *Crit Care Clin* 1998; 14(4):743–773.

Initial AILV settings should include minute ventilation (rate and V_T), FIO_2, and PEEP level in each circuit. Because most patients are on conventional mechanical ventilation prior to instituting ILV, previous FIO_2 and minute ventilation requirements can be used as the starting point for AILV. Patients are heavily sedated, sometimes requiring the use of neuromuscular blockade while on CMV, so the ventilation mode will be one that provides total support.

Utilizing recommendations from the ARDS Network study, lung-protective strategies using smaller V_Ts (6 mL/kg) and lower plateau pressures (less than 30 cm H_2O) should be considered. Newer case reports incorporate HFOV with ILV to decrease barotrauma to the lungs. The delivery of sufficient PEEP during ILV was the subject of several clinical studies. One study reported using progressive increments of PEEP applied to the involved lung until the compliance in both lungs matched. Some studies use pressure-volume curves and compliance data to allocate PEEP. Others cite that continuous monitoring and trending of pressure, volume, and flow data can assist in determining V_T and PEEP settings. Another study reports utilizing PEEP trials of 0 to 5 cm H_2O in the noninvolved lung and PEEP levels of 10 to 20 cm H_2O in the involved lung with subsequent changes based on oxygenation and gas-exchange responses. Trend monitoring of individual lung compliance (C_t), peak plateau pressures, and peak inspiratory and expiratory airway resistance values evaluate the effect of therapy on each lung. When the lung mechanics between the two lungs are nearly equal, the DLT may be replaced with a single-lumen tube (Box 12-5). Deflation of the bronchial cuff and use of a Y-adapter attached to the two lumens allows for a trial application of conventional ventilation before reintubation with a conventional ETT.

Advantages of Independent Lung Ventilation in Asymmetric Lung Disease

ILV is a physiologically directed therapy aimed at correcting $\dot{V}/\dot{Q}$ abnormalities caused by pathologic changes in the lung and exacerbated by conventional ventilation. The increase in V_D (dead-space volume)/V_T in the normal lung that was caused by hyperinflation and shunting of blood to the diseased lung is decreased through the delivery of a VT that places it in a more optimal position on the pressure-volume curve. The percentage of $\dot{Q}s/\dot{Q}T$ in the diseased lung is decreased by the recruitment of more air spaces through the selective application of PEEP. ILV can reverse persistent atelectatic changes by applying a sufficient level of PEEP to reexpand these atelectatic areas.

ILV generally produces a higher combined total compliance by achieving optimal compliance of each lung through a more appropriate distribution of ventilation. The healthier lung is no longer hyperinflated and pushed beyond its limits of elasticity. The diseased lung is ventilated with higher PEEP levels, which opens air spaces, gradually leading to an improvement in compliance.

With ILV, caution must be used to protect against a larger net VT delivery when the VTs of the two lungs are combined, in comparison with what can be delivered by a single-lumen tube. This larger net VT delivery is achieved with lower airway pressures in the more compliant lung, which places it at a much lower risk of barotrauma.

Another definite benefit of ILV is that because the percentage of shunt is decreased, the FIO_2 required to maintain adequate oxygenation is often much less than was needed with conventional ventilation. High levels of oxygen are toxic to pulmonary tissue and can lead to fibrosis, especially if used for a prolonged period. Finally, tissue oxygen delivery is also improved because of a reduction in the pulmonary vascular resistance (PVR) and an increase in the cardiac output (CO). Under the conditions of asymmetric lung disease and conventional ventilation, PVR is high because of hyperinflation of the compliant lung and transmission of high alveolar pressures to the pulmonary capillary bed. When PVR is reduced, CO increases because the stroke volume of the right side of the heart improves.

Finally, with placement of an endobronchial tube, transbronchial contamination is reduced. The spillage of secretions and purulent drainage from the diseased lung to the healthier lung are diminished or prevented.

Patient Care Considerations for the Patient Undergoing Independent Lung Ventilation

DOUBLE-LUMEN TUBE PLACEMENT

Insertion of a DLT is similar to regular intubation with a few modifications. Determining appropriate sizing of the DLT depends on the patient's size and the largest DLT able to pass through the glottis to decrease the chance of tube migration down the main-stem bronchus and provide the best endobronchial seal. In cases of bronchial obstruction, smaller tube sizes may be needed.

Prior to intubation, one should check for cuff air leaks by instilling 10 mL of air into the proximal tracheal cuff port and 3 mL of air into the distal endobronchial cuff port. Intubation is accomplished under direct visualization with a stylet guide passage of the tube through the vocal cords. Once past the cords, the stylet is removed and the tube is rotated 90 degrees to place the endobronchial cuff toward the desired bronchus. The rotation is either counterclockwise for left-sided DLT placement or clockwise for right-sided DLT placement. When moderate resistance is met with passage, both distal and proximal cuffs can be inflated.

Correct DLT placement should be confirmed by an end-tidal carbon dioxide ($ETCO_2$) monitor, auscultation of breath sounds, and fiberoptic bronchoscopy. Auscultation is achieved through sequential clamping of the tracheal and bronchial lumens while listening for breath sounds during assisted ventilation. Clamping of the bronchial lumen produces ipsilateral loss of chest movement and breath sounds. The opposite side has loss of chest expansion and breath sounds when the tracheal lumen is clamped. The reliability of auscultation for correct DLT placement has been the subject of several thoracic surgery studies. In one study when tube placement was determined by auscultation, 48% to 83% of the time the DLT required repositioning when placement was confirmed by bronchoscopy. Another study reported that only 2% of DLTs auscultated for placement required repositioning with bronchoscopy. To visualize the left-sided bronchial cuff placement distal to the carina, the bronchoscope is passed through the tracheal lumen. With right-sided placement of DLT, the bronchoscope is passed through the bronchial lumen to visualize the ventilation slot in relation to the right upper lobe opening.

Because the affected lung is going to have decreased breath sounds relative to the healthier lung, auscultation of breath sounds is not the only ongoing assessment that should be performed to assess tube placement. Inspired VT and expired VT should be frequently recorded for each lung. Tube misplacement may be noted or discovered by a sudden change in volume returns, airway pressures, or lung compliance. If the exhaled tidal volume (EVT) of one lung acutely changes, assess the EVT of the other lung to see whether the volume is shifting to the other side. Volume lost from an endobronchial cuff leak will escape to the other lung. Volume lost from a tracheal cuff leak will likely vent to the atmosphere. Maintaining the correct position of the endobronchial tube is of prime importance. A tube that is too small may slip downward, whereas one that is too large is associated with tube migration in an upward direction. When one is turning or tilting the patient, the tube must be held stationary because up to a reported 32% of cases experience DLT displacement with patient repositioning. The ventilator tubing should be suspended close to the DLT to prevent gravitational displacement. Tube placement at the teeth should be marked on the tube and noted in the medical record after chest radiograph confirmation. A readily available bronchoscope is essential to exclude DLT displacement and to reposition if necessary. Patients are usually heavily sedated, and infrequently neuromuscular blockade is used to prevent tube malposition. As discussed earlier, sedation and paralytics place the patient at risk for complications related to DVT, reduced gastric motility, and skin breakdown. See HFOV patient care considerations for further details.

PATIENT-VENTILATOR SYSTEM MONITORING

The patient-ventilator system monitoring performed for the patient undergoing ILV is the same for the patient undergoing conventional ventilation except that twice the monitoring is required. Each ventilator's control panel should be labeled "left" or "right" and checked for correctness of settings, and the display panel should be checked for the patient data on airway pressures and exhaled VTs. Before ILV is instituted, the risk of pulmonary barotrauma is greatest to the healthier lung. However, after ILV initiation, the lung with reduced compliance is at greater risk because of higher peak opening pressures. The exhaled VT should be monitored to determine VT in pressure modes and whether the set VT is actually being delivered in volume-targeted modes. Dynamic compliance (CDYN) monitoring is helpful to determine individual lung status. EVT is also useful in confirming tube placement.

ENDOBRONCHIAL CUFF PRESSURES

Similar to single ETTs with the development of low-volume, high-compliance cuffs, measuring cuff pressures on DLT cuffs should be done as per institutional policy, usually every 8 to 12 hours. Excessive cuff pressure may result in tracheal or bronchial damage with granuloma formation on healing. Bronchial scarring may result in significant morbidity in that ventilation to the left or right lung may be persistently impaired. Interventions to the scarred bronchial segment, such as dilation, stent placement, or surgical repair, may eventually be required to correct the ventilation problem. Overinflation of cuffs may also result in cuff rupture, distortion, or herniation.

AIRWAY CLEARANCE

Some aspects of bronchial hygiene are facilitated by the DLT, but new problems are also created. Because of the smaller lumen, a smaller suction catheter is required. A larger catheter is difficult to pass and can also lead to obstruction of airflow. A No. 10 French catheter is generally acceptable. A disadvantage of the smaller catheters is that retrieval of plugs and tenacious secretions may become more difficult. Suction catheter length is another consideration when an endobronchial tube is used. Standard adult suction catheters are 22 inches in length. Endobronchial tubes are usually packaged with four or five suction catheters that are 24 inches in length. These should be reserved for use in the longer bronchial lumen. Use of the longer catheters, however, is not required because, provided the suctioning procedure is not being performed through lengthy adapters and the full length of the catheter is inserted, standard catheters reach beyond the tip of the bronchial lumen.

The actual depth of insertion of a suction catheter tip must be governed by clinical judgment. Adequate depth through either lumen is necessary to achieve secretion removal and prevent airway occlusion by accumulated mucus. Vigorous insertion of a suction catheter should be avoided, and when resistance is met, the catheter should be withdrawn. Suctioning through the proximal lumen generally results in slightly more resistance to catheter insertion, compared with suctioning through the bronchial lumen, possibly because of the location and shape of the side opening of the proximal lumen. Resistance, however, may indicate some obstruction of the proximal lumen by the tracheal wall, a potential complication.

Summary and Future Direction

The use of a DLT and ILV is not common, but it can be a lifesaving technology for supporting patients with ULD. Critical care clinicians must be versed in the indications, application, physiology, and troubleshooting associated with ILV. Early studies indicated that ILV should be done with synchronized ventilators. However, newer literature demonstrates that this is not necessary. Once the DLT is placed, the ventilator settings for each lung can be tailored to individual pathophysiology, resistance, and compliance. Treating each lung individually is the essence of ILV. Care must be taken to monitor treatment and changing lung conditions.

Reports demonstrate successful ILV using HFOV in one or both lungs. This is a major advancement in ILV because it demonstrates the primary focus of lung protection incorporated with providing adequate gas exchange. Supporting patients with ULD is time consuming and requires a great deal of technical and physiologic understanding. The use of ILV is accompanied by increased demand for intensive care unit (ICU) care, resource utilization, and continuous monitoring. The future of ILV should focus on advancements in equipment used during the procedure and further understanding of $\dot{V}/\dot{Q}$ relationships within each lung.

HELIOX

History and Physiology

Helium and oxygen mixtures (heliox) have been used for medicinal purposes since 1934. Since that time, heliox has been studied and reported in a variety of respiratory conditions such as upper airway obstruction, status asthmaticus, chronic obstructive pulmonary disease (COPD), decompression sickness, postextubation stridor, bronchiolitis, and ARDS. Barach first described the positive effects of heliox for treating patients with asthma and airway obstruction. The observation of reduced work of breathing (WOB) immediately after treatment with heliox is the basis for today's protocols. From the 1930s until the 1980s, heliox all but faded from medical literature. An increased death rate for patients with status asthmaticus in the 1980s brought heliox back to the clinical arena.

By itself, helium, an inert gas, is odorless and tasteless, and it does not support combustion or react with biologic membranes. Helium is a third as dense (0.179 g/L) as room air (1.293 g/L), seven times lighter than nitrogen, and eight times less dense than oxygen (Table 12-6). The only other gas with a lower density is hydrogen. When helium is combined with room air to make an 80%/20% HeO_2 heliox product, it has a density approximately a third of air. These physical properties reduce the Reynolds number associated with flow through the airways. The Reynolds number represents

TABLE 12-6	Gas Density and Viscosity: Physical Properties of Nitrogen, Oxygen, Air, and Helium	
Gas	Density (ρ) (g/L)	Viscosity (η) (micropoises)
Nitrogen	1.251	167.4
Oxygen	1.429	192.6
Air	1.293	170.8
Helium	0.179	188.7

(From Michael Gentile, RRT, AARC Professor's Rounds, Getting the most out of alternative gas therapies, Jan 15, 2004.)

the relationship between the airway radius and the velocity, density, and viscosity of the gas. The Reynolds number is expressed as follows:

$$\frac{[2(\text{airway radius}) \, (\text{velocity}) \, (\text{density of the gas})]}{\text{gas viscosity}}$$

Heliox, therefore, should convert some areas of turbulent flow to areas of laminar flow. When gas flow is laminar, the Poiseuille equation can be used to calculate resistance to flow:

$$\text{Airway resistance} = \frac{[8 \, (\text{tube length}) \, (\text{gas viscosity})]}{3.14 \, (\text{tube radius}^4)}$$

Heliox mixtures have the potential to decrease the WOB in patients with increased airway resistance. Heliox does not treat airway resistance. It reduces the inspiratory pressure of the patient or ventilator. Helium enhances the effect on carbon dioxide elimination, which diffuses approximately four times faster with a HeO_2 mixture than nitrogen oxygen. Heliox therapy improves alveolar ventilation by improving ventilation-perfusion relationships. The effort required to move a volume of gas to the alveolus is reduced by a third when breathing helium rather than nitrogen.

Indications

Note that heliox has no therapeutic benefit to treat an underlying disease. Instead, heliox is used solely to reduce the resistance of the airways and WOB until other therapies (e.g., oxygen, bronchodilators, steroids, antibiotics) can be effective. Several studies demonstrated a rapid reduction in symptoms with the institution of heliox but an equally quick return to baseline when the heliox was withdrawn.

The use of heliox to manage upper airway obstructions is well described. Since the first described benefits of heliox by Barach in 1934, several other studies have highlighted the rapid and dramatic response to heliox in cases of upper airway obstruction. Fleming and colleagues studied normal subjects breathing through resistors and found significant improvement in pulmonary function tests when heliox was introduced into the system. This study demonstrated that heliox increases gas flow rates past airway obstruction. For postextubation stridor, Smith and colleagues showed significant benefit by reducing respiratory distress by 38% as compared to air-and-oxygen mixtures. Most reports describe an almost immediate response and reduction in symptoms of upper airway obstruction once heliox is started.

Several studies investigated the use of heliox in patients with exacerbations of COPD. A common theme in all studies is that hypoxic patients were excluded, with the focus of research being on hypercarbia. Benefits were found in reductions in $Paco_2$, inspiratory time, respiratory rate, peak pressures, plateau pressures, and intrinsic PEEP. Multiple studies demonstrated the benefits of heliox on respiratory mechanics in decompensated COPD patients. Heliox consistently improves inspiratory and expiratory flow, producing a reduction in dynamic hyperinflation. The amount of improvement is proportional to the degree of compromise in patients with COPD breathing heliox. The use of heliox may reduce the need for endotracheal intubation for patients with COPD, especially when used in combination with noninvasive positive-pressure ventilation (NPPV). Whether heliox aids in weaning COPD patients from CMV remains unclear.

To date, no data exist for the use of heliox in ARDS in the adult population. Theoretically, CMV settings of peak inspiratory pressure, plateau pressure, and minute volume are all reduced while V_T and peak expiratory flow are increased with the application of heliox in ARDS patients. Resulting gas exchange benefit may yield a reduced $PaCO_2$ and improvement in oxygenation. Because these trials have yet to be conducted, the benefits of heliox and ARDS are only speculative.

Heliox is recommended as a useful adjunct in patients with severe asthma, both for spontaneous breathing and those on mechanical ventilation. Gluck and colleagues administered heliox to seven patients with status asthmaticus intubated for respiratory failure. All patients experienced significant reduction in $PaCO_2$ and peak airway pressures within 20 minutes. Also observed was an increased V_T for all patients. The authors concluded that heliox may help reduce the risk of barotrauma and improvement in overall ventilation. The theorized physiology of heliox and asthma is that improved alveolar ventilation promotes rapid washout of alveolar carbon dioxide and enhanced removal of arteriolar carbon dioxide.

Heliox also increases the deposition of inhaled particles to the distal airways in patients with severe asthma. In one study, Anderson and colleagues found that radiographically labeled particles delivered with heliox are better retained in asthmatics when compared to healthy volunteers. They believed that differences in particle deposition occur because of a decreased turbulent flow when heliox is administered. They also suggested that deposition of these particles would be more pronounced in patients with a greater degree of obstruction. Severe asthmatics may be better served by delivering aerosolized medications with heliox rather than air or oxygen.

Delivery Systems

Heliox is commercially available and supplied in medical gas cylinders in sizes H, G, and E. Helium and oxygen typically are blended to percentage concentrations of 80/20, 70/30, and 60/40, respectively. Clinicians must never use 100% helium for safety reasons of delivering less than 0.21 FIO_2 to any patient. Gas regulators manufactured specifically for helium must be used to deliver the gas safely and accurately.

Caution must also be used with heliox and medical devices. Oxygen and airflow meters do not reflect heliox flow rates correctly because of the variation in gas density. Clinicians should calculate predicted heliox flow rates for accuracy. For example, 80/20 heliox is 1.8 times more diffusible than oxygen. For every 10 L/min gas indicated on a standard flowmeter, the actually delivered gas is 16 or 18 L/m.

Multiple studies demonstrated that the use of heliox can affect the function of nebulizers and mechanical ventilators. Heliox can affect nebulizer function, resulting in smaller particle size, reduced output, and longer nebulization time. When heliox is used to power the nebulizer, the flow should be increased by 50% to 100% to ensure adequate output from the nebulizer. Heliox also improves aerosolized medication delivery during mechanical ventilation. Most mechanical ventilators are designed and calibrated only to deliver gas mixtures of oxygen with the balance being air. The density, viscosity, and thermal conductivity of heliox may interfere with the function

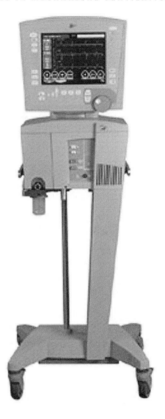

FIGURE 12-7

AVEA heliox delivery system. *(From Viasys Critical Care Operator's Manual [www.Viasyscriticalcare.com].)*

of some mechanical ventilators. Caution must be used by clinicians prior to using heliox with any mechanical ventilator because some devices malfunction with the introduction of any gases other than air and oxygen. Care should also be exercised in delivering heliox through mechanical ventilators because the delivered and exhaled V_T measurement can be severely altered. A mechanical ventilator must be bench-tested first to ensure safe operation when used in conjunction with heliox. Consulting the device's operation manual along with contacting the manufacturer are good steps to guarantee safe delivery of heliox through mechanical ventilators.

Only one mechanical ventilator is specifically designed and calibrated to deliver heliox. The AVEA (Viasys Critical Care, Palm Springs, Calif) (Fig. 12-7) is the first reliable device for heliox delivery. The AVEA's internal blending system automatically compensates for the gas mixture, providing accuracy in all delivered and monitored settings.

Advantages

The unique physical properties of helium promote greater and less turbulent gas flow, decreased airway resistance, and decreased WOB in specific patients. Because helium is an inert gas, not known to interact with human metabolism, it can be used on any patient. No known complications have resulted from the use of heliox.

Disadvantages

Heliox therapy should be a short-term adjunct to assist a patient through a fragile clinical period. Heliox is only a temporizing measure and produces no treatment on its own. It is relatively expensive when compared to other medical gases (up to four times that of oxygen), and its benefits are only realized while the patient is breathing heliox. Therefore, heliox treatment must be continuous and not delivered intermittently. If a patient needs heliox for greater than 48 hours, a reevaluation of the underlying disease state and other therapies should take place. Because heliox is delivered via gas cylinder, steps must be taken to conserve or reduce gas consumption. The number of tanks available at any institution is limited by space, consumption, and ordering practice.

Patient Care Considerations

Patients receiving heliox therapy are usually located in the emergency department, ICU, or a monitored step-down unit. Because of the severity of illness for heliox administration, patients must be closely monitored. Usual monitoring includes pulse oximetry, peak expiratory flow, heart rate, respiratory rate (RR), ABGs, pulsus paradoxus, peak inspiratory pressures (PIPs), and V_T. Great attention must be given to the amount of heliox available because unexpected disruption in gas delivery can have serious consequences. When heliox is stopped abruptly, the patient may decompensate, quickly leading to respiratory arrest. Nonintubated patients must be educated on the importance of continuously wearing the mask delivering heliox. Patients become less anxious, more comfortable, and more cooperative because of the decreased WOB related to heliox. This comfort can quickly be reversed at the sudden stopping of heliox inhalation. Unfortunately, weaning usually takes place by simply turning the heliox off and assessing the patient for signs of respiratory distress, elevated PIPs, or decreased V_Ts. The weaning and discontinuation must be done after other therapeutic agents have had adequate time to work. If the patient tolerates a brief interruption of heliox without any respiratory compromise, a long trial may lead to complete discontinuation. Keeping intubation equipment and personnel nearby is imperative when patients are receiving heliox treatment in case of sudden decompensation that may lead to respiratory distress or arrest.

Summary and Future Direction

Heliox is a safe and rapidly acting gas that reduces airway resistance and WOB and improves gas exchange in a variety of respiratory conditions. The therapeutic benefit lies solely in its low density. Published research using heliox dates back to 1934 and suggests the gas may be useful in airway obstruction, COPD, asthma, and a variety of other circumstances. The ultimate goal of heliox therapy is to reduce respiratory distress and therefore avoid endotracheal intubation or emergent cricothyrotomy. Once patients are placed on mechanical ventilation, heliox may assist in improving gas exchange, reducing ventilator settings, and aiding in liberation from positive-pressure ventilation. Delivery of heliox can be problematic at times because of limited equipment options. Further studies are needed to determine the role of heliox for patients with ARDS on mechanical ventilation. Future investigations should examine the effect of heliox on specific outcome of length of time on mechanical ventilation, hospital stay, and mortality.

INHALED NITRIC OXIDE

History and Physiology

Nitric oxide is a naturally occurring substance found in the human body that acts as a neurochemical transmitter. It also occurs naturally in the atmosphere in concentrations of 10 to 100 parts per billion (ppb) in human airways, 10 to 1000 ppb in smog, and in cigarette smoke at levels of 400 to 1000 parts per million (ppm). Medical dosing for inhaled nitric oxide (iNO) is much lower at 1 to 80 ppm.

The role of iNO for clinical use has increased remarkably over the last decade. It was first described in 1987 as "endothelial-derived growth factor." Since that time, iNO has been the subject of incredible study for the physiologic response in patients with impaired gas exchange and hemodynamics. The discovery of iNO's role in pulmonary vascular tone led to a flood of research from basic science to large randomized clinical trials, resulting in thousands of publications. In 1992, the journal *Science* named nitric oxide the "Molecule of the Year." Several researchers received a Nobel Prize in Medicine and Physiology for their work with nitric oxide in 1998.

Nitric oxide activates guanylate cyclase, which converts into cyclic guanosine monophosphate (cGMP). The presence of cGMP at the smooth muscle causes relaxation (Fig. 12-8). When this occurs in the pulmonary vasculature, the result is reduced pulmonary vascular resistance, redistribution of pulmonary blood flow, and a reduction in right heart work. When nitric oxide is inhaled, redistribution of pulmonary blood is moved to areas of the lung where ventilation is more efficient, thus improving ventilation-perfusion matching and therefore oxygenation. Once nitric oxide enters the circulation, it quickly combines with hemoglobin and forms methemoglobin, preventing any systemic effects and making it a potent and selective pulmonary vasodilator. This property makes iNO an appealing research topic for pulmonary disorders.

Indications

The only FDA-approved indication for iNO is for the treatment of term neonates with hypoxic respiratory failure associated with pulmonary hypertension as a means to improve oxygenation and therefore avoid ECMO or death. All other uses are considered "off label." An important component of ARDS is pulmonary hypertension and accompanying hypoxemia. The rationale for delivery of iNO in ARDS patients is reducing pulmonary hypertension and directing blood flow toward ventilated alveoli. In 1993, Rossaint and colleagues first described improved oxygenation and reduced pulmonary artery hypertension in patients with ARDS. iNO produces vasodilatation in ventilated lung units and decreases pulmonary hypertension,

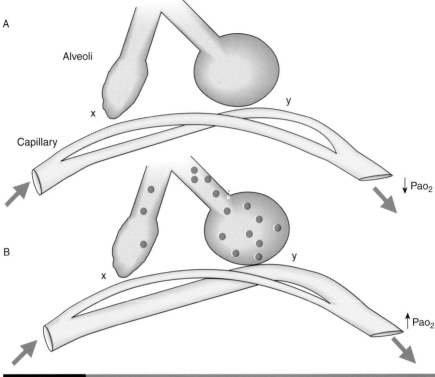

FIGURE 12-8

Proposed mechanism for improvements in oxygenation in patients with acute respiratory distress syndrome (ARDS) treated with inhaled nitric oxide. *(Top)* **A,** inhomogeneous lung injury in ARDS creates two theoretical populations of alveolar-capillary units (x and y). Blood flow to those regions with decreased ventilation produces areas of low $\dot{V}/\dot{Q}$ ratios. Admixture of blood perfusing low $\dot{V}/\dot{Q}$ regions (x) with blood from areas with more normal $\dot{V}/\dot{Q}$ ratios (y) creates hypoxemia ($\downarrow$ Pao$_2$). *(Bottom)* **B,** inhaled nitric oxide *(blue dots)* distributes preferentially to those areas with greater ventilation, stimulating localized vasodilation and enhanced blood flow to well-ventilated lung units while simultaneously "stealing" perfusion from more poorly ventilated areas. The net effect is improved $\dot{V}/\dot{Q}$ matching and reduced hypoxemia ($\uparrow$ Pao$_2$). *(From Hart C: Nitric oxide in adult lung disease. Chest 1999; 5:1407-1417.)*

thereby reducing $\dot{V}/\dot{Q}$ mismatch by redistributing pulmonary perfusion toward ventilated regions and enhancing oxygenation. At least 30 studies of patients with ARDS treated with iNO have been published. Collectively, 60% to 80% of ARDS patients respond to iNO with a 20% improvement in oxygenation and a 10% reduction in pulmonary artery pressure. Despite the impressive improvements in oxygenation, in several randomized, controlled trials in adult patients with ARDS, iNO was found to have no effect on mortality or the duration of mechanical ventilation. However, the improvement in oxygenation allows for the reduction in possibly harmful ventilator settings such as high concentrations of F$_{IO_2}$ and elevated peak

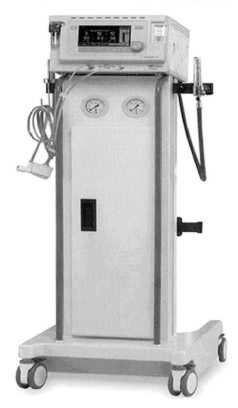

FIGURE 12-9

INOvent nitric oxide delivery system. *(From www.Datex-Ohmeda.com.)*

inspiratory and plateau pressures. In addition to the positive effect of iNO on pulmonary blood flow and gas exchange, iNO plays a role in other processes during ARDS, inhibiting platelet aggregation and inflammatory mediators.

Delivery System

The delivery system currently used to provide iNO to patients is the INOvent (Datex-Ohmeda, Madison, Wis) (Fig. 12-9). The system's sole purpose is to deliver iNO, and it is specifically designed to work with most mechanical ventilators, both conventional and high frequency. The INOvent maintains a constant concentration of nitric oxide in the ventilator circuit and continuously monitors nitrogen dioxide and FIO_2 for all modes and ventilator settings. Alarms are adjustable for iNO delivery, FIO_2, and nitrogen dioxide. The system is configured to accomplish inter- and intra-hospital transports with a battery option and manual bagging capability. The INOvent is not a mechanical ventilator but rather a gas delivery and monitoring system. In the event of a system failure or a wall-outlet power failure, a backup power supply and reserve nitric oxide delivery system should be available.

Advantages

The importance of iNO as a pulmonary vascular muscle relaxant rests on its characteristic of being delivered as a gas directly to the pulmonary circulation, without systemic side effects. When iNO is delivered to better ventilated regions of the lung, blood flow is redistributed to maximize gas exchange. iNO is instantly inactivated by hemoglobin, which leads to rapid results after inhalation of gas begins. With the introduction of new iNO delivery systems, the gas is relatively easy to deliver. Injector module and sample lines are placed into the mechanical ventilator circuit. The dosing, F_{IO_2}, and nitrogen dioxide are continuously monitored and titrated.

Disadvantages

Nitric oxide is an industrial pollutant and has toxic side effects at high concentrations (greater than 1000 ppm). Abrupt discontinuation of iNO may result in worsening Pa_{O_2} and increased pulmonary artery hypertension. Increasing doses of iNO may lead to methemoglobinemia.

Patient Care Considerations

REBOUND HYPOXEMIA AND PULMONARY HYPERTENSION

Abrupt discontinuation of iNO can precipitate a rapid increase in intrapulmonary right to left shunting, a decrease in Pa_{O_2}, and cause severe rebound pulmonary hypertension. The reasons for this rebound phenomenon are not entirely known, but it may relate to feedback inhibition of nitric oxide synthase activity and/or elevated endothelin-1 (ET-1) levels. With some patients, the hypoxemia and pulmonary hypertension can be worse after discontinuation of iNO then prior to instituting treatment. Hess recommends the following guidelines that may help avoid the deleterious effects of rebound during withdrawal of iNO. First, use the lowest effective iNO dose (5 ppm or less). Second, do not withdraw iNO until the patient's clinical status improves sufficiently (e.g., $F_{IO_2} = 0.40$; PEEP = 5 cm H_2O; hemodynamic stability). Third, set the iNO dose at 1 ppm for a short time (30 minutes to 1 hour) before discontinuing iNO. Fourth, increase the F_{IO_2} to 0.60 to 0.70 before withdrawal of iNO, and prepare to support the patient's hemodynamics if necessary.

Reported administration of the nucleotide phosphodiesterase (PDE) inhibitor dipyridamole has been used to prevent rebound pulmonary hypertension. Atz and colleagues suggested that the use of sildenafil, a selective inhibitor of a cGMP-specific phosphodiesterase, can improve the harmful effects related to discontinuation of iNO. Sildenafil is reported to possibly potentiate and/or prolong the pulmonary vasodilating effects of iNO. Further studies on dipyridamole and sildenafil are warranted.

NITROGEN DIOXIDE

In the presence of oxygen, iNO is rapidly oxidized to nitrogen dioxide. The conversion rate of nitric oxide to nitrogen dioxide is related to inspiratory oxygen concentration (F_{IO_2}), the square of nitric oxide concentration, and the residence time of these gases. To minimize production of nitrogen dioxide, both the concentration of oxygen and nitric oxide and the contact between them should be kept to the minimal amount. The Occupational Safety and Health Administration (OSHA) in 1988 set safety limits for nitrogen dioxide at 5 ppm. Increased airway reactivity and parenchymal lung injury is reported in humans with inhalation of 2 ppm or less. Toxicity is unlikely with inhaled nitric oxide at less than 40 ppm.

The INOvent Delivery System (Datex-Ohmeda, Madison, Wis) includes a continuous gas monitoring of nitrogen dioxide for intubated patients. The clinician should set the nitrogen dioxide gas delivery alarm at 2 ppm, with the goal being no nitrogen dioxide detected.

METHEMOGLOBINEMIA

Methemoglobinemia toxicity occurs when inhaled nitric oxide at higher doses binds with hemoglobin in red blood cells. This results in the reduction of the oxygen-carrying capacity of the blood, which, in turn, decreases oxygen delivery and creates a functional anemia. The oxyhemoglobin dissociation curve is also affected and leads to a shift to the left, diminishing the release of oxygen from red blood cells. Methemoglobin reductase within erythrocytes can convert methemoglobin back to hemoglobin. The incidence of methemoglobin (metHb) is low when iNO is administered within the accepted dose range of less than 40 ppm. Doses of iNO are usually 20 or less ppm. Methemoglobinemia can also be caused by certain substances, including nitrates, prilocaine, benzocaine, dapsone, and metoclopramide. MetHb is usually reported with ABG values and can be monitored every 4 hours if rising metHb is suspected. Normal metHb is less than 2%; levels below 5% do not require treatment. If metHb levels are gradually increasing, a lower but still effective iNO dose may be used. If metHb levels are significant, then iNO should be discontinued, and methylene blue, which increases reduced nicotinamide adenine dinucleotide-methemoglobin reductase, should be infused. Ascorbic acid is also used to treat methemoglobinemia.

INHIBITION OF PLATELET FUNCTION

Rarely does iNO exert platelet inhibitory effects such as blocking (ADP) and collagen-induced aggregation and altering platelet adhesions. Platelet counts and coagulation laboratory tests such as prothrombin time (PT) and international normalized ratio (INR) can be obtained if there is a suspicion. Consideration of coagulopathy is important; however, the clinical importance is unclear. An increased incidence in bleeding times was not substantiated in clinical trials.

LEFT VENTRICULAR DYSFUNCTION

Inhaled nitric oxide may have adverse hemodynamic effects in patients with pre-existing severe left ventricular dysfunction. Inhaled nitric oxide increases pulmonary vascular resistance and increases pulmonary capillary occlusive pressures at higher doses (40 to 80 ppm) in some patients with severe left ventricular dysfunction. The acute reduction in right ventricular afterload may lead to an increase in pulmonary venous return to the left heart, thereby increasing left ventricular filling pressures and worsening pulmonary edema.

IMMUNOSUPPRESSANT PROPERTIES

Nitric oxide has immunosuppressant properties that theoretically could increase the risk of nosocomial infection and can cause DNA strand breaks and/or base alterations that are potentially mutagenic. Additional studies are warranted to understand the clinical implications.

Summary and Future Direction

The role of iNO as an adjunct to mechanical ventilation in patients with ARDS remains unclear. Although iNO has scientific and physiologic merits by increasing PaO_2 and reducing pulmonary artery hypertension, no study has ever demonstrated its role for improving outcomes in patients with ARDS. More than 30 human studies reported iNO use in ARDS. An estimated 60% to 80% of the patients who respond to iNO demonstrated a 20% increase in oxygenation. In selected patients, iNO can be used to minimize FIO_2 and reduce lung distention pressures. Although the increase in PaO_2 may allow for patients to overcome a critical phase of ARDS, the determination of whether the iNO strategy affects survival or outcome is not yet determined.

Long-term effects of iNO are still under investigation. The most promising area of iNO research is new clinical applications in patients with sickle cell disease and those with thoracic (heart and lung) transplants. Future iNO research will evaluate the role of iNO in injury and inflammation of the lungs as well as other diseases. Lowson cited a number of other agents being studied that may have similar physiologic effects as iNO. They include inhaled prostanoids (prostacyclin and iloprost) and novel therapies such as phosphodiesterase inhibitors and neuropeptides. As more knowledge is gained about the role of iNO and other agents on the human body, new and promising therapies will emerge to treat cardiopulmonary diseases.

EXTRACORPOREAL MEMBRANE OXYGENATION

History and Indications

Despite maximal supportive care with mechanical ventilation, some patients with ARDS experience unmanageable gas exchange, leading clinicians to consider a more advanced form of cardiopulmonary support. ECMO is an invasive and complex form of cardiopulmonary bypass for patients with severe reversible cardiac and/or pulmonary failure when maximum conventional therapy is not effective. During ECMO, blood is removed from the right side of the circulation and pumped through a machine with a membrane oxygenator, at which point oxygen is added and carbon dioxide is removed, and then the blood is heated and pumped back to the arterial side of the patient. In patients with ARDS, ECMO can reduce right-to-left shunt adequately to reduce mechanical ventilator support and possible volume/pressure-induced lung injury. This technique was once used exclusively in the operating room for short-term support during cardiothoracic surgery. The use of ECMO allows for blood circulation and gas exchange outside the body while theoretically resting the heart and lungs. The advantages of extracorporeal techniques are providing adequate gas exchange with a lower inspired FIO_2 concentration and reducing ventilation pressures. Potential complications involve clot formation; extensive bleeding caused by systemic anticoagulation, including intracranial hemorrhage; seizures; air emboli; sepsis; disseminated intravascular coagulation (DIC); renal failure; decubitus ulcers; and technical failure.

The technology used during ECMO is not new. Extracorporeal circulation was first devised as a tool to be utilized during cardiac surgery. As early as 1936, Gibbon was attempting to research and develop a roller pump that could sustain life during surgical procedures of the heart and great vessels. In 1944, Kolff and Berk reported the oxygenation of venous blood during dialysis. An open heart surgical procedure technology was advanced in the 1950s, as was the use of cardiopulmonary bypass. The first membrane oxygenator was developed by Clowes and colleagues in 1956. This was a substantial technical advancement, but it could not support life for more than a few hours. Common complications of cardiopulmonary bypass at that time were thrombocytopenia, coagulopathy, hemolysis, organ dysfunction, and significant bleeding. Soon it was discovered that silicone rubber had uncommon gas transfer characteristics.

The 1960s was a time of intensive laboratory research to prolong the time that cardiopulmonary bypass could be performed and to improve the membrane lungs. A silicone membrane similar to the one commonly used today was developed in 1963. With such a device it was possible to perform extended bypass procedures in animals up to 1 week. Several premature neonates were supported with ECMO, but all expired from intraventricular hemorrhage. The first successful ECMO case was reported in 1972 in which a man 24 years of age with multiple trauma injuries was supported for 75 hours.

In 1974, the NIH sponsored a multicenter, randomized trial that compared venoarterial ECMO with conventional therapy in adult patients with respiratory failure. The results failed to show an improvement in outcome. Both ECMO and conventional therapies demonstrated a dismal survival rate with no significant difference between the two (9.5% in ECMO patients and 8.3% in the conventional therapy group).

Meanwhile, Bartlett was treating the neonatal population successfully. Throughout the 1980s, more centers started to use ECMO technology for neonates with reversible lung disease who were failing conventional support. In the following decade, ECMO moved into the ICU and become a standard of care for days and even weeks in the support of patients of many age-groups with severe cardiopulmonary dysfunction. Currently, more than 100 centers throughout the world have provided ECMO to over 17,500 patients since 1986. In the 1990s, other therapies became available and reduced the number of patients requiring ECMO. Some of these alternative approaches are HFOV and iNO.

Although criteria for ECMO vary from center to center and patient to patient, there are several agreed-upon recommendations. In the ICU, several diagnoses are commonly associated with ECMO (Table 12-7). Numerous techniques are currently available in the clinical environment, and a number of others are undergoing experimental work.

General guidelines for neonatal ECMO include the following: a disease process that is deemed reversible, gestational age of more than 36 weeks, weight more than

TABLE 12-7	Adult Extracorporeal Life Support Diagnoses and Survival Rates	
Diagnosis	**No. of Cases**	**Survival (%)**
Bacterial pneumonia	186	52
Viral pneumonia	87	62
Aspiration pneumonia	32	56
Adult respiratory distress syndrome	328	52
Acute respiratory failure, non-ARDS	167	64
Others	55	49
Total	1005	63

Data from ELSO Adult ECLS Registry, Extracorporeal Life Support Organization. Ann Arbor, Mich, 1986-2004.

2 kg, mechanical ventilation for no more than 7 to 10 days prior to extracorporeal life support (ECLS), no significant immunosuppression, absence of intraventricular hemorrhage, and no severe neurologic dysfunction or chromosomal abnormality. For adults, the guidelines for ECMO are similar to younger populations: disease processes deemed reversible, mechanical ventilation for no more than 7 to 10 days, and no intraventricular hemorrhage.

For all age-groups, ECMO is usually considered after failure of other available therapies (e.g., HFV, iNO, and permissive hypercapnia). Persistent air leak is also a possible indication for ECMO. Some centers use an oxygen index (OI) of more than 40, and an alveolar-arterial oxygen difference (A-aDo$_2$) of more than 500 for 4 hours as an ECMO criterion; other centers use lower thresholds. If the OI is between 25 and 40, there is a 50% chance of survival. If the OI is more than 40, the mortality is 80%.

For cardiac patients, ECMO criteria include severe and reversible cardiac dysfunction where maximum supportive therapy has failed. A majority of cardiac ECMO is performed in the postoperative period when the patient cannot be weaned from cardiopulmonary bypass or assistance is needed for poor ventricular performance. Patients with severe myocarditis may also be supported with ECMO until the condition resolves or as a bridge to transplantation. ECMO is also an option for patients with complicated posttransplant courses.

Types of Extracorporeal Life Support

VENOARTERIAL ECMO

Venoarterial ECMO (Fig. 12-10) is complete cardiopulmonary bypass that supports both the cardiac and pulmonary functions. The system consists of six components: an extracorporeal circuit, a blood-circulating pump, a membrane oxygenator, a heat exchanger, monitoring and safety devices, and patient cannula. The extracorporeal circuit consists of a series of Super Tygon tubes and access adapters to circulate

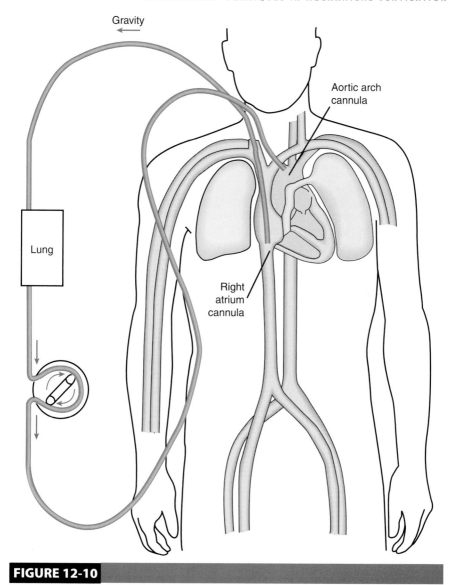

Gravity

Aortic arch
cannula

Lung

Right
atrium
cannula

FIGURE 12-10

Venoarterial extracorporeal life support. *(http://www.med.umich.edu/ecmo/guides/AdultECMO.pdf.)*

venous blood from the patient through the blood-circulating pump and membrane lung back to the patient. The membrane lung is a hollow-fiber silicone oxygenator highly permeable to carbon dioxide and oxygen gas exchange. The surface area of the lung, selected according to patient size, and the flow of ventilating gases across the membrane determine the rate of gas exchange. The blood pump provides the driving pressure from the patient's venous circulation across the membrane lung and back to the arterial circulation.

Two types of extracorporeal pumps are commonly used: the roller-head displacement pump and a centrifugal pump. The circuit cardiac output is a function of blood volume and the speed of pump revolutions. A heat exchanger placed proximal to the patient's arterial return warms the circulating blood volume to body temperature to help prevent hypothermia from ambient cooling of extracorporeal blood volumes.

Appropriate-sized cannulas access the circuit to the patient. Specific monitors within the circuit provide information on circuit safety, function, and performance.

The common carotid artery on both neonatal and pediatric patients is cannulated for blood return to the body. Adult patients typically require alteration of this technique, either by direct transthoracic access to the right atrium and aorta or by femoral access. Venoarterial ECMO is almost complete cardiopulmonary bypass, draining venous blood from the right atrium, circulating the blood through the extracorporeal circuit, and then returning the blood to the aortic arch. Because it is very effective, the patient can be supported for several days to several weeks.

The major advantages of venoarterial ECMO are complete control over the patient's cardiac output and gas exchange. The disadvantages of venoarterial ECMO are the requirement to ligate a major artery and the existence of possible air emboli or clots traveling to the central nervous system.

VENOVENOUS ECMO

Venovenous ECMO (Fig. 12-11) takes only a portion (e.g., 30% to 60%) of the cardiac output from the venous circulation, passes it through a membrane oxygenator, and returns it to the major veins. Venovenous ECMO is reserved for patients with adequate cardiac output. If cardiac insufficiency develops, the patient must be supported by inotropic support or surgically converted to venoarterial ECMO. Venovenous ECMO accesses venous return in neonatal and some pediatric patients by placement of a double-lumen cannula into the right atrium through the internal jugular vein. Venous return circulates from the right atrium through the extracorporeal circuit and returns to the right atrium. Cannula outflow is placed proximal to the tricuspid valve to minimize recirculation of the oxygenated blood from the extracorporeal system. This technique is gaining popularity for patients who were previously considered for venoarterial ECMO. The reasons for the rising interest in the technique are that no arterial ligation or repair is needed, and all debris, clots, and air are routed to the pulmonary circulation and not to the cerebral or systemic circulation (Table 12-8).

Potential Complications Associated with ECMO

Complications of ECMO are usually related to anticoagulation, preexisting hypoxic or hypotensive injury to organ function, and technical/mechanical complications within the ECMO circuit. Bleeding is the most common and potentially disastrous complication of ECMO. Bleeding can occur in one of three places: intracranial, operative site, and gastrointestinal. The most devastating of these occurs in the brain. Proper patient selection can help minimize the probability of intracranial hemorrhage. Maintaining activated clotting times (ACTs) between 180 and 220 seconds can also decrease the incidence of bleeding complications.

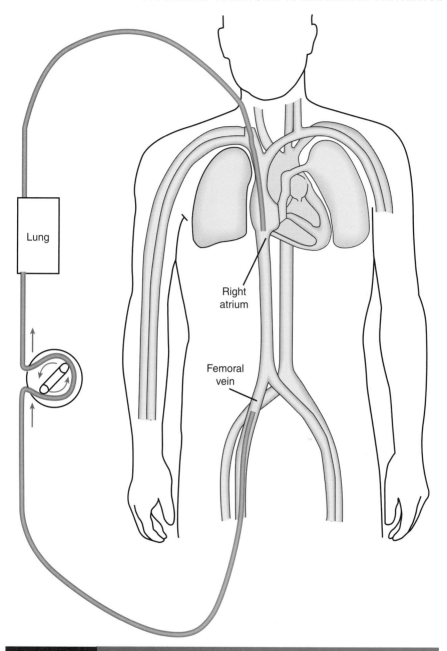

Lung

Right
atrium

Femoral
vein

FIGURE 12-11

Venovenous extracorporeal life support. *(http://www.med.umich.edu/ecmo/guides/AdultECMO.pdf.)*

TABLE 12-8	Differences Between Venoarterial and Venovenous Extracorporeal Membrane Oxygenation	
Venoarterial ECMO	**Venovenous ECMO**	
Higher Pao_2 is achieved.	Lower Pao_2 is achieved.	
Lower perfusion rates are needed.	Higher perfusion rates are needed.	
Bypasses pulmonary circulation.	Maintains pulmonary blood flow.	
Decreases pulmonary artery pressures.	Elevates mixed venous Po_2.	
Provides cardiac support to assist systemic circulation.	Does not provide cardiac support to assist systemic circulation.	
Requires arterial cannulation.	Requires only venous cannulation.	

From Aggarwal S. Extracorporeal membrane oxygenation. eMedicine; http//emedicine.com/ped/topic2895.htm. Most recent update: Oct 21, 2002. Retrieved Oct 21, 2004.

Seizures are also a widely reported complication during ECMO. These are associated with withdrawal of muscle paralysis and the fluid and electrolyte abnormalities often seen at the time of cannulation and early hours of being on ECMO.

Other problems, including renal failure caused by the nonpulsatile flow of venoarterial ECMO performed with a centrifugal pump, hemolysis, hypotension, hypertension, pneumothorax, infection, and cardiac dysrhythmias, should be recognized early and appropriate actions taken.

Mechanical and technical complications of ECMO are rare but equally potentially hazardous. Oxygenator failure is the most commonly reported event, which is corrected by placing a new oxygenator into the circuit. The chance of oxygenator fatigue rises in linear fashion to the length of time on ECMO. Another common complication related to length of time on ECMO is clots formed in the circuit. Other mechanical complications commonly reported are tubing rupture, pump failure, cannulation kinks, heat exchanger malfunction, air in circuitry, and cracks in connectors.

Patient Care Management During ECMO

A patient on ECMO requires collaboration among multiple health care team members to provide the complex care these critically ill patients need. The ECMO specialist remains at the patient's bedside during the ECMO support. In different institutions, the ECMO specialist may be a cardiopulmonary perfusionist, respiratory therapist, or a registered nurse who has received additional ECMO education and training. The role of the ECMO specialist is to maintain, treat, support, and monitor the patient and equipment continuously, physically staying at the bedside during ECMO therapy. In addition to the ECMO specialist, other members of the ECMO team include the physician, respiratory therapist, and the ICU nurse. The physician is responsible for the overall ICU patient management, the respiratory therapist oversees the ventilator management, and the nurse monitors and assesses the patient's response to treatment.

VENTILATOR AND RESPIRATORY CARE

The main intent of ECMO is cardiopulmonary support without iatrogenic complications associated with high ventilation pressures and oxygen toxicity. With these intentions in mind, ventilatory support may be significantly reduced during ECMO. Gas exchange is accomplished by function of the oxygenator. Therefore, keeping PEEP levels of 8 to 10 cm H_2O and a low VT or PIP maintains lung expansion while minimizing barotrauma. Measurement of lung compliance may be helpful in assessment of recovery. SpO_2 can be valuable with venovenous ECMO. During venoarterial ECMO, the SpO_2 depends on ECMO flow. Chest physiotherapy, endotracheal suctioning, and bronchoscopy may be performed to remove retained pulmonary secretions. Once pulmonary function has improved (as evident by chest radiograph, ABG, and SvO_2), the ECMO pump flow rate is decreased slowly over several days. When the ECMO cannula is removed, principles of conventional mechanical ventilation and weaning standards are employed.

ANTICOAGULATION

Continuous heparin infusion is adjusted to keep ACTs from 180 to 220 seconds. If the ACT is less than 180 seconds, the risk of clot formation in the ECMO circuit increases. The ACT level is influenced by blood products and other substances injected into the circuit. Also reported is using activated partial thromboplastin times (APTTs) as a more reliable value in the ECMO patient. The APTT is maintained between 55 and 80 (1.8 to 2.5 × control). The patient is at risk for bleeding not only with the heparin infusion and the potential for heparin-induced thrombocytopenia but also because of platelet loss with the ECMO circuit. Other laboratory values to monitor include fibrinogen (maintain at approximately 150 mg%), platelet count (more than 100,000/mm^3), and hematocrit (approximately 35%). ACTs and APTTs should be drawn every hour from the ECMO circuit. Fibrinogen and blood counts should be done every 4 hours. The frequency of blood draws resulting in patient blood loss is a concern; however, not monitoring coagulation lab values could lead to clot formation, intraventricular hemorrhage, or disseminated intravascular coagulation (DIC). The patient should be frequently monitored for signs and symptoms of active bleeding. Cannulation and other access sites should be monitored for oozing and hematoma. With large-bore ECMO catheters, sites and distal pulses should be assessed every hour.

SEDATION AND ANALGESIA

A patient on ECMO does not need to be continuously chemically paralyzed with the exception of the initial catheter placement or other surgical procedures. Frequent neurologic function examinations and observations of seizures are required for a patient on ECMO. Commonly used medications for ECMO include morphine sulfate, fentanyl, lorazepam (Ativan), and midazolam (Versed). Patients should be sedated to a specific objective level on a sedation scale that correlates with calm and comfortable so they are not at risk of moving cannulas. Daily attempts to wean off sedatives and paralytics should be considered to minimize the risk of prolonged muscle weakness and persistent paralysis.

INFECTION CONTROL

The normal febrile response to infection may go unrecognized in the ECMO patient secondary to the continuous warming of the blood returning from the ECMO circuit. Daily WBCs, chest radiograph, culture results, assessment of cannula site, and signs and symptoms of infection should be reviewed by the ECMO team daily during patient rounds. Serial blood cultures can be drawn from both the patient and the ECMO circuit. Some centers use broad-spectrum antibiotics for prophylaxis and others wait until a positive culture is reported; however, most centers do not use prophylactic antibiotics for fear of selecting resistant organisms. The cannula site is cleansed with chlorhexidine gluconate 2%, and then a sterile gauze sponge dressing is applied. The frequency of dressing changes depends on the amount of bleeding around the cannulation site. Once the cannula is removed under sterile surgical technique, site checks should be done every hour to monitor for bleeding and possible hematoma formation. Temporary fevers and hypotension secondary to systemic inflammatory response after ECMO discontinuation have been reported.

FLUID BALANCE

The possibility exists for the patient to develop acute renal failure while on ECMO; therefore it is important to monitor the patient's fluid status, daily weight, blood urea nitrogen (BUN) and creatinine, drug levels, and intake and output. Hemodynamic monitoring to evaluate cardiac function and volume status may be considered. If hemodialysis and ultrafiltration are needed, a filter can be attached to the ECMO circuit.

NUTRITION

Nutritional support for ECMO patients needs to be catered to the specific caloric and supplement requirements of the patient. Parenteral nutrition (PN) is usually started within 24 hours of initiation of ECMO. PN infused directly into the ECMO circuit is reported. The infusion is placed in the circuit postoxygenation and pre–bubble trap to minimize risk of possible air embolus. Some centers report using enteral feeding via a small-bore enteral feeding tube or gastric tube as tolerated.

MOBILITY

Patient movement while on ECMO is minimal secondary to the risk of cannula displacement and bleeding. Elevating the HOB is patient dependent and as tolerated. Using a low-air-loss pressure-relieving bed surface as well as using continuous lateral rotation therapy with minimal bed rotation is recommended to protect the skin and decrease the risk of breakdown.

Summary and Future Direction

ECMO supports gas exchange while providing a reduction in possible toxic mechanical settings for patients with ARDS and other cardiopulmonary impairments. ECMO is an aggressive treatment for patients who are unresponsive to maximal therapy with CMV, HFOV, iNO, and optimized pharmaceutical support. For patients with severe ARDS, ECMO is a therapeutic option. However, ECMO requires a tremendous commitment of personnel and hospital resources and should only be undertaken when there is a reversible lung process. The factors that most limit the usefulness of ECMO are really not technical but relate to the ability of the lung to recover from its underlying insult. Starting and maintaining an ECMO program is both expensive and labor intensive. Placing a patient on ECMO after failure of other modalities of gas exchange support makes physiologic sense. Many ECMO centers describe survival rates in excess of 50% in uncontrolled reports. The science, technique, and equipment associated with ECMO have improved over time. However, the question of whether ECMO can really challenge the advancement in mechanical ventilation treatment of adult ARDS is unanswered and will need evaluation by future randomized, controlled trials.

RECOMMENDED READINGS

MacIntyre NR, Branson RD. *Mechanical Ventilation*. Philadelphia: Saunders, 2001.

The Acute Respiratory Distress Syndrome Network: Ventilation with lower tidal volumes as compared with traditional tidal volumes for acute lung injury and the acute respiratory distress syndrome. *N Engl J Med* 2000; 342:1301–1308.

High-Frequency Oscillatory Ventilation

Adams AB, Simonson BA, Dries DJ. Ventilator-induced lung injury. *Respir Care Clin* 2003; 9:343–362.

Chan KPW, Stewart TE. Clinical use of high-frequency oscillatory ventilation in adult patients with acute respiratory distress syndrome. *Crit Care Med* 2005; 33(Suppl.):S170–S174.

Chang HK. Mechanisms of gas transport during ventilation by high-frequency oscillation. *J Appl Physiol* 1984; 56:553–563.

Cartotto R, Ellis S, Smith T. Use of high-frequency oscillatory ventilation in burn patients. *Crit Care Med* 2005; 33(Suppl.):S175–S181.

Derdak SD. High-frequency oscillatory ventilation for acute respiratory distress syndrome in adult patients. *Crit Care Med* 2003; 31(4):S317–S323.

Derdak SD. High-frequency oscillatory ventilation for adult acute respiratory distress syndrome: A decade of progress. *Crit Care Med* 2005; 33(Suppl.): S113–S114.

Derdak S, Mehta S, Stewart T, et al. High-frequency oscillatory ventilation for acute respiratory distress syndrome in adults: A randomized, controlled trial. *Am J Respir Care Med* 2002; 166:801–808.

Fan E, Mehta S. High-frequency oscillatory ventilation and adjunctive therapies: Inhaled nitric oxide and prone positioning. *Crit Care Med* 2005; 33(Suppl.): S182–S187.

Ferguson ND. The use of high-frequency oscillatory ventilation in adults with acute lung injury. *Respir Care Clin* 2001; 7(4):647–661.

Ferguson ND, Stewart TE. New therapies for adults with acute lung injury: High-frequency oscillatory ventilation. *Crit Care Clin* 2002; 18(1):91–106.

Fort P, Farmer C, Westerman J. High-frequency oscillatory ventilation for adult respiratory distress syndrome—A pilot study. *Crit Care Med* 1997; 25(6):937–947.

Froese AB. High frequency oscillatory ventilation for adult respiratory distress syndrome: Let's get it right this time. *Crit Care Med* 1997; 25(6):906–908.

Haas CF. Lung protective mechanical ventilation in acute respiratory distress syndrome. *Respir Care Clin* 2003; 9:363–396.

Hess D, Mason S, Branson R. High-frequency ventilation. *Respir Care Clin* 2001; 7(4):577–598.

Hynes-Gay P, MacDonald R. Using high-frequency oscillatory ventilation to treat adults with acute respiratory distress syndrome. *Crit Care Nurse* 2001; 21(5):38–47.

Imai Y, Slutsky AS. High-frequency oscillatory ventilation and ventilator-induced lung injury. *Crit Care Med* 2005; 33(Suppl.):S129–S134.

Kress JP, Pohlman AS, O'Conner MF, et al. Daily interruption of sedative infusions in critically ill patients undergoing mechanical ventilation. *N Engl J Med* 2000; 342:1471–1477.

Krishnan JA, Brower RG. High-frequency ventilation for acute lung injury and ARDS. *Chest* 2000; 118(3):795–807.

MacIntyre NR. High-frequency ventilation. *Crit Care Med* 1998; 26(12):1955–1956.

Marini JJ. Recruitment maneuvers to achieve an "open lung"—Whether and how? *Crit Care Med* 2001; 29(8):1647–1648.

Mehta S, MacDonald R. Implementing and trouble shooting high-frequency oscillatory ventilation in adults in the intensive care unit. *Respir Care Clin* 2001; 7(4):683–695.

Mehta S, Granton J, MacDonald RJ, et al. High-frequency oscillatory ventilation in adults: The Toronto experience. *Chest* 2004; 126:518–527.

Milder R, Cox P. The preclinical history of high-frequency ventilation. *Respir Care Clin* 2001; 7(4):523–534.

Pillow JJ. High-frequency oscillatory ventilation: Mechanisms of gas exchange and lung mechanics. *Crit Care Med* 2005; 33(Suppl.):S135–S141.

Santos C, Slutsky A. Overview of high-frequency ventilation modes, clinical rationale, and gas transport mechanisms. *Respir Care Clin* 2001; 7(4):549–575.

SensorMedics Critical Care Corporation. *3100B High Frequency Oscillatory Ventilator Operator's Manual.* SensorMedics Critical Care Corporation, Yorba Linda, Calif. 2002.

Sessler CN. Sedation, analgesia, and neuromuscular blockade for high-frequency oscillatory ventilation. *Crit Care Med* 2005; 33(Suppl.):S209–S216.

Slutsky AS, Drazen JM. Ventilation with small tidal volumes. *N Engl J Med* 2002; 347(9):630–631.

Sweeny A, Lyle J, Ferguson ND. Nursing and infection control issues during high-frequency oscillatory ventilation. *Crit Care Med* 2005; 33(Suppl.):S204–S208. .

Wunsch H, Mapstone J. High-frequency ventilation versus conventional ventilation for treatment of acute lung injury and acute respiratory distress syndrome. *Cochrane Database Syst Rev* 2004; 2(1):CD004085.

Independent Lung Ventilation

Anatham D, Jagadesan R, Eng Cher Tiew P. Clinical review: Independent lung ventilation in critical care. *Crit Care* 2005; 9:594–600.

Graciano AL, Barton P, Luckett PM. Feasibility of asynchronous independent lung high-frequency oscillatory ventilation in the management of acute hypoxemic respiratory failure: A case report. *Crit Care Med* 2000; 28(8):3075–3077.

Mays LC, Eckert S. Synchronous independent lung ventilation. *Dimens Crit Care Nurs* 1994; 13(5):249–255.

Ost D, Corbridge T. Independent lung ventilation. *Clin Chest Med* 1996; 17(3):591–601.

Strange C. Double-lumen endotracheal tubes. *Clin Chest Med* 1991; 2(3):497–506.

Thomas AR, Bryce TL. Ventilation in the patient with unilateral lung disease. *Crit Care Clin* 1998; 14(4):743–773.

Twomey CR. Preventing complications in double-lumen endotracheal tubes with independent lung ventilation. *Dimens Crit Care Nurs* 1994; 13(6):309–314.

Heliox

Auston F, Polise M. Management of respiratory failure with noninvasive positive pressure ventilation and heliox adjunct. *Heart Lung* 2002; 31(3):214–218.

Barach AL. The use of helium in the treatment of asthma and obstructive lesions in the larynx and trachea. *Ann Intern Med* 1935; 9:739–765.

Gerbeaux P, Gainnier M, Boussuges A. Use of heliox in patients with severe exacerbation of chronic obstructive pulmonary disease. *Crit Care Med* 2001; 29(12): 2322–2324.

Gluck EH, Onoranto DJ, Castriotta R. Helium-oxygen mixtures in intubated patients with status asthmaticus and respiratory acidosis. *Chest* 1990; 98:693–698.

Jolliet P, Tassaux D. Helium-oxygen ventilation. *Respir Care Clin* 2002; 8:295–307.

Kass JE. Heliox redux. *Chest* 2003; 123:673–676.

Kass JE, Castriotta RJ. Heliox therapy in acute severe asthma. *Chest* 1995; 107:757–760.

Kass J, Terregino C. The effect of heliox in acute severe asthma: A randomized controlled trial. *Chest* 1999; 116(2):296–300.

Rodrigo GJ, Rodrigo C, Pollack CV, et al. Use of helium-oxygen mixtures in the treatment of acute asthma: A systematic review. *Chest* 2003; 123:891–896.

Inhaled Nitric Oxide

Atz AM, Wessel DL. Sildenafil ameliorates effects of inhaled nitric oxide withdrawal. *Anesthesiology* 1999; 91:307–310.

Dellinger RP, Zimmerman JL, Taylor RW, et al. Effects of inhaled nitric oxide in patients with acute respiratory distress syndrome: Results of a randomized, phase II trial. *Crit Care Med* 1998; 26(1):15–23.

Hart CM. Nitric oxide in adult lung disease. *Chest* 1999; 115(5):1407–1417.

Hess DR. Adverse effects and toxicity of inhaled nitric oxide. *Respir Care* 1999; 44(3):315–330.

Hurford WE. Inhaled nitric oxide. *Respir Care Clin* 2002; 8:261–279.

Ichinose F, Roberts JD, Zapol WM. Inhaled nitric oxide. A selective pulmonary vasodilator: Current uses and therapeutic potential. *Circulation* 2004; 109:3106–3111.

Jindal N, Dellinger RP. Inhalation of nitric oxide in acute respiratory distress syndrome. *Lab Clin Med* 2000; 136(1):21–28.

Klinger JR. Inhaled nitric oxide in ARDS. *Crit Care Clin* 2002; 18(1):45–68.

Lopez BL, Christopher TA, Griswold SK, Ma XL. Bench to bedside: Nitric oxide in emergency medicine. *Acad Emerg Med* 2000; 7(3):285–293.

Lowson SM. Inhaled alternatives to nitric oxide. *Crit Care Med* 2005; 33(Suppl.): S188–S195.

Mehta S, MacDonald R, Hullett DC, et al. Acute oxygenation response to inhaled nitric oxide when combined with high-frequency oscillatory ventilation in adults with acute respiratory distress syndrome. *Crit Care Med* 2003; 31(2):383–389.

Sokol J, Jacobs SE, Bohn D. Inhaled nitric oxide for acute hypoxemic respiratory failure in children and adults [review]. *Cochrane Database Syst Rev* 2004; 2. Most recent update: November 26, 2003. Retrieved October 27, 2004.

Taylor RW, Zimmerman JL, Dellinger RP, et al. Low-dose inhaled nitric oxide in patients with acute lung injury: A randomized controlled trial. *JAMA* 2004; 291:1603–1609.

Weinberger B, Laskin DL, Heck DE, et al. The toxicology of inhaled nitric oxide. *Toxicol Sci* 2001; 59(1):5–16.

Extracorporeal Membrane Oxygenation

Aggarwal S, Walters HL, Rodriquez E. Extracorporeal membrane oxygenation. eMedicine; http://emedicine.com/ped/topic2895.htm. Most recent update: October 21, 2002. Retrieved October 21, 2004.

Gay SE, Ankney N, Cochran JB, Highland KB. Critical care challenges in the adult ECMO patient. *Dimens Crit Care Nurs* 2005; 24(4):157–162.

Hemmila MR, Rowe SA, Boules TN, et al. Extracorporeal life support for severe acute respiratory distress syndrome in adults. *Ann Surg* 2004; 240(4):595–607.

Meyers BF, Sundt TM, Henry S, et al. Selective use of extracorporeal membrane oxygenation is warranted after lung transplantation. *J Thorac Cardiovasc Surg* 2000; 120(1):20–28.

Mols G, Loop T, Hermle G, et al. Extracorporeal membrane oxygenation: A ten year experience. *Am J Surg* 2000; 180(2):144–154.

Pulmonary Symbols and Abbreviations

SYMBOLS

C	Content of a gas in blood phase
F	Fractional concentration (or percentage) of a gas
P	Partial pressure of a gas
Q	Blood volume
$\dot{Q}$	Blood volume per unit of time
S	Saturation of hemoglobin with oxygen
V	Gas volume
$\dot{V}$	Gas volume per unit of time

Secondary or Qualifying Symbols

GAS PHASE

A	Alveolar
B	Barometric
D	Dead-space gas
E	Expired
I	Inspired
T	Tidal gas

BLOOD PHASE

a	Arterial
v	Venous
$\bar{v}$	Mixed venous
c	Capillary
p	Pulsatile

EXAMPLES

CaO_2	Content of oxygen in arterial blood
$C\bar{v}O_2$	Content of oxygen in mixed venous blood
FIO_2	Fraction of oxygen in inspired gas
PaO_2	Partial pressure of oxygen in arterial blood

Pa_{CO_2}	Partial pressure of carbon dioxide in arterial blood
PA_{O_2}	Partial pressure of oxygen in alveolar gas
P_B	Barometric pressure
PI_{O_2}	Partial pressure of oxygen in inspired gas
Sa_{O_2}	Saturation of hemoglobin with oxygen in arterial blood
Sp_{O_2}	Saturation of hemoglobin with oxygen measured by pulse oximetry
$S\bar{v}_{O_2}$	Saturation of hemoglobin with oxygen in mixed venous blood
$\dot{V}_A$	Volume of alveolar gas per unit of time (alveolar ventilation)
$\dot{V}_E$	Volume of expired gas per unit of time (minute ventilation)
V_D	Dead-space volume
V_T	Tidal volume

ABBREVIATIONS

Lung Volumes

V_T	Tidal volume
IRV	Inspiratory reserve volume
ERV	Expiratory reserve volume
RV	Residual volume

Lung Capacities

NOTE: When two or more volumes are added together, they are known as a *capacity.*

IC	Inspiratory capacity (IRV + V_T)
VC	Vital capacity (IRV + V_T + ERV)
FRC	Functional residual capacity (ERV + RV)
TLC	Total lung capacity (IC + FRC)

Pulmonary Mechanics

C_{ST}	Static compliance
C_{DYN}	Dynamic compliance
C_{TL}	Total compliance (chest wall + lung)
Raw	Airway resistance
WOB	Work of breathing
$\dot{V}_E$	Volume of expired gas per unit of time (minute ventilation)
MVV	Maximum voluntary ventilation
V_T	Tidal volume
VC	Vital capacity
MIP	Maximum inspiratory pressure
f	Respiratory frequency
RR	Respiratory rate
$f{:}V_T$	Ratio of respiratory frequency to tidal volume

Perfusion

$\dot{Q}$	Blood flow
QT	Cardiac output; also abbreviated CO
PVR	Pulmonary vascular resistance
SVR	Systemic vascular resistance
$\dot{V}O_2$	Volume of oxygen consumed per unit of time (oxygen consumption per minute)
$\dot{V}CO_2$	Volume of carbon dioxide produced per minute

Ventilation/Perfusion Relationships

$\dot{V}/\dot{Q}$	Ratio of ventilation to perfusion
$\dot{Q}s/\dot{Q}T$	Ratio of shunted blood flow to total blood flow (physiologic shunt)
VD/VT	Ratio of dead space to tidal volume ventilation (physiologic dead space)

Airway Pressures

PIP	Peak inspiratory pressure
Paw	Pressure in the airway
mPaw	Mean airway pressure
pPlat	Plateau pressure (end-inspiratory)

Drugs Used in Intensive Respiratory Care

Lisa Riggs

Medications used in respiratory care assist mechanical ventilation in the management of respiratory disease processes. Respiratory medications are used to decrease secretions, decrease inflammation, control bronchospasm or improve bronchodilation, and, in specific situations, manage pulmonary hypertension. The goals for the patient are improved oxygenation, improved ventilation, and decreased fatigue, with the ultimate goal being liberation from mechanical ventilation.

ROUTE OF ADMINISTRATION

Respiratory agents are administered as inhaled, oral, subcutaneous, or intravenous. The inhaled route is the preferred route of administration. The inhaled route targets the lung and offers local effects with a lower incidence of often-undesirable systemic side effects. The systemic effects that occur with administration via the inhaled route in the nonventilated patient are caused by swallowing of oropharyngeal-deposited medication. It is imperative that the patient and clinicians properly administer the inhaled medication to decrease the amount of oropharyngeal deposition, therefore maximizing the local effects and minimizing the systemic effects. Systemic effects of inhaled medication are less prominent in the mechanically ventilated patient because of the lack of oropharyngeal deposition.

The three ways to deliver inhaled or aerosolized medications are the metered-dose inhaler (MDI), small-volume nebulizer (SVN), and dry powder inhaler (DPI). Studies demonstrate that different delivery devices deliver different percentages of medication to the lungs in the nonventilated and ventilated patient. Medication delivery ranges from 15% to 30% in the nonventilated patient. The amount of inhaled medication delivered is affected by the endotracheal tube (ETT) in the mechanically ventilated patient. The percentage of drug that reaches the airway and lungs via the ETT decreases to less than 10%. The size of the ETT further affects the amount of drug reaching the lungs. The smaller the ETT diameter, the lesser amount of the drug is actually delivered.

BRONCHODILATORS

Bronchodilators relax smooth muscle of the airways, affording the patient decreased airway resistance, decreased fatigue, decreased sensation of dyspnea, and lowered airway pressures during mechanical ventilation. Bronchodilators fall into one of three categories: β-agonists, anticholinergic agents, or methylxanthines. A review of the lung response to autonomic nervous system stimulation will assist in understanding the role and indications for the use of two of the three categories of bronchodilators. The third category, methylxanthines, is not well understood (Fig. II-1).

No sympathetic nerve fibers are found in the lungs. Epinephrine and norepinephrine stimulate the β_2 receptor sites. Through a cascade of target enzymes, cyclic adenosine monophosphate (cAMP) is activated when the β_2 receptors are stimulated, leading to muscle relaxation and bronchodilation. β-Agonists such as albuterol,

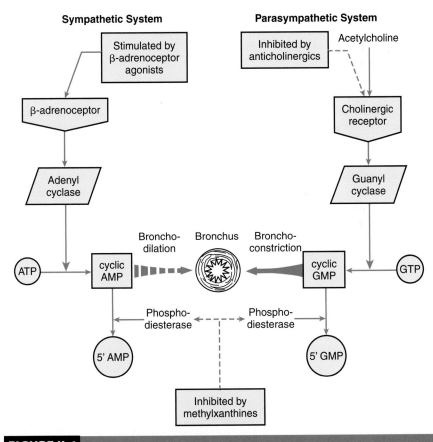

FIGURE II-1

Action of adrenergic and anticholinergic bronchodilating drugs. *(Modified from Shenfield GM. Combination bronchodilator therapy. Drugs 1982; 24:414–439.)*

metaproterenol, and salmeterol stimulate the β_2 receptors and are referred to as sympathomimetic agents. In other words, they mimic the sympathetic nervous system and the subsequent lung response to its stimulation.

The parasympathetic stimulation to the lungs is via the tenth cranial nerve or the vagus nerve. Transmission of stimulation is via the neurotransmitter acetylcholine on the lungs' muscarinic receptors. Parasympathetic transmission of acetylcholine causes normal bronchomotor tone. Anticholinergics (e.g., atropine, ipratropium bromide, and tiotropium bromide) serve as antagonists and bind to the muscarinic receptors to block the action of acetylcholine, causing decreased bronchomotor tone and improved bronchodilation. Increased bronchomotor tone is thought to be a component of airflow obstruction in chronic obstructive pulmonary disease (COPD). Anticholinergic bronchodilators, therefore, are most useful in patients with COPD.

Methylxanthines such as theophylline derivatives have been available since the beginning of the 20th century and at one time were widely used for bronchodilation. It is surprising to find that the mechanism of action is not well understood. Methylxanthines were believed to be a nonselective phosphodiesterase (PDE) inhibitor. Phosphodiesterase enzymes were thought to degrade cAMP levels in COPD and asthma. The theory was that methylxanthines inhibited PDE, thus increasing cAMP levels needed for bronchodilation. Newer studies of methylxanthines do not demonstrate inhibition of PDE in airway smooth muscle, and recent interest is in the possible antiinflammatory properties of PDE inhibitors. The lack of understanding of the mechanism of action and the undesirable side effects of cardiac arrhythmias, tremors, sleep disturbance, and seizures has decreased the earlier popularity of this category of bronchodilators.

In contrast, combination therapy of anticholinergic and β_2-agonist agents is raising interest again. It appears that they produce better bronchodilation in COPD than either agent alone. The drawback to combination therapy is the inability to individualize the dose of each agent. One such combination therapy is Combivent, which contains albuterol sulfate and ipratropium bromide. Table II-1 outlines β-agonists and the anticholinergic method of administration, clinical implications, and side effects.

MUCUS-CONTROLLING AGENTS

Mucus-controlling agents, in theory, decrease volume and viscosity of secretions that impair airway clearance in the mechanically ventilated patient who may be sedated or paralyzed. These agents were once very popular, but this has waned. They liquefy secretions in vitro, but clinical outcomes in patients other than those with cystic fibrosis have not been realized.

Mucus production occurs in the conducting airways and nasal passages and is absent from the more distal terminal airways. Most of the mucus production is from the submucosal glands and surface goblet cells. Mucus is a complex macromolecule made up of a protein backbone with carbohydrate side chains. The macromolecule is a very flexible, threadlike strand that has cross-links of disulfide bonds. The result of this cross-linking is the formation of a gelatin-like state that is hydrophilic and

TABLE II-1 Bronchodilators

Drug Class	Agent	Side Effects	Clinical Implications	Route
Short-acting β-agonist	Albuterol sulfate: Proventil Ventolin Metaproterenol Alupent	Palpitations Tachycardia Arrhythmia Headache Tremors Agitation	Smooth muscle relaxation of the distal airways such as in asthma Onset of action within minutes for rapid symptom relief Duration of 4-6 hr	Inhaled or oral Inhaled
Long-acting β-agonist	Salmeterol (Serevent)	Same as short-acting β-agonist	Smooth muscle relaxation of the distal airways such as in asthma Onset of action: 20 min Duration: 12 hr	Inhaled or oral
Short-acting anticholinergic	Ipratropium bromide (Atrovent)	Negligible side effects	Decreases broncho-motor tone	Inhaled
	Atropine	Tachycardia Dry mouth Dry secretions Pupil dilation	Blocks acetylcholine neurotransmission Bronchodilation of distal airways Indicated in bronchitis and bronchospasm such as in COPD Onset is 15-30 min with therapeutic effect in 30-90 min Duration: 6-8 hr	Inhaled
Long-acting anticholinergic	Tiotropium bromide (Spiriva)	Tachycardia Dry mouth Urinary retention	Indicated in bronchitis and bronchospasm such as in COPD Duration: 24 hr	Inhaled
β-Agonist and anticholinergic	Combivent		Combination of albuterol sulfate and ipratropium bromide Bronchodilation	Inhaled

spongelike. Mucus-controlling agents target either the mucus production or the structure of the macromolecule.

Bland aerosols of normal, hypotonic, or hypertonic saline were used historically as mucolytics. As described earlier, the chemical structure of mucus is hydrophilic and repels liquid. Saline solutions serve more as an expectorant and stimulate cough rather than actually breaking down mucus or inhibiting its production.

The internal support of the mucous macromolecule is the disulfide bond. This is the primary target of acetylcysteine. N-Acetylcysteine, or Mucomyst, breaks the disulfide bond and replaces it with a sulfhydryl radical that reduces the viscosity and elasticity of the gel layer of the macromolecule. N-Acetylcysteine is the most frequently used mucus-controlling agent and can be administered via aerosol or by direct tracheal instillation. It is known to cause bronchospasm; administration, therefore, is preceded by or given in conjunction with a bronchodilator.

Proteolytic enzymes are used to break down the protein component of the mucus macromolecule in an attempt to liquefy secretions. The earlier agent, pancreatic dornase, was not selective to attacking proteins in the lungs and is no longer available. However, dornase alfa (Pulmozyme) is an enzymatic agent now available to decrease the viscosity of secretions and increase mucociliary transport.

The anticholinergic agent atropine is an antagonist for submucosal gland mucus production. Atropine does decrease the amount of secretions, but it increases the viscosity of secretions as well as compromises ciliary activity. Ipratropium bromide has similar actions as atropine but without the compromised ciliary activity.

CORTICOSTEROIDS

Corticosteroids are indicated for inflammatory processes that cause airway obstruction or hypoventilation states associated with pleural disease. They have the ability to prevent histamine release, diminish hypersensitivity reactions, decrease edema, and reduce excessive mucus production that contributes to airway obstruction. They are not indicated for rapid response, but rather the onset of action is hours to days. Corticosteroids are also indicated for pleural disease to decrease the inflammation associated with rheumatoid pleurisy, lupus pleuritis, postcardiac injury syndrome, and sarcoidosis. An added benefit of corticosteroids is potentiation of smooth muscle relaxation by β-agonists. The number of β_2 receptor sites is increased, and their threshold to respond to sympathetic stimulation is lowered in the presence of corticosteroids. The use of corticosteroids in asthma shows improved peak flow, improved symptoms scores, decreased airway responsiveness, and decreased need for rescue therapy.

Corticosteroids are administered orally, intravenously, or by aerosol. Aerosolized corticosteroids should be given 10 to 15 minutes after administration of a β-agonist agent to potentiate smooth muscle relaxation. Side effects of corticosteroids are numerous and can be categorized by systemic or local effects (Table II-2).

PULMONARY ANTIHYPERTENSIVE AGENTS

Pulmonary hypertension can be a primary disease process or secondary to disease processes ranging from collagen vascular disease to thromboembolic obstruction of the pulmonary arteries. It is associated with left-sided heart disease, portal hypertension, and pulmonary vasculitis, to name just a few. The pathophysiology of pulmonary hypertension is complex and not always well understood. It is known that pulmonary arterial vasoconstriction is an important component of that pathophysiology. Pulmonary arterial vasoconstriction is expressed as an elevated mean pulmonary artery pressure (PAP) and an elevated pulmonary vascular resistance

TABLE II-2 Corticosteroid Side Effects	
Local Effects	Fungal infection of oropharynx
	Dysphonia
	Cough
	Bronchospasm
Systemic Effects	Protein wasting
	Osteoporosis
	Hyperglycemia
	Fluid retention
	Sodium retention
	Potassium loss
	Gastrointestinal distress and peptic ulcers
	Steroid psychosis
	Impaired healing
	Acute adrenal insufficiency with rapid withdrawal

(PVR). An increase in mean PAP and PVR increases right ventricular afterload and substantially lowers cardiac output.

The approach to treatment of pulmonary arterial vasoconstriction consists of symptomatic treatment of right heart failure, anticoagulation, and vasodilation. The desired positive response to pulmonary vasodilators is a 20% reduction in mean PAP and PVR. One possible vasodilator is high-dose calcium channel blockers. Calcium channel blockers are only beneficial in a small number of patients. These agents are nonselective and offer a greater vasodilatory effect on the systemic circulation than on the pulmonary arteries. Patients often are unable to tolerate the systemic vasodilation, experiencing problems with hypotension and syncope. Calcium channel blockers have a negative inotropic effect that compromises right ventricular contractility and cardiac output and compounds the hypotension and syncope. Development of pharmacologic agents such as prostacyclin, endothelin-1 (ET-1) antagonist, nitric oxide, and PDE inhibitors, which have relative selectivity for the pulmonary circulation, has led to a reduction in morbidity and mortality in pulmonary hypertension.

Prostacyclin is a potent vasodilator and platelet aggregation inhibitor produced by the vascular endothelium. Patients with primary pulmonary hypertension have a reduction in the ratio of prostacyclin to the potent vasoconstrictor thromboxane A. This is believed to lead to elevation in PAP and PVR. Epoprostenol is a synthetic form of prostacyclin administered intravenously. Studies show an improvement in hemodynamic measurements, exercise capacity, quality of life, and survival at 3 months. Epoprostenol is expensive, and its short half-life (3 to 5 minutes) dictates that the patient be on a continuous infusion. The infusion is initiated slowly. The most serious complication occurs with interruption of the infusion and acute right heart failure. Treprostinil is another prostacyclin that can be administered subcutaneously. It improves hemodynamic measurements and exercise capacity, but studies do not show that it improves survival rates.

ET-1 is a potent vasoconstrictor found in elevated levels in patients with pulmonary hypertension. It is mediated by two receptors, ET-A and ET-B, located in the pulmonary vasculature. ET-A receptor stimulation results in vasoconstriction; ET-B receptor stimulation results in production of nitric oxide and vasodilation. Bosentan is an oral ET-1 antagonist blocking both ET-A and ET-B receptor stimulation. In 2002, the BREATHE (Bosentan Randomized Trial of Endothelin Antagonist Therapy) trial showed an improvement in exercise capacity and hemodynamic measurements as well as prolonging the time to clinical worsening. On the horizon is selective ET-A antagonist agents. Sitaxsentan, a selective ET-1 antagonist, is being investigated as treatment for pulmonary hypertension.

The choice to treat pulmonary hypertension with a calcium channel blocker, epoprostenol, or bosentan is determined by two factors: functional status and hemodynamic measurements. Patients with less severe disease are evaluated for vasodilation therapy during a right heart catheterization. Patients that are responders to nitric oxide, an endogenous potent vasodilator, or adenosine during right heart catheterization proceed to treatment with a calcium channel blocker. Severe pulmonary hypertension requires epoprostenol. It is unclear whether responder patients should be considered for bosentan. Finally, emerging evidence suggests that sildenafil may be effective in the treatment of pulmonary hypertension. Sildenafil, a PDE inhibitor, increases cyclic guanine monophosphate (cGMP) levels, resulting in vasodilation. Human anecdotal reports and animal studies showed a decrease in PVR and PAP without affecting the systemic pressure.

RECOMMENDED READINGS

Booker R. Pharmacology of bronchodilators. *Nurs Times* 2004; 100(6):54–59.

Burke-Martindale C. Inhaled nitric oxide therapy for ARDS. *Crit Care Nurse* 1998; 18(6):21–27.

Chami H, Tapson V. What's new in treatment of pulmonary arterial hypertension. *J Respir Dis* 2004; 25(1):14–26.

Gerger-Bronsky M. Anticholinergic therapy in the critically ill patient with bronchospasm. *AACN Clin Issues* 1995; 6(2):287–296.

Guillaume P. Drugs used in intensive respiratory care. In L Pierce (ed.), *Guide to Mechanical Ventilation and Intensive Respiratory Care* (pp. 346–355). Philadelphia: WB Saunders, 1995.

Rau J. Recent developments in respiratory care pharmacology. *J Perianesth Nurs* 1998; 13(6):359–369.

Sterling L. Beta adrenergic agonists. *AACN Clin Issues* 1995; 6(2):271–278.

Taylor R, Zimmerman JL, Dellinger RP, et al. Low dose inhaled nitric oxide in patients with acute lung injury. *JAMA* 2004; 291(13):1603–1609.

Chest Drainage Systems

Chest drainage systems provide a mechanism to reestablish normal physiology of the pleural space. The disruption in the pleural space may be caused by air, fluid, or blood. When occupied with air, such as a pneumothorax, the chest drainage system works to pull the air out from the pleural space, thereby reexpanding the lung. Fluid, such as a pleural effusion or blood from a hemothorax, requires a chest tube drainage system to drain the collection of fluid and reexpand the lung. A combined process may be occurring with both air and fluid, such as a hemopneumothorax. Chest drainage systems use gravity, suction, or both to remove air or fluid from the thoracic cavity and restore the normal negative pressure in the intrapleural space.

Mediastinal chest tubes drain fluid from the mediastinal space. This is indicated for the patient after heart surgery.

CHEST TUBE INSERTION

Insertion Materials
The following items are necessary for implementation of chest drainage systems:
- Chest tube: for drainage of air, a No. 16 to 24 French tube is adequate; for drainage of fluid or blood, a larger tube, such as a No. 28 to 36 French is needed
- Drainage collection system
- Local anesthetic, such as 1% lidocaine with epinephrine
- Antiseptic skin preparation, such as povidone-iodine (unless contraindicated by allergy)
- Sterile gloves, gowns, and drapes; clean masks
- Chest tube insertion or tube thoracostomy tray
  - Sterile towels and 4 × 4 gauze
  - Scalpel with No. 11 blade
  - Large hemostats and a needle holder
  - 2–0 or 3–0 silk suture with a cutting needle
  - Syringe and needle to administer anesthetic
- Dressing material: petrolatum-impregnated gauze, 4 × 4 gauze pads, tape

Site of Insertion
To drain air, a chest tube is placed in the second, third, or fourth intercostal space in the midclavicular line. This higher placement is indicated to promote the drainage of air, which rises. For fluid, a chest tube is placed in the fifth or sixth intercostal space in the midaxillary line. Fluid is heavier and warrants a lower tube to use the principle of gravity for drainage.

Insertion Process

Initiation of a chest tube drainage system begins with the insertion of the chest tube. The steps for insertion are as follows:

- Clean site with antiseptic, such as povidone-iodine.
- Inject local anesthetic to anesthetize insertion site.
- Incise skin between ribs and dissect to pleural space. Incision site is one rib below insertion site.
- Insert chest tube into pleural space (between parietal and visceral pleura).
- Clamp chest tube close to the chest wall until connected to drainage system.
- Pull suture in place around tube.
- Connect drainage system to chest tube.
- Release clamp from chest tube.
- Apply dressing around chest tube insertion site:
  - Apply petrolatum gauze around site
  - Place split drain sponge from above and below
  - Cover with 4 × 4 as needed
- Tape to create occlusive dressing
- Secure all connections; assess system.
- Obtain chest radiograph film for placement.

ASSESSMENT AND TROUBLESHOOTING

From the time of insertion until discontinuation, the patient and system must be assessed for effectiveness. All components of a chest tube drainage system are assessed to determine proper functioning: patient, chest tube site, tubing, and all three chambers of the drainage system. Figure III-1 shows a typical three-chamber chest tube drainage system, which is the commercial equivalent to a three-bottle system. A variety of chest drainage systems are on the market. Depending on the particular chest drainage system, it may have all or some of the features discussed in this section. It is critical for patient safety that clinicians are thoroughly familiar with the setup and management of the chest drain units used in their facility.

Patient

- Assess respiratory rate and breathing pattern.
- Auscultate lung sounds.
- Assess use of accessory muscles or abdominal breathing.
- Assess patient's comfort and anxiety level.

Site

- Assess dressing for drainage and change every 48 hours or more often as necessary.
- Palpate patient's skin around chest tube insertion site for subcutaneous emphysema. Subcutaneous emphysema indicates that air has escaped into the tissue under the skin. An increase in size of subcutaneous emphysema could indicate an air leak. Air may be escaping from the pleural space around the tube and into the tissue.

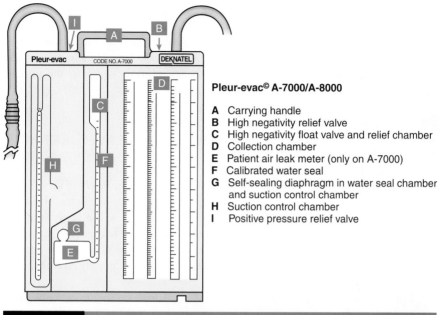

Pleur-evac© A-7000/A-8000

A Carrying handle
B High negativity relief valve
C High negativity float valve and relief chamber
D Collection chamber
E Patient air leak meter (only on A-7000)
F Calibrated water seal
G Self-sealing diaphragm in water seal chamber
   and suction control chamber
H Suction control chamber
I Positive pressure relief valve

FIGURE III-1

Three-chamber chest tube drainage system. Component parts are labeled. *(Courtesy of Telefex Medical, Research Triangle Park, NC.)*

Tubing

The tubing should provide a straight passage down to the chest tube drainage system. There should be no kinks or dependent loops in the tubing. All tubing connections should be securely taped if they are not a snap-lock connection.

Assess tubing for the presence of drainage and/or clots. Passively empty any drainage in the tubing into the collection chamber. Clots may be dislodged by milking or stripping the chest tube. Stripping is controversial and should not be done without a physician's order because it is known to create transient high levels of negative pressure within the pleural space. Stripping of the chest tube requires anchoring the tubing with one hand while vigorously squeezing the length of the chest tube with the other hand. This process can create negative pressures in the pleural space up to –400 cm H_2O pressure and cause barotrauma to the lungs. The cardiac patient with mediastinal tubes who presents with signs of cardiac tamponade may require vigorous milking or stripping of the mediastinal tubes to evacuate the cardiac effusion. Milking a chest tube is less stressful on the pleura. It is performed by gently squeezing the chest tube between the fingers and performing this process down the length of the tube.

Clamping of a chest tube is not recommended because it prevents the escape of air in the pleural space, which could result in a tension pneumothorax. A more commonly recommended practice is to place the patient on water seal when there is a need to discontinue suction, such as during transport or during weaning from a chest drainage system.

A sterile 4×4 pad with petrolatum-impregnated gauze should always be in the room in case a chest tube inadvertently comes out. Immediately placing the petrolatum gauze covered by a 4×4 pad over the insertion site decreases the amount of air let into the pleural space.

Suction Control Chamber

The level of suction regulates the amount of negative pressure applied to the pleural space to facilitate lung expansion. Generally, –20 cm H_2O pressure is used for the adult patient. There are two types of suction available, wet and dry.

With wet suction, the amount of suction is regulated *by the height of water in the suction control chamber*. This level must be routinely assessed to verify that the water is filled to the appropriate level. When this chamber is assessed, it is necessary to pinch the suction line to stop movement in this column. This chamber should be refilled with sterile normal saline solution or distilled water. Water in the suction control chamber should gently bubble. More vigorous bubbling only contributes to noise and evaporation.

With *dry suction*, the amount of suction is regulated by a spring or screw valve mechanism attached to an external suction control dial. When the dial is turned, both mechanisms apply pull on a diaphragm in the drainage system, thereby controlling the level of negative pressure. There is visual confirmation of the level of suction on the front panel of the suction control chamber. The degree of pull determines the level of suction. Although no water is used in these systems, they still require connection to a suction source to work. The level of suction must be routinely assessed to confirm the appropriate setting.

In either the wet or dry suction setup, there is a potential for increased positive-pressure buildup within the system if the suction tubing is inadvertently clamped (e.g., by the rolling of a bed over the tubing). When positive pressure accumulates in the chest drainage system, a relief valve opens on the drainage system, allowing the positive pressure to be vented.

Water Seal Chamber

The water in the water seal chamber acts as a seal between the thoracic cavity and the environment. As air comes from the pleural space, it bubbles through the water in the water seal chamber and vents to the atmosphere. This prevents air from being pulled back into the pleural space from the chest drainage system every time the patient inhales. The water in this chamber is filled to the 2-cm line and must be assessed routinely for evaporation.

Tidaling is indicated by fluctuations in the water seal chamber that correlate with the respiratory cycle. This action reflects the changes in the pleural pressures that occur with respirations. Tidaling can be assessed only when the patient is not connected to suction. Absence of tidaling is observed if the patient's chest tube or tubing is kinked or clotted, there is a loss of negative pressure because of fluid-filled dependent loops, or the lung has fully expanded.

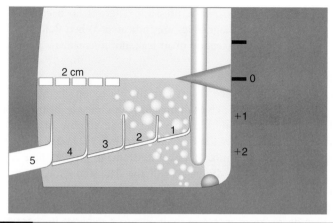

FIGURE III-2

Patient air leak can be quantified by the numbered scale in the air leak meter. *(Courtesy of Atrium Medical, Hudson, NH.)*

High negativity is indicated by a rising water level in the water seal chamber. Excess negative pressure in the drainage system can result if the patient takes deep breaths before coughing or from stripping of the chest tube. This excess negative pressure can be relieved by depressing the high-negativity relief valve. This valve allows filtered air to enter the system, relieving the pressure. Caution should be exercised when using this valve. If the patient is not on suction or the suction is not operating properly, depressing the high-negativity relief valve could reduce negative pressure to zero (atmospheric) and possibly result in a pneumothorax.

Air leaks are evidenced by bubbling in the water seal chamber. One reason that an air leak may occur is the natural escape of air from the pleural space as the lung reexpands. This is generally seen right after insertion of the tube. A second reason that an air leak may be present is that air may be leaking into the drainage system from a loose connection or a cracked drainage system. To locate the source of the air leak, clamp the chest tube close to the patient. If there is no bubbling in the water seal chamber, the air is leaking either from around the dressing or internally from the pleural space. If the bubbling does not cease when the tube is clamped, somewhere along the chest drainage system there is a leak. If the air leak persists after all tubing connections are checked, consider replacing the chest drainage system. Many units have a calibrated air leak meter that indicates the approximate degree of air leak from the chest cavity (Fig. III-2). By documenting the degree of air leak indicated by the meter, the caregiver can assess increase or reduction in a leak.

One-Way Valve

Some chest drainage systems are waterless and a one-way valve replaces the traditional water seal. This is known as a dry-dry system. The one-way valve protects the intrathoracic cavity from atmospheric pressure. There is no need to add water to the chamber unless air leak diagnostics are indicated. When fluid is placed to the indicated level, it is used for detection of air leak, not to create a water seal.

Collection Chamber

Excess fluid in the pleural space drains into the collection chamber as a result of gravity. For gravity to work, the chest drainage system must be below the level of the patient's chest. After insertion of a chest tube, the volume of drainage should be assessed hourly for 2 hours then advanced to every 2 hours if the amount of drainage is within normal limits. In general, drainage greater than 200 mL/hr is significant. Mark the level of drainage with the date and time, minimally every 8 hours on the write-on surface of the collection chamber. The volume of drainage should gradually taper down. However, trends should be monitored for each patient because sudden decreases or increases in drainage or a change in character can also be significant.

If the collection columns are only partially filled, the unit may have tipped over and allowed spillage from one column to the next. Mark the level of drainage in each column and add the volumes to calculate the total drainage. Assess whether drainage entered the water seal chamber, and aspirate excess fluid until the proper water seal level is achieved.

Overall System

In the event that the entire chest drainage system tips over, reassess the fluid levels in each chamber. The unit does not need to be replaced unless it was cracked in the process.

If the chest drainage system does need to be replaced because it is broken or the collection chamber is full, follow this process:

1. Prepare new chest drainage system by filling the suction and water seal chamber appropriately as indicated.
2. *Briefly* double-clamp the chest tube close to the patient.
3. Disconnect old chest drainage system and reconnect new system.
4. Release clamps.
5. Retape all connections and assess system for proper function.

DISCONTINUATION

Before the chest drainage system is discontinued, an assessment for patient readiness should be done. This assessment includes the following:

1. Auscultation of lung sounds
2. Assessment of patient's respiratory rate and breathing pattern
3. Absence of fluctuations in the water seal chamber
4. Absence of an air leak in the water seal chamber
5. Absence of or minimal drainage in the collection chamber
6. Confirmation of lung expansion by chest radiograph film

After assessment of the readiness of the patient, the chest tube may be removed as follows:

1. Medicate before procedure if needed.
2. Remove dressing around chest tube.
3. Cut anchoring suture.
4. Instruct patient to perform Valsalva maneuver by exhaling and bearing down while the tube is pulled. This will increase the intrathoracic pressure and decrease the potential for air to enter during the removal process.
5. Secure with purse string suture. Cleanse area with normal saline.
6. Apply dressing with petrolatum-impregnated gauze on pleural chest tube site. Petrolatum gauze is not indicated if purse string suture is present at a pleural chest tube site or at mediastinal chest tube sites. Cover with 4 × 4 pads and tape.
7. Monitor patient closely for changes in respiratory assessment, especially an increase in respiratory rate and decrease in breath sounds and for complaints of shortness of breath.
8. Confirm lung expansion with chest x-ray film.

ALTERNATIVE SYSTEMS: FLUTTER OR DRY VALVE

The flutter valve is an optional chest drainage system indicated primarily for treating pneumothorax. It is also known as a Heimlich valve and was named after Henry Heimlich, the physician who originated the abdominal thrust mechanism used to rescue a choking victim. The flutter valve consists of rubber leaflets encased in a transparent plastic chamber tapered at both ends (Fig. III-3). One end attaches to the chest tube, and the other end can be left alone (but this may compromise sterility) or attached to a vented drainage bag. The flutter valve allows air or fluid to escape from the pleural space in one direction only with normal respirations (Fig. III-4). On exhalation the rubber leaflets open and allow air or fluid to escape, and on inhalation the leaflets close to prevent air from entering into the pleural space. This function mimics the water seal chamber in a traditional chest drainage system.

The advantages of the flutter valve are that it is less expensive than a three-chamber chest drainage system, and it allows easy mobility by the patient. In some cases the patient may even be discharged with this tube in place. The disadvantages include the potential for occlusion caused by clots, the inability to detect an air leak, difficulty connecting to small chest drain or a radiology pigtail, and the absence of suction.

In caring for a patient with a flutter valve, consider the following:

- Secure chest tube to dressing to prevent dislodgment.
- Ensure that drainage bag is vented to prevent pressure buildup within drainage compartment.
- Monitor valve for fluttering, which corresponds to closure of the valve before inhalation. The absence of fluttering could mean that the lung has fully expanded or the valve has become obstructed by drainage.

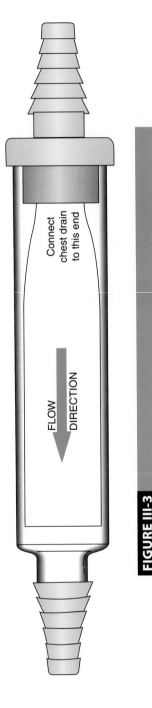

Connect
chest drain
to this end

FLOW
DIRECTION

FIGURE III-3

Heimlich chest drain (flutter) valve. *(Courtesy of Becton Dickinson AcuteCare, Franklin Lakes, NJ.)*

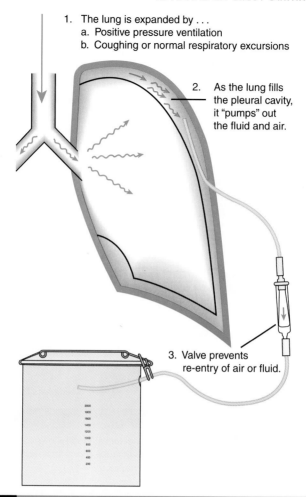

1. The lung is expanded by . . .
   a. Positive pressure ventilation
   b. Coughing or normal respiratory excursions

2. As the lung fills the pleural cavity, it "pumps" out the fluid and air.

3. Valve prevents re-entry of air or fluid.

FIGURE III-4

Flow of air and fluid with Heimlich valve connected to a vented drainage bag. Normal respiration promotes evacuation of the pleural space. *(Modified from Heimlich HJ. Heimlich valve for chest drainage. Medical Instrumentation 1983; 17:1 [Association for the Advancement of Medical Instrumentation, Arlington, Va]).*

Dry Valve

Figure III-5 shows a dry one-way valve system. The valve is a mechanical disk that prevents leakback. The Pneumostat chest drain valve consists of a closed, emptyable 30-mL collection chamber containing a dry seal valve. The system is very portable because it does not have to be connected to a drainage bag. Multiple connection adaptors allow the system to be securely connected to any size thoracic catheter. This prevents the nurse from having to create a secure connection by piecing together equipment available on the patient care unit. Air leak can be detected by placing 1 mL of water in the air leak well. Bubbling in water confirms a patient air leak. The air leak well should be emptied after use.

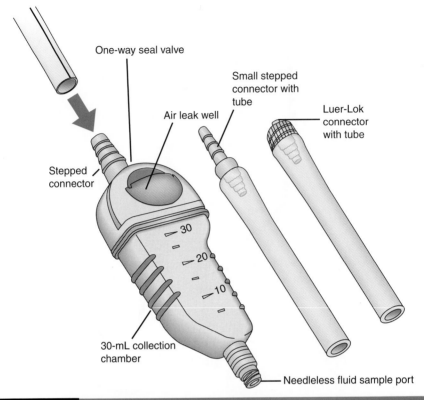

FIGURE III-5

Dry valve portable chest drain. The small stepped connector with tube allows connection to
No. 8–20 French chest drains. The Luer-Lok connector with tube allows for a secure connection to
radiology or pigtail catheters. *(Courtesy of Atrium Medical, Hudson, NH.)*

RECOMMENDED READINGS

Carroll P. Exploring chest drain options. *RN* 2000; 63(10):50–58.

Conner P. When and how do you use a Heimlich flutter valve? *Am J Nurs* 1987;
87(3):288–290.

Heimlich H. Heimlich valve for chest drainage. *Med Instrum* 1983; 17(1):29–31.

Lawrence DM, Carlson KK. Chest tube placement (assist). In DJ Lynn-McHale,
KK Carlson (eds.), *AACN Procedure Manual for Critical Care* (pp. 134–139).
St. Louis: Elsevier Saunders, 2005.

Lazzara D. Eliminate the air of mystery from chest tubes. *Nursing* 2002; 32(6):36–43.

Pickett JD. Closed chest drainage systems. In DJ Lynn-McHale, KK Carlson (eds.),
AACN Procedure Manual for Critical Care (pp. 151–169). St. Louis: Elsevier
Saunders, 2005.

Telefex Medical. *Understanding Chest Drainage.* Research Triangle Park, NC: Telefex
Medical, 2004.

Removal of Mechanical Ventilation at End of Life

Margaret L. Barnett

Removing mechanical ventilation (RMV) or the decision to forgo life-prolonging medical treatment occurs in 75% of deaths in U.S. hospitals. Because of the frequency, serious nature, and emotional impact of RMV, a well-defined interdisciplinary process must be in place that provides a standardized approach to this medical procedure. Withdrawal of life support is defined as removal of artificial ventilatory support with or without extubation and forgoing of additional life-prolonging treatments such as cardiopulmonary resuscitation, vasopressors, blood products, hemodialysis, artificial nutrition/hydration, or antibiotics, thus allowing natural death to occur from the patient's underlying disease process. Clinical considerations that influence the decision of the health care team regarding RMV at the end of life include patient characteristics such as age, functional status prior to illness, ability to participate in decisions, and the patient's preference about the use of life support. Also, severity of illness and the physician's clinical judgments influence the health care team's decision making. Some of the most common factors contemplated by the surrogate decision makers for patients are as follows: current therapies that would be deemed unacceptable by the patient/surrogate, quality of life beyond therapies that would be deemed unacceptable by the patient/surrogate, poor prognosis, advance directives or patient's known wishes, and the perception that the patient is suffering.

The goal of RMV at the end of life is to transition from treatments no longer desired by the patient to treatments designed to maximize comfort and quality of the patient's remaining time. This transition may be either initiated by the patient with decisional capacity or by a designated surrogate decision maker or described in an advance directive.

Because RMV is not commonly an emergency situation, time should be taken to form consensus between the patient's family and the health care team. A palliative care team consult is appropriate at this time. The team usually consists of physicians, nurses, social workers, chaplains, and other interdisciplinary specialties as needed. Palliative care services often help manage patients with a poor prognosis whose decisions for end-of-life (EOL) care may not be known and whose families are hesitant to make decisions about RMV. The palliative care team also plays a role in working with the critical care clinicians and other services pre- and post-ventilator removal as well as during the procedure. Consulting the palliative care consult service is recommended if one is available.

ETHICAL CONSIDERATIONS

Removal of life-sustaining therapies such as ventilators usually arises when medical therapy and interventions fail to improve the condition of the patient significantly and the patient's death is imminent and unavoidable. Also, RMV may become an issue when the quality of life is not or will not be acceptable to the patient and/or the patient is seen as suffering. Sometimes the continued use of ventilation merely prolongs the dying process instead of improving the patient's condition. Ethical principles that support the consideration of EOL ventilator withdrawal should be familiar to all health care professionals who participate in the procedure. Some of these principles include autonomy, nonmaleficence, beneficence, and justice as fairness.

Self-determination or the right of autonomy is an important ethical consideration in EOL removal of mechanical ventilation. Patients of decision-making capacity have the right to make decisions about the course of their treatment and life for themselves or delegate that responsibility to a family member or significant other. The principle of autonomy includes the concept of informed consent, the patient's right to be adequately informed, and the right to authorize or refuse any medical treatment.

Nonmaleficence is one of the most established principles of health care ethics, which directs providers to avoid or minimize harm to patients. Health care professionals need to weigh the burdens and risks associated with any proposed treatment. If a treatment is becoming more of a burden than a benefit, the treatment needs to be reevaluated and stopped. The principle of beneficence is the obligation to promote the good of the patient. Generally speaking, extending life usually promotes the good of the patient. However, sometimes the patient may be experiencing a great deal of pain and suffering and the patient may prefer to stop the treatment even if it means death will occur sooner. To promote the good of the patient, the possible benefits the current treatment provides must be determined from the patient or surrogate's perspective. If the patient or surrogate concludes that the current treatment is no longer providing benefits, it should be stopped.

The principle of justice as fairness involves the decisions about accepting or deferring/removing treatment. This type of decision making should involve the health care team and the patient or designated surrogate. Open and ongoing dialogue with all parties involved in the decision making allow for due process to occur as well as the appropriate respect for everyone involved in the decision-making process. Sustained dialogue also provides an opportunity for careful consideration of all options, appropriate consultation, and review of the current situation. Continued discussions also provide mechanisms for addressing differences of opinion between the primary health care team and consultants, within the family, and between the family and the health care providers.

Family meetings provide a forum to discuss the patient's wishes and directives along with the description of what quality of life means to the person who is seriously ill or dying. The health care team, the patient, and/or family share information that leads to decisions that respect the wishes of the patient regarding the risk versus the benefit of ongoing treatment. When a decision is reached to remove mechanical ventilation, the health care team and the institution have a continuing obligation to provide a comprehensive range of supportive care and treatment including consideration of alternative methods of care such as palliative care and/or hospice programs.

THE FAMILY MEETING

Once it is decided that further aggressive medical care is incapable of meeting the desired goals of care for a ventilator-dependent patient, discussing RMV to allow natural death is appropriate. When the patient cannot make his or her wishes known, it is important to determine who holds the durable power of attorney for health care decisions or is the surrogate decision maker. If there is no formal legal decision maker, consensus must be attained whenever possible among the individuals participating in the family meeting. Laws and guidelines may vary from state to state regarding who is the surrogate decisionmaker and what are their responsibilities for the patient. The health care providers should be familiar with the state laws and guidelines where they practice.

The purpose of the family meeting is to discuss and/or determine the patient's goals of care. The meeting provides a forum that facilitates the discussion of the family's understanding of the patient's condition, the risks and benefits of various treatment options, and the probable outcomes and prognosis with or without ventilator support. The discussion should focus on the patient's hopes, goals, and concerns utilizing open-ended questions. It is also important to establish what the patient finds meaningful in life and what the patient would consider as an acceptable quality of life. Options of care for the patient to be discussed are not only the issue of RMV but also include other treatments such as vasopressors, artificial hydration/nutrition, antibiotics, blood products, and any other treatment not directly related to the goals of care. If RMV is part of the decision, other treatments should be discussed in light of how they may or may not support the patient's goal of comfort care.

Communication style is very important during this difficult and emotional decision-making time. It is important for the family/surrogate to understand that they are not making decisions for their loved one. Their role is to honor the decision that the patient has already made or would make if he or she could do so. It is also important for the family/surrogate to know that the illness is what is causing the death of the patient, not the process of determining how to best to support their loved one's goals. All members of the health care team should participate in the discussion and support the decision-making process. Reaching a decision to RMV may take hours, days, or weeks depending on the needs of the patient and the family. Occasionally, a time-limited trial for a few days of a particular intervention is needed before the family/surrogate feels that enough information is available to allow transition to the expressed goals. It is not unusual to see a time-limited ventilator, dialysis, or antibiotic trial.

Documentation of the family meeting should include those present, the goals that were identified, concerns or issues that were discussed, and the outcomes and the plan of care including date and time of interventions. A "do not resuscitate, do not reintubate" order should be documented in the patient's chart. Other orders may include discontinuation of radiograph examinations, laboratory evaluations, and other tests that increase the patient's discomfort but do not help with assessment of comfort. Frequency of vital signs may be decreased or discontinued altogether. Medications that do not provide comfort for the patient should also be discontinued. It is also important to notify other services involved in the care of the patient when the decision is made to remove ventilator support. Organ transplant coordinators may need to be notified depending on institution policy.

If the patient/surrogate decides to remove mechanical ventilation, the procedure should be explained step by step. Some family members choose to be present during the removal procedure and others prefer to come into the room afterward. Potential outcomes following RMV need to be discussed because families may be anticipating death to occur quickly or may expect the patient to be awake and conversive. Family members begin to second-guess decisions that have been made if death does not occur as soon as the family anticipates that it will. Patients who are removed from the ventilator at the end of life survive an average of 48 hours; however, most die within the first day. Family members need intensive support during this time of watching and waiting for the death of the patient.

RMV PROCEDURE

Preprocedure Reduction in Ventilator Support

Decide if the patient can be immediately removed from the ventilator or if the patient will need a rapid terminal weaning process by analyzing the current ventilator settings. Patients on minimal settings can be removed immediately without any reduction in support. Patients on higher settings require rapid reduction in ventilator support, a procedure that decreases the ventilator rate, oxygen saturation, and/or positive end-expiratory pressure (PEEP) over a short period of time. The purpose of a rapid reduction in ventilator support is to ensure that adequate symptom management is obtained prior to RMV.

Indications for rapid reduction in support are patients on levels of PEEP greater than 7 cm H_2O, FIO_2 greater than 0.5, pressure support (PS) greater than 12 cm H_2O, or pressure control (PC) ventilation. The process can occur over a 10- to 15-minute period. The procedure for rapid terminal reduction involves simultaneous performance of each of the following three steps:

1. Decrease the FIO_2 in increments of 0.3 every 2 to 5 minutes until patient is on an FIO_2 of 3. Monitor patient for signs of discomfort such as tachypnea, increasing accessory muscle usage, increased agitation, or increased heart rate, and bolus opiates as necessary to maintain patient comfort. Hold further weaning until patient is again comfortable, and then continue the process.

2. Decrease PEEP in increments of 5 cm H_2O every 2 to 5 minutes until at a level of 5 cm H_2O. Monitor for symptoms as just listed and bolus opiates as necessary to maintain patient comfort.

3. Decrease PS in increments of 5 cm H_2O every 2 to 5 minutes until a PS of 5 cm H_2O is reached. Again, monitor for symptoms and bolus opiates as necessary to maintain patient comfort.

Once on extubation settings, the extubation procedure may proceed. The endotracheal tube (ETT) is removed in almost every situation, except when the patient would be expected to have a catastrophic airway collapse because of tumor encroachment, tracheal stenosis, or airway burns. Overwhelming secretions, which are not under control with antisecretory agents, is another indication for keeping the ETT in place.

PRIOR TO END-OF-LIFE VENTILATOR REMOVAL

Physician orders prior to EOL RMV should include the following: discontinue the ventilator and specify medications such as opiate, sedative, antisecretory medications, and any other medications that provide comfort to the patient. Discontinue any neuromuscular blocking agent and allow time for the effects to dissipate prior to extubation. When neuromuscular blockade is present, signs of pain or other symptoms cannot be observed or monitored because of the effect of the agent. The individual responsible for RMV should contact the patient's nurse, respiratory therapist, and the chaplain to discuss the plan of RMV and the time that extubation will occur.

WITHIN 30 MINUTES OF RMV

Verify the time of RMV with the family, and make sure that all who wish to be present have arrived. Discuss with the patient's nurse the plan of care and ascertain what role she or he is able to assume and what role the palliative care nurse will play if one is available. Discontinue tube feeding and place the nasogastric (NG) tube to suction. Place scopolamine patches on the patient and administer intravenous (IV) glycopyrrolate at this time if excessive oral and airway excretions are a problem or anticipated to be a problem. The IV glycopyrrolate is faster acting to get secretions under control while awaiting action of the scopolamine patch. Notify respiratory therapy and discuss their role during and after RMV including what respiratory equipment will be needed postextubation such as oxygen equipment. Consider use of octreotide (Sandostatin) if the patient has a diagnosis of bowel obstruction or has had significant gastrointestinal (GI) secretions. Octreotide, which shuts down most GI secretions, may be administered either as a continuous infusion or as intermittent intravenous/subcutaneous dosing, up to 1200 mcg per 24-hour period.

TEN MINUTES PRIOR TO RMV

The patient should be premedicated with the appropriate opiate and benzodiazepine to prevent pain, air hunger, anxiety, or other symptoms during the RMV procedure. The patient parameters for dosing include keeping the respiratory rate less than 30/minute, heart rate less than 100/minute, and elimination of grimacing and agitation. It is important to explain to the family when and why the medications are being given to avoid the perception of euthanasia. Severely brain-injured patients may not require sedating medication prior to extubation, but opiates may be useful to control agonal or labored breathing or tachypnea (rate >30/min). If the patient appears restless or agitated, benzodiazepines may be given.

Continuous-Infusion Sedative and Opiates

If the patient is already receiving opiate/benzodiazepine drips, they should be continued. To keep the patient comfortable, bolus the patient with 10% of the prior 24-hour usage or 1.5 to 2.5 times the current hourly rate of each of the medications. When initiating an opioid drip, it is common to start at 50% of the amount of medication administered prior to extubation. The medications may be repeated by doubling the dose every 10 to 15 minutes until the patient is comfortable.

Intermittent-Dosing Sedative and Opiates

If the patient is not currently on an opiate, initial bolus doses of morphine may range from 2 to 10 mg depending on the assessment and cognitive function of the patient. If the patient is not on a sedative, lorazepam is a common choice because it can usually be administered both in and out of the intensive care unit (ICU) setting. The starting dose varies from 1 to 2 mg IV. To prevent interruptions in the procedure, it is important to have extra syringes of medication at the bedside.

While waiting for the medications to take effect, the patient is removed from the monitoring equipment, unnecessary arterial or IV access lines, leg compression devices, and restraints. The electrocardiogram (ECG) monitor is usually removed from the patient if allowed by ICU policy. By removing the ECG and turning off the monitor in the patient's room, the family can focus more on the patient instead of the information on the monitors. Unnecessary equipment is also removed from the bedside.

AT THE TIME OF RMV

The physician, nurse, and respiratory therapist should all be present in the room. For the family members who are present, review the procedure and what may or may not happen when the ventilator is removed. Place a towel on the patient's chest to use as a shield in front of the face of the patient during the removal of the ETT and also as a wrap for the ETT and/or NG tube. Have warm washcloths available to wipe the patient's face after extubation.

Respiratory therapy will turn off the ventilator alarms, suction the patient, deflate the ETT cuff, and remove the ETT as well as the nasogastric/orogastric tube. The respiratory therapist then turns off the ventilator and removes it from the room. The nurse washes the patient's face and positions the head to allow for the best possible air movement. If the patient begins snoring loudly, reposition the head to the right or left or elevate or lower the head of bed position. If the family was not in the room during the procedure, let them join the patient at this time. Lower the bedside railings and allow the family to touch, hug, and kiss their family member. Document the procedure, noting who was present, medications used, outcome, and plan of care to follow.

AFTER RMV

Stay at the bedside to assess the patient's symptoms as well as the family's reaction to what has occurred. Monitor the patient closely for excessive secretions, rapid radial pulse, increasing respiratory rate, grimacing, agitation, and so on, and bolus first with opiates every 10 minutes then benzodiazepines until you are confident the patient is comfortable. As the patient is monitored and assessed, keep the family informed about how the patient is doing. Many families have never witnessed a natural death and they may interpret a peaceful demise as a horrible struggle. Describe peaceful as a relaxed forehead or facial expression or relaxed body position. Anticipate frequently asked questions, and provide the family information on what to expect during the dying process.

One frequently asked question is "How long will it be?" The dying process can be rapid, only a few minutes or longer, lasting up to several days. It is very difficult to predict each person's course. Assure the family that the care team will continue to monitor the patient very closely to maintain comfort for whatever time remains. Another question that often arises is "What do we expect to see now?" Changing respiratory patterns will occur. It is very common to see the patient's breathing become irregular, shallow, even with pauses. Describe to the family the Cheyne-Stokes pattern of respiration. As death nears and agonal respirations occur, many family members see this as distressing to the patient as well as themselves. Be sure to inform the family about changing respiration patterns, reflex shrugging of the shoulders, color changes, and temperature changes. It is also important for the family to know that as professional health care providers we see these changes as normal, peaceful signs of death. It is helpful to point out the relaxed tone of the face and any signs of peaceful demise that are present.

The family may also ask about practical matters such as what arrangements will they need to make when death occurs. Inform them about what arrangements need to be considered after their family member dies. Encourage the family to talk to the patient about the family's good times, about forgiveness, the expression of love, and saying good-bye. Individual family members may need private one-on-one time with the patient. Provide a comfortable environment for the family and food and drink when possible. Some families are hesitant to leave the room for fear that the patient may die while they are gone. Talk with the family about their fears and concerns surrounding their grief and bereavement.

If the patient stabilizes after RMV, the patient may be moved out of the ICU to a private room. It is important to reinforce with the family that attentive comfort care will continue outside of the ICU. Many families want to participate in the care of their family member. Provide the families with the needed equipment and instruction for frequent mouth care, bathing, or turning if they wish to provide some of the care.

After the patient dies, allow the family all the time they need with the deceased patient. When possible it is helpful for the physicians and nurses to express to the family what a privilege it has been to care for their family member. Bereavement care is an important part of the follow-up care that is often done by the palliative care team. Bereaved family members who participate in the decision to RMV at the EOL may have feelings of doubt and guilt in addition to the expected grieving process. Careful evaluation for complicated bereavement is important with referral to bereavement services to assist the family member after the death of the patient.

DEBRIEFING PROCESS

The EOL RMV procedure is an emotionally charged and stressful process. The health care team of physicians, nurses, and respiratory therapists support the patient and family before, during, and after the process. The health care team should allow some time to debrief about the procedure. It is important to discuss what was done well and what could have been improved, but it is also essential that the team members discuss how it felt for them. When this procedure has been done well and the eventual outcome is a comfortable death, it poses a dilemma over feeling accomplished for the technical and supportive aspect going well even though the outcome is death. The teams that participate in EOL RMV have helped the patient and family meet the goal of comfort care in a caring and compassionate manner. Death is not an enemy but a fact of life, and it is important to remain focused on the outcome of meeting and honoring the patient's goal. If immediate debriefing cannot take place, the palliative care team weekly staff/team meeting is another forum for exploring the ventilator removal experience. Not too much time should elapse between the RMV process and debriefing when there are concerns by any member of the health care team.

SUMMARY

RMV at the end of life allows a more natural dying process. Ethical guidelines and principles for decision making and forgoing life-sustaining treatment provide health care teams support when they are involved in EOL for the seriously ill and or dying patient. Open and frequent communication with the patient and/or the patient's surrogate is essential to relay clinical information, identify the goals of care, and build trust. Communication with the patient and family also helps establish the definition of quality of life for the patient and how that relates to the current illness and prognosis. A standardized clinical approach to RMV improves the care of the patient. Supporting the family before, during, and after the RMV procedure is essential to help allay any feelings of doubt about implementation of the goals of care. A quote by Dan Tobin, MD, says it so well: "Just because dying is natural doesn't mean it's easy." Providing debriefing for team members and for ourselves is essential so that we may continue to serve patients and families who participate in the procedure of RMV.

RECOMMENDED READINGS

Ambuel B, Weissman D. *Conducting a Family Conference*. Fast Fact and Concept #016. Available at http://www.eperc.mcw.edu. Accessed June 20, 2005.

Diringer MN, Edwards DF, Aiyagari V, et al. Factors associated with withdrawal of mechanical ventilation in a neurology/neurosurgery intensive care unit. *Crit Care Med* 2001; 29(9):1792–1797.

Kirchhoff KT, Anumandla PR, Foth KT, et al. Documentation on withdrawal of life support in adult patient in the intensive care unit. *Am J Crit Care* 2004; 13(4):328–334.

Kristjanson LJ. Establishing goals: Communication traps and treatment lane changes. In BR Ferrell, N Coyle (eds.), *Palliative Nursing*. New York: Oxford University Press, 2001.

Marr L, Weissman D. Withdrawal of ventilatory support from the dying adult patient. *J Support Oncol* 2004; 2(3):283–288.

Miller PA, Forbes S, Boyle DK. End-of-life care in the intensive care unit: A challenge for nurses. *Am J Crit Care* 2001; 10(4):230–237.

O'Mahony S, McHugh M, Zallman L, et al. Ventilator withdrawal: Procedures and outcomes. Report of a collaboration between a critical care division and a palliative care service. *J Pain Symptom Manage* 2003; 26(4):954–961.

Puntillo K, Stannard D. The intensive care unit. In BR Ferrell, N Coyle (eds.), *Palliative Nursing*. New York: Oxford University Press, 2001.

Rubenfeld GD, Crawford SW. Principles and practice of withdrawing life-sustaining treatment in the ICU. In JR Curtis, GD Rubenfeld (eds.), *Managing Death in the ICU: The Transition from Cure to Comfort*. New York: Oxford University Press, 2001.

Stanley KJ, Zoloth-Dorfman L. Ethical considerations. In BR Ferrell, N Coyle (eds.), *Palliative Nursing*. New York: Oxford University Press, 2001.

Tasota FJ, Hoffman LA. Terminal weaning from mechanical ventilation: Planning and process. *Crit Care Nurs Q* 1996; 19(3):36–51.

Treece PD, Engelberg RA, Crowley L, et al. Evaluation of a standardized order form for the withdrawal of life support in the intensive care unit. *Crit Care Med* 2004; 32(5):1141–1147.

Truog RD, Cist AF, Brackett SE, et al. Recommendations for end-of-life care in the intensive care unit: The ethics committee of the society of critical care medicine. *Crit Care Med* 2001; 29(12):2332–2346.

VonGunten C, Weissman DE. *Ventilator Withdrawal Protocol: Part 1*. Fast Fact and Concept #033. Available at http://www.eperc.mcw.edu. Accessed June 20, 2005.

VonGunten C, Weissman DE. *Information for Patients and Families About Ventilator Withdrawal: Part III*. Fast Fact and Concept #035. Available at http://www.eperc.mcw.edu. Accessed June 20, 2005.

VonGunten C, Weissman DE. *Symptom Control for Ventilator Withdrawal in the Dying Patient: Part II*. Fast Fact and Concept #034. Available at http://www.eperc.mcw.edu. Accessed June 20, 2005.

VonGunten C, Weissman DE. *Morphine and Hastened Death*. Fast Fact and Concept #008. Available at http://www.eperc.mcw.edu. Accessed June 20, 2005.

Index

Note: Page numbers followed by "b," "f" or "t" refer to boxes, figures and tables respectively.